Practice **G**

for

ACUTE CARE
NURSE
PRACTITIONERS

Practice Guidelines
for
ACUTE CARE NURSE PRACTITIONERS

THOMAS W. BARKLEY, JR., DSN, RN, CS, ACNP
Associate Professor
California State University, Los Angeles
School of Nursing
Los Angeles, California

CHARLENE M. MYERS, MSN, RN, CS, ACNP, CCRN
Clinical Assistant Professor
University of South Alabama
College of Nursing
Mobile, Alabama

W.B. SAUNDERS COMPANY
A Harcourt Health Sciences Company
Philadelphia   London   New York   St. Louis   Sydney   Toronto

W.B. SAUNDERS COMPANY
A Harcourt Health Sciences Company

The Curtis Center
Independence Square West
Philadelphia, Pennsylvania 19106

Library of Congress Cataloging-in-Publication Data

Barkley, Thomas W.
Practice guidelines for acute care nurse practitioners / Thomas W. Barkley, Jr.
and Charlene M. Myers.—1st ed.

p.; cm.

ISBN 0–7216–8536–6

1. Emergency nursing. 2. Intensive care nursing. 3. Nurse practitioners.
  I. Myers, Charlene M.   II. Title.
  [DNLM: 1. Acute Disease—nursing. 2. Critical Care. 3. Nurse
  Practitioners.   WB 105 B254p 2001]

RT120.E4 B53 2001   610.73'61—dc21

DNLM/DLC   00–033811

Vice President and Publishing Director—Nursing: Sally Schrefer
Executive Editor: Barbara Nelson Cullen
Editorial Assistant: Adrienne Simon
Manuscript Editor: Jeffrey L. Scheib
Production Manager: Natalie Ware
Illustration Specialist: Lisa Lambert

PRACTICE GUIDELINES FOR
ACUTE CARE NURSE PRACTITIONERS   ISBN 0–7216–8536–6

Printed in the United States of America.

Last digit is the print number: 9   8   7   6   5   4   3   2   1

To my parents, who always encouraged me to be the best that I could be, and my family and friends who provided support, reassurance and encouragement.

To the emerging nurse practitioners and faculty in acute care, may this book guide you in successfully meeting your career goals.

THOMAS W. BARKLEY, JR.

In memory of my parents, who provided me with the love, support, and encouragement to succeed in life.

To the most special people in my life, my children Garrett and Courtney, and sister, Kathryn, who bring me such joy, happiness and laughter.

CHARLENE M. MYERS

CONTRIBUTORS

JUDITH AZOK, MSN, RN, ARNP, GNP-C
Assistant Clinical Professor, Adult Health Nursing
University of South Alabama
College of Nursing
Mobile, Alabama
DIAGNOSTIC CONCEPTS OF OXYGENATION AND VENTILATION;
PNEUMOTHORAX

THOMAS W. BARKLEY, JR., DSN, RN, CS, ACNP
Associate Professor
California State University, Los Angeles
Los Angeles, California
CARDIOVASCULAR ASSESSMENT; HYPERTENSION; CORONARY ARTERY
DISEASE; ANGINA/MYOCARDIAL INFARCTION; ADJUNCT
EQUIPMENT/DEVICES; PERIPHERAL VASCULAR DISEASE; INFLAMMATORY
CARDIAC DISEASES; CONGESTIVE HEART FAILURE; VALVULAR DISEASE;
CARDIOMYOPATHY; ECTOPY AND DYSRHYTHMIA EMERGENCIES;
DIABETES MELLITUS; DIABETIC EMERGENCIES; THYROID DISEASE;
CUSHING'S SYNDROME; PRIMARY ADRENOCORTICAL INSUFFICIENCY
(ADDISON'S DISEASE) AND ADRENAL CRISIS; PHEOCHROMOCYTOMA;
SYNDROME OF INAPPROPRIATE ANTIDIURETIC HORMONE; DIABETES
INSIPIDUS

ALICE S. BOHANNON, PhD, ARNP
Associate Professor
University of South Alabama
College of Nursing
Mobile, Alabama
PAIN

JOANN BROADUS, MSN, RN, CS, FNP
Assistant Professor of Nursing
University of South Alabama
College of Nursing
Mobile, Alabama
ECTOPIC PREGNANCY AND SEXUALLY TRANSMITTED DISEASES

BARBARA S. BROOME, PhD, RN
Chair, Community–Mental Health Nursing
University of South Alabama
College of Nursing
Mobile, Alabama
MAJOR CAUSES OF MORTALITY IN THE UNITED STATES

R. MICHAEL CULPEPPER, MD, FACP
Professor of Medicine
Director, Division of Nephrology
University of South Alabama
Attending Physician
University of South Alabama Hospitals
Mobile, Alabama
FLUID, ELECTROLYTE, AND ACID-BASE IMBALANCES

JASON A. JONES, EdD, RN, CS, ARNP
Former Assistant Professor
Community–Mental Health Nursing
University of South Alabama
College of Nursing
Mobile, Alabama
Psychiatric Nurse Practitioner
Lake View Center
Pensacola, Florida
PSYCHOSOCIAL PROBLEMS IN ACUTE CARE

SYLVIA R. LOVE, MED, MSN, RN, CS, ACNP, ANP
Clinical Assistant Professor
University of South Alabama
College of Nursing
Mobile, Alabama
**ANEMIAS; SICKLE CELL DISEASE/CRISIS; COAGULOPATHIES; LEUKEMIAS;
LYMPHOMA; OTHER COMMON CANCERS; INTEGUMENTARY DISORDERS;
HEADACHE**

SARA C. MAJORS, PhD, CRNA
Clinical Assistant Professor
University of South Alabama
College of Nursing
Mobile, Alabama
PAIN

JOHN P. MCGUINNESS, MD
Medical Director
Clinica del Migrante, Inc.
Summerdale, Alabama
**MEASURES OF OXYGENATION AND VENTILATION; THE CHEST X-RAY;
OXYGEN SUPPLEMENTATION; MECHANICAL VENTILATORY SUPPORT**

TEENA M. MCGUINNESS, PhD, RN, CS
Assistant Professor
Community–Mental Health Nursing
University of South Alabama
College of Nursing
Mobile, Alabama
IMMUNIZATION RECOMMENDATIONS

DAVID A. MILLER, MD, FCCP
Adjunct Professor of Nursing
Nurse Practitioner Programs
Texas A&M University—Corpus Christi
Private Practice, Pulmonary Disease and Internal Medicine
Corpus Christi, Texas
THE CHEST X-RAY; DIFFERENTIAL DIAGNOSIS OF PULMONARY DISORDERS;
  PULMONARY FUNCTION TESTING; OBSTRUCTIVE (VENTILATORY) LUNG
  DISEASES; RESTRICTIVE (INFLAMMATORY) LUNG DISEASES AND
  CONGESTIVE HEART FAILURE/PULMONARY EDEMA;
  PATHOPHYSIOLOGICALLY DERIVED THERAPY FOR RESPIRATORY
  DYSFUNCTION; PULMONARY HYPERTENSION AND PULMONARY VASCULAR
  DISORDERS; CHEST WALL AND SECONDARY PLEURAL DISORDERS;
  RESPIRATORY FAILURE; LOWER RESPIRATORY TRACT PATHOGENS;
  OBSTRUCTIVE SLEEP APNEA; HIV/AIDS AND OPPORTUNISTIC INFECTIONS

DIANTHA D. MILLER, MSN, RN, CS, ACNP, ANP, CEN
Nurse Practitioner
Premier Medical Management, Inc.
Mobile, Alabama
EYE, EAR, NOSE, AND THROAT DISORDERS

SALLY K. MILLER, MS, RN, CS, ACNP, ANP, GNP, CCRN
Adjunct Lecturer, Rutgers—The State University of New Jersey
College of Nursing
Newark
Nurse Practitioner
Atlantic County Justice Facility
Mays Landing, New Jersey
AUTOIMMUNE DISEASES; MANAGING THE SURGICAL PATIENT

CHARLENE M. MYERS, MSN, RN, CS, ACNP, CCRN
Clinical Assistant Professor
University of South Alabama
College of Nursing
Mobile, Alabama
CEREBROVASCULAR ACCIDENTS: BRAIN ATTACK; STRUCTURAL
  ABNORMALITIES; PERIPHERAL NEUROPATHIES; NEUROLOGIC TRAUMA;
  CENTRAL NERVOUS SYSTEM DISORDERS; SEIZURE DISORDERS;
  DEMENTIA; PEPTIC ULCER DISEASE; LIVER DISEASE; BILIARY
  DYSFUNCTION; INFLAMMATORY GASTROINTESTINAL DISORDERS;
  ANATOMIC INTESTINAL DISORDERS; GASTROINTESTINAL BLEEDING;
  URINARY TRACT INFECTIONS; RENAL INSUFFICIENCY/FAILURE; BENIGN
  PROSTATIC HYPERTROPHY; RENAL ARTERY STENOSIS; NEPHROLITHIASIS;
  MANAGEMENT OF THE PATIENT IN SHOCK

JULIE T. SANFORD, MSN, RN
Springhill College
Mobile, Alabama
CHEST, ABDOMINAL, AND EYE TRAUMA

AMY E. SAYLER, MSN, RN, CS, ACNP
Nurse Practitioner
Alton Oschner Medical Foundation Hospital
New Orleans, Louisiana
FEVER

MARTHA N. SURLINE, MS
Clinical Assistant Professor of Nursing and Director of Student Affairs
University of South Alabama
College of Nursing
Mobile, Alabama
NUTRITIONAL CONSIDERATIONS

JEAN SMITH TEMPLE, MSN, BSN, RN
Clinical Assistant Professor
University of South Alabama
College of Nursing
Mobile, Alabama
WOUND MANAGEMENT

ELIZABETH A. VANDE WAA, PhD
Associate Professor of Adult Health Nursing
University of South Alabama
College of Nursing
Mobile, Alabama
POISONING AND DRUG TOXICITIES

JOHN A. VANDE WAA, DO, PhD
Assistant Professor of Medicine
Division of Infectious Diseases
University of South Alabama
Mobile, Alabama
INFECTIONS

COLLEEN R. WALSH, MSN, RN, ONC, CS, ACNP
Faculty, Graduate Nursing
University of Southern Indiana
Evansville, Indiana
Adjunct Assistant Professor
University of South Alabama
College of Nursing
Mobile, Alabama
Acute Care Nurse Practitioner
Free Clinic of Owensboro
Owensboro, Kentucky
ARTHRITIS; SUBLUXATIONS AND DISLOCATIONS; SOFT TISSUE INJURY; FRACTURES; COMPARTMENT SYNDROME; BACK PAIN SYNDROMES

CAROLYN G. WHITE, MSN, RN, CS, FNP, PNP, CCRN
Clinical Assistant Professor and Program Coordinator
Advanced Child Health Specialty
University of South Alabama
College of Nursing
Mobile, Alabama
Clinic Manager and Nurse Practitioner Provider
Clinica del Migrante, Inc.
Summerdale, Alabama
**EYE, EAR, NOSE, AND THROAT DISORDERS; GUIDELINES FOR
HEALTH PROMOTION AND SCREENING**

PREFACE

Practice Guidelines for Acute Care Nursing Practitioners is a succinct and comprehensive pocket text for advanced practice nurses. The text is organized in a systematic fashion, addressing over 230 of the most common conditions experienced by adult patients in acute care. Using an easy-to-read outline format, coverage of each condition includes defining terms, incidence/predisposing factors, subjective and physical examination findings, diagnostic tests, and management strategies.

The text has been written to provide the practitioner with a quick overview of research-based practice guidelines. In this light, the text builds on previous knowledge of anatomy, physiology, and pathophysiological concepts, which have not been separately emphasized. While many practitioners may be highly specialized, this text was designed as a useful tool for the entire scope of acute care nursing practice, including settings such as clinics, emergency departments, medical/surgical departments in hospitals, as well as critical care units. Although this text was developed based on research and expertise, we also feel strongly that collaborative practice with other experts and clinicians is essential to successfully meeting patient goals.

Thomas W. Barkley, Jr.
Charlene M. Myers

ACKNOWLEDGMENTS

We gratefully acknowledge the outstanding contributors and reviewers for this text. Without the expertise of these scholars, this work would not have been possible.

We express sincere appreciation to our secretaries, Sharon Jones and Sarrah Loggins, who offered so much reassurance and humor while this project was in progress.

We also thank the following people at W.B. Saunders: former editor Thomas Eoyang, editor Barbara Nelson Cullen, production manager Natalie Ware, and editorial assistant Adrienne Simon, whose combined efforts have produced an excellent resource for the profession.

THOMAS W. BARKLEY, JR.
CHARLENE M. MYERS

REVIEWERS

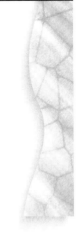

MAXINE BERNREUTER, DSN, RN, CNAA
University of Texas Health Science Center
San Antonio, Texas

LORAINE A. BRZOZOWSKI, MSN, RN, ACNP-CS, CCRN
Acute Care Nurse Practitioner
Chest Medicine Consultants
Chicago, Illinois

DONNA CHARLEBOIS, MSN, RN, CCRN, ACNP-CS
University of Virginia Health System
Charlottesville, Virginia

REBECCA COHEN, EdD, RN, MSN, MPA, CPHQ
Rockford College Department of Nursing
Rockford, Illinois

JEANNE FLANNERY, DSN, ARNP, CNRN, CRRN, CCH
Florida State University
Tallahassee, Florida

DIANE M. FORD, MSN, RN, CCRN
Andrews University
Berrien Springs, Michigan

PHILIP M. GOLD, MD, MACP
Professor of Medicine
Loma Linda University
Loma Linda, California

DENISE GUAGLIANONE, RN, CS, CCRN, APRN
Acute Care Nurse Practitioner—Cardiology
Bridgeport Hospital
Bridgeport, Connecticut

JANE M. HARTSOCK, MA, RN, AOCN, CNS
Trinity College of Nursing
Moline, Illinois

JANIE HEATH, MS, RN, CS, ACNP, ANP, CCRN
Clinical Assistant Professor
Georgetown University
Department of Nursing
Washington, DC

MARCIA J. HILL, MSN, RN
Associate Manager
Bertek Pharmaceuticals, Inc.
Morgantown, West Virginia

LYNN A. KELSO, MSN, RN, ACNP-CS, CCRN
University of Kentucky
Lexington, Kentucky

JOAN E. KING, PhD, RN, ACNP, ANP
Specialty Director for Acute Care Nurse Practitioner Track
Vanderbilt University School of Nursing
Nashville, Tennessee

RUTH KLEINPELL, PhD, RN-CS, ACNP, CCRN
Rush University College of Nursing
Chicago, Illinois

JUDI L. KURIC, MSN, RN, CRRN-A, CCRN, CNRN
University of Southern Indiana
Evansville, Indiana

CAROL S. LADDEN, MSN, CRNP
University of Pennsylvania
Philadelphia, Pennsylvania

ANN BUTLER MAHER, MS, RN, FNPC, ONC
Family Nurse Practitioner
Jersey Battered Women's Service
Morris Plains, New Jersey

DENISE G. MAX, MSN, ACNP, NP-C
Mercer-Bucks Cardiology
Trenton, New Jersey

BARBARA MCKEEHEN, MSN, ARNP, DNC
VAMC—Bay Pines
Bay Pines, Florida
Clinical Instructor
College of Medicine
University of South Florida
Tampa, Florida

SALLY K. MILLER, MS, RN, CS, ACNP, ANP, GNP, CCRN
Adjunct Lecturer, Rutgers—The State University of New Jersey
College of Nursing

Newark
Nurse Practitioner
Atlantic County Justice Facility
Mays Landing, New Jersey

CANDIS MORRISON, PhD, CACNP
Johns Hopkins University
Baltimore, Maryland

MARY B. NEIHEISEL, EdD, BSN, MSN, CNS, CFNP
University of Louisiana at Lafayette College of Nursing
Lafayette, Louisiana

KATHLEEN M. POWERS, BSN, RN, NP
University of Virginia
Charlottesville, Virginia

LAURIE QUINN, PhD, RN, CDE
University of Illinois at Chicago
Chicago, Illinois

GAYLE M. ROUX, PhD, RN, CNS
University of Southern Indiana
Evansville, Indiana

BARBARA RYAN, MSN
University of Ottawa
Ottawa, Ontario
Canada

DENISE A. SADOWSKI, MSN, RN
Independent Consultant and Educator—Burns and Wounds
Cincinnati, Ohio

ANNE W. SALOMONE, MS, RN-C, CNM
Private Practice with Dr. George Stankevych
McHenry, Illinois

BARBARA SCHAEFER, MS, RN, CS-ACNP
Kaiser Permanente Medical Center
Anaheim, California

LINDA S. SMITH, DSN, RN
Oregon Health Sciences University School of Nursing
Klamath Falls, Oregon

WENDY J. SMITH, MSN, RN, CS, ACNP, AOCN
North Mississippi Hematology and Oncology Associates, Ltd.
Tupelo, Mississippi

DONNA AYERS SNELSON, MSN, RN, CS
College Misericordia
Dallas, Pennsylvania

CHRIS STEWART-AMIDEI, MSN, RN, CNRN, CCRN
Clinical Nurse Specialist—Neurosurgery
University of Chicago
Chicago, Illinois

THOMAS D. SUNNENBERG, MD
Sacred Heart Hospital
Hematology–Oncology Associates
Pensacola, Florida

LAURA B. SUTTON, PhD, RN, CS
West Liberty State College
West Liberty, West Virginia

HAROLD M. SZERLIP, MD
Tulane University School of Medicine
New Orleans, Louisiana

KATHLEEN H. TOTO, MSN, RN, CS, ACNP, CCRN
Parkland Memorial Hospital
Dallas, Texas

DENISE A. TUCKER, DSN, RN, MSN, BSN, BA
Florida State University School of Nursing
Tallahassee, Florida

CONTENTS

Management of Patients with Neurologic Disorders

CEREBROVASCULAR ACCIDENTS: BRAIN ATTACK

Charlene M. Myers, MSN, RN, CS, ACNP, CCRN

I. TIA—TRANSIENT ISCHEMIC ATTACKS

A. Definition[21]

A sudden or rapid onset of neurologic deficit caused by focal ischemia that lasts for a few minutes and resolves completely within 24 h

B. Etiology/Incidence/Prevalence[1, 8, 9, 15, 21]

1. Incidence is 160/100,000; prevalence is 135/100,000.
2. Carotid or vertebral artery disease
3. Cardiac emboli as seen in arrhythmias (atrial fibrillation), myocardial infarction, congestive cardiomyopathies, and valvular disease
4. Hematologic causes

   a. RBC disorders
      i. Increased sludging
      ii. Decreased cerebral oxygenation such as in severe anemia
      iii. Polycythemia, sickle cell anemia
   b. Platelet disorders: thrombocytosis and thrombocytopenia
   c. Myeloproliferative disorders, leukemias with WBCs >150,000
   d. Increased viscosity/hypercoagulable conditions, such as antiphospholipid antibody syndromes (e.g., lupus anticoagulant and anticardiolipin antibody), oral contraceptives, and antithrombin III deficiency, protein S & C deficiency, and tissue-type plasminogen activator (t-PA) and plasminogen deficiencies
      i. Patients who are particularly at risk for a hypercoagulable state are those <45 years of age and those with a history of thrombolytic events, spontaneous abortions, related autoimmune conditions (e.g., lupus), stroke of unknown cause, or a family history of thrombotic events.
5. Intracranial causes: Brain tumor, focal seizure, and hemorrhages (subdural hematoma [SDH], subarachnoid hemorrhage [SAH], intracerebral hemorrhage [ICH]), which may cause cerebrovascular dysfunction due to leakage of blood outside the normal vessels

6. Subclavian steal syndrome: Localized stenosis or occlusion of a subclavian artery proximal to the source of the vertebral artery, so that blood is stolen from that artery. Blood pressure is significantly lower in the affected arm compared with the opposite arm.
7. Others: Transient hypotension, osteophytes that cause compression of neck vessels, kinking of neck vessels during rotation of the head, cocaine abuse, hypoglycemia

C. Risk factors[1, 2, 8, 13, 15, 17, 21]

1. Individuals are at risk for stroke in months immediately following the initial TIA, as well as years; therefore, proper treatment of attacks is important. Approximately one third of stroke patients have a history of TIAs.
2. Hypertension
3. Cardiac disease, such as mitral valve disease, anterior wall myocardial infarction, congestive myopathies, and arrhythmias (e.g., atrial fibrillation)
4. Smoking
5. Obesity
6. Hyperlipidemia
7. Advanced age
8. Diabetes
9. Alcohol and recreational drug abuse

D. Clinical manifestations[2, 6, 21]

1. Carotid artery syndrome

   a. Ipsilateral monocular blindness (amaurosis fugax)
   b. Paresthesia/weakness of contralateral arm, leg, and face
   c. Dysarthria, transient aphasia
   d. Ipsilateral, vascular-type headache
   e. Carotid bruit may be present.
   f. Microemboli, hemorrhages, and exudates may be visualized in the ipsilateral retina.

2. Vertebrobasilar artery syndrome

   a. Visual disturbances bilaterally (blurred vision, diplopia, complete blindness)
   b. Vertigo, ataxia, tinnitus
   c. Nausea and/or vomiting
   d. Sudden loss of postural tone of all extremities without loss of consciousness ("drop attacks")
   e. Dysarthria
   f. Perioral or facial paresthesia
   g. Acute confusional state

E. Diagnostics/Laboratory findings[1, 6, 9, 14, 18, 21, 22]

1. Laboratory evaluation should include

   a. CBC, platelet count, prothrombin time (PT), partial thromboplastin time (PTT)—Detect anemia, polycythemia, leukemia, thrombocytopenia, hypercoagulopathies

   b. Anticardiolipin antibodies (IgG, IgM, IgA) and assay for lupus anticoagulant for suspected antiphospholipid antibody syndromes

   c. Assays for antithrombin III, protein S & C, plasminogen, and t-PA

   d. Electrolytes, glucose—Detect hyponatremia, hypokalemia, hypoglycemia, or hyperglycemia

   e. Sedimentation rate—Detects vasculitis, infective endocarditis, hyperviscosity

   f. Lipid profile—Detects hyperlipidemia

   g. In selected patients: ANA, VDRL, toxicology screen

2. CT scan of the head: May reveal "silent" ischemia or ischemic images as well as hemorrhage or infarct and SDH; 10–20% of patients with TIAs have an infarct in the territory relevant to their symptoms.

3. MRI, particularly diffusion-weighted imaging (DWI) and perfusion-weighted imaging (PWI), is more sensitive than CT scan to early pathologic changes of ischemic infarction because of its excellent detection of brain edema. MRI is also preferred for the dectection of lacunar or vertebrobasilar TIAs, or when vascular territory is not well defined.

4. Duplex ultrasonography: 85% sensitivity and 90% specificity, useful in identifying hemodynamically-significant carotid stenosis

5. Magnetic resonance angiography (MRA): Alternative to ultrasound studies; no contrast medium is needed and can be obtained at the same time as an MRI scan; good means for assessment of both extra- and intracranial vessels

6. Carotid Doppler ultrasound has limited usefulness.

7. Echocardiography and a 24-h Holter monitor are used to evaluate for a cardiac source of emboli.

8. Transesophageal echocardiography (TEE): Detects vascular tree abnormalities and stenosis

9. Cerebral angiography: For patients whose symptoms suggest involvement of the carotid circulation and are candidates for carotid endarterectomy (CEA)

10. Chest x-ray: Note for enlarged heart.

11. Blood cultures: Monitor for infective endocarditis.

12. Temporal artery biopsy: To detect giant cell arteritis

13. Cardiac enzymes: To detect an acute myocardial infarction

14. EEG: To detect seizure activity

F. Management[1, 6, 8, 10, 13, 15, 21]

1. Address underlying risk factors: hypertension (HTN), diabetes mellitus (DM), obesity, hyperlipidemia, smoking
2. Carotid TIAs: >70% obstruction—CEA is indicated for those who are a good surgical risk. Surgery is not indicated for those with a <30% obstruction.
3. Anticoagulation: May prevent recurrent cardioembolic events. Begin with heparin (a loading dose of 5000–10,000 units for those not at risk for hemorrhagic transformation and a maintenance infusion of 1000–2000 U/h). The target PTT should be 1.5 times control. Follow with warfarin (Coumadin), 5–15 mg p.o., which is indicated for TIAs caused by embolism arising from a mural thrombus following a myocardial infarction (MI) or from an embolus in patients with mitral stenosis or prosthetic heart valves, and in those with recurrent TIAs despite platelet antiaggregant agents. An international normalized ratio (INR) of 2.0–3.0 is considered therapeutic.
4. Antiplatelet therapy is useful for patients who are not candidates for surgery or warfarin therapy (patients with GI bleeding, bleeding tendencies, or severe hypertension, elderly patients who fall frequently, or uncooperative patients).

   a. Aspirin (ASA) decreases the incidence of subsequent stroke by 15–30% in male patients with TIAs; a dose of 75–325 mg/day is as effective as higher doses and has fewer side effects.
   b. Ticlopidine (Ticlid): 250 mg b.i.d. for those who cannot tolerate ASA or who have recurrent TIAs on ASA therapy: Inhibits platelet aggregation, blocks the platelet-release action, and prolongs bleeding time; reduces the risk of stroke in both men and women, but is very costly and has serious side effects (neutropenia). Use necessitates blood monitoring every 2 weeks for the first 3 months of therapy.
   c. Clopidogrel (Plavix) 75 mg/day p.o.
   d. A combination of dipyridamole (Persantine), 75–100 mg q.i.d., and ASA has been effective in some studies, although is not standard treatment.

II. STROKE/BRAIN ATTACK

A. Definition[1, 18, 21]

1. The rapid onset of a neurologic deficit involving a certain vascular territory and lasting longer than 24 h.
2. A stroke in evolution is an enlarging infarction manifested by neurologic defects that increase over 24 to 48 h.
3. Stroke remains the leading cause of disability and the third leading cause of death in the United States today.

4. Stroke can be classified as ischemic and hemorrhagic.
5. Eighty percent of strokes are caused by blood clots that result in ischemic areas in the brain, and the remaining strokes are caused by intracerebral hemorrhage.

B. Etiology and risk factors

1. Same as for TIAs
2. Cocaine-related stroke is increasing in frequency.
3. Women who use oral contraceptives and who smoke are at high risk.

III. ISCHEMIC STROKE[5, 6, 9, 18, 21, 24]

A. Etiology

1. Caused by a thrombus (30%)

   a. Progression of symptoms over hours to days
   b. Patients often have a history of TIAs.
   c. Often occurs during the night while the patient is sleeping. Patient may completely infarct and be unarousable in the morning.
   d. The patient may awaken with a slight neurologic deficit that gradually progresses.
   e. Atherosclerosis, HTN, DM, arteritis, vasculitis, hypotension, and trauma to the head and neck are all predisposing factors.

2. Caused by embolism (25%)

   a. Very rapid onset
   b. History of prior TIAs uncommon
   c. Patient is usually involved in an activity when the symptoms occur.
   d. Atrial fibrillation, mitral stenosis and regurgitation, endocarditis, and mitral valve prolapse are all predisposing factors.

B. Clinical manifestations (depend on the cerebral vessel involved)[3, 17]

1. Middle cerebral artery

   a. Hemiplegia (involves upper extremity and face more often than lower extremity)
   b. Hemianesthesia
   c. Hemianopia (blindness of half the field of vision)
   d. Eyes may deviate to the side of the lesion.
   e. Aphasia if dominant hemisphere is involved
   f. Occlusions of different branches of the middle cerebral artery may cause different findings (involvement of the anterior division may cause expressive aphasia and involve-

ment of the posterior branch may produce receptive aphasia).

2. Anterior cerebral artery

   a. Hemiplegia (lower extremity more often than upper extremity)
   b. Primitive reflexes (such as thumb-sucking)
   c. Urinary incontinence
   d. Bilateral anterior infarction may cause behavioral changes and disturbance in memory.

3. Vertebral and basilar arteries

   a. Ipsilateral cranial nerve findings
   b. Contralateral (or bilateral) sensory and motor deficits

4. Deep penetrating branches of major cerebral arteries (lacunar infarction)

   a. Most common, <5 mm in diameter
   b. Associated with poorly controlled HTN or diabetes
   c. Contralateral pure motor or sensory deficit
   d. Ipsilateral ataxia with crural (pertaining to the leg or thigh) paresis
   e. Dysarthria with clumsiness of the hand
   f. Prognosis for recovery is high, with partial or complete resolution occurring over 4–6 weeks.

C. Diagnostics/Laboratory findings[6, 9, 11, 14, 18, 21, 22]

1. CT scan of the head without contrast is important to rule out cerebral hemorrhage (especially when considering anticoagulation), when signs and symptoms cannot be explained by one lesion, in patients who present with a stroke on anticoagulation therapy, and to rule out abscess, tumor, and SDH.

   a. Appears as an area of decreased density
   b. Lacunar infarcts appear as small, punched-out, hypodense areas.
   c. The initial CT scan may be negative, and the infarct may not be visible for 2–3 days after the infarct.

2. Chest radiography

   a. May reveal cardiomegaly or valvular calcification
   b. Neoplasm may suggest metastasis rather than stroke as the cause for neurologic deficits.

3. CBC, sedimentation rate, blood glucose, VDRL, lipid profile
4. ECG
5. Blood cultures if endocarditis is suspected
6. Echocardiography
7. Holter monitor

8. Lumbar puncture (LP)—Not always necessary but may be helpful if cause of stroke is uncertain. Obtain a CT scan first to rule out cerebral hemorrhage or any expanding mass that could lead to herniation if LP is performed.

D. Management[1, 4, 7, 10, 12, 24]

1. Blood pressure (BP) control: Acute lowering of systemic BP is not recommended because it may lead to further damage in the ischemic penumbra, in which autoregulation may be defective, and clinically worsen the stroke. Most patients with acute cerebral infarction have an elevated BP, which usually returns to baseline within 48 h without any special treatment. BP control may be warranted, however, in the following conditions:

   a. Systolic BP (SBP) >220 mmHg and diastolic BP (DBP) >120 mmHg (malignant hypertension)
   b. Hypertensive encephalopathy is present.
   c. Vital organs are compromised.
   d. Aortic dissection
   e. Symptomatic cardiac disease
   f. Patients receiving t-PA therapy. (Some experts recommend decreasing BP in those receiving intravenous heparin therapy as well, although this is not universally accepted.)
   g. When indicated, BP should be lowered gradually to 170–180 mmHg systolic and 95–100 mmHg diastolic.
   h. Sublingual nifedipine (Procardia) is inappropriate because of its precipitous lowering of BP and possible worsening of a stroke.
   i. Sodium nitroprusside (Nipride), nitroglycerin, and calcium channel blockers should be avoided as well, particularly with large infarcts that may cause the brain to swell and herniate, because these agents increase intracranial pressure.
   j. Esmolol (Brevibloc [5 g/500 mL IVF titrated to desired BP; maintenance dose should not exceed 200 $\mu g/kg/$min]), labetalol (Trandate [20 mg IV push initially; additional doses of 40–80 mg may be given q10min as needed, not to exceed 300 mg total dose, or 200 mg/250 mL of solution begun at 2 mg/min and titrated to desired response]), or enalapril (enalaprilat) IV

2. Anticoagulation: Heparin does not decrease the severity of a stroke that has occurred, but may prevent recurrent cardioembolic strokes. It may also be used in patients with stroke-in-evolution and in hypercoagulable states. Heparin may increase the risk of transformation from ischemic stroke to hemorrhagic stroke and therefore is not recommended

for massive strokes. The loading dose of heparin is 5000–10,000 units IV followed by a maintenance infusion of 1000–2000 U/h—PTT should be 1.5 times control. Heparin followed by warfarin (5–15 mg/day p.o.) is indicated in suspected cerebral embolism from

a. Mural thrombus
b. Mitral stenosis
c. Atrial fibrillation
d. CT scan may be necessary after 48 h to determine whether there is any hemorrhaging.
e. Anticoagulation is absolutely contraindicated if CT scan or LP suggests cerebral hemorrhage, tumor, abscess, SDH, or epidural hematoma.
f. Use cautiously in patients with a history of GI bleeding, bleeding tendencies, severe HTN, or a large cerebral infarct.
g. May use in a completed stroke *if* embolization is determined to be the cause.

3. Platelet therapy may be used with nonhemorrhagic stroke victims who are not candidates for surgery or warfarin therapy.

a. ASA 75–325 mg/day p.o.
b. Ticlopidine (Ticlid), 250 mg b.i.d.; has reported side effects such as agranulocytosis, thrombotic thrombocytopenic purpura (TTP), and GI intolerance. The cost tends to be higher than that of other platelet therapies. Necessitates blood monitoring every 2 weeks for the first 3 months of therapy.
c. Clopidogrel (Plavix), 75 mg/day p.o., does not have as many side effects as ticlodipine and is being prescribed in place of ticlodipine by many practitioners.
d. Combination of dipyridamole (Persantine), 75–100 mg q.i.d., plus ASA, 25–325 mg/day, has been more effective than ASA alone in some studies, although it is not a standard treatment to date.

4. Mannitol and/or furosemide (Lasix) can be used for cerebral edema that may occur on the second or third day.

5. Corticosteroids have been used in an attempt to reduce vasogenic cerebral edema, but the benefits are conflicting.

6. Tissue plasminogen activator (TPA), 0.9 mg/kg up to a maximum of 90 mg, is now being used, if appropriate conditions are met, as thrombolytic therapy for acute stroke if the patient is brought in less than 3 h after the stroke. Such conditions include:

a. A physician with appropriate expertise to diagnose the stroke must be available.

  b. Twenty-four hour availability to provide CT scanning to assess for hemorrhage
  c. The facility must have the capability to manage intracranial hemorrhage and other complications of thrombolytic therapy.
  d. Patients must seek help early and have a well-defined onset of their symptoms.
  e. The patient's condition must be carefully examined for contraindications (e.g., previous and/or current hemorrhage, previous stroke or head trauma within 3 months, major surgery within 14 days, urinary or gastrointestinal hemorrhage within 24 days, seizure at stroke onset, arterial puncture at noncompressible site within 7 days, elevated PTT, PT > 15 s, oral anticoagulants or heparin with elevated PTT within 48 h, serum glucose level <50 or >400 mg/dL, and SBP >185 mmHg or DBP >110 mmHg).
  f. The patient must have a CT scan and interpretation to exclude hemorrhage.
  g. The drug must be administered within 3 h of the onset of symptoms.
  h. Ten percent of the dose should be administered as a bolus, followed by a 60-min infusion.
  i. There is a serious risk of intracerebral hemorrhage: therefore, the patient must be monitored very closely.

7. The use of calcium channel blockers such as nimodipine (30 mg p.o. q6h for 4 weeks) is under study, suggesting that these agents may reduce the deficit produced by cerebral ischemia and the morbidity and mortality rates from stroke.
8. Surgery, carotid endarterectomy (CEA), may be indicated for those with high grade extracranial carotid artery disease (70–99% stenosis) if they are not high risk.
9. Rehabilitation should take a multidisciplinary approach.
10. Correct treatment depends on a correct diagnosis of the type of stroke; therefore it is imperative to have quick completion of diagnostic tests. The report from the National Institute of Neurological Disorders and Stroke advocates the following goals, based on the time of arrival:

1. Perform an initial emergency department evaluation within 10 min.
2. Notify the stroke team or neurologist within 15 min.
3. Start a CT scan within 25 min.
4. Obtain a CT scan interpretation within 45 min.
5. Administer thrombolytics, if appropriate, within 60 min.
6. Transfer the patient to an inpatient bed within 3 h.

IV. HEMORRHAGIC STROKE[3–5, 18, 21]

A. Definition

1. Condition resulting from bleeding into the subarachnoid space or brain parenchyma
2. Accounts for approximately 14% of all cerebral infarctions

B. Etiology

1. ICH is usually associated with HTN and may occur during activity. ICH is much more likely to result in death or major disability than cerebral infarction or SAH. Hypertension, use of anticoagulants or thrombolytics, use of illicit street drugs (e.g., cocaine), heavy use of alcohol, or hematologic disorders may predispose the patient to ICH.
2. SAH: caused by ruptured saccular aneurysm (85%), arteriovenous malformation (AVM) (8%), or cryptogenic.

C. Clinical manifestations (SAH)

1. Sudden headache of intense severity that radiates into the posterior neck region and is worsened by neck and head movements
2. Vomiting may follow.
3. May have no loss of consciousness or a loss or impairment of consciousness varying from confusion to deeply comatose
4. Twenty-five percent of patients have seizures at onset.
5. Diplopia, dilated pupil, pain above or behind an eye
6. Fever, nuchal rigidity, and other signs of meningeal irritation
7. Fundi may show papilledema and/or retinal hemorrhage.
8. The Hunt and Hess scale grades the clinical severity of SAH and is the best predictor of survival. Overall mortality is 50%.

   a. Grade I: Asymptomatic or slight headache
   b. Grade II: Moderate to severe headache, stiff neck, no focal signs other than cranial nerve palsy
   c. Grade III: Drowsy, mild focal deficit
   d. Grade IV: Stupor, hemiparesis
   e. Grade V: Deep coma, decerebration

D. Clinical manifestations (ICH)[6, 9, 14, 17]

1. Elevation in BP, often to very high levels (90% of patients)
2. Headache (40%)
3. Vomiting is an important diagnostic sign, particularly if the bleed lies in the cerebral hemisphere (49%).
4. Sudden onset of neurologic deficits that can rapidly progress to coma or death, depending on area involved (50%).
5. Putamen hemorrhage

   a. Eyes deviate conjugately to the side of the lesion.
   b. PERRL (pupils equal, round, reactive to light)

    c. Contralateral hemiplegia
    d. Hemisensory disturbance

6. Thalamic hemorrhage

    a. Downward deviation of the eyes, looking at the nose
    b. Pupils pinpoint with a positive reaction
    c. Coma is common.
    d. Flaccid quadriplegia

7. Cerebellar hemorrhage

    a. Ipsilateral lateral conjugate gaze paresis
    b. PERRL
    c. Inability to stand or walk
    d. Facial weakness
    e. Ataxia of gait, limbs, or trunk
    f. Vertigo and dysarthria

E. Diagnostics/Laboratory findings (SAH)[5, 6, 14, 18, 21]

1. CT scan of the head will assist in differentiating between an ischemic and a hemorrhagic stroke in 75% of patients; the scan may be normal, however, if obtained 48 h after the SAH, or if the bleed is small. An aneurysm itself may be seen in 50% of the cases when contrast material is given, depending on site and size, the CT scan quality, and whether fine cuts were obtained.
2. LP if CT scan is unavailable or negative and suspicion is high

    a. *Contraindicated* in any expanding mass as it may cause herniation
    b. A funduscopic examination must be performed to rule out papilledema prior to the procedure.
    c. The CSF will be uniformly grossly bloody; however, it may not be if the bleed is small. In a true SAH, LP reveals 10^3 to 10^6 RBCs/mm^3.
    d. The opening pressure is elevated.
    e. Xanthochromia will be present—yellowish discoloration of CSF produced by blood breakdown products. Xanthochromia appears no earlier than 2–4 h after bleeding.

3. Cerebral angiography: This study is used to determine the source of bleed, the presence of an aneurysm, and the best source of treatment (medical or surgical), and it may also demonstrate vasospasm. The procedure should be performed after the patient has been stabilized.

F. Diagnostics/Laboratory findings (ICH)[3, 5, 6, 18, 21]

1. CT scan without contrast: To confirm a bleed and determine the size and site. CT scan may reveal structural abnormalities such as aneurysms, AVMs, and brain tumors that may

have caused the bleed as well as complications such as herniation, intraventricular hemorrhage, or hydrocephalus.

2. Cerebral angiography may be performed to determine whether the source is an aneurysm or an AVM. It should be considered for all patients without a clear cause of hemorrhage who are surgical candidates, particularly young, normotensive patients who are clinically stable. Timing depends on the patient's clinical state and the neurosurgeon's judgment about the urgency of surgery, if needed.

3. Magnetic resonance imaging (MRI) and magnetic resonance angiography (MRA) may be useful for detecting structural abnormalities (i.e., AVMs and aneurysms).

4. CBC, platelet count

5. Electrolytes

6. ECG

7. Chest x-ray

8. Bleeding time

9. PT/PTT

10. Liver enzymes

11. Renal studies

12. *LP is contraindicated:* it may cause a herniation in the presence of a large hematoma.

G. Management (SAH)[5, 6, 16, 18–21, 23]

1. Strict bed rest in a quiet, stress-free environment

2. Cardiac monitoring

3. Treat symptomatically for headache or anxiety (acetaminophen [Tylenol] and codeine)

4. Have the patient avoid all forms of straining and exertion.

5. Order stool softeners and laxatives (docusate [Colace], 1–2 tablets p.o. q.i.d.).

6. Phenobarbital (Luminal), 30–60 mg p.o. t.i.d.

7. Maintain SBP 140–160 mmHg

8. In severe hypertension, lower the BP gradually, rather than extreme reduction, but not below a DBP < 100 mmHg. Modest hypotension in these patients can produce global cerebral ischemia.

9. Cerebral edema can be reduced with mannitol and/or furosemide (Lasix).

10. Cerebral vasospasms:

   a. Vasospasms occur in approximately 30% of patients.

   b. Symptoms, which include headache, ischemia, and increased ICP, may or may not be present.

   c. Vasospasm commonly occurs 4–14 days after bleeding and is associated with the presence of a thick clot in the subarachnoid space.

d. Calcium channel blockers (nimodipine) may be used to treat cerebral blood vessel spasm after SAHs from ruptured aneurysms (60 mg q4h for 3 weeks).

e. If symptomatic vasospasms occur, the patient is usually treated with IV fluid loading (hypervolemic hemodilution) and induced hypertension.

   i. Aim for a hematocrit of about 30%.

   ii. Monitor cardiac output, pulmonary wedge pressure, central venous pressure, pulmonary arterial pressure, and systemic blood pressure.

   iii. The goal is to optimize the low shear-rate viscosity of the whole blood and to ensure adequate cerebral perfusion pressure in order to restore the regional cerebral blood flow in perfusion areas beyond the vasospastic vessels.

f. Treatment is less risky if the aneurysm has been clipped.

g. Angioplasty or papaverine may be used for vasospasms resistant to the preceding treatments.

h. A new treatment being studied for refractory cerebral spasms is the use of intrathecally delivered sodium nitroprusside.

   i. 1–4 mg/mL, admixed with the patient's CSF (draw off 5–10 mL from the catheter before administration and mix medication with a portion).

   ii. Dosing in patients with established vasospasms varies and is intermittent, based on the clinical response of the patient. End points of the intervention may include an angiographic reversal of vasoconstriction, failure of treatment to alleviate vasoconstriction within 30 min, and adverse effects (e.g., systemic hypotension, intracranial hypertension).

   iii. The recommended dosing for patients being treated prophylactically is 4 mg/mL, 1–2 mL in two divided doses via ventriculostomy.

11. Rebleeding

a. Rebleeding is unpredictable, but often occurs between days 2 and 19 after initial rupture and is thought to originate from fibrinolysis of the clot at the site of the ruptured aneurysm.

b. Forty percent of patients rebleed, with approximately half of these rebleeds being fatal; therefore, efforts to seal off an aneurysm should be made as soon as possible.

c. Neurologic deterioration is generally abrupt.

d. A repeat CT scan, and occasionally a repeat LP, is needed to confirm rebleeding.

e. Research is being conducted on the use of antifibrinolytic therapy in combination with anti-ischemic medications (calcium channel blockers) to determine whether this treatment reduces the rate of rebleeds and results in decreased morbidity and mortality.

12. Surgery may be indicated for aneurysms, depending on the size of the aneurysm, the patient's age and clinical condition, and the neurosurgeon's opinion.

   a. Because the brain is acutely swollen and ischemic, early surgery may trigger more severe vasospasm than may occur without surgery.
   b. One approach is to take grade I and II patients immediately to angiography and surgery to evacuate the clot and clip the aneurysm as soon as possible.
   c. In the case of patients in grades III–IV, whose prognosis is worse, the surgeon should wait until they are grade I or II, if they are to be operated on at all.

H. Management (ICH)[3–6, 17, 18, 21]

1. Initial management should be directed toward the basic airway, breathing, and circulation as well as toward the focal neurologic deficits.
2. Intubation is indicated for insufficient ventilation, for hypoxia (Po_2 <60 mmHg or Pco_2 >50 mmHg) or obvious risk of aspiration.
3. Oxygen should be administered to all patients with possible ICH.
4. Control severe HTN: Should not exceed 20% reduction and should be achieved through short-acting agents (sodium nitroprusside 50 mg/250 mL D_5W titrated to maintain BP).

   a. The goal is to decrease the risk of ongoing bleeding from ruptured small arteries and arterioles.
   b. Overaggressive treatment of high blood pressure may decrease the cerebral perfusion pressure (CPP) and therefore worsen brain injury, particularly in the setting of increased intracranial pressure.
   c. Maintaining a mean arterial blood pressure (MAP) of 130 mmHg is recommended.

5. CPP (MAP − ICP) should be kept >70 mmHg.
6. Some suggested medications for elevated BP

   a. Labetalol (Trandate), 5–100 mg/h IV by intermittent bolus doses every 10 min of 10–40 mg or continuous drip (2–8 mg/min), not to exceed 300 mg total for both intermittent and continuous dose. Avoid in patients with asthma.
   b. Esmolol (Brevibloc), 500 μg/kg as a load (IV); maintenance use, 50–200 μg/kg/min
   c. Sodium nitroprusside, 0.5–10 μg/kg/min IV

    d. Hydralazine (Apresoline), 10–20 mg q4–6h IV

    e. Enalapril, 0.625–1.2 mg q6h as needed

7. Guidelines for antihypertensive therapy in patients with acute stroke may be used in the first few hours of ICH.

    a. If SBP is >230 mmHg or DBP is >140 mmHg on two readings taken 5 min apart, institute nitroprusside.

    b. If SBP is 180–230 mmHg, DBP is 105–140 mmHg, or MAP is >130 mm Hg on two readings 20 min apart, institute IV labetalol, esmolol, enalapril, or other small doses of easily titratable IV medications such as diltiazem, lisinopril, or verapamil.

    c. If SBP is <180 mmHg and DBP is <105 mmHg, defer antihypertensive therapy.

    d. In the immediate postoperative period, a MAP >110 mmHg should be avoided.

    e. If BP falls below 90 mmHg, pressors should be given (dopamine 2–20 μg/kg/min; phenylephrine [epinephrine], 2–10 μg/kg/min; or norepinephrine [Levophed], 0.05–0.2 μg/kg/min).

8. Maintain ICP <20 mmHg and CPP >70 mmHg.

    a. Mannitol for cerebral edema (0.25–0.5 g/kg of a 20% solution) given IV q4h. Due to its rebound phenomenon, mannitol is recommended for ≤5 days. To maintain the osmotic gradient, furosemide (Lasix) (10 mg q2–8 h) may be administered with mannitol. Serum osmolality should be measured twice a day for those receiving osmotherapy and should be kept ≤310 mOsm/L.

    b. Ventricular drain for secondary hydrocephalus: Use should not exceed 7 days because of possible infectious complications, and IV antibiotic prophylaxis is recommended.

    c. If hyperventilation is used, P_{CO_2} should be maintained at 30–35 mmHg.

9. Steroids are not recommended.

10. Supportive measures.

    a. IVFs: Excessive administration can worsen cerebral edema. The goal is euvolemia. Fluid balance is calculated by measuring daily urine production and adding 500 mL for insensible losses plus 300 mL per degree in febrile patients.

    b. Phenytoin (Dilantin) if seizure activity is noted.

    c. Nutritional support

    d. Maintain body temperature with acetaminophen (Tylenol), 650 mg, for temperature >38.5°C (101.3°F).

e. Physical therapy (PT)

f. Skin care/turning

11. Surgery

a. Indicated for patients with cerebellar hemorrhage

b. Indicated for those with surgically accessible cerebral hematomas that show signs of temporal herniation.

References

1. Alberts, M.J. (1999). Diagnosis and treatment of ischemic stroke. *American Journal of Medicine, 106*, 211–221.
2. Bennett, J.C. & Plum, F. (1996). *Cecil textbook of medicine* (20th ed.). Philadelphia: W.B. Saunders.
3. Broderick, J.P., Adams, H.P., Barsan, W., Feinberg, W., Feldmann, E., Grotta, J., Kase, C., Krieger, D., Mayberg, M., Tilley, B., Zabramski, J.M., & Zuccarello, M. (1999). Guidelines for the management of spontaneous intracranial hemorrhage: A statement for healthcare professionals from a special writing group of the stroke council, American Heart Association. *Stroke, 30*, 905–915.
4. Clochesy, J.M., Breu, C., & Dossey, B. (1997). *AACN handbook of critical care nursing*. Stamford, CT: Appleton & Lange.
5. Devinsky, O., Feldmann, E., Weinreb, H.J., & Wilterdink, J.L. (1997). *The resident's neurology book*. Philadelphia: FA Davis.
6. Ferri, F.F. (1998). *Practical guide to the care of the medical patient* (4th ed.). St. Louis: Mosby.
7. Fisher, M. & Bogousslavsky, J. (1998). Further evolution toward effective therapy for acute ischemic stroke. *Journal of the American Medical Association, 279*, 1298–1303.
8. Gilman, S. (1998). Medical progress: Imaging the brain: First of two parts. *New England Journal of Medicine, 338*, 812–820.
9. Hankey, G. (1999). Stroke: How large a public health problem, and how can the neurologist help. *Archives of Neurology, 56*, 748–754.
10. Horowitz, S.H. (1998). Thrombolytic therapy in acute stroke: Neurologists, get off your hands! *Archives of Neurology, 55*, 155–157.
11. Keiser, M.M. (1999). Neurologic disorders. In A. Gawlinski & D. Hamwi (Eds.), *Acute care nurse practitioner: Clinical curriculum and certification review*. Philadelphia: WB Saunders.
12. Luisi, A. & Hume, A.L. (1998). Thrombolysis in acute ischemic stroke. *Journal of the American Board of Family Practice, 11*, 145–151.
13. Miller, SK (1999). Chapter 13 In V.L. Millonig & S.K. Miller (Eds.), *Adult nurse practitioner certification review guide* (3rd ed.). Potomac, MD: Health Leadership Associates, Inc.
14. Phillips, P. (1999). Improved stroke imaging techniques. *Journal of the American Medical Association, 281*, 2073–2074.
15. Rakel, R.E. (1996). *Saunders manual of medical practice*. Philadelphia: WB Saunders.
16. Roos, Y., Vermeulen, M., Rinkel, G., Algra, A., Van Gijn, J., & Algra, A. (1998). Systemic review of antifibrinolytic treatment in aneurysmal subarachnoid haemorrhage. *Journal of Neurology, Neurosurgery and Psychiatry, 65*, 942–943.
17. Schwarz, S., Schwab, S., Bertram, M., Aschoff, A., & Hacke, W. (1998). Effects of hypertonic saline hydroxyethyl starch solution and mannitol

in patients with increased intracranial pressure after stroke. *Stroke, 29,* 1550–1555.

18. Stein, J.H. (1998). *Internal medicine* (5th ed.). St. Louis: Mosby.
19. Stobo, J.D., Hellmann, D.B., Ladenson, P.W., Petty, B.G., & Traill, T.A. (1990). *Principles and practice of medicine* (23rd ed.). Stamford, CT: Appleton & Lange.
20. Thomas, J.E., Rosenwasser, R.H., Armonda, R.A., Harrop, J., Mitchell, W., & Galaria, I. (1999). Safety of intrathecal sodium nitroprusside for the treatment and prevention of refractory cerebral vasospasm and ischemia in humans. *Stroke, 30,* 1409–1416.
21. Tierney, L.M., McPhee, S.J., & Papadakis, M.A. (1999). *Current medical diagnosis & treatment* (38th ed.). Stamford, CT: Appleton & Lange.
22. van Everdingen, K.J., van der Grond, J., Kappelle, L.J., Ramos, L.M.P., & Mali, W.P.T.M. (1998). Diffusion-weighted magnetic resonance imaging in acute stroke. *Stroke, 29,* 1783–1790.
23. Vermeij, F.H., Hasan, D., Bijvoet, H., & Avezaat, C. (1998). Impact of medical treatment on the outcome of patients after aneurysmal subarachnoid hemorrhage. *Stroke, 29,* 924–930.
24. Wilson, E.M. (1998). Strokes, CVAs, or brain attacks: By any name they need quick attention. *Journal of Emergency Nursing, 24,* 251–252.

STRUCTURAL ABNORMALITIES

Charlene M. Myers, MSN, RN, CS, ACNP, CCRN

I. ANEURYSM

A. Definition

1. An abnormal dilatation of an arterial wall in which the intima bulges outward
2. Usually caused by an abnormal weakening
3. Usually a sudden increase in systolic blood pressure caused by events such as straining or sexual intercourse will precipitate a rupture.

B. Types[3, 13]

1. Berry (saccular)—Congenital aneurysm of a cerebral vessel

    a. Tend to occur at arterial bifurcations
    b. More common in adults
    c. Frequently multiple
    d. Usually asymptomatic
    e. May be associated with polycystic kidney disease or coarctation of the aorta

2. Fusiform—An aneurysm that is tapered at both ends, spindle-shaped, and in which all walls of the blood vessel dilate more or less equally, creating tubular swelling
3. Mycotic—Caused by or infected by microorganisms (bacterial)
4. Traumatic

C. Location

1. The majority of intracranial aneurysms (80–85%) are located in the anterior circulation.

    a. Most commonly at the junction of the internal carotid artery and the posterior communicating artery
    b. At the anterior communicating artery complex
    c. At the trifurcation of the middle cerebral artery

2. Aneurysms of the posterior circulation are most frequently located at the bifurcation of the basilar artery or at the junction of a vertebral artery and the ipsilateral posterior inferior cerebellar artery.
3. Multiple intracranial aneurysms, usually two or three in number, are found in 20–30% of patients.

4. Rupture results in

   a. Subarachnoid hemorrhage (SAH)—Most common (see Chapter 1).
   b. Intracerebral hemorrhage (ICH)—Less common (see Chapter 1).
   c. Subdural hematoma (SDH)—Rare (see Chapter 4).

D. Risk Factors

1. There is evidence to support the association of intracranial aneurysm with heritable connective-tissue disorders (e.g., polycystic kidney disease, Ehlers-Danlos syndrome type IV, neurofibromatosis type I, Marfan's syndrome) and their familial occurrence.
2. Seven percent to twenty percent of patients with aneurysmal SAH have a first- or second-degree relative who has had a confirmed intracranial aneurysm.
3. Cigarette smoking has been identified as an environmental factor.

   a. The risk of an aneurysmal SAH is about 3–10 times higher among smokers.
   b. The risk increases with the number of cigarettes smoked.
   c. Smoking has been shown to decrease the effectiveness of α_1-antitrypsin, the main inhibitor of proteolytic enzymes (proteases) such as elactase, and the imbalance between proteases in smokers may result in the degradation of a variety of connective tissues, including the arterial wall.

4. The risk is higher among women than among men after age 50. This suggests the role of hormonal factors. Premenopausal women have a low risk of aneurysmal SAH, postmenopausal women have a relatively high risk, and postmenopausal women receiving hormone-replacement therapy have an intermediate risk.
5. A moderate to high level of alcohol consumption is an independent risk factor for aneurysmal SAH. Recent, heavy use of alcohol in particular appears to increase the risk of SAH.

E. Clinical manifestations[13]

1. Most aneurysms are asymptomatic until they rupture, at which time SAH results (see signs and symptoms in Chapter 1, under SAH).
2. There may be some focal neurologic deficit related to compression of adjacent structures.
3. A small amount of blood from the aneurysm ("warning leaks") may precede the major hemorrhage by a few hours or days. These may cause the patient to have headaches, nausea, and neck stiffness.

4. Ophthalmologic examination may reveal unilateral or bilateral subhyaloid hemorrhages in approximately one fourth of patients with aneurysmal SAH. These hemorrhages are venous in origin, located between the retina and vitreous membrane, and convex at the bottom and flat on the top.

5. Some aneurysms may have a mass effect, causing the patient to become symptomatic. These aneurysms are generally large or giant ($\geq$25 mm).

   a. The most common symptom of mass effect is headache.
   b. The most common sign is palsy of cranial nerve III (pupils).
   c. Brain stem dysfunction, visual field defects, trigeminal neuralgia, a cavernous sinus syndrome, seizures, and hypothalamic-pituitary dysfunction may also occur, depending on the location of the aneurysm.
   d. These aneurysms carry a high risk of rupture (approximately 6% per year).

F. Diagnostics [3, 9, 10, 13]

1. CT scan or magnetic resonance angiography to obtain a base line of ventricular size and rule out infarct/hemorrhage. These studies are noninvasive and carry a lower complication rate than conventional catheter angiography.

   a. CT scans are sensitive in detecting acute hemorrhage, and they can demonstrate the presence of SAH in 90–95% of patients who undergo scanning within the first 24 h after hemorrhage.
   b. The sensitivity of CT scanning, however, decreases to 80% at 3 days after hemorrhage, 70% at 5 days, 50% at 1 week, and 30% at 2 weeks because blood is cleared rapidly from the subarachnoid space.
   c. CT scans are also useful in detecting any associated intracranial hemorrhage or hydrocephalus, and the distribution of blood may offer important clues to the location of the ruptured aneurysm.

2. Cerebral angiography to obtain size, shape, location, and number of aneurysms, and occurrence of arterial spasm. The risk of permanent neurologic complications is lower than previously recognized, and cerebral angiography has high diagnostic accuracy. Angiography has superior spatial resolution and lacks the flow-related artifacts that affect magnetic resonance angiography.

3. MRI angiography does not require contrast material and can detect intracranial aneurysms as small as 2–3 mm in diameter.

4. Standard MRI is the best method for detecting the presence of a thrombus within the aneurysmal sac.

5. Beginning in the late 1990s helical CT angiography has been used to detect intracranial aneurysms, and preliminary re-

ports indicate that the detection rate with this technique is similar to that with MRI angiography. Helical CT angiography has the ability to demonstrate the relation of the aneurysm to the bony structures of the skull base and can be performed safely in patients who have been treated with ferromagnetic clips, which are a contraindication to MRI angiography.

6. Lumbar puncture: If there is a negative CT scan but a strong clinical suspicion of SAH, then lumbar puncture should be performed. There is a risk of herniation if intracranial pressure is increased (see Chapter 1).

7. Elevated WBC count and sedimentation rate are indicators of a ruptured aneurysm.

G. Management[4, 8, 10, 13]

1. Surgery

    a. Choosing surgery for patients with an unruptured intracranial aneurysm involves weighing the risk of intracranial rupture against the risks associated with brain surgery.

    b. Size, location, and previous SAH are the most important features that predict aneurysmal rupture.

        i. As noted in the cooperative Study of Intracranial Aneurysms and Subarachnoid Hemorrhage, which involved 6038 ruptured aneurysms, the critical size for rupture was 7–10 mm. Many studies support the critical size as being >10 mm.

        ii. Major compressive symptoms (i.e., headache, neurologic signs and symptoms) should lead to the consideration of surgery.

        iii. Coexisting medical problems or factors that favor the need for surgery need to be considered (i.e., hypertension, poorly controlled hypertension) to prevent the risk of bleeding.

    c. Early (within 72 h of the bleed) surgery is desirable to eliminate risk of rebleed and to allow aggressive treatment for vasospasm should it occur.

    d. Late: More than 7 days post bleed.

    e. Methods

        i. Clipping

        ii. Wrapping

        iii. Embolization

        iv. Endovascular treatment is emerging. Soft metallic coils are inserted within the lumen of the aneurysm. The goal is complete obliteration of the aneurysmal sac.

2. Medical management if surgery is not feasible, as outlined for SAH in Chapter 1, is continued for about 6 weeks.

H. Possible Complications[3, 8, 9, 10]

1. Vasospasm

   a. Occurs several days to 3–4 weeks after treatment
   b. Calcium channel blockers (nimodipine 60 mg q4h for 21 days) have been shown to reduce the incidence of ischemic deficit from cerebral spasms.
   c. Intravascular volume expansion, induced hypertension, intra-arterial papaverine infusion, or transluminal balloon angioplasty of involved cranial vessels may also be used after obliteration of the aneurysm.

2. Rebleeding

   a. Greatest within a few days of first hemorrhage
   b. Approximately 20% of patients will have further bleeding within 2 weeks, and 40% within 6 months.
   c. Prevent hypertensive episodes (see Chapter 1).
   d. Antifibrolytic agents—Aminocaproic acid used during the first 2 weeks after hemorrhage has been shown to reduce the risk of rebleeding. It is controversial, however, as it has been associated with an increase in cerebral ischemia, and there is no significant decrease in mortality rate or in degree of disability among survivors.

3. Hydrocephalus (see below—Communicating hydrocephalus)

   a. Caused by interference with the flow of CSF
   b. Generally occurs after 2 or more weeks
   c. May be relieved by shunting

4. Seizures
5. Increased ICP

II. HYDROCEPHALUS

A. Definition[3, 8, 12]

1. A condition in which there is an excessive amount of CSF that accumulates within the cerebral ventricles. The human brain makes approximately 500 mL of CSF per day, most of which is generated by the choroid plexus within the ventricular system. CSF circulates around the brain and spinal cord and is reabsorbed in the venous system.
2. Hydrocephalus is a common neurosurgical problem that leads to changes in cerebral blood flow by displacement, deformation, stretching, or decrease in the caliber of cerebral vessels. Change in the vessels causes a change in vascular resistance and cerebral perfusion pressure, which is important for cerebral microcirculation.
3. Normal pressure hydrocephalus is an unusual cause of dementia occurring as a late complication of intracerebral infection or SAH. The CSF pressure in some cases may not be ele-

vated, but is almost always above 100 cm H_2O, and is usually at the upper-normal limit. The syndrome develops subacutely over a few weeks, and in some patients no predisposing reason is identified.

B. Etiology[2, 3, 8]

1. Oversecretion/production of CSF
2. Obstruction of CSF (lesions or tumors)
3. Impaired absorption
4. Normal pressure hydrocephalus may follow head injury, SAH, or meningoencephalitis.

C. Classification[2, 3]

1. Communicating

    a. Ventricles are patent; obstruction is beyond the fourth ventricle.
    b. Caused by impaired absorption or overproduction
    c. Usually occurs 4–20 days after aneurysmal rupture, although it may occur at any time.

2. Noncommunicating

    a. Obstruction is within or next to the ventricular system, preventing CSF made in the lateral and third ventricles from circulating normally, so that this fluid no longer communicates with the subarachnoid space.
    b. Related to lesion or tumors

D. Clinical Manifestations (Adults)[3, 12]

1. Normal pressure hydrocephalus

    a. Lethargy and mental failure
    b. Gait disorder
    c. Incontinence
    d. Frequent falls and failure in the pursuit of usual activities
    e. Moderate dementia
    f. Language may be affected.
    g. Abulic (slow to respond), but, if given time, often responds with the correct answers to questions.
    h. Slow EEG
    i. Enlarged ventricles

2. Post-traumatic

    a. Progressive enlargement of ventricles
    b. Gait disturbances
    c. Memory difficulty
    d. Urinary incontinence

3. Nausea and vomiting may be present.
4. Choked disks may be found.
5. Atrophy of the optic nerve

E. Management[3, 12]

1. Acute: Intraventricular catheter
2. Chronic: Ventricular shunt
3. Endoscopic third ventriculostomy (Mixter's surgery) has been used in noncommunicating hydrocephalus to enable the surgeon to control the condition without the need for ventricular shunting and without long-term complications associated with shunts. The advantage of endoscopic surgery is that, when feasible, it can be performed with minimal disruption of neural tissue, thus frequently allowing patients to be mobilized rapidly, resulting in shorter hospitalizations and reduction in costs.

III. SPACE-OCCUPYING LESIONS (BRAIN TUMORS)

A. Definition[1, 3, 7, 9, 13]

1. Consists of primary neoplasms (originating in the brain) or secondary neoplasms (originating from sites other than the brain, such as the lung, the breast, the genitourinary tract, and the gastrointestinal tract) that are located within the intracranial vault
2. Glioblastoma multiforme is the most common primary tumor, followed by meningioma and astrocytoma.
3. The cause is unknown; however, genes and viruses may be associated with these lesions.

B. Types and characteristics[8]

See Table 2–1 for a description of tumor types and characteristics.

C. Clinical Manifestations[1-4, 7, 9, 13]

1. Vary, depending on the type, location, and growth of the tumor. Most symptoms do not develop until the tumor is well advanced.
2. Headache
3. Nausea and vomiting; vomiting may not be preceded by nausea.
4. Weakness
5. Hemiparesis
6. Sensory disturbances
7. Irritability, emotional lability, forgetfulness, drowsiness, lethargy
8. Impaired gait
9. Aphasia
10. Agraphia
11. Papilledema (10%)
12. Visual disturbances: amaurosis fugax (temporary blindness), diplopia, diminished visual acuity
13. Generalized or focal seizure activity (30%)

D. Diagnostics[1, 3–6, 11]

1. MRI is the procedure of choice for imaging all types of brain tumors because of its high sensitivity; its capacity to delineate small tumors in sites near bone; its sensitivity to tissue edema; and its inherent multiplanar capability that allows accurate localization of tumors and identification of their relation to normal structures.
2. CT scan may be useful for screening in patients with known cancers elsewhere in the body, or in patients with atypical headache. Contrast medium may be needed. If CT scan is negative, but there is high suspicion, an MRI should be performed. CT scan is effective for following progression of a diagnosed tumor.
3. Cerebral angiography can help to determine vascularity of lesions and/or proximity to blood vessels.
4. EEG can detect the presence and the location of seizure activity.
5. Open brain biopsy (craniotomy) or CT- or MRI-directed stereotactic needle biopsy will provide a definitive diagnosis.
6. Metastatic workup (chest x-ray, mammogram, bone scan, prostate examination, chest/abdominal/pelvic CT) is necessary.

E. Management[1, 3, 4, 8, 11, 13]

1. Chemotherapy, depending on type and stage of tumor (carmustine [BCNU], lomustine [CCNU], cisplatin, and procarbazine are the most commonly used agents for malignant gliomas in adults.)
2. Radiation therapy, depending on type of tumor. Malignant gliomas are not radiosensitive; however, radiation will lengthen survival rate in affected patients.
3. Corticosteroids

    a. Dexamethasone (Decadron)
       i. Standard dose at initiation of therapy is 4–6 mg IV/ p.o. q.i.d.
       ii. Monitor for side effects.
       iii. Taper slowly, and discontinue if possible.
       iv. Patients with incompletely treated tumors may not tolerate the decrease in dosage (e.g., continue to show neurologic deterioration/cerebral edema) and therefore may require chronic steroid use during their last months of life.
       v. Prescribe a concurrent H_2 blocker to prevent gastric irritability associated with steroid use: ranitidine (Zantac), 150 mg p.o. b.i.d, cimetidine (Tagamet), 200 mg p.o. b.i.d., or famotidine (Pepcid), 20 mg p.o. b.i.d.

TABLE 2-1. TUMOR TYPES AND CHARACTERISTICS

TUMOR	CLINICAL FEATURES	TREATMENT AND PROGNOSIS
Glioblastoma multiforme	Commonly, nonspecific complaints and increased intracranial pressure. As it grows, focal deficits develop.	Course is rapidly progressive, with poor prognosis. Total surgical removal is usually not possible, and response to radiation therapy is poor.
Astrocytoma	A glioma whose presentation is similar to that of glioblastoma multiforme, but its course is more protracted, often over several years. Cerebellar astrocytoma, especially in children, may have a more benign course.	Prognosis is variable. By the time of diagnosis, total excision is usually impossible; tumor often is not radiosensitive. In cerebellar astrocytoma, total surgical removal is often possible.
Medulloblastoma	A glioma seen most frequently in children. Generally arises from roof of fourth ventricle and leads to increased intracranial pressure accompanied by brain stem and cerebellar signs. May seed subarachnoid space.	Treatment consists of surgery combined with radiation therapy and chemotherapy.
Ependymoma	Glioma arising from the ependyma of a ventricle, especially the fourth ventricle; leads early to signs of increased intracranial pressure. Arises also from central canal of spinal cord.	Tumor is not radiosensitive and is best treated surgically if possible.
Oligodendroglioma	Slow-growing glioma. Usually arises in cerebral hemisphere in adults. Calcification may be visible on skull x-ray.	Treatment is surgical, which is usually successful.
Brain stem glioma	Occurs during childhood with cranial nerve palsies and then with long-tract signs in the limbs. Signs of increased intracranial pressure occur late.	Tumor is inoperable; treatment is by irradiation and shunt for increased intracranial pressure.
Cerebellar hemangioblastoma	Presents with disequilibrium, ataxia of trunk or limbs, and signs of increased intracranial pressure. Sometimes familial. May be associated with retinal and spinal vascular lesions, polycythemia, and hypernephromas.	Treatment is surgical.

Pineal tumor	Manifests with increased intracranial pressure, sometimes associated with impaired upward gaze (Parinaud's syndrome) and other deficits indicative of midbrain lesion.	Ventricular decompression by shunting is followed by surgical approach to tumor; irradiation is indicated if tumor is malignant. Prognosis depends on histopathologic findings and extent of tumor.
Craniopharyngioma	Originates from remnants of Rathke's pouch above the sella, depressing the optic chiasm. May occur at any age but usually in childhood, with endocrine dysfunction and bitemporal field deficits.	Treatment is surgical, but total removal may not be possible.
Acoustic neuroma	Ipsilateral hearing loss is most common initial symptom. Subsequent symptoms may include tinnitus, headache, vertigo, facial weakness or numbness, and long-tract signs. (May be familial and bilateral when related to neurofibromatosis). Most sensitive screening tests are MRI and brain stem auditory evoked potential.	Treatment is excision by translabyrinthine surgery, craniectomy, or a combined approach. Outcome is usually good.
Meningioma	Originates from the dura mater or arachnoid; compresses rather than invades adjacent neural structures. Increasingly common with advancing age. Tumor size varies greatly. Symptoms vary with tumor site (e.g., unilateral exophthalmos [sphenoidal ridge]; anosmia and optic nerve compression [olfactory groove]). Tumor is usually benign and readily detected by CT scanning; may lead to calcification and bone erosion visible on plain x-rays of skull.	Treatment is surgical. Tumor may recur if removal is incomplete. Patients may receive radiation if removal is incomplete to decrease risk of recurrence.
Primary cerebral lymphoma	Associated with AIDS and other immunodeficient states. Presentation may be with focal deficits or with disturbances of cognition and consciousness. May be indistinguishable from cerebral toxoplasmosis.	Treatment is by whole-brain irradiation; chemotherapy may have an adjunctive role. Prognosis depends upon CD4 count at diagnosis.

(Adapted from Aminoff, M.J. [1996]. Nervous system. In L.M. Tierney, S.J. McPhee, & M.A. Papadakis [Eds.]. *Current Medical Diagnosis and Treatment*. Stamford, CT: Appleton & Lange, with permission.)

   b. Methylprednisolone (Solu-Medrol), 120–200 mg IV, in 4–6 divided doses to decrease tumor-associated edema

   c. Decrease tumor-associated edema

4. For patients with severe cerebral edema, or in situations where intracranial pressure becomes life threatening, an osmotic diuretic may be necessary. Mannitol (Osmitrol) in the usual dose of 1g/kg of a 20% solution IV over 3–5 min can reduce intracranial pressure.

5. In patients with recurrent seizures caused by tumor location and/or edema, anticonvulsants may be necessary. The agent of choice by many practitioners is phenytoin (Dilantin), 1 g IV or p.o., as a loading dose, followed by 300 mg/day in divided doses as a maintenance dose.

6. Brachytherapy (the stereotactic implantation of interstitial radionuclide sources [wafer]) may have a positive effect on survival in patients with glioblastomas.

7. The modified linear accelerator with stereotactic guidance, the gamma knife, and the proton beam are other noninvasive stereotactic radiosurgical methods that have had some success.

8. If obstructive hydrocephalus is present, surgical shunting can produce dramatic benefit.

References

1. Borkowski-Benoit, C. (1999). Neurological problems. In P. Logan (Ed.), *Principles of practice for the acute care nurse practitioner.* Stamford, CT: Appleton & Lange.

2. Clochesy, J.M., Breu, C., & Dossey, B. (1997). *AACN handbook of critical care nursing.* Stamford, CT: Appleton & Lange.

3. Devinsky, O., Feldmann, E., Weinreb, H.J., & Wilterdink, J.L. (1997). *The resident's neurology book.* Philadelphia: FA Davis.

4. Ferri, F.F. (1998). *Practical guide to the care of the medical patient* (4th ed.). St. Louis: Mosby.

5. Gilman, S. (1998). Medical progress: Imaging the brain: First of two parts. *New England Journal of Medicine, 338,* 812–820.

6. Gilman, S. (1998). Medical progress: Imaging the brain: Second of two parts. *New England Journal of Medicine, 338,* 889–898.

7. Hector Dunphy, L.M. (1999). *Management guidelines for adult nurse practitioners.* Philadelphia: FA Davis.

8. Keiser, M.M. (1999). Neurologic disorders. In A. Gawlinski & D. Hamwi (Eds.), *Acute care nurse practitioner: Clinical curriculum and certification review.* Philadelphia: WB Saunders.

9. Rakel, R.E. (1996). *Saunders manual of medical practice.* Philadelphia: WB Saunders.

10. Schievink, W.I. (1997). Medical progress: Intracranial aneurysms. *New England Journal of Medicine, 336,* 28–40.

11. Shapiro, W.R. (1999). Current therapy for brain tumors: Back to the future. *Archives of Neurology, 56,* 429–432.

12. Stein, J.H. (1998). *Internal medicine* (5th ed.). St. Louis: Mosby.

13. Tierney, L.M., McPhee, S.J., & Papadakis, M.A. (1999). *Current medical diagnosis & treatment* (38th ed.). Stamford, CT: Appleton & Lange.

PERIPHERAL NEUROPATHIES

Charlene M. Myers, MSN, RN, CS, ACNP, CCRN

I. GUILLAIN-BARRÉ SYNDROME (GBS)

A. Definition[3, 14]

1. An acute, usually rapidly progressive form of inflammatory polyneuropathy of the peripheral nerves
2. Characterized by muscular weakness, mild distal sensory loss, and autonomic dysfunction that, in about two thirds of cases, begins 5 days to 3 weeks after an ordinary infectious disorder, surgery, or an immunization
3. GBS is the most frequently acquired demyelinating neuropathy.

B. Etiology[1, 5, 6, 7, 8, 14]

1. Unknown, although an autoimmune basis is probable
2. Triggered by antecedent infection; described after upper respiratory infection, infectious mononucleosis, cytomegalovirus infections, herpes zoster, influenza A, mycoplasma, mumps, AIDS, Lyme disease, lymphoma (especially non-Hodgkin's), serum sickness, surgery, and heat stroke
3. In 50–75% of all cases, GBS is associated with *Campylobacter jejuni* enteritis. Culture studies have shown that a high proportion of patients with GBS have *C. jejuni* in their stools at the time of onset of neurologic symptoms.

C. Significance[5]

1. Incidence/prevalence in the United States: 1.3–1.9 cases per 100,000 annually; nonseasonal, nonepidemic in nature
2. Systems affected: Nervous, endocrine/metabolic
3. Predominant age/sex: All ages; occurs with equal frequency in males and females

D. Clinical manifestations[2, 4, 7, 9]

1. Symmetrical distal muscle weakness and paresthesia, beginning in the legs, ascending rapidly to the arms, face, and oropharynx
2. Weakness is more prominent than sensory signs and symptoms and may be more prominent proximally.
3. Hypotonia; sphincters are spared
4. Reduced reflexes, followed by loss of deep tendon reflexes—100% of patients

5. "Stocking" distribution sensory loss; may have hyperesthesia
6. Bulbar involvement—Bilateral facial and oropharyngeal paresis
7. Difficulty swallowing
8. Urinary retention
9. Respiratory paralysis
10. Autonomic dysfunction, including blood pressure fluctuations, inappropriate antidiuretic hormone secretion, cardiac arrhythmias, and pupillary changes

E. Laboratory findings[2, 3, 5]

1. CSF—Elevation of CSF protein (especially IgG) without increased cells. Elevation begins a week after symptoms and peaks in 4–6 weeks. Protein elevation may be very high (>1000 mg/dL).
2. CBC—Can see early leukocytosis with a left shift that resolves during the course of illness
3. If diagnosis is strongly suspected, repeat lumbar puncture is indicated.

F. Pathologic findings[2, 3, 12]

1. Segmental demyelination of peripheral nerves; axonal degeneration
2. Inflammatory lesion—Lymphocyte and macrophage invasion of myelin sheath
3. Special tests: Electromyography—Reveals slowed conduction velocities and prolonged motor, sensory, and F-wave latencies; decreased nerve conduction related to demyelination

G. Management[2, 4, 7, 12, 13]

1. Severe acute polyneuropathy is a medical emergency.
2. Admit to the intensive care unit for constant monitoring and vigorous support of vital functions.
3. Anticipate respiratory support by mechanical ventilation.
4. Measure vital capacity (VC) and arterial blood gases. VC < 1000 mL and Pao_2 < 70 indicate need for assisted ventilation.
5. Plasmapheresis: Perform in severe cases. Shortens course and reduces time on ventilator. Treatment of choice in those who are acutely ill, and should be performed within 7 days after onset. Very beneficial in preventing paralytic complications. Patients reportedly improve more quickly, can be weaned from assisted ventilation earlier, and can ambulate earlier.

   a. Recommendations are to use two plasma-exchange treatments for mild GBS.

   b. Use four or five plasma-exchange treatments for severe GBS.

   c. Start as soon as possible on alternating days.

6. IgG—Therapy that has been traditionally used as an alternative to plasmapheresis (0.4 g/kg IV for 5 consecutive days). It was recognized in 1999 that the use of high-dose intravenous immune globulin G (IVIgG) may promote remyelination in demyelinating disease.

7. New insights in GBS pathophysiology have emphasized the role of cellular immune reaction and the role of proinflammatory and anti-inflammatory cytokines (especially tumor necrosis factor [TNF] and tumor growth factor [TGF]). A research study suggests the potential usefulness of interferon beta-1a (Ribif, 6 mIU subcutaneously on alternate days) in decreasing motor deficit. Effects may be related to a decrease in TNF production, decrease of T-cell activation and proliferation, decrease of gelatinase B production, and increase of TGF production.

8. Prevention of thrombophlebitis: Thromboembolic disease stockings (TEDS) and heparin, (5000 U subcutaneously q12h)

9. Encourage fluid intake to maintain urine volume of 1 to 1.5 L/day.

10. Monitor serum and electrolytes to prevent water intoxication.

11. Protect extremities from trauma and pressure.

12. Apply moist heat to relieve pain and to permit early physical therapy.

13. Passive range of motion exercises immediately; active range of motion exercises when the acute symptoms subside

14. Emotional support and social counseling

15. No drug therapy is recommended.

16. Steroids have not been shown to be of benefit in GBS.

17. Prednisone is used in the chronic form of the disease, chronic relapsing polyneuropathy.

18. Pressors such as dopamine may be necessary for blood pressure support.

H. Follow-up[2, 4]

1. Patient will require physical rehabilitation to regain strength.

2. Subsequent development of chronic course: Chronic inflammatory demyelinating polyradiculoneuropathy (CIDP).

   a. CIDP has an insidious onset following GBS and may continue for years.

   b. Plasmapheresis benefits one third of these patients as well as immunosuppressive agents (azathioprine).

I. Expected course and prognosis[2-4]

1. Weakness and paralysis progress over a 2-week period, stabilize, and then gradually improve. Improvement over a period of months is common.
2. Ten percent to 23% of patients require ventilatory support.
3. Seven percent to 22% of patients are left with mild disability, mild weakness, or reflex loss.
4. About 10% of patients—those with a more prolonged course—have severe residual defects.
5. Axonal regeneration requires 6–18 months.
6. Mortality is approximately 3–5%.

II. MYASTHENIA GRAVIS (MG)

A. Definition[2]

1. A disorder of the neuromuscular junction resulting in a pure motor syndrome characterized by weakness and fatigue, particularly of the extraocular, pharyngeal, facial, cervical, proximal limb, and respiratory musculature
2. Caused by an autoimmune attack on the acetylcholine receptor of the postsynaptic neuromuscular junction, resulting in dysfunction of acetylcholine receptors and jeopardizing normal muscular transmission
3. Onset may be sudden or severe (myasthenic crisis) but, more typically, is mild and intermittent over many years.

B. Significance[4]

1. Incidence/prevalence in the United States: 2–5 million cases/year; 3/100,000
2. Predominant age: 20–40, but can occur at any age (1–80). Incidence in females peaks in the third decade, in males in the fifth and sixth decades.
3. Predominant sex: Females > males

C. Clinical manifestations[2, 3, 5, 6]

1. Ptosis—Ocular muscles are affected first in 40% of patients and eventually in 80%.
2. Diplopia
3. Facial weakness
4. Fatigue on chewing
5. Dysphagia
6. Dysarthria
7. Dysphonia
8. Neck weakness
9. Fatigue after exercise
10. Proximal limb weakness
11. Respiratory weakness

12. Generalized weakness
13. Sensory modalities and deep tendon reflexes normal
14. Severe generalized quadriparesis may develop, especially in relapse.

C. Diagnostics/Laboratory findings[2, 4, 12]

1. Acetylcholine receptor antibody (AChRAb)

   a. Generalized myasthenia—80% positive
   b. Ocular myasthenia—50% positive
   c. Myasthenia plus thymoma—100% positive
   d. Congenital myasthenia—0% positive
   e. There is no correlation between antibody titer and disease severity.

2. Thyroid function test: MG patients have a higher incidence of thyroid disease.
3. Vitamin B_{12} levels may be low because of associated pernicious anemia.
4. Muscle electron microscopy: Receptor infolding and the tips of the folds are lost; synaptic clefts are widened.
5. Immunofluorescence—IgG antibodies and complement in receptor membranes
6. Antinuclear antibodies, antithyroid, and rheumatoid arthritis factor are often present.
7. Repetitive nerve stimulation: In 60% of affected patients, there is a decremental response at 3 Hz which is seen more frequently in the proximal, cervical, or facial muscles. The decrement is less pronounced 30 s after a 30-s maximal voluntary contraction (postsynaptic facilitation) and most pronounced 120 s after the contraction (post-tetanic depression).
8. Single fiber electromyography (SFEMG): Highly sensitive but less specific, technically difficult to perform, limited availability. SFEMG assesses the temporal variability between two muscle fibers within the same motor unit (jitter). MG is one condition that increases jitter.
9. Edrophonium (Tensilon) test: Short duration (<5 min) and used in testing MG for differentiating between myasthenic and cholinergic crises

   a. Two mg IV, followed in 30 s by 3 mg, followed in 30 s by 5 mg, to a maximum dose of 10 mg.
   b. In MG there is a sudden, brief improvement in muscle function.
   c. Patients in myasthenic crises improve, whereas those in cholinergic crises worsen.
   d. Dangerous cardiorespiratory depression can occur, and atropine and equipment to maintain respiration must be available during the test.

e. CT scan of the chest may document an associated thymoma.

E. Management[2–4]

1. Typically outpatient
2. Inpatient care includes plasmapheresis, IV gamma globulin, and management of pulmonary infections and myasthenic or cholinergic crises.
3. General measures: Management is difficult and should be carried out by a neurologist who specializes in the field.

   a. Symptomatic approach
      i. Reversal of weakness with anticholinesterase inhibitor.
      ii. An overdose of these agents may induce severe weakness, known as a cholinergic crisis. A cholinergic crisis should be suspected if there are other signs of cholinergic overactivity.
   b. Immunosuppressive approach
      i. Immunosuppressive therapy in some form is necessary for patients with MG.
      ii. Thymectomy is the treatment for patients with thymoma.
      iii. Corticosteroids (see dosing following, under 6. Medications, b. Prednisone)
      iv. Plasmapheresis is more consistently effective and is used for rapid improvement of severe weakness.
      v. Immunosuppressive drugs such as azathioprine (Imuran), 2–3 mg/kg/day, or cyclosporine, 5 mg/kg/day, are often used in patients with severe generalized weakness and may reduce the need for steroids. Many require lifelong immunosuppressive therapy.
      vi. IV immune globulin G (IVIgG) has been used in myasthenics with severe disease and poor responses to other treatments. IVIgG therapy appears to improve strength rapidly, within 5 days of initiation, and lowers anti–acetylcholine-receptor antibodies, but the response is short-lived and is not uniformly observed.
   c. Supportive approach
      i. May include intubation
      ii. Tracheostomy
      iii. Artificial ventilation
      iv. Respiratory therapy
      v. Antibiotic administration
      vi. Nasogastric tube or gastrostomy

4. Activity: As tolerated. Heat and exercise both temporarily exacerbate symptoms.
5. Diet: As tolerated

6. Medications

   a. Cholinesterase inhibitors

      i. Pyridostigmine bromide (Mestinon): 30–60 mg p.o. q4–6h initially. Onset of effect is 30 min, duration 4 h. A longer-acting preparation (Mestinon Timespan 180 mg sustained release tablets) can be given q.i.d. or b.i.d. The longer-acting preparation is beneficial for those patients who have symptoms first thing in the morning. Titrate dosage to clinical need. An average requirement would be 600 mg/day.

      ii. Neostigmine methylsulfate (Prostigmin): 0.25, 0.5, and 1 mg/mL concentrations. Titrate to clinical need. A starting dose would be 0.5 mg SC or IM q3h. For oral administration, usual dose is 7.5–30 mg q.i.d.

      iii. Monitor for cholinergic side effects such as nausea and vomiting, diarrhea, increased salivation and bronchial secretions, and cramps. These side effects can be controlled with atropine and glycopyrrolate.

      iv. Overmedication may temporarily increase weakness, which is enhanced by intravenous edrophonium.

   b. Prednisone should be administered to those who have responded poorly to anticholinesterase drugs and, if indicated, have already had a thymectomy. The dose is determined on an individual basis, but a high initial dose (60–100 mg) can gradually be tapered to a low maintenance dose. Switch to q.o.d. within 2 weeks. Continue to taper very slowly, attempting to establish the minimum dosage necessary to maintain remission. A typical maintenance dosage would be 35 mg q.o.d.

   c. Azathioprine is an effective treatment (2–3 mg/kg p.o. q.i.d.), alone or in combination with prednisone, but weakness may take several months to improve.

   d. Cyclophosphamide may be used in a fashion similar to azathioprine, but usually takes effect within months.

   e. Immune globulin

F. Associated conditions[2, 4]

1. Thymoma
2. Thymic hyperplasia
3. Thyrotoxicosis
4. Other autoimmune diseases

References

1. Allen, A., & Antony, S. (1999). Severe Guillain-Barré syndrome associated with campylobacter jejuni infection with failure to respond to plasmapheresis and immunoglobulin. *Journal of the American Board of Family Practice, 12*, 249–252.

2. Boonyapisit, K., Kaminski, H., & Ruff, R. (1999). Disorders of neuromuscular junction ion channels. *American Journal of Medicine, 106*, 97–113.

3. Clochesy, J.M., Breu, C., & Dossey, B. (1997). *AACN handbook of critical care nursing.* Stamford, CT: Appleton & Lange.

4. Creange, A., Lerat, H., Meyrignac, C., Degos, J., Gherardi, R., & Cesaro, P. (1998). Treatment of Guillain-Barré syndrome with interferon-β. *The Lancet, 352*, 368–369.

5. Devinsky, O., Feldmann, E., Weinreb, H.J., & Wilterdink, J.L. (1997). *The resident's neurology book.* Philadelphia: FA Davis.

6. Ferri, F.F. (1998). *Practical guide to the care of the medical patient* (4th ed.). St. Louis: Mosby.

7. Hahn, A. (1998). Guillain-Barré syndrome. *The Lancet, 352*, 635–641.

8. Hartung, H. (1999). Infections and the Guillain-Barré syndrome. *Journal of Neurology, Neurosurgery, and Psychiatry, 66*, 277.

9. Keiser, M.M. (1999). Neurologic disorders. In A. Gawlinski & D. Hamwi (Eds.), *Acute care nurse practitioner: Clinical curriculum and certification review.* Philadelphia: WB Saunders.

10. Pfeiffeir, G. & Steffen, W. (1999). Guillain-Barré syndrome after heat stroke. *Journal of Neurology, Neurosurgery, and Psychiatry, 66*, 408.

11. Rakel, R.E. (1996). *Saunders manual of medical practice.* Philadelphia: WB Saunders.

12. Stein, J.H. (1998). *Internal medicine* (5th ed.). St. Louis: Mosby.

13. Stangel, M., Klaus, V., & Gold, R. (1999). Mechanisms of high-dose intravenous immunoglobulins in demyelinating diseases. *Archives of Neurology, 56*, 661–663.

14. Tierney, L.M., McPhee, S.J., & Papadakis, M.A. (1999). *Current medical diagnosis & treatment* (38th ed.). Stamford, CT: Appleton & Lange.

NEUROLOGIC TRAUMA

Charlene M. Myers, MSN, RN, CS,
ACNP, CCRN

4

I. HEAD TRAUMA/TRAUMATIC BRAIN INJURY[1, 2, 4, 5, 7, 9, 10, 14, 17]

A. Head trauma accounts for two thirds of all casualties of motor vehicle accidents.

1. Head trauma is the leading cause of death in all trauma cases.
2. The anatomic structures and physiologic functions of the head provide protection for the brain.

    a. Scalp
    b. Skull
    c. Cerebral meninges ("PAD"—pia mater, arachnoid, dura mater)
    d. CSF

3. The brain is dependent upon glucose (25%) and oxygen (20%) for functioning.

B. Mechanism of injury

1. Acceleration
2. Deceleration
3. Deformation

C. Type of injury

1. Blunt trauma
2. Penetrating injuries

    a. High-velocity objects
    b. Low-velocity objects

3. Coup-contrecoup injuries: Brain tissue injury directly at the site of impact (coup) and at the pole opposite the site of impact (contrecoup), which may be caused by movement of cranial contents within the skull

D. Categories of injury

1. Primary head injuries

    a. Scalp laceration
        i. Most common head injury seen
        ii. Can result in profuse bleeding secondary to the great vascular supply to the scalp (monitor for signs and

symptoms of hypovolemia, such as increased heart rate and decreased blood pressure)

   iii. Apply direct pressure to control bleeding (first assess for skull fracture)

   iv. Suture/staple laceration after thorough examination and cleansing. Lidocaine 1% with epinephrine should be used on the scalp lacerations to help control the bleeding. Do not use lidocaine with epinephrine on lacerations located on the nose or ears.

b. Skull fractures

   i. Simple: No displacement of bone. Observe for scalp laceration, protect the cervical spine; may indicate underlying brain injury

   ii. Depressed: Bone fragment depressing the thickness of the skull

- Often have a scalp laceration
- May be asymptomatic or have altered level of consciousness
- Requires surgery to elevate and debride wound
- Prophylactic broad-spectrum antibiotics
- Tetanus toxoid if indicated
- Institute seizure precautions.

   iii. Basilar: Fracture in the floor of the skull

- Raccoon eyes—periorbital ecchymosis
- Battle's sign—mastoid ecchymosis
- Otorrhea and/or rhinorrhea (positive Dextrostix test result, halo or target sign, and salty taste in mouth). *Do not* obstruct the flow.
- Prophylactic antibiotic coverage
- Oral intubation and oral gastric tube are indicated instead of nasal intubation and nasogastric tube.

c. Brain injuries

   i. Concussion: Transient, reversible alteration in brain functioning

- Brief loss of consciousness, amnesia of events
- Lethargy, headache, nausea, dizziness
- Do not give narcotics—Evaluate for changes in level of consciousness.
- May need to admit to hospital if unconsciousness lasted longer than 2 min

   ii. Contusion: Bruising to the surface of the brain with varying degrees of edema, contrecoup injury; skull is rough and jagged, and the brain may be damaged as it moves across the underlying structures.

- Variable level of consciousness and amnesia
- Nausea and vomiting, dizziness
- Visual disturbances
- Institute seizure precautions.
- Brain stem contusion: Posturing, variable temperature, variable vital signs

2. Secondary head injuries

   a. Epidural hematoma: Collection of arterial blood between the skull and the dura mater in the epidural space
      i. Loss of consciousness, followed by a lucid interval, then rapid deterioration
      ii. Stupor progresses to coma.
      iii. Ipsilateral pupil dilation
      iv. Hemiplegia
      v. Obtain CT scan.
      vi. Mannitol may be given to "buy time."
      vii. Immediate surgical intervention is necessary.
   b. Subdural hematoma: Venous bleeding between the dura mater and the brain tissue
      i. Most frequently seen type of intracranial bleeding
      ii. Acute: Develops over minutes to hours

      - Drowsiness, agitation, confusion
      - Headache
      - Unilateral or bilateral pupil dilation
      - Late hemiparesis
      - Obtain a CT scan.
      - Surgery is required.

      iii. Chronic: Develops over days or weeks

      - Headache
      - Memory loss
      - Personality changes
      - Incontinence
      - Ataxia
      - Obtain a CT scan.
      - Surgery is usually required, but close monitoring may be sufficient if the hematoma is small.

   c. Infections
      i. Meningitis
      ii. Brain abscess
   d. Brain swelling or edema

E. Clinical manifestations[1, 2, 5, 7, 9, 10, 14]

1. Many have been discussed previously under specific types of head injuries.

2. When the patient is beginning to decompensate, symptoms of Cushing's triad may develop.

   a. Widening pulse pressure (The systolic blood pressure will increase in an attempt to maintain a constant cerebral perfusion pressure [CPP].)

$$CPP = MAP - ICP$$

   where MAP = mean arterial pressure and ICP = intracranial pressure

   b. Decreased respiratory rate
   c. Decreased heart rate

3. Neurologic examination

   a. AVPU—A = awake, V = responds to verbal stimuli, P = responds to painful stimuli, U = unresponsive
   b. Glasgow coma scale (Individuals with subdural hematoma and a score of 8 or less have a poor prognosis.)
   c. Posturing
     i. Decorticate: Flexion of upper extremities with extension of lower extremities
     ii. Decerebrate: Extension of both upper extremities and lower extremities (more of the brain stem is involved)

4. Laboratory findings in patients with diabetes insipidus

   a. Electrolytes: Increased sodium, decreased potassium, and so forth
   b. Increased serum osmolality (>275–285 mOsm/kg)
   c. Decreased urine osmolality (N = 300–900 mOsm/kg)
   d. Decreased urine specific gravity (N = 1.010–1.030)
   e. CBC; hemoconcentration (hematocrit and hemoglobin may be falsely high)

F. Management[1, 2, 4, 5, 7, 9, 10, 13–16]

1. Consult a neurosurgeon.
2. Prevent hypotension and hypoxemia.

   a. According to the Brain Trauma Foundation guidelines, resuscitation should be aimed at maintaining a systolic blood pressure (SBP) greater than 90 mmHg and a partial pressure of arterial oxygen (Pao_2) greater than 60 mmHg.
   b. Attempt to maintain a mean arterial blood pressure (MAP) greater than 90 mmHg.

$$MAP = (2[DBP] + SBP) \div 3$$

   where DBP is diastolic blood pressure

   c. If the patient is hypotensive, administer 1–2 L of isotonic crystalloid solution immediately. Avoid overhydration as attempts are made to restore adequate blood pressure (MAP > 90 mmHg).

d. As of the end of the 1990s literature is beginning to recommend small-volume resuscitation with hypertonic/hyperosmolar solutions (e.g., hypertonic saline, dextran) because of the findings that these solutions increase the intracranial compliance, resulting in a smaller increase in intracranial pressure (ICP).

e. Administration of blood is another way to improve tissue perfusion to the brain by optimizing the oxygen-carrying capacity of the intravascular fluid. The goal is to maintain hematocrit at 30–33%.

3. Hyperventilation/hyperoxia

a. Hyperventilation (Pa_{CO_2} 25–30 mmHg) has been used for decades to cause cerebral vasoconstriction and thereby lower ICP. Cerebral vasoconstriction secondary to hyperventilation has also been known to cause cerebral ischemia.

b. Experts now recommend that hyperventilation not be used routinely, especially in the first 24 h after injury, unless ICP is severely high, or when the patient requires suctioning. The Brain Trauma Foundation's guidelines specifically recommend that hyperventilation to bring Pa_{CO_2} < 35 mmHg be undertaken only if there is a measured increase in ICP, or if increased ICP is suspected because of physical signs, and intracranial hypertension is refractory to other interventions. Other methods to control ICP should be be instituted first (elevating the head of the bed, sedation, paralysis, mannitol, and CSF drainage).

c. Other studies support that hyperoxia during acute hyperventilation improves oxygen delivery to the brain, as indicated by improved jugular venous bulb saturation and arteriovenous oxygen content difference. Moderate hyperventilation to a Pa_{CO_2} of 30 mmHg in combination with a higher Pa_{O_2} may be beneficial in patients with head injury.

d. Nasal intubation and an NGT are preferred over oral intubation, taking into consideration the possibility of cervical spine injury, with the exception of basilar skull fractures.

4. CNS depressants

a. Narcotic sedatives help lower ICP by reducing metabolic demand and relieving anxiety and pain. Naloxone (Narcan) can reverse the effects of a narcotic sedative when performing a neurologic assessment.

b. Short-acting narcotics are the best choices (IV fentanyl, 2–20 μg/kg over 1–2 min, up to 50 μg/kg, or sufentanil [Sufenta], 1–8 μg/kg/min). These may be supplemented with propofol (Diprivan) or benzodiazepines (diazepam [Valium] or lorazepam [Ativan]) if the patient remains agitated or ICP remains elevated.

c. Neuromuscular blocking agents (vecuronium [Norcuron, .04–.1 mg/kg IV] or doxacurium [Nuromax, .05 mg/kg]) can be used to help lower ICP in patients in whom confusion, posturing, or severe agitation is interfering with treatment or diagnostic testing. Patients must be sedated, intubated with an adequate set rate on the ventilator. Paralytic agents also may be needed to help oxygenate and ventilate the patient.

5. Steroids

a. Corticosteroids remain controversial. Theoretically, these drugs work by preventing fluid from entering the cells and by increasing blood vessel diameter, thereby increasing cerebral blood flow.

b. Many practitioners feel the risks of steroids (e.g., compromise of immune function, infections, delayed wound healing, gastric distress) far outweigh the benefits. It is reported that no significant improvement or reduction in ICP has been noted with the use of steroids.

6. Osmotherapy (mannitol):

a. Very useful in certain patients, and is the drug of choice in an emergency situation when brain herniation is pending

b. Mannitol creates an osmotic gradient across the blood-brain barrier that pulls water from the CNS into the intravascular space.

c. Mannitol may enhance cerebral oxygen delivery via decreased blood viscosity, increased CPP, or both.

d. Mannitol may also provide some cytoprotective effects through oxygen-free radical scavenging.

e. Administer as a bolus (0.25–1.0 g/kg). Results are quick, usually within 10–20 min, and can last up to 6 h.

f. Monitor serum osmolarity, and keep lower than 320 mOsm. Monitor electrolytes as well, and replace as needed.

g. Monitor blood pressure closely, as hypotension is a side effect resulting from dehydration as a result of diuresis. The goal is to gain beneficial effects without inducing dehydration.

h. Volume replacement may be necessary to keep the patient euvolemic and to prevent hypotension (e.g., replace urinary output volume-for-volume each hour, or one half volume-for-volume each hour with isotonic crystalloids).

i. An indwelling urinary catheter should be in place with urine output recorded each hour.

j. Some investigators are replacing mannitol with loop diuretics such as furosemide (Lasix) and ethacrynic acid (Edecrin) to control ICP, believing that these drugs are less likely to cause severe dehydration.

7. ICP monitoring, CSF drainage, and CPP management

    a. ICP monitoring is appropriate for
        i. Comatose patients (Glasgow coma scale score of 3–8) with an abnormal CT scan
        ii. Comatose patients with a normal CT scan and two of the following: (1) age >40 years; (2) unilateral or bilateral motor posturing; (3) or hypotension.

    b. ICP monitoring is not routinely appropriate for patients with mild or moderate head injuries.

    c. A ventricular catheter will allow the practitioner to measure ICP and also drain CSF.

    d. The guideline threshold for ICP is 20–25 mmHg.

    e. Monitoring ICP allows the practitioner to calculate CPP (CPP = MAP − ICP).

    f. Ideally, the CPP should be maintained at >70 mmHg.

8. The patient must have an ongoing neurologic assessment in order to evaluate treatment effectiveness as well as the need for further interventions.

    a. Evaluating the Glasgow coma scale score may be necessary every 30–60 min the first 24 h. Note whether the patient is receiving sedation and/or paralytics, as they may lower the score.

    b. Pupil size and reaction

    c. Vital signs

9. All patients with a head injury are presumed to have a cervical spine injury until proven otherwise. Once the patient is stabilized, order a cervical spine series.

10. Avoid any condition that increases metabolic rate and therefore increases the demand for O_2 and glucose (e.g., fever, pain, shivering).

11. Prospective treatment

    a. Polyethylene glycol superoxide dismutase is a drug being studied to determine whether it can decrease the toxicity to the brain of the free radicals that are released during trauma. This drug appears to improve clinical outcome in head trauma victims.

b. Lazaroids, synthetic nonglucocorticoids, are a group of experimental drugs that may slow cellular membrane breakdown after head injury by inhibiting lipid peroxidation.

c. N-methyl-D-aspartates (NMDAs) are potentially useful in that they inhibit the harmful effects of certain excitatory amino acids found at the site of injury that, when released during ischemia, create a hypermetabolic state that makes the injury worse. The ultimate goal of NMDAs is to help minimize the extent of brain damage by controlling the metabolic rate.

d. Hypothermia may possibly improve clinical outcomes by controlling ICP. Lowering the temperature to 89.6°–91.4° F has shown improved outcomes in animals and is now being tested in humans.

G. Major complications

1. Post-traumatic seizures
2. Stress ulcers
3. Diabetes insipidus
4. Acute hydrocephalus

H. Brain death criteria

1. No spontaneous movement
2. No spontaneous respiration after receiving 100% O_2 for 10 min and tested for a period of 4–6 min, with a P_{CO_2} reaching 60 mmHg
3. Absence of brain stem reflexes

   a. Fixed and dilated pupils
   b. No corneal reflexes
   c. Absent doll's eyes
   d. Absent gag reflex
   e. Absent vestibular response to caloric stimulation

4. Demonstration of "no flow" state to the brain using arteriography
5. A flat EEG repeated over a 12–24 h period
6. Rudimentary spinal reflexes, when present, should not influence the determination of brain death.
7. Hypothermia, barbiturate poisoning, and metabolic imbalances must be ruled out as the cause of CNS lesions.

I. Information specific to the Guidelines for Management of Severe Head Injury can be found on the website of the Aitken Neuroscience Center at http://www.aitken.org.

II. SPINAL CORD TRAUMA[1, 2, 5, 6, 8, 9, 11, 12, 14, 17]

A. Mechanisms of injury

1. Motor vehicle accidents account for the largest number of spinal cord injuries (SCIs) (40%).

2. Falls or falling objects (10–20%)
3. Acts of violence (15%)
4. Sports-related injuries (13%)
5. Penetrating wounds (12%)

B. Spinal cord injuries (SCIs)

1. Rapid acceleration/deceleration

   a. Hyperextension—Usually occurs as a result of a fall onto the face, forehead, or chin. Rear-end collisions may also result in rupture of the anterior longitudinal ligament. Hyperextension may cause the cord to stretch and result in central cord syndrome (described hereafter at I. Spinal cord lesions [syndromes], 3).
   b. Hyperflexion—Greatest stress occurs at C5–C6, causing bilateral facet dislocations.
   c. Vertical column loading (compression)—Occurs in diving accidents or falls when the patient lands on the feet or buttocks. The vertebral body is compressed and/or shattered, resulting in a "burst" fracture, and bone fragments may become embedded in the cord. Injuries may occur at the level of C1 with diving accidents.
   d. "Whiplash"—A sudden hyperextension of the spine that causes stretching of the ligaments as a result of the force of the lower body moving forward and by the backward and downward course of the head

2. Distraction injuries—A result of hanging
3. Penetrating trauma

   a. Gunshot wound
   b. Stab wound
   c. Bony fragments

4. Hematoma
5. Pathologic fractures—Occur in patients with osteoporosis or metastatic disease

C. Epidemiology

1. Incidence

   a. Sixty percent of SCIs involve the cervical spine.
   b. Approximately 8000 SCIs per year, or 32.1 per million
   c. Approximately 40% of SCI patients die before reaching the hospital or during the initial resuscitation phase.
   d. Average hospital cost: $80,200 for quadriplegics and $72,000 for paraplegics
   e. Average lifetime care of a young adult with an SCI exceeds $1 million.

D. Age

1. More common in young males (82% males compared with 18% females)
2. More frequent in younger persons (80% younger than 40 years, and 50% between 15 and 25 years)

E. Anatomy and physiology

1. 33 Vertebrae

   a. Cervical spine (C1–C7)—Very flexible in nature, smaller in diameter, therefore many fractures occur here
   b. Thoracic spine (T1–T12)—Articulate with the ribs, therefore less common site for fractures because of their stability
   c. Lumbar spine (L1–L5)—Very mobile, yet large in diameter, requiring a greater amount of force to fracture
   d. Sacral spine (S1–S5)
   e. Coccygeal vertebrae (3–5 coccyx)

2. Spinal cord

   a. Gray matter
   b. White layer
   c. Meningeal layer (pia mater, arachnoid, dura mater)

F. Assessment

1. History

   a. Mechanism of injury (e.g., speed of impact; blunt vs. penetrating forces; whether flexion, extension, rotation, or distraction to the spine occurred; height of fall; use of restraints or deployed airbag; extent of vehicular damage; position of patient in vehicle)
   b. Patient complaints (e.g., back pain, neck pain, numbness, paresthesia)
   c. Motor response/sensory response
   d. Prehospital treatment

2. Physical assessment

   a. ABCs and life-threatening injuries are treated first.
   b. Pulmonary complications account for most of the early deaths following acute traumatic quadriplegia.
   c. Assess respiratory ability.
      i. Chest excursion
      ii. Use of intercostal muscles or diaphragm
      iii. Cervical cord injury above C3 results in respiratory arrest. C5–C6 spare the diaphragm, and diaphragmatic breathing occurs. T1–L2 lesions cause loss of intercostal muscle use.

d. Intubation—If necessary
    i. Jaw thrust maneuver
    ii. Apnea
    iii. Breathing difficulty
    iv. Diaphragmatic fatigue
e. Arterial blood gases should be monitored closely.
f. Monitor for pneumonia, pulmonary edema, and pulmonary emboli.

3. Motor assessment

a. Inability to perform the function listed in the following indicates that the lesion is above the level indicated.
    i. Deltoids (C4): Apply pressure to shoulders and ask patient to shrug shoulders.
    ii. Biceps (C5): Have patient flex arm (gravity), then apply pressure by trying to straighten arm. Tell patient not to let you straighten extremity (resistance).
    iii. Wrist (C6): Have patient hyperextend the wrist (gravity) and apply pressure by trying to straighten wrist. Tell patient not to let you push down (resistance).
    iv. Triceps (C7): Have patient extend arm (gravity) and try to pull arm up to the flexed position. Tell patient not to let you bend arm (resistance).
    v. Intrinsic (C8): Have patient abduct (fan) fingers and try to push them together.
    vi. Hip flexion: Have patient bend knee and apply pressure to determine resistance (L2–L4).
    vii. Knee extension: While hip is flexed and knee bent, have patient try to extend the knee (L2–L4).
b. Grade the strength using the following scale:
    i. 5 = Normal movement against gravity and full resistance
    ii. 4 = Full range of motion against moderate resistance and gravity
    iii. 3 = Full range of motion against gravity, not against resistance
    iv. 2 = Extremity can move, but not against gravity (can roll but not lift)
    v. 1 = Muscle contracts, but extremity cannot move
    vi. 0 = No visible or palpable muscle contraction or movement of extremity (flaccid)
c. All motor groups need to be comprehensively assessed.
d. Complete lesion: The patient lacks sensory function, proprioception, and voluntary motor activity below the level of spinal cord damage; worse prognosis for recovering neurologic function.
e. Incomplete lesion: Parts of the spinal cord at the level of the lesion are intact. There is sacral sparing. Note sensory

perception and voluntary contraction of the anus around the examiner's finger.

4. Sensory function

a. Begin at the area of no feeling and proceed to the area of feeling.
b. Assess response to pain.

- Great toe: L4
- Back of leg: S1–S3
- Perianal area: S4–S5
- Umbilicus: T10
- Nipple line: T4
- Ring and little fingers: C8
- Middle finger: C7
- Thumb: C6
- Top of shoulder: C4

c. If the patient is unable to feel pain, the lesion is at or above the spinal nerve level indicated.

5. Evaluate the patient's back, performing a well-coordinated log-roll maneuver. Maintain in-line spinal stabilization.

a. Gently palpate spine for pain, tenderness, or gaps between spinous processes.
b. Observe for entrance/exit wounds, impaled objects, and other signs of injury.

G. Key signs of various levels of injury

1. C2–C3

a. Respiratory paralysis
b. Flaccid paralysis
c. Areflexia (deep tendon reflexes [DTRs])
d. Loss of sensation below the mandible

2. C5–C6

a. Diaphragmatic breathing
b. Paralysis of intercostal and abdominal muscles
c. Quadriplegia
d. Anesthesia below the clavicle and ulnar half of the arms
e. Areflexia (with possible exception of the biceps reflex)
f. Fecal and urinary retention
g. Priapism (spontaneous erection)

3. T12–L1

a. Paraplegia
b. Anesthesia in the legs
c. Areflexia in the legs

    d. Fecal and urinary retention

    e. Priapism (spontaneous erection)

4. L1–L5

    a. Flaccid paralysis to partial flaccid paralysis

    b. Abdominal and cremasteric reflexes present

    c. Ankle and plantar reflexes absent

H. Multisystem impact of SCIs

1. Cardiovascular

    a. Hypotension

        i. Caused by loss of sympathetic tone in patients with high thoracic or cervical injuries with pooling of blood into the periphery

        ii. If associated with a neurologic deficit, normal or decreased heart rate, and warm, vasodilated extremities, *spinal shock* is suspected.

        iii. Initial fluid resuscitation with 2–3 L of lactated Ringer's solution (Do not overload—possible loss of cardiac contractility puts the patient at risk for CHF and pulmonary edema.)

        iv. Rule out hypovolemia as cause of hypotension.

        v. Vasopressors (dopamine) and hemodynamic monitoring may be indicated if patient is unresponsive to intravenous fluids.

    b. Bradycardia

        i. Caused by sympathetic blockade, and may lead to arrhythmias (junctional or ventricular escape)

        ii. Be alert for conditions that promote bradycardia in patients with SCIs: hypoxia, hypothermia, and vagal stimulation

        iii. Be sure the patient is well-oxygenated.

        iv. Maintain body temperature at >96.8°F.

        v. Administer atropine for symptomatic bradycardia (decreased level of consciousness, urinary output, and blood pressure).

    c. Vasovagal reflex

        i. Induced by any straining, coughing, bearing down

        ii. Frequently induced by suctioning, which leads to hypoxia, and by vagal stimulation (bradycardia—cardiac arrest)

        iii. Oxygenate and hyperventilate with 100% O_2 prior to suctioning.

        iv. Limit suctioning to 10 s.

        v. Monitor cardiac rate and rhythm.

    d. Poikilothermy

        i. Patient's temperature is dependent on temperature of the environment, resulting from interruption of the sympathetic pathways to the temperature-regulating centers in the hypothalamus.

    ii. Maintain temperature of the environment.

  e. Venous thrombosis

    i. Venous stasis in the legs and pelvis resulting from a decreased blood flow and flaccid paralysis

    ii. Administer deep venous thrombosis prophylaxis (heparin, 5000 U SC b.i.d.), antiembolic stockings, range of motion, vena cava filters.

    iii. Measure thighs and calves for swelling from deep venous thromboses.

  f. Orthostatic hypotension

    i. Occurs when patients moved from supine to sitting position; related to venous pooling in the legs and abdomen due to loss of skeletal muscle pump and impaired sympathetic nervous system control.

    ii. Use thigh high stockings and abdominal binders to promote venous return.

2. Gastrointestinal

  a. Abdominal injuries resulting from trauma

    i. Difficult to diagnosis in SCI because abdominal pain and muscular rigidity, the telltale signs of internal bleeding, are absent if the patient has sensory and motor deficits.

    ii. Assess patient for abdominal distention; monitor hematocrit and hemoglobin and blood volume.

    iii. Perform a diagnostic peritoneal lavage.

  b. Curling's ulcer

    i. Patients with CNS injury may have this type of stress ulcer as a result of vagal-stimulated gastric production and/or release of adrenocorticotropic hormone.

    ii. Assess gastric pH and administer antacids and H_2 antagonists for prevention and treatment.

    iii. Warm- and cold-water lavage may be used to treat bleeding.

    iv. Monitor patient for coagulation defects.

    v. Vasopressin may be used.

    vi. Gastrectomy may be necessary in severe cases.

  c. Gastric atony and ileus

    i. Related to loss of central control

    ii. Leads to severe gastric distention that in turn can lead to respiratory compromise, vomiting, and aspiration

    iii. Place an NGT to low wall suction—Note amount and quality of aspirate.

  d. Loss of bowel function

    i. Patient cannot sense when the bowel is full or perform the Valsalva maneuver to aid in evacuation.

    ii. May lead to obstruction or autonomic dysreflexia (described immediately following under 3. Genitourinary)

    iii. Initiate a bowel program—Suppository same time every day either AM or PM

3. Genitourinary
   a. Autonomic dysreflexia
      i. Distended bladder is the most common cause, although it can result from any noxious stimuli (e.g., distended bowel, wrinkled sheets, pressure ulcers, constrictive clothing, constrictive devices such as foot splints, shoes that are tied too tightly).
      ii. A hypertensive crisis that may occur from a noxious stimulus in injuries above T6, the sympathetic outflow level
      iii. SCI may result in denervation of the bladder, which may become overdistended.
      iv. A noxious stimulus below the level of injury triggers the sympathetic nervous system, causing massive release of catecholamines.
      v. The result of catecholamine release is vasoconstriction.
      vi. Vasodilation occurs above injury—red, flushed, warm skin, headache, nasocongestion, diaphoresis.
      vii. Piloerection occurs below the injury.
      viii. Place a urinary catheter to monitor urinary output and to decompress the bladder.
      ix. Do not drain bladder rapidly if cardiovascular system suggests autonomic dysreflexia (no more than 600 mL at a time).
   b. Urinary tract infection
      i. May result from urinary retention or catheterization
      ii. Intermittent catheterization is recommended.
      iii. Early detection is essential to prevent sepsis or prolonged spinal shock.

4. Musculoskeletal
   a. Impaired skin integrity related to abnormal nerve supply and poor circulation
   b. Paralysis
      i. Muscle atony and wasting
      ii. Contractures
      iii. Perform passive range of motion and positioning, and use handsplints and boots to prevent footdrop.

5. Psychological devastation
   a. Effect on the patient
      i. Disturbance of self-concept
      ii. Ineffective coping

      iii. Feelings of powerlessness

      iv. Denial, anger, depression

  b. Practitioner's response

      i. Be honest, with a positive attitude.

      ii. Include patient in his/her care.

      iii. Set limits of behavior, and be consistent with care.

      iv. Take an interdisciplinary approach—e.g., social services, psychiatry, physical therapy, occupational therapy, pastoral care.

I. Spinal cord lesions (syndromes)

1. Anterior cord syndrome

  a. Probably the most devastating of the syndromes

  b. Disruption of blood flow through the anterior spinal artery

  c. Flexion injuries

  d. Weakness or paralysis with loss of sense of pain and temperature

  e. Proprioception intact

2. Posterior cord syndrome

  a. Rare injury resulting from disruption of the posterior column

  b. Decrease in touch proprioception, vibration

3. Central cord syndrome

  a. Hyperextension injuries with stretching of the cord and subsequent hemorrhaging in the center of the cord

  b. Greater motor loss and sensation in the upper extremities than in the lower extremities because the upper extremities are controlled by the central portion of the cord

4. Brown-Séquard syndrome

  a. Stab wounds, gunshot wounds, fracture of the vertebral process, and spinal cord tumors

  b. One side of the spinal cord is damaged.

  c. Ipsilateral motor loss and contralateral loss of pain and temperature sensation

  d. The extremities that can move have no feeling, and those that have feeling cannot move.

J. Diagnostic procedures

1. Cervical vertebrae

  a. Cross table lateral position first. All seven vertebrae must be seen. To do so may require

      i. Firmly pulling the patient's shoulders down

      ii. Lateral swimmer's view

    b. Obtain anteroposterior x-ray if lateral x-ray is abnormal.
    c. Obtain open-mouth odontoid x-ray for conscious patient to visualize C2.
    d. Failure to obtain basic radiographic studies is the primary reason for missed diagnosis of cervical spine injuries.

2. Thoracic vertebrae

    a. Lateral and anteroposterior x-rays
    b. View all 12 vertebrae.

3. Lumbar vertebrae

    a. Lateral and anteroposterior views
    b. View all five lumbar vertebrae.

4. CT may be helpful to clearly identify normal cervical spine anatomy or presence of bony fragments.
5. Films in flexion/extension position or oblique films at times for further delineation of suspected fractures
6. Myelogram detects compression of the cord by herniated disks, bone fragments, or foreign matter that needs surgical intervention.
7. MRI can add further information regarding cord impingement, hematomas, and infarcts. Cord contusions or hemorrhage cannot be visualized by any other technique.

K. Management[1-3, 5, 6, 8, 11, 14, 17, 18]

1. Consult neurosurgeon.
2. Airway maintenance

    a. Nasotracheal intubation or cricothyrotomy if necessary
    b. *Do not* hyperextend or rotate the neck.
    c. Administer oxygen.

3. Immobilization

    a. Protective devices (e.g., cervical collar, spine board)
    b. Do not remove device until x-rays are obtained and cleared.
    c. Log-roll only.

4. Intravascular fluids (limit to appropriate levels)

    • Distinguish neurogenic shock (warm, dry extremities, bradycardia) from hypovolemic shock (cool, clammy skin, tachycardia).

5. Bladder catheterization
6. Nasogastric intubation
7. Corticosteroids (controversial)

    a. May be useful in early treatment of spinal cord injury to reduce swelling if administered within the first 6 h

   b. Methylprednisolone (Solu-Medrol), 30 mg/kg, as an intravenous bolus, followed by a maintenance infusion of 5.4 mg/kg/h for 23 h

   c. The improvement is in 6 weeks to 6 months after injury.

   d. Monitor for elevation in blood glucose levels.

   e. Monitor for other side effects such as immunosuppression, fluid and electrolyte disturbances, adrenocortical insufficiency, impaired wound healing, and gastrointestinal disturbances.

8. Antibiotics for penetrating injuries: Nafcillin, 200 mg/kg/day IV in 4–6 divided doses

9. Maintain room temperature—Avoid poikilothermy.

10. Meticulous skin care: Order rotating bed for respiratory therapy (postural drainage) and skin therapy.

11. Prepare for insertion of skeletal tongs and traction—Stryker frame, kinetic bed, or halo vest, used to assist in restoration of the spine to a normal position (reduction).

   a. At least 10 lb of weight are initially applied.

   b. Weight is applied based on the 5 lb per interspace formula (i.e., a C5–C6 injury would require 25–30 lb of traction).

   c. Muscle relaxants are helpful.

   d. Lateral x-rays are taken to assess vertebral alignment as weights are applied.

   e. Too much weight can pull the spine apart, resulting in distraction injury.

   f. If paralytics are needed, weight may need to be reduced.

12. Fixation: Involves stabilizing vertebral fracture with wires, plates, and other types of hardware

13. Fusion: Involves attaching injured vertebrae to uninjured vertebrae with bone grafts and steel rods

14. Surgery for removal of bony fragments or to drain hematomas that compress the cord may be indicated.

15. Rehabilitation begins upon admission. Follow an interdisciplinary approach.

References

1. Clochesy, J.M., Breu, C., & Dossey, B. (1997). *AACN handbook of critical care nursing.* Stamford, CT: Appleton & Lange.
2. Devinsky, O., Feldmann, E., Weinreb, H.J., & Wilterdink, J.L. (1997). *The resident's neurology book.* Philadelphia: FA Davis.
3. Ferri, F.F. (1998). *Practical guide to the care of the medical patient* (4th ed.). St. Louis: Mosby.
4. Grant, I.S. & Andrews, P.J. (1999). ABC of intensive care: Neurological support. *British Medical Journal, 319,* 110–113.
5. Haskell, R.M. (1999). Trauma. In P. Login (Ed.), *Principles of practice for the acute care nurse practitioner* (pp. 347–377). Stamford, CT: Appleton & Lange.

6. Iida, H., Tachibana, S., Kitahara, T., Horiike, S., Ohwada, T., & Fujii, K. (1999). Association of head trauma with cervical injury, spinal cord injury or both. *Journal of Trauma, 46,* 450–452.

7. Jastremski, C. (1998). Head injuries. *RN, 61,* 40–44.

8. Jastremski, C.A. (1999). Spinal cord injury. In L. Bucher & S. Melander (Eds.), *Critical care nursing* (pp. 869–898). Philadelphia: WB Saunders.

9. Keiser, M.M. (1999). Neurologic disorders. In A. Gawlinski & D. Hamwi (Eds.), *Acute care nurse practitioner: Clinical curriculum and certification review.* Philadelphia: WB Saunders.

10. March, K. (1999). Acute head injury. In L. Bucher & S. Melander (Eds.), *Critical care nursing* (pp. 843–865). Philadelphia: WB Saunders.

11. Mattera, C. (1998). Spinal trauma: New guidelines for assessment and management in the out-of-hospital environment. *Journal of Emergency Nursing, 24,* 523–538.

12. Rakel, R.E. (1996). *Saunders manual of medical practice.* Philadelphia: WB Saunders.

13. Shackford, S., Bourguignon, P., Wald, S., Rogers, F., Osler, T., & Clark, D. (1998). Hypertonic saline resuscitation of patients with head injury: A prospective, randomized clinical trial. *Journal of Trauma, 44,* 50–58.

14. Stein, J.H. (1998). *Internal medicine* (5th ed.). St. Louis: Mosby.

15. Talbert, S. & Talbert, P. (1998). Summary of strategies for managing severe traumatic brain injury during the early posttraumatic phase. *Journal of Emergency Nursing, 24,* 254–258.

16. Thiagarajan, A., Goverdan, P.D., Chari, P., & Somasunderam, K. (1998). The effect of hyperventilation and hyperoxia on cerebral venous oxygen saturations in patients with traumatic brain injury. *Anesthesia & Analgesia, 87,* 850–853.

17. Tierney, L.M., McPhee, S.J., & Papadakis, M.A. (1999). *Current medical diagnosis & treatment* (38th ed.). Stamford, CT: Appleton & Lange.

18. White, R. & Likavec, M. (1999). Spinal shock–Spinal man. *Journal of Trauma, 46,* 979–980.

CENTRAL NERVOUS SYSTEM DISORDERS

Charlene M. Myers, MSN, RN, CS, ACNP, CCRN

I. MENINGITIS

A. Definition[3, 5, 10]

An inflammation of the pia mater and arachnoid of the brain or spinal cord

B. Etiology/Predisposing factors[2-5, 10]

1. Predisposing factors for the development of community-acquired meningitis include pre-existing diabetes mellitus, otitis media, pneumonia, sinusitis, and alcohol abuse.
2. Bacterial meningitis: Profound and life-threatening

   a. *Haemophilus influenzae:* Most common cause of acute bacterial meningitis (50%), generally occurring in infancy and childhood
   b. *Neisseria meningitidis:* May occur in schools, colleges, and other group settings; spread by contact with drainage of the nasopharynx or with blood
   c. *Streptococcus pneumoniae* (pneumococcal meningitis): Occurs frequently in infants and the elderly
   d. *Escherichia coli, Enterobacter, Klebsiella,* and *Proteus* spp. May occur in infants and immunosuppressed patients
   e. Other bacterial meningitides: Staphylococci (*S. aureus* and *S. epidermidis*) and streptococci are less common.
   f. Meningitis may follow an upper respiratory infection or head trauma.

3. Aseptic meningitis

   a. Much more benign and self-limited than bacterial meningitis
   b. Caused by viruses: Mumps, enterovirus, herpes, adenovirus, Epstein-Barr virus
   c. Fungal: Found most commonly in the immunocompromised: *Candida albicans, Coccidioides immitis, Cryptococcus neoformans*
   d. Tuberculosis: *Mycobacterium tuberculosis*
   e. Syphilis

C. Clinical manifestations[1-6, 9, 10]

1. Fever of 101°–103°F (38°–40°C)
2. Stiff neck (nuchal rigidity) related to meningeal irritation
3. Altered sensorium

4. Severe headache
5. Photophobia
6. Chills, myalgias
7. Kernig's sign: Flex the patient's leg at the knee, then at the hip, to a 90-degree angle, and extend the knee. In a patient with meningitis, this maneuver will trigger pain and spasms of the hamstring muscles due to the inflammation of the meninges and spinal nerve roots.
8. Brudzinski's sign: Flex the patient's head and neck to the chest. The legs will flex at both the hips and knees in response to this movement.
9. Nausea and vomiting
10. Purpura or petechiae

D. Laboratory findings/Diagnostics[1–4, 6, 7, 10]

1. Lumbar puncture should be performed as soon as a diagnosis is suspected.
2. Lumbar puncture in bacterial meningitis
   a. Appearance of CSF: Cloudy
   b. Opening pressure: Elevated (>180 mm H_2O)
   c. Cells: Increased WBCs (1000–2000/mm, mostly polymorphonuclear cells)
   d. Total protein: Increased (100–500 mg/dL) (normal 15–45 mg/dL)
   e. Glucose: Decreased (<40 mg/dL or 40% of glucose) (normal 60–80%)
   f. Culture: Bacteria present on Gram's stain and culture

3. Lumbar puncture in viral meningitis
   a. Appearance of CSF: Clear, occasionally cloudy
   b. Opening pressure: Variable
   c. Cells: Increased WBCs (300/mm, mostly mononuclear cells)
   d. Total protein: Normal or sightly increased
   e. Glucose: Normal
   f. Culture: No bacteria present; demonstration of virus requires special technique.

4. CT scan of the head is indicated in patients with focal neurologic signs or diminished level of consciousness.
5. In patients who have signs and symptoms and cerebrospinal fluid findings typical of bacterial meningitis, but in whom no organisms are found, follow-up CT scans should be obtained, even if clinical improvement occurs, because such patients may have a brain abscess, necessitating neurosurgical intervention.
6. An additional maneuver in assessing for meningitis is to elicit jolt accentuation of the patient's headache by asking

the patient to turn his or her head horizontally at a frequency of two to three rotations per second.

   a. Worsening of a baseline headache represents a positive sign.

   b. Include an examination of the cranial nerves, the motor and sensory systems, the reflexes, and testing for Babinski's reflex.

7. Assess the ears, sinuses, and respiratory system.
8. Obtain blood cultures.
9. Obtain CBC, electrolytes, liver/renal panel.
10. Chest, skull, and sinus films or chest CT scan may be necessary to help identify primary infection.

E. Management[2–5, 8–10]

1. Antibiotics must be initiated immediately in those suspected to have meningitis. Empiric treatment:

   a. Cefotaxime (Claforan), 200 mg/kg/day IV

   b. Ampicillin (Ampicin), 200 mg/kg/day IV, is added for adults over age 50, and for the immunocompromised.

   c. In those allergic to penicillin and a third-generation cephalosporin, other medications must be considered. One drug that is excellent for infections of the CNS is chloramphenicol. It has been found to be effective, although it has also been associated with the incidence of aplastic anemia in approximately 1 in 40,000 patients.

2. Meningococcal meningitis: (patients 18–60 years of age) aqueous penicillin G (3–4 million units IV q4h), or ampicillin (2 g q6h); continue until 5–7 days after the patient becomes afebrile.

3. *Haemophilus influenzae* meningitis: Third-generation cephalosporin (ceftriaxone [Rocephin], 50 mg/kg IV q12h), or ampicillin plus chloramphenicol (Chlorofair), 50–100 mg/kg/day IV in divided dosages

4. Pneumococcal meningitis: Aqueous penicillin IV for 12–15 days. Chloramphenicol is an alternative drug.

5. Postsurgical or post-traumatic meningitis: Third-generation cephalosporin (cefotaxime, ceftizoxime [Cefizox], ceftriaxone), with or without nafcillin (Nafcil), 2 g IV q4h

6. Aseptic meningitis: Supportive therapy. Treat the severely ill empirically with antibiotics.

7. Tuberculosis: Isoniazid (INH) 15–20 mg/kg/day (maximum 500 mg), rifampin 15–20 mg/kg/day (maximum 600 mg)

8. Corticosteroids remain controversial; however, they may be prescribed when there is evidence of cerebral edema or herniation.

9. Anticonvulsants for seizure control (phenytoin [Dilantin], 300 mg/day)

10. Acetaminophen, 325–1000 mg q4h (not to exceed 4 g/day)
11. IV hydration with lactated Ringer's solution or normal saline. Avoid hypotonic solutions such as D_5W.

II. ENCEPHALOPATHY

A. Definition[10]
A dysfunction of the brain secondary to a disease or disease process

B. Etiology[1–3, 10]

1. Hepatic
2. Hypertensive
3. Metabolic (lactic acidosis, metabolic acidosis)
4. Electrolytes (hyponatremia, hypoglycemia, hypercalcemia)
5. Uremic
6. Anoxic-ischemic
7. Hypercapnic
8. Endocrine (hyperparathyroidism, Cushing's disease)
9. AIDS
10. Thiamine deficiency (Wernicke's disease)

C. Clinical manifestations[2–4, 9, 10]

1. Depends on cause and can include
   a. Headache
   b. Inattentiveness, impaired judgment
   c. Motor incoordination
   d. Drowsiness
   e. Confusion
   f. Stupor
   g. Coma

D. Diagnosis[3, 4, 10]

1. Depends on clinical event
   a. Physical presentation
   b. Serum laboratory analysis (ammonia)
   c. CSF analysis
   d. EEG activity
   e. MRI

E. Management[3, 4, 10]

1. ABCs of emergency care
2. Prevention of irreversible neurologic injury
3. Anticonvulsant therapy for seizures (phenytoin, 300 mg/day)
4. Correction of underlying cause

References

1. Attia, J., Hatala, R., Cook, D.J., & Wong, J.G. (1999). Does this adult patient have acute meningitis? *Journal of the American Medical Association, 282,* 175–181.

2. Clochesy, J.M., Breu, C., & Dossey, B. (1997). *AACN handbook of critical care nursing*. Stamford, CT: Appleton & Lange.
3. Devinsky, O., Feldmann, E., Weinreb, H.J., & Wilterdink, J.L. (1997). *The resident's neurology book*. Philadelphia: F.A. Davis.
4. Ferri, F.F. (1998). *Practical guide to the care of the medical patient* (4th ed.). St. Louis: Mosby.
5. Keiser, M.M. (1999). Neurologic disorders. In A. Gawlinski & D. Hamwi (Eds.), *Acute care nurse practitioner: Clinical curriculum and certification review*. Philadelphia: W.B. Saunders.
6. Rakel, R.E. (1996). *Saunders manual of medical practice*. Philadelphia: W.B. Saunders.
7. Ruttimann, S. (1999). Clinical problem-solving: A balancing act. *New England Journal of Medicine, 341*, 129–130.
8. Saha, S., Saint, S., & Tierney, L.M. (1999). A balancing act. *New England Journal of Medicine, 340*, 374–378.
9. Stein, J.H. (1998). *Internal medicine* (5th ed.). St. Louis: Mosby.
10. Tierney, L.M., McPhee, S.J., & Papadakis, M.A. (1999). *Current medical diagnosis & treatment* (38th ed.). Stamford, CT: Appleton & Lange.

SEIZURE DISORDERS

Charlene M. Myers, MSN, RN, CS,
ACNP, CCRN

I. SEIZURE DISORDERS

A. Definition

A transient disturbance of cerebral function caused by an abnormal paroxysmal neuronal discharge in the brain

B. Etiology[1-4, 7, 9, 10]

1. Cause may be unknown
2. Metabolic disorders

   a. Acidosis
   b. Electrolyte imbalance (e.g., hyponatremia, hypocalcemia)
   c. Hypoglycemia
   d. Hypoxia
   e. Alcohol or barbiturate withdrawal—the most common cause of new-onset seizures in adults

3. CNS infections
4. Head trauma
5. Tumors and other space-occupying lesions
6. Vascular diseases (common in advancing age and the most common cause of the onset of seizure disorder at age 60 or older)
7. Degenerative disorders, such as Alzheimer's disease in later life
8. Natural reaction to physiologic stress or transient systemic injury
9. The most common cause of seizures is noncompliance with a drug regimen on the part of a diagnosed epileptic.

C. Clinical manifestations[1, 3, 5, 7-11]

1. Partial seizures: Only a restricted part of one hemisphere has been activated.

   a. Simple partial seizure
      i. Consciousness is preserved; rarely lasts >1 min
      ii. Jacksonian march movements: Convulsive jerking or paresthesias/tingling that spreads to different parts of the limb or body
      iii. Sensory symptoms: Flashing lights, simple hallucinations, tingling, or buzzing

      iv. Autonomic symptoms: Abnormal epigastric symptoms, pallor, sweating, flushing, pupillary dilation, piloerection

      v. Speech arrest or vocalization

      vi. Nausea

      vii. Psychic symptoms: Déjà vu; dreamy states, fear, distortion of time perception

  b. Complex partial seizure

      i. Any simple partial seizure onset followed by impairment of consciousness

      ii. Automatisms may occur (lip smacking, chewing, swallowing, sucking, picking at clothes)

      iii. May begin with a stare at the time consciousness is impaired

      iv. May have an aura

2. Secondary generalized partial seizures: Simple or complex seizures progressing to generalized seizures, with loss of consciousness and motor activity that is often convulsive

3. Generalized seizures

  a. Absence (petit mal)

      i. Sudden loss of consciousness (5–30 s), with eye or muscle flutterings at a rate of three per second; begins and ends so quickly that it may not be apparent

      ii. Common in children (6–14 years old)

      iii. Occasionally accompanied by mild clonic, tonic, or atonic components

      iv. Autonomic components (enuresis)

      v. Can accompany automatisms

      vi. If the seizure occurs during conversation, the patient may miss a few words or may break off for a few seconds.

      vii. Often occur several times a day, often when the patient is sitting quietly; infrequent during exercise

  b. Tonic-clonic (grand mal)

      i. Usually preceded by an aura and followed by an outcry

      ii. Loss of consciousness and falling

      iii. Tonic, then clonic contractions of the muscles of the extremities, trunk, and head

      iv. Urinary and fecal incontinence may occur.

      v. Usually lasts 2–5 min

      vi. May be preceded by a prodromal mood change and followed by a postictal state (deep sleep, headache, muscle soreness, amnesia of events, nausea, confusion, or a combination of these)

4. Status epilepticus: A series of grand mal seizures that may occur when the patient is awake or asleep, but the patient never gains consciousness between attacks.

    a. Aggressive treatment is required for a patient with continuing seizures lasting over 10 min, or seizures without intervening consciousness.

    b. Most uncommon, but most life-threatening

D. Diagnosis[2, 3, 7, 9, 10]

1. Obtain a thorough history from the patient, the family, and/or observers of the event.
2. EEG is the most important test to differentiate between the types of seizures.

    a. Focal abnormalities indicate partial seizures.

    b. Generalized abnormalities indicate primary generalized seizures.

    c. A normal EEG does not rule out a seizure.

3. CT or MRI of the head—for all new-onset seizures, especially after age 30, because of the possibility of an underlying neoplasm
4. Chest x-ray of patients over age 30 as well
5. Lumbar puncture to assess for an infectious process
6. Twenty-four hour EEG to document seizure activity
7. Blood analysis: CBC, glucose, liver and renal function tests, VDRL, electrolytes, magnesium, calcium, antinuclear antibody, erythrocyte sedimentation rate, arterial blood gases
8. Urinalysis, drug screen
9. Serum prolactin—Rises two to three times above normal for 10–60 min after 80% of tonic-clonic or complex partial seizures.

E. Management[1–4, 6, 7, 9, 10]

1. Initial management is supportive.
2. Most seizures are self-limiting.

    a. Maintain open airway.

    b. Protect the patient from injuries.

    c. Administer oxygen if the patient is cyanotic.

    d. Do not force airways or objects (e.g., tongue blade) between the teeth until the muscles have relaxed, as this could cause the tongue to occlude the airway or teeth to break off and cause a partial obstruction.

    e. Start IV with normal saline.

    f. Perform ECG and monitor respiration and blood pressure.

3. For status epilepticus

    a. The preceding, plus

    b. 100 mg thiamine IM

    c. 50-mL bolus injection of 50% glucose

TABLE 6–1. PHARMACOLOGIC MANAGEMENT FOR SEIZURE DISORDERS*

SEIZURE TYPE	MEDICATIONS	USUAL DAILY DOSAGE	THERAPEUTIC LEVEL
Generalized tonic-clonic	**Drugs of Choice**		
	Carbamazepine (Tegretol)	800–1600 mg	6–12 μg/mL
	Phenytoin (Dilantin)	300–400 mg	10–20 μg/mL
	Alternates/Adjuncts		
	Phenobarbital (Luminal)	90–150 mg	15–35 μg/mL
	Primidone (Mysoline)	750–1250 mg—not to exceed 2 g/day	6–12 μg/mL
	Lamotrigine (Lamictal)	50–75 mg bid—not to exceed 200 mg/day	Not established
Absence	**Drugs of Choice**		
	Ethosuximide (Zarontin)	750–1250 mg	40–100 μg/mL
	Valproate (Depakene)	1000–3000 mg—not to exceed 60 mg/kg/day	50–120 μg/mL
	Alternates/Adjuncts		
	Clonazepam (Klonopin)	1.5–20 mg	20–80 μg/mL
	Lamotrigine (Lamictal)	50–75 mg bid—not to exceed 200 mg/day	Not established
Atonic or myoclonic	**Drug of Choice**		
	Valproate (Depakene)	1–3 g—not to exceed 60 mg/kg/day	50–120 μg/mL
	Alternates/Adjuncts		
	Clonazepam (Klonopin)	1.5–20 mg—not to exceed 20 mg/day	20–80 μg/mL
	Felbamate (Felbatol)	1200–3600 mg	Not established

Simple partial	**Drugs of Choice**	
	Carbamazepine (Tegretol)	800–1600 mg	6–12 μg/mL
	Phenytoin (Dilantin)	300–400 mg	10–20 μg/mL
	Lamotrigine (Lamictal)	50–75 mg bid—not to exceed 200 mg/day	Not established
	Phenobarbital (Luminal)	90–150 mg	15–35 μg/mL
	Alternates/Adjuncts		
	Primidone (Mysoline)	750–1250 mg—not to exceed 2 g/day	6–12 μg/mL
	Clonazepam (Klonopin)	1.5–20 mg	20–80 μg/mL
	Gabapentin (Neurontin)	900–1800 mg/day	Not established
	Felbamate (Felbatol)	1200–3600 mg	Not established
Complex partial	**Drugs of Choice**		
	Phenytoin (Dilantin)	300–400 mg	10–20 μg/mL
	Carbamazepine (Tegretol)	800–1600 mg	6–12 μg/mL
	Lamotrigine (Lamictal)	As above	Not established
	Gabapentin (Neurontin)	900–1800 mg/day	Not established
	Alternates/Adjuncts		
	Phenobarbital (Luminal)	90–150 mg	15–35 μg/mL
	Primidone (Mysoline)	750–1500 mg—not to exceed 2 g/day	6–12 μg/mL
	Valproate (Depakene)	1000–6000 mg—not to exceed 60 mg/kg/day	50–120 μg/mL
	Clonazepam (Klonopin)	1.5–20 mg—not to exceed 20 mg/day	20–80 μg/mL
	Felbamate (Felbatol)	1200–3600 mg	Not established

* All anticonvulsant medications must be tapered up and down while carefully monitoring drug levels and other pertinent diagnostic tests (laboratory and radiologic) to avoid serious side effects. Patients should be maintained on the lowest effective dose.

(From Keiser, M.M. [1999]. Neurologic disorders. In A. Gawlinski & D. Hamwi [Eds.], *Acute care nurse practitioner: Clinical curriculum and certification review* [p. 309]. Philadelphia: W.B. Saunders, with permission; Deglin, J.P., & Vallerand, A.H. [1999]. *Davis's Drug Guide for Nurses* [6th ed.]. Philadelphia: F.A. Davis.)

    d. Lorazepam (Ativan), 0.1 mg/kg at 2 mg/min (maximum 10 mg), or IV diazepam (Valium), 0.2 mg/kg at 5 mg/min (maximum 20 mg)

    e. Monitor for respiratory depression after the medications; intubation may be necessary.

    f. Increase normal saline if the patient becomes hypotensive.

    g. Phenytoin (Dilantin) administered simultaneously with lorazepam or diazepam and saline at a rate of 50 mg/min until a loading dose of 18 mg/kg is reached

    h. If the above measures are unsuccessful, intubate and administer phenobarbital (Luminal), 100 mg/min IV, to a maximum of 20 mg/kg, or diazepam (100 mg in 500 mL D_5W) at 40 mL/h.

TABLE 6–2. SIDE EFFECTS OF NEW ANTIEPILEPTIC DRUGS

DRUG	PRINCIPAL SIDE EFFECTS	SERIOUS BUT RARE SIDE EFFECTS
Gabapentin	Somnolence, fatigue, ataxia, dizziness, gastrointestinal upset	
Lamotrigine	Rash, dizziness, tremor, ataxia, diplopia, headache, gastrointestinal upset	Stevens-Johnson syndrome
Felbamate	Irritability, insomnia, anorexia, nausea, headache	Aplastic anemia, hepatic failure
Clobazam	Sedation, dizziness, irritability, depression, disinhibition	
Vigabatrin	Behavioral changes, depression, sedation, fatigue, weight gain, gastrointestinal upset	Psychosis
Oxcarbazepine	Dizziness, diplopia, ataxia, headache, weakness, rash, hyponatremia	
Zonisamide	Somnolence, headache, dizziness, ataxia, renal calculi	
Tiagabine	Confusion, dizziness, gastrointestinal upset, anorexia, fatigue	
Topiramate	Cognitive difficulties, tremor, dizziness, ataxia, headache, fatigue, gastrointestinal upset, renal calculi	

(From Dichter, M., & Brodie, M.J. [1996]. Drug therapy: New antiepileptic drugs. *New England Journal of Medicine, 334*, 4, with permission. Copyright © 1996 Massachusetts Medical Society. All rights reserved.)

TABLE 6–3. INTERACTIONS BETWEEN NEW AND CONVENTIONAL ANTIEPILEPTIC DRUGS

NEW DRUG	EFFECT OF CONVENTIONAL DRUGS ON NEW DRUG	EFFECT OF NEW DRUG ON CONVENTIONAL DRUGS
Gabapentin	None known	None known
Lamotrigine	Phenobarbital, phenytoin, and carbamazepine increase metabolism by 50%	Does not induce cytochrome P-450
	Valproic acid decreases metabolism by 50%*	When added to carbamazepine, may induce neurotoxicity because of pharmacodynamic interactions
Felbamate	Valproic acid decreases clearance	Decreases metabolism of phenytoin and valproic acid (increases serum phenytoin levels by approximately 20% and increases serum valproic acid levels by 18–31%)
	Phenytoin and carbamazepine increase clearance	Decreases serum carbamazepine levels but increases serum carbamazepine epoxide levels
Clobazam	Target for enzyme inducers or inhibitors	May precipitate toxic effects of phenytoin and increase serum carbamazepine epoxide levels
Oxcarbazepine	Not affected by enzyme inducers	Induces cytochrome P-450, 3A isoform family (but less so than carbamazepine)
		May increase serum phenytoin and valproic acid levels by 20–30% if oxcarbazepine is substituted for carbamazepine
		Increases metabolism of oral contraceptives
Tiagabine	Phenobarbital, phenytoin, and carbamazepine increase clearance	Does not induce cytochrome P-450
Topiramate	Phenytoin and carbamazepine increase clearance	Does not affect serum phenytoin, carbamazepine, or valproic acid levels
	Valproic acid has no marked effect	Weak inducer of cytochrome P-450
Vigabatrin	None known	May increase serum phenytoin levels in some patients (mechanism unknown)
		May decrease serum phenytoin levels by 20% (mechanism unknown)
Zonisamide	Phenobarbital increases clearance	May increase serum phenytoin and carbamazepine levels (not in all studies)

(From Dichter, M., & Brodie, M.J. [1996]. Drug therapy: New antiepileptic drugs. *New England Journal of Medicine, 334*, 4, with permission. Copyright © 1996 Massachusetts Medical Society. All rights reserved.)

TABLE 6-4. INVESTIGATIONAL ANTIEPILEPTIC DRUGS

DRUG	INDICATIONS	STARTING DOSE	MAINTENANCE DOSE	PLASMA HALF-LIFE (H)	PLASMA BINDING (%)
Clobazam	Partial and generalized seizures	10 mg at bedtime or 10 mg b.i.d.	20–30 mg/day Up to 60 mg/day	30–46	85
Oxcarbazepine	Partial and tonic-clonic seizures	300 mg b.i.d.	1200–2400 mg/day	8–24 (for active metabolite)	40
Tiagabine	Partial and secondary generalized seizures	Not available	32–56 mg/day	6–8	96
Topiramate	Partial and secondary generalized seizures	100 mg/day, with the dose increased by 100 mg/day at weekly intervals	400–1000 mg/day	20–24	10–20
Vigabatrin	Partial and secondary generalized seizures and possibly infantile spasms	500 mg b.i.d.	Up to 3 g/day	4–8 (effect lasts ≥3 days)	Minimal
Zonisamide	Partial and secondary generalized seizures	100–200 mg/day	400–600 mg/day	50–68 (27–38 with enzyme-inducing drugs)	38–40

(From Dichter, M., & Brodie, M.J. [1996]. Drug therapy: New antiepileptic drugs. *New England Journal of Medicine, 334,* 4, with permission. Copyright © 1996 Massachusetts Medical Society. All rights reserved.)

    i. If still unsuccessful after 60 min, institute general anesthesia with isoflurane and neuromuscular blockade.

4. Pharmacologic management for seizure disorders (Table 6–1)
5. Side effects of new antiepileptic drugs (Table 6–2)
6. Interactions between new antiepileptic drugs and conventional drugs (Table 6–3)
7. Investigational antiepileptic drugs (Table 6–4)
8. Titrate dosages to achieve adequate serum levels. If a first drug partially controls the seizures at a maximal therapeutic level, add a second drug to achieve therapeutic levels.
9. Never abruptly withdraw an anticonvulsant from a patient; these drugs should be tapered.

References

1. Clochesy, J.M., Breu, C., & Dossey, B. (1997). *AACN handbook of critical care nursing.* Stamford, CT: Appleton & Lange.
2. Devinsky, O. (1999). Current concepts: Patients with refractory seizures. *New England Journal of Medicine, 340,* 1565–1570.
3. Devinsky, O., Feldmann, E., Weinreb, H.J., & Wilterdink, J.L. (1997). *The resident's neurology book.* Philadelphia: F.A. Davis.
4. Dichter, M., & Brodie, M.J. (1996). Drug therapy: New antiepileptic drugs. *New England Journal of Medicine, 334,* 1583–1590.
5. Ferri, F.F. (1998). *Practical guide to the care of the medical patient* (4th ed.). St. Louis: Mosby.
6. Grant, I.S., & Andrews, P.J. (1999). ABC of intensive care: Neurological support. *British Medical Journal, 319,* 110–113.
7. Keiser, M.M. (1999). Neurologic disorders. In A. Gawlinski & D. Hamwi (Eds.), *Acute care nurse practitioner: Clinical curriculum and certification review.* Philadelphia: W.B. Saunders.
8. Miller, S. (1999). Neurological disorders. In V.L. Millonig, & S.K. Miller (Eds.). *Adult Nurse Practitioner Certification Review Guide* (3rd ed.) (pp. 568–574). Potomac, MD: Health Leadership Associates, Inc.
9. Rakel, R.E. (1996). *Saunders manual of medical practice.* Philadelphia: W.B. Saunders.
10. Samuels, M. (1998). Update in neurology. *Annals of Internal Medicine, 129,* 878–885.
11. Tierney, L.M., McPhee, S.J., & Papadakis, M.A. (1999). *Current medical diagnosis & treatment* (38th ed.). Stamford, CT: Appleton & Lange.

DEMENTIA

Charlene M. Myers, MSN, RN, CS,
ACNP, CCRN

I. DEMENTIA

A. Definition[3, 6, 10]

1. A broad (global) acquired impairment of intellectual function (cognition) that usually is progressive and that interferes with normal social and occupational activities.
2. Key features of dementia are intact arousal state with impairment of memory, intellect, and personality.
3. Refer to Chapter 74 for differentiating dementia from delirium.

B. Etiology[1–3, 6, 8, 9]

1. Degenerative: Alzheimer-type, Parkinson's disease (50–60%)
2. Vascular: Multi-infarct, arteritis (15–20%)
3. Infectious: HIV, syphilis, meningitis, encephalitis, abscess, Creutzfeldt-Jakob disease
4. Postencephalitic syndrome, CNS anoxia (drug overdose, cardiac arrest)
5. Vitamin B_{12} deficiency
6. Other vitamin deficiency
7. Chronic alcoholism
8. Subdural hematoma
9. Hydrocephalus
10. Chronic seizures
11. Hypothyroidism/hyperthyroidism
12. Hearing loss
13. Blindness
14. Depression
15. Electrolyte imbalances

C. Clinical manifestations[2, 3, 5–8, 11]

1. Onset may be slow, over a period of months or years.
2. Memory deficits (usually short-term), impaired abstract reasoning
3. Higher cognitive functions may be impaired (aphasia, apraxia, agnosia).
4. Patients may become easily lost or wander.
5. Patients may have difficulty with learned tasks, such as dressing or cooking.
6. Poor judgment

7. Clouding of consciousness and orientation is not present until the terminal stages.
8. Emotional problems such as depression, lability, or flattened affect
9. Agitation
10. Sleeplessness
11. Paranoid ideation
12. Patients often lose insight into their deficits.

D. Diagnosis[2–4, 6, 8, 9]

1. Attempt the Folstein Mini-Mental State Examination to screen for dementia (a score of ≤20 indicates cognitive impairment), and also document the progression of disease over time by repeating at 3- to 6-month intervals.
2. Examination should include observations of memory, thinking, concentration, attention, judgment, insight, and behavior.
3. Screening laboratory examination:

   a. Glucose
   b. Electrolytes
   c. Magnesium
   d. Calcium
   e. Liver tests
   f. BUN/creatinine
   g. Thyroid function tests
   h. Vitamin B_{12} level, folate
   i. VDRL
   j. HIV (selected patients)
   k. CBC with differential, clotting studies
   l. Arterial blood gases
   m. Serum levels of ingested drugs
   n. Illicit drugs and alcohol levels in selected patients
   o. Albumin

4. Other tests, depending on patient history and findings of physical examination

   a. CT of head/MRI—Note: For tumors, subdural hematoma, infarction, hemorrhage, hydrocephalus, atrophy
   b. Lumbar puncture—Rule out neurosyphilis, chronic meningitis, normal-pressure hydrocephalus
   c. EEG
   d. Chest x-ray—Note: For malignancy or infection
   e. ECG

5. Identification of treatable causes is very important.

   a. Drug-induced
   b. Depression
   c. Hypothyroidism/hyperthyroidism

    d. Hypoglycemia
    e. Vitamin B_{12} or folate deficiency
    f. Subdural hematoma
    g. Liver failure
    h. Normal-pressure hydrocephalus
    i. Stroke
    j. CNS infections
    k. Generalized infections
    l. Cerebral neoplasms
    m. Renal failure
    n. Alcohol abuse
    o. Hypoxia
    p. Hypercalcemia
    q. Vasculitis
    r. Cardiopulmonary disorders
    s. Anemia

E. Management[2–5, 6, 8, 9, 11]

1. Supportive care
2. Treat underlying precipitating illnesses.
3. Attempt to withdraw, reduce, or stop all nonessential medications.
4. Maintain nutrition.
5. Avoid restraints, except for safety.
6. Because there is a cholinergic deficiency in Alzheimer's disease, recent research has focused on medications to increase cholinergic activity.

    a. Tacrine tetrahydroaminoacridine (THA): A reversible cholinesterase inhibitor used for treatment of cognitive deficits
    b. Administration of 80–160 mg/day in four divided doses has improved cognition in 25–42% of patients.
    c. Monitor alanine transaminase (alanine aminotransferase) levels, which are increased in 50% of patients on therapy.

7. Medications that affect serotonin have been useful in controlling aggression and agitation.

    a. Lithium
    b. Trazodone
    c. Buspirone
    d. Clonazepam

8. Dopamine blockers have been used for many years to treat aggression—Haloperidol, 0.5–1 mg nightly.
9. Carbamazepine, 100–400 mg/day, has recently been shown to reduce agitation in patients with Alzheimer's disease.
10. Emotional lability has been decreased with medication in some cases.

11. Two small doses of imipramine (25 mg po b.i.d. or t.i.d.) or fluoxetine (5–20 mg/day)

12. Depression responds to the usual doses of antidepressants. Selective serotonin reuptake inhibitors and monoamine oxidase inhibitors have the fewest anticholinergic side effects.

References

1. Carr, D.B., Goate, A., Phil, D., & Morris, J.C. (1997). Current concepts in the pathogenesis of Alzheimer's disease. *American Journal of Medicine, 103* (supplement), 3S–10S.

2. Clark, S. (1999). Mental health disorders. In A. Gawlinski & D. Hamwi (Eds.), *Acute care nurse practitioner: Clinical curriculum and certification review.* Philadelphia: W.B. Saunders.

3. Devinsky, O., Feldmann, E., Weinreb, H.J., & Wilterdink, J.L. (1997). *The resident's neurology book.* Philadelphia: F.A. Davis.

4. Eccles, M., Clarke, J., Livingston, M., Freemantle, N., & Mason, J. (1998). North of England evidence based guidelines development project: Guideline for the primary care management of dementia. *BMJ (Clinical Research Ed.), 317*, 802–808.

5. Ferri, F.F. (1998). *Practical guide to the care of the medical patient* (4th ed.). St. Louis: Mosby.

6. Kennnedy-Malone, L., Fletcher, K.R., & Plank, L.M. (2000). *Management guidelines for gerontological nurse practitioners.* Philadelphia: F.A. Davis.

7. Rakel, R.E. (1996). *Saunders manual of medical practice.* Philadelphia: W.B. Saunders.

8. Richards, S.S., & Hendrie, H.C. (1999). Diagnosis, management, and treatment of Alzheimer disease: A guide for the internist. *Archives of Internal Medicine, 159*, 789–798.

9. Small, G.W., et al. Diagnosis and treatment of Alzheimer's disease and related disorders. *Journal of the American Medical Association, 278*, 1363–1371.

10. Stein, J.H. (1998). *Internal medicine* (5th ed.). St. Louis: Mosby.

11. Tierney, L.M., McPhee, S.J., & Papadakis, M.A. (1999). *Current medical diagnosis & treatment* (38th ed.). Stamford, CT: Appleton & Lange.

Management of Patients with Cardiovascular Disorders

CARDIOVASCULAR ASSESSMENT

Thomas W. Barkley, Jr., DSN, RN, CS, ACNP

I. CARDIOVASCULAR ASSESSMENT[1-8]

A. Cardiac cycle review

1. Atrioventricular (AV) valves close.
2. Aortic/pulmonic (semilunar) valves open.
3. Aortic/pulmonic valves close.
4. AV valves open.
5. Rapid ventricular filling (70% fill of ventricles)
6. Atrial kick (atria pushing out remaining blood to the ventricles)

B. Auscultatory areas of the precordium—Characterized by location where valvular activity may usually be heard best

1. Aortic—2nd right ICS at the right sternal border (S_2 heart sound louder than S_1)
2. Pulmonic—2nd left ICS at the left sternal border (S_2 heard louder than S_1)
3. Erb's point—3rd ICS at the left sternal border
4. Tricuspid—left lower sternal border at the 5th ICS (closure of AV valves)
5. Mitral—5th ICS midclavicular line (S_1 heard louder than S_2)

C. S_1 heart sound

1. Denotes closure of the mitral and tricuspid (atrioventricular) valves
2. Occurs almost simultaneously with the apical and carotid impulses
3. Coincides with the R wave on ECG
4. More easily heard than S_2 at the apex

D. S_2 heart sound

1. Denotes closure of the aortic and pulmonic (semilunar) valves
2. Occurs at the onset of ventricular diastole (Note: Ventricular systole occurs between S_1 and S_2)
3. Heard louder than S_1 at the base of the heart

E. Split S_2 heart sound

1. A normal event heard at end-inspiration in some patients
2. Located in the pulmonic auscultatory area

3. If the patient holds his or her breath, the sound will disappear.
4. Occurs approximately every fourth heartbeat

F. S₃ heart sound

1. Referred to as a *ventricular* gallop
2. Caused by resistance to ventricular filling
3. Occurs immediately after S_2 (early diastole) at the left lower sternal border (apex)
4. Occurs with such conditions as fluid overload, congestive heart failure, and cardiomyopathy
5. Normal sound associated with pregnancy (i.e., hyperdynamic state of increased volume)
6. Sounds like the word "Ken-tuc'-ky"

G. S₄ heart sound

1. Referred to as an *atrial* or *presystolic* gallop
2. Caused by increased ventricular diastolic pressure
3. Occurs immediately before S_1 (late diastole)
4. Most clearly heard at the left lower sternal border (apex)
5. Occurs with such conditions as myocardial infarction, hypertension, ventricular hypertrophy
6. Sounds like the word "Ten-nes-see' "

H. Murmur

1. "Blowing" or "swooshing" sound as a result of turbulent blood flow. Identified by the following variables:
   a. *Timing*—Is the murmur systolic or diastolic, pansystolic or holosystolic, pandiastolic or holodiastolic?
   b. *Loudness*—Graded I–VI

      • Grade I: Barely audible
      • Grade II: Clearly audible but faint
      • Grade III: Moderately loud, easily heard
      • Grade IV: Loud, associated with a thrill
      • Grade V: Very loud; heard with one corner of stethoscope off the chest wall
      • Grade VI: Loudest; no stethoscope needed

   c. *Pitch*—Is the pitch high, low, or medium, crescendo, decrescendo, plateau, or crescendo-decrescendo?
   d. *Quality*—Is the quality musical, blowing, rumbling, or harsh?
   e. *Location*—At what area is the murmur heard best?
   f. *Radiation*—Is the murmur heard at other auscultatory areas, e.g., neck, back, axilla?
   g. *Posture*—Does the murmur disappear or become louder with changes in posture?

2. *Early diastolic murmurs:* Due to incompetent semilunar valves (e.g., aortic or pulmonic regurgitation)
3. *Diastolic rumbling murmurs:* Due to mitral stenosis (low-pitched, noted at apex better in the left lateral position, and does not radiate) and tricuspid stenosis (heard louder with inspiration)
4. *Midsystolic ejection murmurs:* Due to forward flow through semilunar valves, namely, aortic stenosis (loud, harsh, crescendo-decrescendo sound that radiates) and pulmonic stenosis (mostly systolic, medium-pitched, crescendo-decrescendo sound that also radiates)
5. *Pansystolic regurgitant murmurs:* Due to backward flow, such as with mitral regurgitation (loud, blowing, heard best at apex, and radiates to axilla) and tricuspid regurgitation (soft, blowing, heard best at left lower sternal border, louder with inspiration)

I. Clicks

1. *Midsystolic click:* Most common type; associated with mitral valve prolapse
2. *Aortic ejection click:* Related to stenosis; occurs during early systole; audible at apex and base of the heart
3. *Pulmonic ejection click:* Occurs during early systole; audible at the base of the heart only

J. Friction rub

1. "Scratchy," high-pitched sound
2. Classic sound of pericarditis (inflammation)
3. Usually heard best at the apex with the patient leaning forward

K. Peripheral pulse amplitude
(Graded on a scale from zero to four)

1. Bounding = +4
2. Full = +3
3. Normal = +2
4. Diminished = +1
5. Absent = 0

L. Electrocardiographic changes associated with electrolyte disturbances

1. *Hyperkalemia:* Tall, peaked T waves, widening of the QRS complex, and prolongation of the P wave/PR interval. Increased levels of K^+ decrease ventricular depolarization and slow AV conduction.
2. *Hypokalemia:* U waves and appearance of new or additional premature ventricular contractions. Less common changes in-

clude bradycardia, atrial flutter, AV blocks, and increased effects of digitalis toxicity.

3. *Hypercalcemia:* AV blocks, bundle branch block, and bradycardia related to increased contractility of the heart and shortening of the period of ventricular repolarization. Hypercalcemia is also associated with potentiated effects of digitalis toxicity.

4. *Hypocalcemia:* Bradycardia to ventricular dysrhythmias, and asystole as low calcium levels decrease contractility. Reductions in cardiac output including hypotension and decreased effectiveness of digitalis may also be seen.

5. *Hypermagnesemia:* Rarely evident in the acute care setting. Hypermagnesemia is usually related to renal failure or over-administration of magnesium during replacement therapy.

6. *Hypomagnesemia:* Changes similar to those associated with hypokalemia and hypocalcemia, including U wave appearances, prolonged PR/QT intervals, widened QRS complexes, flattened T waves, supraventricular tachycardia (SVT), ventricular dysrhythmias, and torsades de pointes. (Note: Hypomagnesemia may cause hypertension and coronary/systemic vasospasms. Hypomagnesemia usually must be corrected before replacement therapy for hypokalemia and hypocalcemia is effective.)

References

1. Bradley, E.G. (1999). Cardiovascular assessment. In L. Bucher & S. Melander (Eds.), *Critical care nursing* (pp. 129–141). Philadelphia: W.B. Saunders.
2. Braunwald, E. (1998). The clinical examination. In L. Goldman & E. Braunwald (Eds.), *Primary cardiology* (pp. 27–43). Philadelphia: W.B. Saunders.
3. Estes, M.E. (1998). *Health assessment and physical examination.* Cincinnati: Delmar Publishers.
4. Garrett, A.P. (1997). Assessing cardiovascular status in the older adult with cognitive impairments. *Journal of Cardiovascular Nursing, 11,* 1–11.
5. Jarvis, C. (2000). *Physical examination and health assessment* (3rd ed.). Philadelphia: W.B. Saunders.
6. Ludwig, L.M. (1998). Cardiovascular assessment for home healthcare nurses. Part II: Assessing blood pressure and cardiac function. *Home Healthcare Nurse, 16,* 547–554.
7. Talbot, L. & Curtis, L. (1996). Cardiovascular assessment of the patient with renal problems. *ANNA Journal, 23,* 445–454.
8. Thelan, L.A., Urden, L.D., Lough, M.E., & Stacy, K.M. (Eds.). (1998). *Critical care nursing: Diagnosis and management* (3rd ed.). St. Louis: Mosby.

HYPERTENSION

Thomas W. Barkley, Jr., DSN, RN,
CS, ACNP

I. HYPERTENSION (HTN)

A. Definition[3-7]

1. Sustained elevation of systolic blood pressure
   (SBP) $\geq$ 140 mmHg, or diastolic blood pressure (DBP)
   $\geq$ 90 mmHg at least *three times on two different occasions*
2. Includes individuals currently taking antihypertensive pharmacologic agents

B. Incidence/predisposing factors[4-6, 9]

1. Affects 20–30% of African Americans
2. Affects 10–15% of whites in the United States
3. Affects approximately 60 million Americans
4. Hypertension is a leading risk factor for coronary artery disease, stroke, congestive heart failure, renal failure, and retinopathy.

C. Types and theories[1, 4, 5, 9]

1. *Primary*—Referred to as "essential" or "idiopathic"
   a. Cause is unknown.
   b. Represents 95% of all cases of HTN
   c. Onset is usually between 25 and 55 years of age.
   d. Exacerbating factors include obesity, excessive alcohol consumption (more than 2 drinks a day), cigarette smoking, and the use of nonsteroidal anti-inflammatory drugs.
   e. Theories of etiology include genetic and environemntal factors, elevated intracellular calcium and sodium levels, sympathetic nervous system hyperactivity, and high renin-angiotensin activity causing vascular dysfunction; among others.

2. *Secondary*—Secondary to other known causes or disease processes

   a. Represents 5% of all cases of HTN
   b. Etiology includes estrogen use (via oral contraceptives or hormone replacement therapy), renal disease, pregnancy, and endocrine disorders, such as pheochromocytoma.

3. *Isolated systolic hypertension*—Common with aging

   a. Poorly understood
   b. May account for 65–75% of hypertension in the elderly

   c. Systolic BP > 160 mmHg and diastolic BP < 90 mmHg
   d. Effectively treated with diuretics and long-acting calcium channel blockers

D. Subjective and physical examination findings[5, 10]

1. Often none; known as the "silent killer"
2. Elevated blood pressure ($\geq$140/90)
3. May complain of classic suboccipital "pulsating" headache, usually in the early morning and resolving throughout the day
4. May complain of epistaxis, lightheadedness, and visual disturbances, among others
5. S_4 heart sound may be present, related to left ventricular hypertrophy.
6. Retinal changes are present with severe, chronic disease.
7. Rare findings, such as hematuria

E. Diagnostic/Laboratory testing[5, 6]

1. Laboratory data are usually unremarkable with uncomplicated disease.
2. Consider ordering

   a. CBC and electrolytes with hemoglobin levels (establish base line)
   b. Urinalysis
   c. Blood urea nitrogen and creatinine concentrations
   d. Fasting glucose level
   e. Lipid panel
   f. Electrocardiogram (establish base line and rule out dysrhythmias)
   g. Chest x-ray (rule out cardiomegaly, for example)
   h. Echocardiogram (if left ventricular hypertrophy is suspected)
   i. Captopril stimulation test (if indicated, to rule out renovascular hypertension)
   j. Overnight 1-mg dexamethasone suppression test (if indicated to rule out Cushing's syndrome)
   k. Aldosterone level (if indicated, to rule out aldosteronism)
   l. Plasma catecholamine level (if indicated, to rule out pheochromocytoma)

F. Classification[6] (Table 9–1)

G. Follow-up recommendations for initial hypertensive measurements (Table 9–2)

H. Determining risk stratification and treatment recommendations (Fig. 9–1)

TABLE 9–1. CLASSIFICATION OF BLOOD PRESSURE FOR ADULTS AGE 18 AND OLDER*

CATEGORY	SYSTOLIC (mmHg)		DIASTOLIC (mmHg)
Optimal†	<120	and	<80
Normal	<130	and	<85
High-normal	130–139	or	85–89
Hypertension‡			
Stage 1	140–159	or	90–99
Stage 2	160–179	or	100–109
Stage 3	≥180	or	≥110

* Not taking antihypertensive drugs and not acutely ill. When systolic and diastolic blood pressures fall into different categories, the higher category should be selected to classify the individual's blood pressure status. For example, 160/92 mmHg should be classified as stage 2 hypertension, and 174/120 mmHg should be classified as stage 3 hypertension. Isolated systolic hypertension is defined as SBP of 140 mmHg or greater and DBP below 90 mmHg and staged appropriately (e.g., 170/82 mmHg is defined as stage 2 isolated systolic hypertension). In addition to classifying stages of hypertension on the basis of average blood pressure levels, clinicians should specify presence or absence of target organ disease and additional risk factors. This specificity is important for risk classification and treatment.

† Optimal blood pressure with respect to cardiovascular risk is below 120/80 mmHg. However, unusually low readings should be evaluated for clinical significance.

‡ Based on the average of two or more readings taken at each of two or more visits after an initial screening.

(From National Institutes of Health Publication #98–4080 [1997]. Sixth Report of the Joint National Committee on Prevention, Detection, Evaluation, and Treatment of High Blood Pressure [p. 11].)

I. Management[2, 5, 6, 7, 8, 9]

1. Principle—in *sequential order*

   a. Analyze base line studies.
   b. See algorithm for the treatment of hypertension (Fig. 9–2).
   c. Utilize nonpharmacologic strategies.
   d. Employ pharmacologic measures.

2. Nonpharmacologic strategies

   a. Restriction of dietary sodium (no more than 100 mmol per day—2.4 g sodium or 6 g salt)
   b. Weight loss, if overweight
   c. Exercise (aerobic exercise 30–45 min each day on most days of the week)
   d. Stress management planning
   e. Reduction or elimination of alcohol consumption
   f. Smoking cessation
   g. Maintenance of adequate potassium, calcium, and magnesium intake
   h. Reduction of dietary saturated fats

TABLE 9–2. RECOMMENDATIONS FOR FOLLOW-UP BASED ON INITIAL BLOOD PRESSURE MEASUREMENTS FOR ADULTS

INITIAL BLOOD PRESSURE (mmHg)*		FOLLOW-UP RECOMMENDED†
Systolic	**Diastolic**	
<130	<85	Recheck in 2 years
130–139	85–89	Recheck in 1 year‡
140–159	90–99	Confirm within 2 months‡
160–179	100–109	Evaluate or refer to source of care within 1 month
≥180	≥110	Evaluate or refer to source of care immediately or within 1 week, depending on clinical situation

* If systolic and diastolic categories are different, follow recommendations for shorter time follow-up (e.g., 160/86 mmHg should be evaluated or referred to source of care within 1 month).

† Modify the scheduling of follow-up according to reliable information about past blood pressure measurements, other cardiovascular risk factors, or target organ disease.

‡ Provide advice about lifestyle modifications.

(From National Institutes of Health Publication #98–4080 [1997]. Sixth Report of the Joint National Committee on Prevention, Detection, Evaluation, and Treatment of High Blood Pressure [p. 13].)

3. Pharmacologic measures[1, 5, 6]

  a. Based on degree of blood pressure elevation and/or the presence of end-organ damage, cardiovascular disease, or other risk factors

  b. Goal of therapy—To prescribe the least number of medications possible at the lowest dosage to provide acceptable blood pressure

  c. Special considerations—Neither age nor gender usually affects agent responsiveness. However, the following may be helpful in making prudent pharmacologic choices:

  d. Beta blockers—Particularly effective with African Americans; part of first-line therapy or in combination with diuretics; especially useful in patients with angina, previous myocardial infarction, atrial fibrillation/tachycardia, migraines, or hyperthyroidism; contraindicated in patients with congestive heart failure, symptomatic bronchospasm, severe asthma, and insulin-dependent diabetes (inhibits gluconeogenesis and prolongs hypoglycemia)

    i. Properties

      • Decrease myocardial contractility
      • Decrease heart rate

- Decrease peripheral resistance
- Decrease blood pressure
- Decrease myocardial oxygen demands
- Decrease renin release

ii. Common preparation (Trade name)/Usual daily dosage

- Propranolol hydrochloride (Inderal LA), 40–480 mg p.o. q.d.
- Metoprolol tartrate (Lopressor), 50–300 mg p.o. b.i.d.; Topro XL, 50 mg q.d.
- Atenolol (Tenormin), 25–100 mg p.o. b.i.d.
- Nadolol (Corgard), 40–320 mg p.o. q.d.
- Acebutolol hydrochloride (Sectral); 200–800 mg p.o. q.d.

iii. Major side effects

- Bradycardia
- Bronchospasm
- May mask insulin-induced hypoglycemia
- Hypotension
- May increase triglyceride levels
- Gastrointestinal complaints
- Weight gain
- Depression
- Impotence
- Sudden discontinuation can exacerbate angina.

e. Diuretics—Usually second therapy after initiation of one antihypertensive agent; may enhance the effects of other agents; African Americans may be more responsive than whites; particularly indicated in elderly patients with isolated systolic hypertension and patients with congestive heart failure; may have unfavorable effects in patients with gout

i. Properties

- Decrease venous return (preload).
- Relieve adventitious breath sounds.
- Mobilize fluid from edematous tissue.

ii. Common preparation/(Trade name)/Usual daily dosage/(Side effect/Comment)

(1) Loop diuretics—Short duration of action

(a) Furosemide (Lasix), 40–240 mg p.o. b.i.d. or t.i.d.

(b) Bumetanide (Bumex), 0.5–4 mg p.o. b.i.d. or t.i.d.

(c) Ethacrynic acid (Edecrin), 25–100 mg p.o. b.i.d. or t.i.d. (ototoxicity)

- Determine blood pressure stage.
- Determine risk group by major risk factors and TOD/CCD.
- Determine treatment recommendations (by using the table below).
- Determine goal blood pressure.
- Refer to specific treatment recommendations.

Major Risk Factors

- Smoking
- Dyslipidemia
- Diabetes mellitus
- Age > 60 years
- Gender:
  - Men
  - Postmenopausal women
- Family history:
  - Women < age 65
  - Men < age 55

TOD/CCD (Target Organ Damage/Clinical Cardiovascular Disease)

Heart Diseases
- LVH
- Angina/prior MI
- Prior CABG
- Heart failure

Stroke or TIA
Nephropathy
Peripheral arterial disease
Hypertensive retinopathy

Blood pressure stages (mmHg)	Risk Group A No major risk factors No TOD/CCD	Risk Group B At least one major risk factor, not including diabetes No TOD/CCD	Risk Group C TOD/CCD and/or diabetes, with or without other risk factors
High-normal (130-139/85-89)	Lifestyle modification	Lifestyle modification	Drug therapy for those with heart failure, renal insufficiency or diabetes Lifestyle modification
Stage 1 (140-159/90-99)	Lifestyle modification (up to 12 months)	Lifestyle modification (up to 6 months). For patients with multiple risk factors, clinicians should consider drugs as initial therapy plus lifestyle modifications.	Drug therapy Lifestyle modification
Stage 2 and 3 (≥160/≥100)	Drug therapy Lifestyle modification	Drug therapy Lifestyle modification	Drug therapy Lifestyle modification

Example: A patient with diabetes and a blood pressure of 142/94 mmHg plus left ventricular hypertrophy should be classified as having stage 1 hypertension with target organ disease (left ventricular hypertrophy) and with another major risk factor (diabetes). This patient would be categorized as **Stage 1, Risk Group C**, and recommended for immediate initiation of pharmacologic treatment.

Goal Blood Pressure

<140/90 mmHg	Uncomplicated hypertension, Risk Group A, Risk Group B, Risk Group C except for the following:
<130/85 mmHg	Diabetes; renal failure; heart failure
<125/75 mmHg	Renal failure with proteinuria > 1 gram/24hours

SPECIFIC TREATMENT RECOMMENDATIONS

Lifestyle modification should be definitive therapy for some patients and adjunctive therapy for all patients recommended for pharmacologic therapy.

- Start with a low dose of a long-acting once-daily drug, and **titrate dose**
- Low-dose combinations may be appropriate

INITIAL DRUG CHOICES

Uncomplicated Hypertension	Compelling Indications		Specific Indications for the Following Drugs:
Diuretics	Diabetes type 1 (DDM)	Start with ACE inhibitor if proteinuria is present	(See text)
Beta blockers			ACE inhibitors
	Heart failure	Start with ACE inhibitor or diuretic	Angiotensin II receptor blockers
			Alpha blockers
	Myocardial infarction	Beta blocker (non-ISA) after MI; ACE inhibitor for LV dysfunction after MI	Alpha-beta blockers
			Beta blockers
	Isolated systolic hypertension (older patients)	Diuretics (preferred) or calcium antagonists (long-acting DHP)	Calcium antagonists
			Diuretics

From *The Sixth Report of the Joint National Committee on Prevention, Detection, Evaluation, and Treatment of High Blood Pressure.*
Arch Intern Med 1997, 157-2413-2446 NIH Publication No. 98-4080.

Figure 9-1. JNC VI Guide to Stratification, Prevention, and Treatment of Hypertension. (Redrawn from National Institutes of Health Publication #98-4080 [1997]. For a copy of JNC VI, call the National Heart, Lung, and Blood Institute Information Center at 301-251-1222. Sixth Report of the Joint National Committee on Prevention, Detection, Evaluation, and Treatment of High Blood Pressure.)

Illustration continued on following page

The JNC VI Guide To Prevention and Treatment of Hypertension Recommendations

Blood Pressure Measurement	Patient should: • Rest for 5 minutes before measurement. • Refrain from smoking or ingesting caffeine for 30 minutes prior to measurement. • Be seated with feet flat on floor, back and arm supported, arm at heart level. Clinician should: • Use the appropriate size cuff for the patient; the bladder should encircle at least 80 percent of the upper arm. • Use calibrated or mercury manometer. • Average two or more readings, separated by at least 2 minutes.
Primary Prevention	Encourage patients to make healthy lifestyle choices: • Quit smoking to reduce cardiovascular risk. • Lose weight, if needed. • Restrict sodium intake to no more than 100 mmol per day. • Limit alcohol intake to no more than 1-2 drinks per day. • Get at least 30-45 minutes of aerobic activity on most days. • Maintain adequate potassium intake–about 90 mmol per day. • Maintain adequate intakes of calcium and magnesium for general health.
Goal	Set a clear goal of therapy based on patient's risk. Control blood pressure to below: • 140/90 mmHg for patients with uncomplicated hypertension; set a lower goal for those with target organ damage or clinical cardiovascular disease. • 130/85 mmHg for patients with diabetes. • 125/75 mmHg for patients with renal insufficiency with proteinuria greater than 1 gram per 24 hours.
Treatment	Begin with lifestyle modifications (see primary prevention box) for all patients. Be supportive! • Add pharmacologic therapy if blood pressure remains uncontrolled. • Start with a diuretic or beta blocker unless there are compelling indications to use other agents. Use low dose and titrate upward. Consider low dose combinations. • If no response, try a drug from another class or add a second agent from a different class (diuretic if not already used).
Adherence	• Encourage lifestyle modifications. Be supportive! • Educate patient and family about disease. Involve them in measurement and treatment. • Maintain communications with patient. • Discuss how to integrate treatment into daily activities. • Keep care inexpensive and simple. • Favor once-daily, long-acting formulations. • Use combination tablets, when needed. • Consider using generic formulas or larger tablets that can be divided. This may be less expensive. • Be willing to stop unsuccessful therapy and try a different approach. • Consider using nurse case management.

Figure 9–1. *Continued*

    (2) Potassium-sparing agents—Watch for hyperkalemia
       (a) Spironolactone (Aldactone), 25–100 mg p.o. q.d.
          (gynecomastia)
       (b) Amiloride hydrochloride (Midamor), 5–10 mg
          p.o. q.d.
       (c) Triamterene (Dyrenium), 25–100 mg p.o. q.d.
    (3) Other agents—Watch for elevations in cholesterol
       and glucose levels, reductions in sodium, potassium,
       and magnesium levels, and increases in uric acid and
       calcium levels.
       (a) Hydrochlorothiazide (HydroDIURIL, Micro-
          zide), 12.5–50 mg p.o. q.d.
       (b) Chlorthalidone (Hygroton), 12.5–50 mg
          p.o. q.d.
       (c) Metolazone (Zaroxolyn), 2.5–10 mg p.o. q.d.
       (d) Indapamide (Lozol), 1.25–5 mg p.o. q.d. (less or
          no hypercholesterolemia)
f. Adrenergic inhibitors
  i. Properties

- Central agents prevent sympathetic responses while encouraging ''parasympathetic predominance.''
- Peripheral agents prevent norepinephrine release.

  ii. Common preparation (Trade name)/Usual daily dosage
    (1) Central alpha agonists
       (a) Clonidine hydrochloride (Catapres), 0.2–
          1.2 mg p.o. b.i.d. or t.i.d.
       (b) Methyldopa (Aldomet), 500–3000 mg p.o. b.i.d.
    (2) Peripheral agents—Watch for diarrhea and pos-
       tural hypotension.
       (a) Guanethidine monosulfate (Ismelin), 10–150 mg
          p.o. q.d.
       (b) Guanadrel (Hylorel), 10–75 mg p.o. b.i.d.
    (3) Alpha blockers—Particularly useful in patients
       with benign prostatic hypertrophy and hyperlip-
       idemia
       (a) Prazosin hydrochloride (Minipress), 2–30 mg
          p.o. b.i.d. or t.i.d.
       (b) Doxazosin mesylate (Cardura), 1–16 mg
          p.o. q.d., with dosing in the evening
       (c) Terazosin hydrochloride (Hytrin), 1–20 mg
          p.o. q.d.
g. Combined alpha and beta blockers—Watch for bronchospasm and postural hypotension.
  i. Common preparations (Trade name)/Usual daily dosage

- Labetalol hydrochloride (Normodyne, Trandate), 200–1200 mg p.o. b.i.d.

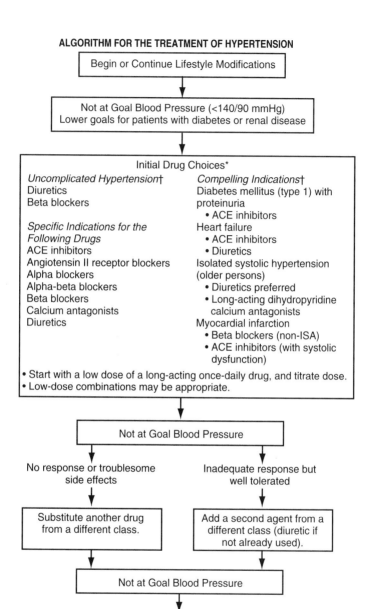

ALGORITHM FOR THE TREATMENT OF HYPERTENSION

Begin or Continue Lifestyle Modifications

Not at Goal Blood Pressure (<140/90 mmHg)
Lower goals for patients with diabetes or renal disease

Initial Drug Choices*

Uncomplicated Hypertension†
Diuretics
Beta blockers

Specific Indications for the Following Drugs
ACE inhibitors
Angiotensin II receptor blockers
Alpha blockers
Alpha-beta blockers
Beta blockers
Calcium antagonists
Diuretics

Compelling Indications†
Diabetes mellitus (type 1) with proteinuria
• ACE inhibitors
Heart failure
• ACE inhibitors
• Diuretics
Isolated systolic hypertension (older persons)
• Diuretics preferred
• Long-acting dihydropyridine calcium antagonists
Myocardial infarction
• Beta blockers (non-ISA)
• ACE inhibitors (with systolic dysfunction)

• Start with a low dose of a long-acting once-daily drug, and titrate dose.
• Low-dose combinations may be appropriate.

Not at Goal Blood Pressure

No response or troublesome side effects

Inadequate response but well tolerated

Substitute another drug from a different class.

Add a second agent from a different class (diuretic if not already used).

Not at Goal Blood Pressure

Continue adding agents from other classes. Consider referral to a hypertension specialist.

*Unless contraindicated. ACE indicates angiotensin-converting enzyme; ISA, intrinsic sympathomimetic activity.
†Based on randomized controlled trials

Figure 9–2. *See legend on opposite page*

- Carvedilol (Coreg), 12.5–50 mg p.o. b.i.d.; also quite effective in patients with heart failure.

h. Angiotensin Converting Enzyme (ACE) Inhibitors— Commonly the drug of choice in patients with diabetes mellitus, particularly effective with whites < 65 years of age or in patients with left ventricular hypertrophy and CHF; indicated for African Americans and may be especially useful in combination with a diuretic or calcium channel blocker; may offer secondary protection from renal complications; watch for cough and bronchospasm.

  i. Properties

   - Inhibit ACE, which decreases levels of angiotensin
   - Vasodilator—Less fluid retention

  ii. Preparations

   - Captopril (Capoten), 25–150 mg p.o. b.i.d. or t.i.d.
   - Enalapril maleate (Vasotec), 5–40 mg p.o. q.d. or b.i.d.
   - Fosinopril sodium (Monopril), 10–40 p.o. q.d. or b.i.d.
   - Benazepril hydrochloride (Lotensin), 5–40 mg p.o. q.d. or b.i.d.
   - Quinapril hydrochloride (Accupril), 5–80 mg p.o. q.d. or b.i.d.
   - Ramipril (Altace), 1.25–20 mg p.o. q.d. or b.i.d.

i. Angiotensin II receptor blockers—Many clinicians now argue that these medications should be considered for first line therapy; watch for hyperkalemia and angioedema (rare).

  i. Properties

   - Block angiotensin-mediated vasoconstriction
   - Decrease aldosterone formation

  ii. Preparations

   - Losartan potassium (Cozaar), 25–100 mg p.o. q.d. or b.i.d.
   - Valsartan (Diovan), 80–320 mg p.o. q.d.
   - Irbesartan (Avapro), 150–300 mg p.o. q.d.
   - Telmisartan (Micardis), 40–80 mg q.d.
   - Candesartan cilexetil (Atacand), 16–32 mg q.d.

Figure 9–2. Algorithm for the Treatment of Hypertension. (Redrawn from National Institutes of Health Publication #98-4080 [1997]. Sixth Report of the Joint National Committee on Prevention, Detection, Evaluation, and Treatment of High Blood Pressure [p. 32].)

j. Calcium channel blockers—Particularly effective as monotherapy, and in elderly whites patients and others with angina when beta blockers may be contraindicated; also effective in patients with atrial fibrillation/tachycardia, diabetes mellitus (types 1 and 2) with proteinuria, and migraines

  i. Properties

- Depress myocardium by blocking movement of calcium
- Decrease automaticity by slowing sinoatrial node
- Slow conduction through atrioventricular node
- Systemic vasodilation with decreased systemic vascular resistance
- Decreased myocardial contractility
- Coronary vasodilation

  ii. Common preparations (Trade name)/Usual daily dosage

    (1) Nondihydropyridines—More cardioselective than dihydropyridines. When prescribed for hypertension, use with caution in patients with coronary disease, conduction defects, and/or dysrhythmias.

      (a) Diltiazem hydrochloride (Cardizem SR), 120–360 mg p.o. b.i.d. (may cause nausea, headache)

      (b) Diltiazem hydrochloride (Cardizem CD), 120–360 mg p.o. q.d.

      (c) Verapamil hydrochloride (Calan SR, Isoptin SR), 90–480 mg p.o. b.i.d.; not used post-MI.

      (d) Verapamil hydrochloride (Verelan, Covera-HS), 120–480 mg p.o. q.d.; not used post-MI.

    (2) Dihydropyridines—More vascular-selective than nondihydropyridines; therefore, less concern about cardioselective effects. Watch for ankle edema, headache, flushing, and gingival hypertrophy.

      (a) Amlodipine (Norvasc), 2.5–10 mg p.o. q.d.

      (b) Nicardipine hydrochloride (Cardene SR), 60–90 mg p.o. b.i.d.

      (c) Nisoldipine (Sular), 20–60 mg p.o. q.d.

      (d) Felodipine (Plendil), 2.5–20 mg p.o. q.d.

k. Direct vasodilators—Watch for headache, flushing, and fluid retention.

  i. Properties

- Relax arterioles independent of sympathetic interactions
- Increase renal blood flow

ii. Common preparations (Trade name)/Usual daily dosage

- Minoxidil (Loniten), 5–100 mg p.o. q.d.
- Hydralazine hydrochloride (Apresoline), 50–300 mg p.o. b.i.d.

4. Combination preparations—While not used as first line treatment, to enhance patient compliance, several antihypertensives have been formulated as combination agents (Table 9–3).
5. Selected drug interactions with antihypertensive therapy (Table 9–4)

J. Hypertensive urgencies and emergencies[5, 7]

1. Hypertensive urgencies

a. Situations where blood pressure must be controlled within a few hours
b. Examples
   i. Asymptomatic severe HTN: SBP > 240 mmHg and DBP > 130 mmHg
   ii. Symptomatic moderately severe HTN: SBP > 200 mmHg and DBP > 120 mmHg (or lower) with accompanying headache, angina, heart failure
c. Parenteral therapy is rarely required.
d. Oral therapy may include
   i. Clonidine (Catapres): Alpha-adrenergic stimulant; dosage = 0.2 mg p.o., then 0.1 mg q1h until BP is controlled or total of 0.8 mg is given; patient may experience sedation; rebound HTN is possible if drug is discontinued.
   ii. Captopril (Capoten): ACE inhibitor; dosage = 12.5–25 mg p.o.
   iii. Nifedipine (Procardia): Calcium channel blocker; dosage = 10 mg p.o. Use with caution: sublingual administration may result in excessive hypotension and reflex tachycardia, resulting in angina. For these reasons, should not be used with suspected or actual heart disease.

2. Hypertensive emergencies[5, 7]

a. Situations requiring rapid (within 1 h) reduction in blood pressure to avoid morbidity or death
b. Generally classified when DBP > 130 mmHg
c. Examples
   i. Hypertensive encephalopathy: Related to cerebrovascular spasms (headache, confusion, irritability, altered mental status)

Text continued on page 100

TABLE 9–3. COMBINATION DRUGS FOR HYPERTENSION

DRUG	TRADE NAME
Beta adrenergic Blockers and Diuretics	
Atenolol, 50 or 100 mg/chlorthalidone, 25 mg	Tenoretic
Bisoprolol fumarate, 2.5, 5, or 10 mg/hydrochlorothiazide, 6.25 mg	Ziac*
Metoprolol tartrate, 50 or 100 mg/hydrochlorothiazide, 25 or 50 mg	Lopressor HCT
Nadolol, 40 or 80 mg/bendroflumethiazide, 5 mg	Corzide
Propranolol hydrochloride, 40 or 80 mg/hydrochlorothiazide, 25 mg	Inderide
Propranolol hydrochloride (extended release), 80, 120, or 160 mg/hydrochlorothiazide, 50 mg	Inderide LA
Timolol maleate, 10 mg/hydrochlorothiazide, 25 mg	Timolide
ACE Inhibitors and Diuretics	
Benazepril hydrochloride, 5, 10, or 20 mg/hydrochlorothiazide, 6.25, 12.5, or 25 mg	Lotensin HCT
Captopril, 25 or 50 mg/hydrochlorothiazide, 15 or 25 mg	Capozide*
Enalapril maleate, 5 or 10 mg/hydrochlorothiazide, 12.5 or 25 mg	Vaseretic
Lisinopril, 10 or 20 mg/hydrochlorothiazide, 12.5 or 25 mg	Prinzide, Zestoretic
Angiotensin II Receptor Antagonists and Diuretics	
Losartan potassium, 50 mg/hydrochlorothiazide, 12.5 mg	Hyzaar

Calcium Antagonists and ACE Inhibitors

Amlodipine besylate, 2.5 or 5 mg/benazepril hydrochloride, 10 or 20 mg — Lotrel
Diltiazem hydrochloride, 180 mg/enalapril maleate, 5 mg — Teczem
Verapamil hydrochloride (extended release), 180 or 240 mg/trandolapril, 1, 2, or 4 mg — Tarka
Felodipine, 5 mg/enalapril maleate, 5 mg — Lexxel

Other Combinations

Triamterene, 37.5, 50, or 75 mg/hydrochlorothiazide, 25 or 50 mg — Dyazide, Maxide
Spironolactone, 25 or 50 mg/hydrochlorothiazide, 25 or 50 mg — Aldactazide
Amiloride hydrochloride, 5 mg/hydrochlorothiazide, 50 mg — Moduretic
Guanethidine monosulfate, 10 mg/hydrochlorothiazide, 25 mg — Esimil
Hydralazine hydrochloride, 25, 50, or 100 mg/hydrochlorothiazide, 25 or 50 mg — Apresazide
Methyldopa, 250 or 500 mg/hydrochlorothiazide, 15, 25, 30, or 50 mg — Aldoril
Reserpine, 0.125 mg/hydrochlorothiazide, 25 or 50 mg — Hydropres
Reserpine, 0.10 mg/hydralazine hydrochloride, 25 mg/hydrochlorothiazide, 15 mg — Ser-Ap-Es
Clonidine hydrochloride, 0.1, 0.2, or 0.3 mg/chlorthalidone, 15 mg — Combipres
Methyldopa, 250 mg/chlorothiazide, 150 or 250 mg — Aldochlor
Reserpine, 0.125 or 0.25 mg/chlorthalidone, 25 or 50 mg — Demi-Regroton
Reserpine, 0.125 or 0.25 mg/chlorothiazide, 250 or 500 mg — Diupres
Prazosin hydrochloride, 1, 2, or 5 mg/polythiazide, 0.5 mg — Minizide

* Approved for initial therapy.
(From National Institutes of Health Publication #98-4080 [1997]. Sixth Report of the Joint National Committee on Prevention, Detection, Evaluation, and Treatment of High Blood Pressure [p. 28].)

TABLE 9–4. SELECTED DRUG INTERACTIONS WITH ANTIHYPERTENSIVE THERAPY*

CLASS OF AGENT	INCREASE EFFICACY	DECREASE EFFICACY	EFFECT ON OTHER DRUGS
Diuretics	Diuretics that act at different sites in the nephron (e.g., furosemide + thiazides)	Resin–binding agents NSAIDs Steroids	Diuretics raise serum lithium levels. Potassium-sparing agents may exacerbate hyperkalemia due to ACE inhibitors.
Beta blockers	Cimetidine (hepatically metabolized beta blockers) Quinidine (hepatically metabolized beta blockers) Food (hepatically metabolized beta blockers)	NSAIDs Withdrawal of clonidine Agents that induce hepatic enzymes, including rifampin and phenobarbital	Propranolol hydrochloride induces hepatic enzymes to increase clearance of drugs with similar metabolic pathways. Beta blockers may mask and prolong insulin-induced hypoglycemia. Heart block may occur with nondihydropyridine calcium antagonists. Sympathomimetics cause unopposed alpha adrenoceptor-mediated vasoconstriction. Beta blockers increase angina-inducing potential of cocaine.
ACE inhibitors	Chlorpromazine or clozapine	NSAIDs Antacids Food decreases absorption (moexipril)	ACE inhibitors may raise serum lithium levels. ACE inhibitors may exacerbate hyperkalemic effect of potassium-sparing diuretics.
Calcium antagonists	Grapefruit juice (some dihydropyridines) Cimetidine or ranitidine (hepatically metabolized calcium antagonists)	Agents that induce hepatic enzymes, including rifampin and phenobarbital	Cyclosporine levels increase† with diltiazem hydrochloride, verapamil hydrochloride, mibefradil dihydrochloride, or

Alpha blockers		nicardipine hydrochloride (but not felodipine, isadipine, or nifedipine). Nondihydropyridines increase levels of other drugs metabolized by the same hepatic enzyme system, including digoxin, quinidine, sulfonylureas, and theophylline. Verapamil hydrochloride may lower serum lithium levels. Prazosin may decrease clearance of verapamil hydrochloride.
Central alpha$_2$-agonists and peripheral neuronal blockers	Tricyclic antidepressants (and probably phenothiazines) Monoamine oxidase inhibitors Sympathomimetics or phenothiazines antagonize guanethidine monosulfate or guanadrel sulfate Iron salts may reduce methyldopa absorption	Methyldopa may increase serum lithium levels. Severity of clonidine hydrochloride withdrawal may be increased by beta blockers. Many agents used in anesthesia are potentiated by clonidine hydrochloride.

* For initial drug therapy recommendations, see also *Physicians' Desk Reference* (51st edition) and *Cardiovascular Pharmacotherapeutics* (New York: McGraw-Hill), 1997. NSAIDs, nonsteroidal anti-inflammatory drugs; ACE, angiotensin-converting enzyme.

† This is a clinically and economically beneficial drug-drug interaction because it both retards progression of accelerated atherosclerosis in heart transplant recipients and reduces the required daily dose of cyclosporine.

(From National Institutes of Health Publication #98-4080 [1997]. Sixth Report of the Joint National Committee on Prevention, Detection, Evaluation, and Treatment of High Blood Pressure [p. 33].)

      ii. Hypertensive nephropathy: Hematuria, proteinuria, progressive renal dysfunction

     iii. Intracranial hemorrhage

     iv. Unstable angina/myocardial infarction

      v. Aortic dissection

     vi. Pulmonary edema

    vii. Preeclampsia-eclampsia

   viii. Malignant HTN—Characterized by encephalopathy or nephropathy and papilledema accompanying a DBP > 110 (frequently > 130) mmHg.
Patients may also complain of headache, blurred vision, or dyspnea.

d. Acute management possibilities for hypertensive emergencies

      i. Critical care unit nursing care and an arterial line are indicated.

     ii. Blood pressure should be lowered to 160–180 mmHg (systolic) or <105 mmHg (diastolic), and then *gradually lowered over several days* with oral therapy to prevent further complications.

    iii. Sodium nitroprusside: Drug of choice

- Dosage $= 0.25$–10 $\mu g/kg/min$ IV
- May cause rapid, profound hypotension
- Do not give for more than 72 hours because of the risk of cyanide poisoning.

    iv. Nitroglycerin: Used especially in patients with ischemia

- Dosage $= 0.25$–5 $\mu g/min$ IV.

     v. Labetalol hydrochloride (Normodyne, Trandate): Used especially with hypertension associated with pregnancy

- Dosage $= 20$–40 mg q10 min to 300 mg; 2 mg/min infusion IV

    vi. Hydralazine (Apresoline): Dosage $= 5$–20 mg IV; may repeat in 20 min; contraindicated in patients with aortic dissection

   vii. Esmolol hydrochloride (Brevibloc): Dosage 500 $\mu g/kg/min$ IV for 1 min, then 50 $\mu g/kg/min$ over 4 min; if an adequate response is not achieved in 5 min, the loading dose should be repeated, followed by a maintenance infusion of 100 $\mu g/kg/min$. Repeat the titration as necessary, increasing the rate of the maintenance dose in increments of 50 $\mu g/kg/min$. As a desired heart rate is achieved, omit the loading dose and decrease the incremental progression to ≤25 $\mu g/$

kg/min or increase the time between titration steps from 5 to 10 min. Infusion may continue for 24–48 h; especially indicated for aortic dissection and in perioperative care.

References

1. Barden, R.M. (1996). Patient with hypertension. In J.M. Clochesy, C. Breu, S. Cardin, A.A. Whittaker, & E.B. Rudy (Eds.), *Critical care nursing* (2nd ed.), (pp. 519–534). Philadelphia: W.B. Saunders.
2. Bueher, D. (1999). Coronary artery disease. In L. Bucher & S. Melander (Eds.), *Critical care nursing* (pp. 203–226). Philadelphia: W.B. Saunders.
3. Burtner, D.E. (1999). Hypertension, essential. In M.R. Dambro (Ed.), *Griffith's 5 minute clinical consult* (pp. 526–527). Media, PA: Williams & Wilkins.
4. Ferri, F.F. (1999). Hypertension. In F.F. Ferri (Ed.), *Ferri's clinical advisor* (pp. 245–247). St Louis: Mosby.
5. Massie, B.M. (1999). Systemic hypertension. In L.M. Tierney, S.J. McPhee, & M.A. Papadakis (Eds.), *Current medical diagnosis & treatment* (38th ed.), (pp. 430–452). Stamford, CT: Appleton & Lange.
6. NIH Publication #98-4080 (1997). Sixth Report of the Joint National Committee on Prevention, Detection, Evaluation, and Treatment of High Blood Pressure.
7. Oparil, S. (1996). Arterial hypertension. In J.C. Bennett & F. Plum (Eds.), *Cecil textbook of medicine* (20th ed.), (pp. 256–271). Philadelphia: W.B. Saunders.
8. Sullivan, J.A. (1998). Hypertension in the elderly: Don't treat too quickly! *Journal of Emergency Nursing, 24*, 20–26.
9. Thelan, L.A., Urden, L.D., Lough, M.E., & Stacy, K.M. (Eds.). (1998). *Critical care nursing: Diagnosing and management.* St Louis: Mosby.
10. Woolliscroft, J.O. (1996). *Handbook of current diagnosis & treatment.* St. Louis: Mosby.

CORONARY ARTERY DISEASE

Thomas W. Barkley, Jr., DSN, RN, CS, ACNP

I. CORONARY ARTERY DISEASE (CAD)[3, 10, 12, 17, 25, 30, 31]

A. Definition[22, 33]

Partial or complete blockage of the coronary arteries as the result of atherosclerosis

B. Incidence/Predisposing factors/Risk factors[3, 11, 12, 18, 23, 24, 26–29, 32–34]

1. Leading cause of death in the United States
2. Responsible for approximately 646,000 emergency department visits each year
3. Accounts for 4.4 million cardiac procedures annually and 4 million hospital discharges
4. Nonmodifiable risk factors
   1. Age—Increasing age increases risk.
   2. Gender—Men are six to eight times more likely to have CAD than premenopausal women; the incidence in post-menopausal women who are unprotected by estrogen is approximately equal to the incidence in men.
   3. Race—White males die more frequently from CAD than men of other ethnic backgrounds, while women of other ethnic backgrounds die from CAD slightly more frequently than white women.
   4. Heredity—Family history of CAD increases risk.

5. Modifiable risk factors

   a. Smoking—Increases low-density lipoproteins (LDLs) and decreases high-density lipoproteins (HDLs); smokers have a two- to six-times greater risk of death from CAD than non-smokers.
   b. Hypertension—The risk of CAD is three times greater when blood pressure is >160/95 mmHg.
   c. Diabetes—Uncontrolled diabetes increases risk.
   d. Obesity and/or sedentary lifestyle
   e. Increased stress and Type A personality
   f. Use of oral contraceptives (especially if the woman is more than 35 years of age)
   g. Hyperlipidemia—Elevations in triglyceride levels, LDLs, and very low density lipoproteins (VLDLs) are associated with increased risk of CAD; low HDL levels are also associated with increased risk.

C. Laboratory/Diagnostic testing[1, 8, 19, 20, 30, 31]

1. For patients with suspected CAD presenting with intermittent chest pain

   a. 12-lead ECG
   b. See Chapter 11, I. H. Management of angina/Acute MI.
   c. Stress testing

2. 12-lead ECG/Stress testing—Controversy exists regarding screening of asymptomatic patients in terms of a resting ECG or stress testing. Studies have not shown significant differences between asymptomatic individuals with and without CAD.
3. Patients should be screened for hypertension every time they seek health care.
4. Pulse pressure—Recent studies have suggested that the higher the pulse pressure, the greater the risk for CAD. Future studies are needed to quantify such findings.
5. Cholesterol screening should be employed for all adults beginning at age 20 and at least every 5 years thereafter in accordance with the National Cholesterol Education Program.
6. Plasma lipoprotein testing

   a. Normal total cholesterol is <200 mg/dL.
   b. Very low density lipoproteins (VLDLs) contain mostly triglycerides and 10–15% of total serum cholesterol.

      • Normal triglyceride level = <200 mg/dL

   c. Low-density lipoproteins (LDLs) contain 60–70% of total serum cholesterol in combination with HDLs; level is inversely correlated with HDL levels.

      • Normal LDL level without known CAD = <130 mg/dL
      • Normal LDL level with known CAD = <100 mg/dL

   d. High-density lipoproteins (HDLs) contain 20–30% of total cholesterol; level is inversely correlated with LDL levels and directly correlated with risk of coronary disease.

      • Normal HDL level = >35 mg/dL

D. Lifestyle changes to modify risk factors[1, 5, 7, 9, 13, 15, 20]

1. Dietary modification/restriction of fat

   a. Total fat <30% of total calories
   b. Saturated fat <10% of total calories
   c. Cholesterol <300 mg per day

2. Smoking cessation
3. Control of hypertension—See Chapter 9.

4. Control of diabetes
5. Stress management
6 Exercise
7. Discontinuance of oral contraceptives for women at risk for CAD who are more than 35 years of age—Consider other means of birth control.
8. Consider estrogen therapy, as indicated, for postmenopausal women.
9. Control of cholesterol through modifiable means or via pharmacologic therapy—See section E. Management of high blood cholesterol, which follows.

E. Management of high blood cholesterol in adults

1. Acquire fasting or nonfasting total cholesterol and HDL levels. Fingerstick methods may be used.
2. Total cholesterol classification (in patients without evidence of coronary heart disease [CHD])

   - Desirable = <200 mg/dL (<5.2 mmol/L)
   - Borderline-high = 200–239 mg/dL (5.2–6.2 mmol/L)
   - High risk = ≥240 mg/dL (≥6.2 mmol/L)

3. HDL level classification

   - Low = <35 mg/dL (0.9 mmol/L)
   - High = ≥60 mg/dL (≥1.55 mmol/L); "protective"

4. If total cholesterol is in the "desirable" range and HDL cholesterol is low, patients should be rechecked within 5 years.
5. If total cholesterol is not within the "desirable" level, risk for CHD is assessed (Table 10–1).
6. Based on CHD risk factors, total cholesterol, and HDL levels, follow the protocol depicted in Figure 10–1.
7. Management options, as depicted in Figure 10–2, should also be considered based on the patient's LDL cholesterol level.
8. Consider causes of secondary hyperlipidemia.

   a. Diabetes mellitus
   b. Nephrotic syndrome
   c. Chronic renal failure
   d. Hypothyroidism

9. In patients with *known* CHD, follow the protocol shown in Figure 10–3.
10. Dietary and drug treatment: Dietary modification remains the cornerstone of treatment for patients with hyperlipidemia, and therapy should always begin with dietary modification. Table 10–2 summarizes treatment recommendations using diet and pharmacologic treatment based on LDL cholesterol. Note that regular exercise (30 min per day), fat re-

TABLE 10–1. RISK STATUS BASED ON PRESENCE OF CHD RISK FACTORS OTHER THAN LDL CHOLESTEROL

POSITIVE RISK FACTORS

Age
 Male: ≥45 years
 Female ≥55 years, or premature menopause without estrogen
  replacement therapy
Family history of premature CHD (definite myocardial infarction or
 sudden death before 55 years of age in father or other male first-
 degree relative, or before 65 years of age in mother or other female
 first-degree relative)
Current cigarette smoking
Hypertension (≥140/90 mmHg,* or on antihypertensive medication)
Low HDL cholesterol (≤35 mg/dL*)
Diabetes mellitus

NEGATIVE RISK FACTOR†

High HDL cholesterol (≥60 mg/dL)

High risk, defined as a net of two or more CHD risk factors, leads to more vigorous intervention. Age (defined differently for men and for women) is treated as a risk factor because rates of CHD are higher in the elderly than in the young, and in men than in women of the same age. Obesity is not listed as a risk factor because it operates through other risk factors that are implicated (hypertension, hyperlipidemia, decreased HDL cholesterol, and diabetes mellitus), but it should be considered a target for intervention. Physical inactivity is similarly not listed as a risk factor, but it, too, should be considered a target for intervention, and physical activity is recommended as desirable for everyone.

* Confirmed by measurements on several occasions.

† If the HDL cholesterol level is ≥60 mg/dL, subtract one risk factor (because high HDL cholesterol levels decrease CHD risk).

National Cholesterol Education Program, Second Report of the Expert Panel on Detection, Evaluation, and Treatment of High Blood Cholesterol in Adults. www.nhlbi.nih.gov/guidelines/cholesterol/atp-sum.htm

striction, and control of other CHD risk factors are *usually* employed *for at least 6 months* before pharmacologic therapy is initiated.

11. Dietary considerations

  a. About one half of all saturated fat and the majority (70%) of cholesterol in the United States come from the follow-ing foods, which should be restricted: hamburgers/cheese-burgers, meat loaf, whole milk, cheese, other dairy prod-ucts, beef steaks, roast beef, hot dogs, ham, lunch meats, doughnuts, cookies, cakes, and eggs.

  b. Encourage the consumption of poultry (without skin), fish, skimmed/low-fat milk, nonfat/low-fat yogurt, low-fat cheeses, fruits, vegetables, and grains. Preferred oils in-clude canola, soybean, olive, or corn because these repre-

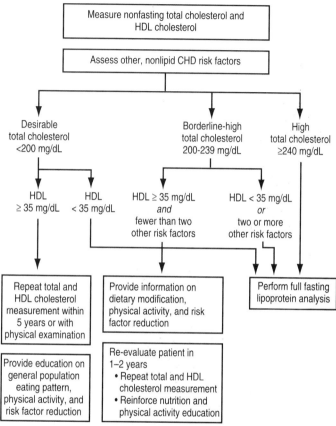

PRIMARY PREVENTION IN ADULTS WITHOUT EVIDENCE OF CHD: INITIAL CLASSIFICATION BASED ON TOTAL CHOLESTEROL AND HDL CHOLESTEROL

Measure nonfasting total cholesterol and HDL cholesterol

Assess other, nonlipid CHD risk factors

Desirable total cholesterol <200 mg/dL

Borderline-high total cholesterol 200-239 mg/dL

High total cholesterol ≥240 mg/dL

HDL ≥ 35 mg/dL

HDL < 35 mg/dL

HDL ≥ 35 mg/dL *and* fewer than two other risk factors

HDL < 35 mg/dL *or* two or more other risk factors

Repeat total and HDL cholesterol measurement within 5 years or with physical examination

Provide information on dietary modification, physical activity, and risk factor reduction

Perform full fasting lipoprotein analysis

Provide education on general population eating pattern, physical activity, and risk factor reduction

Re-evaluate patient in 1–2 years
• Repeat total and HDL cholesterol measurement
• Reinforce nutrition and physical activity education

Figure 10–1. Primary prevention classification by total cholesterol. In patients without coronary heart disease (CHD), initial assessment for dyslipidemia is by total cholesterol and high-density lipoprotein levels (minimal approach). The physician may choose the full fasting lipoprotein analysis as the first assessment. (Redrawn from Goldman, L., & Braunwald, E. [1998]. *Primary cardiology* [p. 453]. Philadelphia: W.B. Saunders; redrawn from Farmer, J.A., & Gotto, A.M., Jr. [1997]. Dyslipidemia and other risk factors for coronary artery disease. In E. Braunwald [Ed.], *Heart disease* [5th ed.] [pp. 1126–1160]. Philadelphia: W.B. Saunders, from Expert Panel on Detection, Evaluation, and Treatment of High Blood Cholesterol in Adults [1993]. Summary of the second report of the National Cholesterol Education Program [NCEP] Expert Panel on Detection, Evaluation, and Treatment of High Blood Cholesterol in Adults [Adult Treatment Panel II]. *Journal of the American Medical Association, 269,* 3015, and National Cholesterol Education Program [1994]. Second report of the Expert Panel on Detection, Evaluation, and Treatment of High Blood Cholesterol in Adults [Adult Treatment Panel II]. *Circulation, 89,* 1329, with permission.)

**PRIMARY PREVENTION IN ADULTS WITHOUT EVIDENCE OF CHD:
SUBSEQUENT CLASSIFICATION BASED ON LDL CHOLESTEROL**

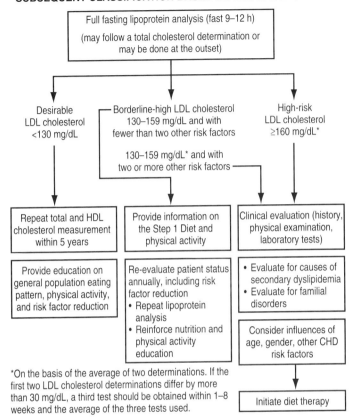

Figure 10–2. Primary prevention classification by low-density lipoprotein (LDL) cholesterol. In patients without coronary heart disease (CHD) or other atherosclerotic disease who have low high-density lipoprotein (HDL) cholesterol, borderline-high total cholesterol in the presence of two or more other risk factors, of high total cholesterol, full fasting lipoprotein analysis is required to determine LDL cholesterol level. (Redrawn from Goldman, L., & Braunwald, E. [1998]. *Primary cardiology* [p. 455]. Philadelphia: W.B. Saunders; redrawn from Farmer, J.A., & Gotto, A.M., Jr. [1997]. Dyslipidemia and other risk factors for coronary artery disease. In E. Braunwald [Ed.], *Heart disease* [5th ed.] [pp. 1126–1160]. Philadelphia: W.B. Saunders, from Expert Panel on Detection, Evaluation, and Treatment of High Blood Cholesterol in Adults [1993]. Summary of the second report of the National Cholesterol Education Program [NCEP] Expert Panel on Detection, Evaluation, and Treatment of High Blood Cholesterol in Adults [Adult Treatment Panel II]. *Journal of the American Medical Association, 269,* 3015, and National Cholesterol Education Program [1994]. Second report of the Expert Panel on Detection, Evaluation, and Treatment of High Blood Cholesterol in Adults [Adult Treatment Panel II]. *Circulation, 89,* 1329, with permission.)

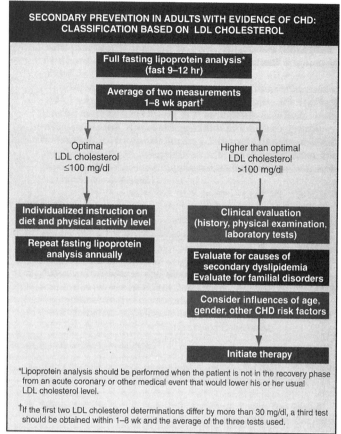

Figure 10–3. Secondary prevention classification by low-density lipoprotein (LDL) cholesterol. In patients with coronary heart disease (CHD) or other atherosclerotic disease, initial assessment for dyslipidemia is by full fasting lipoprotein analysis to determine LDL cholesterol level. (Redrawn from Goldman, L., & Braunwald, E. [1998]. *Primary cardiology* [p. 455]. Philadelphia: W.B. Saunders; redrawn from Farmer, J.A., & Gotto, A.M., Jr. [1997]. Dyslipidemia and other risk factors for coronary artery disease. In E. Braunwald [Ed.], *Heart disease* [5th ed.] [pp. 1126–1160]. Philadelphia: W.B. Saunders, from Expert Panel on Detection, Evaluation, and Treatment of High Blood Cholesterol in Adults [1993]. Summary of the second report of the National Cholesterol Education Program [NCEP] Expert Panel on Detection, Evaluation, and Treatment of High Blood Cholesterol in Adults [Adult Treatment Panel II]. *Journal of the American Medical Association, 269,* 3015, and National Cholesterol Education Program [1994]. Second report of the Expert Panel on Detection, Evaluation, and Treatment of High Blood Cholesterol in Adults [Adult Treatment Panel II]. *Circulation, 89,* 1329, with permission.)

TABLE 10–2. TREATMENT DECISIONS BASED ON LDL CHOLESTEROL

	DIETARY THERAPY	
	Initiation Level	LDL Goal
Without CHD and with fewer than two risk factors	≥160 mg/dL (4.1 mmol/L)	<160 mg/dL
Without CHD and with two or more risk factors	≥130 mg/dL (3.4 mmol/L)	<130 mg/dL
With CHD*	>100 mg/dL (2.6 mmol/L)	≤100 mg/dL
	DRUG TREATMENT	
	Consideration Level	LDL Goal
Without CHD and with fewer than two risk factors	≥190 mg/dL† (4.9 mmol/L)	<160 mg/dL
Without CHD and with two or more risk factors	≥160 mg/dL (4.1 mmol/L)	<130 mg/dL
With CHD	≥130 mg/dL (3.4 mmol/L)	≤100 mg/dL

* In CHD patients with LDL cholesterol levels 100–129 mg/dL (2.6–3.3 mmol/L), the physician should exercise clinical judgment in deciding whether to initiate drug treatment.

† In men under 35 yr of age and premenopausal women with LDL cholesterol levels 190–219 mg/dL (4.9–5.7 mmol/L), drug therapy should be delayed except in high-risk patients such as those with diabetes.

(From Goldman, L., & Braunwald, E. [1998]. *Primary cardiology* [p. 459]. Philadelphia: W.B. Saunders; Schaefer, E.J. [1995]. Overview of the diagnosis and treatment of lipid disorders [p. 17]. Cambridge, MA: Copyright Genzyme Corporation, with permission.)

sent unsaturated vegetable oils that contain polyunsaturated fat and monounsaturated fatty acids.

c. Step 1 diets are encouraged for the entire population.

- *Total fat* = 30% or less of total calories.
- *Saturated fatty acids* = 8–10% of total calories.
- *Polyunsaturated fatty acids* = up to 10% of total calories.
- *Monounsaturated fatty acids* = up to 15% of total calories.
- *Carbohydrates* = 55% or more of total calories.
- *Protein* = approximately 15% of total calories.
- *Cholesterol* = <300 mg/day.
- *Total calories* = to achieve and maintain desirable weight.

d. For patients with elevated LDL levels, the Step 2 diet should be recommended.

- *Total fat* = 30% or less of total calories.
- *Saturated fatty acids* = <7% of total calories.

- *Polyunsaturated fatty acids* = up to 10% of total calories.
- *Monounsaturated fatty acids* = up to 15% of total calories.
- *Carbohydrates* = 55% or more of total calories.
- *Protein* = approximately 15% of total calories.
- *Cholesterol* = <200 mg/day.
- *Total calories* = to achieve and maintain desirable weight.

e. Restriction of fat to 20% of total calories concurrent with exercise (30 min per day) has been shown to decrease the prevalence of age-related weight gain and obesity that are associated with hyperlipidemia, hypertension, and diabetes.

f. Preparations associated with lowering cholesterol

- Dietary fiber supplementation utilizing such preparations as oat bran, oatmeal, psyllium, and soluble/insoluble mixed fiber
- Fish oil
- Vitamin E supplementation
- Diets rich in alpha-linolenic acid

g. Employ the expertise of a registered dietitian for referral/consultation.

12. Pharmacologic therapy[2, 6, 10, 11, 16, 17, 21]

a. Three classes of medications may be used to *lower LDL levels* (Table 10–3).

- HMG CoA reductase inhibitors—Drugs of choice
- Anion-exchange resins
- Other agents (see Table 10–3)

b. LDLs should be checked at 4–6 weeks after the initiation of pharmacologic therapy, and then again at 3 months after initiation. If the optimum goal for LDL has been reached, guidelines suggest that the patient be seen in 4 months, or more frequently if agents require closer following. Long-term follow-up of lipoprotein analysis with LDL may then occur annually.

c. If initial therapy with one medication is inadequate, either change drugs or change to a combination of two agents. Most commonly, the combination of an anion exchange resin (e.g., cholestyramine or colestipol) in combination with either niacin or a "statin" (e.g., lovastatin, atorvastatin) may reduce LDL levels by as much as 40–50%.

F. Complications of CAD—See specific complications

1. Angina—Chapter 11
2. Myocardial infarction—Chapter 11

Text continued on page 116

TABLE 10–3. PHARMACOLOGIC THERAPY TO LOWER LDLs

PREPARATION	INITIAL DOSE	PROGRESSIVE DOSE	MAXIMAL DOSE	MAJOR SIDE EFFECTS	LDL REDUCTION	HDL INCREASE	TRIGLYCERIDE REDUCTION
HMG CoA Reductase Inhibitors/"Statins"							
Lovastatin (Mevacor)	20 mg p.o. in the evening	20–80 mg/day p.o. Adjust at intervals of 4 weeks or more	80 mg/day p.o. Patients receiving immunosuppressants should receive a maximal dose of 20 mg/day p.o.	As a class of medications, the following major adverse effects are possible: Headache, blurred vision, GI complaints, elevations in AST/ALT and creatinine/alkaline phosphatases, liver failure. Possible rhabdomyolysis with acute renal failure or myopathy when combined with erythromycin, cyclosporine, niacin, gemfibrozil, or antifungals. Digitalis toxicity more possible with some agents.	20–40%	5–10%	20%
Pravastatin (Pravachol)	10–20 mg at bedtime	20–30 mg at bedtime	40 mg at bedtime		20–40%	5–10%	20%

Table continued on following page

111

TABLE 10–3. PHARMACOLOGIC THERAPY TO LOWER LDLs *Continued*

PREPARATION	INITIAL DOSE	PROGRESSIVE DOSE	MAXIMAL DOSE	MAJOR SIDE EFFECTS	LDL REDUCTION	HDL INCREASE	TRIGLYCERIDE REDUCTION
Simvastatin (Zocor)	5–10 mg before evening meal or at bedtime	5–10 mg b.i.d.	20 mg b.i.d. or 40 mg before evening meal or at bedtime		20–40%	5–10%	20%
Fluvastatin (Lescol)	20 mg p.o. in the evening	20–40 mg p.o. every day	40 mg p.o. every day		20–40%	5–10%	20%
Atorvastatin (Lipitor)	10 mg p.o. every day	10–80 mg p.o. every day; may be combined with anion-exchange resins.	80 mg p.o. every day		20–40%	5–10%	20%
Cerivastatin (Baycol)	0.3 mg p.o. every day in the evening; effectiveness increased if combined with an anion-exchange resin (give cerivastatin >2 hours after the resin.)	Not documented	Not documented		20–40%	5–10%	20%

Anion-Exchange Resins						
Cholestyramine (Questran)	4 g powder 1–6 times per day			As a class of medications, the following major adverse effects are possible: Constipation to fecal impaction, exacerbation of hemorrhoids, other GI complaints, increased bleeding tendencies, decreased/delayed absorption with warfarin, thiazide diuretics, digitalis preparations, thyroid medications, and corticosteroids. Malabsorption of fat-soluble vitamins.	15–25%	5%	Uncertain
Colestipol (Colestid)	5 g q.i.d. or b.i.d. p.o.	Increase in 5 g p.o. increments per day at 1- to 2-month intervals; maximum = 30 g/day	30 g p.o. per day			

Table continued on following page

TABLE 10–3. PHARMACOLOGIC THERAPY TO LOWER LDLs *Continued*

PREPARATION	INITIAL DOSE	PROGRESSIVE DOSE	MAXIMAL DOSE	MAJOR SIDE EFFECTS	LDL REDUCTION	HDL INCREASE	TRIGLYCERIDE REDUCTION
Other Agents							
Niacin (Niaspan)	375 mg p.o. every day for the 1st week, 500 mg p.o. for the 2nd week, 750 mg p.o. for the 3rd week, then 1 g p.o. every day for weeks 4–7	May increase by 500 mg every 4 weeks until an adequate response is reached	2 g per day	Headache, flushing, GI upset, hypotension, arrhythmias, glucose intolerance, increased risk of rhabdomyolysis with HMG CoA inhibitors, increased effectiveness of antihypertensives	15–25%	May raise by 25% or lower HDL by 35%	Lowers

Drug				Side effects			
Gemfibrozil (Lopid)	1200 mg p.o. every day in two divided doses 30 min before morning and evening meals	900–1200 mg per day	1200 mg per day	Headache, dizziness, blurred vision, vertigo, GI complaints, liver function changes, hyperglycemia, eczema, rash, risk of rhabdomyolysis when combined with HMG CoA inhibitors	0–15%	5–15%	35%
Fish oils	2 capsules t.i.d. with meals	4 capsules t.i.d. with meals	6 capsules t.i.d. with meals				
Probucol (Lorelco)	500 mg p.o. b.i.d.			GI complaints	10–15%	May lower HDL levels 10%	0%

3. Congestive heart failure—Chapter 15
4. Peripheral vascular disease—Chapter 13
5. Hypertension—Chapter 9

References

1. Allison, T.G., Squires, R.W., Johnson, B.D., & Gau, G.T. (1999). Achieving national cholesterol education program goals for low-density lipoprotein cholesterol in cardiac patients: Importance of diet, exercise, weight control and drug therapy. *Mayo Clinic Proceedings, 74,* 466–473.
2. Baron, R.B. (2000). Lipid abnormalities. In L.M. Tierney, S.J. McPhee, & M.A. Papadakis (Eds.). *Current medical diagnosis and treatment 2000* (pp. 1198–1240). New York: Lange Medical Books/McGraw-Hill.
3. Becker, D. (1999). Coronary artery disease. In L. Bucher & S. Melander (Eds.), *Critical care nursing* (pp. 201–226). Philadelphia: W.B. Saunders.
4. Carlson, E., Braun, L.T., Murphy, M.P. (1996). Coronary artery disease. In M.R. Kinney & D. R. Packa (Eds.), *Andreoli's comprehensive cardiac care* (8th ed.) (pp. 256–275). St. Louis: Mosby.
5. Cleeman, J., & Lenfant, C. (1998). The national cholesterol education program. *Journal of the American Medical Association, 280,* 2009.
6. Gregorio G.J., Barbieri, E.J. (1998). *Handbook of commonly prescribed drugs.* Philadelphia: Roche Laboratories.
7. Dracup, K.A., & Cannon, C.P. (1999). Combination treatment strategies for management of acute myocardial infarction: New directions with current therapies. *Critical Care Nurse,* (Suppl.), 3–17.
8. Foxton, J. (1998). Hyperlipidemia. *Nursing Standard, 12,* 49–56.
9. Franklin, S.S., Khan, S.A., Wong, N.D., Larson, M.G., & Levy, D. (1999). Is pulse pressure useful in predicting risk for coronary heart disease? The Framingham heart study. *Circulation, 100,* 354–360.
10. Froom, J., Froom, P., Benjamin, M., & Benjamin, B.J. (1998). Measurement and management of hyperlipidemia for the primary prevention of coronary heart disease. *Journal of the American Board of Family Practice, 11,* 12–22.
11. Gawlinski, A., McCloy, K., Caswell, D., & Quintones-Baldrich, W.J. (1999). Cardiovascular disorders. In A. Gawlinski & D. Hamwi (Eds.), *Acute care nurse practitioner: Clinical curriculum and certification review* (pp. 154–160). Philadelphia: W.B. Saunders.
12. Gaziano, J.M. (1999). Cholesterol reduction and risk of stroke. *Cardiology Review, 16,* 7–8.
13. Grover, S.A., Paquet, S., Levington, C., Coupal, L., & Zowall H. (1998). Estimating the benefits of modifying risk factors of cardiovascular disease: A comparison of primary vs secondary prevention. *Archives of Internal Medicine, 158,* 655–662.
14. Harper, C.R., & Jacobson, T.A. (1999). New perspectives on the management of low levels of high-density lipoprotein cholesterol. *Archives of Internal Medicine, 159,* 1049–1057.
15. Hayes, E.R., & Kee, J.L. (1996). *Pharmacology: Pocket companion for nurses.* Philadelphia: W.B. Saunders.
16. Jacobs, D.S., DeMott, W.R., Grady, H.J., Horvat, R.T., Huestis, D.W., & Kasten, B.L., Jr. (1996). *Laboratory test handbook.* Cleveland: Lexi-Comp Inc.
17. Kannel, W.B. (1998). The worth of controlling plasma lipids. *The American Journal of Cardiology, 81,* 1047–1049.

18. Karch, A.M. (Ed.). (2000). *Lippincott's nursing drug guide 2000*. Philadelphia: J.B. Lippincott.

19. Keen, J.H. (1997). In J.H. Keen & P.L. Swearingen (Eds.), *Mosby's critical care nursing consultant* (pp. 92–93). St. Louis: Mosby.

20. Kozisek, P. (1999). Arteriosclerotic heart disease. In M.R. Dambro (Ed.), *Griffith's 5 minute clinical consult* (pp. 76–77). Media, PA: Williams & Wilkins.

21. Koren, M.J., & Bakker-Arkema, R.G. (1999). Achieving LDL goals: A comparison of four statins. *Cardiology Review, 16,* 34–37.

22. Lacy, C.F., Armstrong, L.L., Ingrine, N.B., & Lauce, L.L. (1998). *Drug information handbook.* Cleveland: Lexi-Comp Inc.

23. Lamborn, M.L., & Moseley, M.K. (1997). Cardiac alterations. In J.C. Hartshorn, M.L. Sole, & M.L. Lamborn (Eds.), *Introduction to critical care nursing* (2nd ed.) (pp. 232–269). Philadelphia: W.B. Saunders.

24. Lip, G.Y.H., & Beevers, D.G. (1997). Can we treat coronary artery disease with antibiotics? *The Lancet, 350,* 378–379.

25. Lowe, A., & Melander, S.D. (1996). In S.D. Melander (Ed.), *Review of critical care nursing* (pp. 50–73). Philadelphia: W.B. Saunders.

26. National cholesterol education program second panel of the expert panel on detection, evaluation, and treatment of high blood cholesterol in adults (Adult treatment II Panel) www.nhlbi.nih.gov/guidelines/cholesterol/atp_sum.htm

27. Penque, S., Halm, M.H., Smith, M., Deutsch, J., Van Roekel, M., McLaughlin, L., Dzubay, S., Doll, N., & Beahrs, M. (1998). Women and coronary disease: Relationship between descriptors of signs and symptoms and diagnostic and treatment course. *American Journal of Critical Care, 7,* 175–182.

28. Pitt, B., & Rubenfire, M. (1999). Risk stratification for the detection of preclinical coronary artery disease. *Circulation, 99,* 2610–2612.

29. Piatek, Y.M., & Atzori, M. (1999). PTMR: When all options are exhausted, percutaneous transmyocardial revascularization can diminish symptoms of angina. *American Journal of Nursing, 99,* 64–65.

30. Thelan, L.A., Urden, L.D., Lough, M.E., & Stacy, K.M. (1998). *Critical care nursing: Diagnosis and management* (3rd ed.). St. Louis: Mosby.

31. Shaefer, E.J. (1998). Lipoprotein disorders. In L. Goldman & E. Braunwald (Eds.), *Primary cardiology* (pp. 445–468). Philadelphia: W.B. Saunders.

32. Sox, H.C. (1998). Screening for coronary artery disease and its risk factors. In L. Goldman & E. Braunwald (Eds.), *Primary cardiology* (pp. 57–69). Philadelphia: W.B. Saunders.

33. Unknown author (1998). Are you one of the few following NCEP guidelines for finding, treating high cholesterol? *Modern Medicine, 66,* 36.

34. Verderber, A., Castelfranco, A.M., Nishioka, D., & Johnson, K.G. (1999). Cardiovascular risk factors and cardiac surgery outcomes in a multiethnic sample of men and women. *American Journal of Critical Care, 8,* 140–148.

ANGINA/MYOCARDIAL INFARCTION

Thomas W. Barkley, Jr., DSN, RN, CS, ACNP

I. ANGINA/MYOCARDIAL INFARCTION (MI)

A. Definition[20, 46]

1. Angina—"Pain in the chest" related to ischemia
2. Myocardial infarction—Death of myocardial tissue
3. Pathology—supply/demand mismatch: the demand for myocardial oxygen is greater than the ability of the coronary arteries to supply oxygen.

B. Incidence/Predisposing factors/General comments[3, 4, 8, 10–12, 19, 31, 32, 42]

1. Incidence

   a. Heart disease is the leading cause of death in the United States.
   b. Approximately 7 million people in the United States suffer from angina.
   c. Over 1.5 million people in the United States experience an acute MI each year.
   d. The majority (55%) of patients experiencing MI are more than 65 years of age.
   e. Eighty percent of deaths related to MI are among individuals more than 65 years of age.
   f. Classically, MI is precipitated by events that increase myocardial oxygen demand.
      i. Physical exertion (e.g., exercise, sex)
      ii. Extremes in weather conditions
      iii. Consumption of a heavy meal
      iv. Stressful events
      v. Smoking

2. Predisposing factors

   a. Coronary artery disease/Hyperlipidemia
   b. Hypertension
   c. Other—such as male gender and family history

3. General comments

   a. Misdiagnosis of MI is the leading cause of liability among emergency room physicians.
   b. National recommendations stipulate that all emergency departments treat acute MI within 30 min after the patient's arrival at the hospital.

c. Peak occurrence of MI and sudden cardiac death is between the hours of 6 AM and noon. A significant number of deaths related to MI also occur between 4 AM and 6 AM.

C. Types of angina[2, 20, 42, 43, 46]

1. Stable (Classic)

   a. Intermittent chest pain over time with the same onset, intensity, and duration
   b. Usually induced by exercise or exertion
   c. Pain at rest is unusual; pain usually lasts 1–5 min to a maximum of 10 min.
   d. ECG usually shows *ST segment depression* (ischemia).
   e. With lifestyle changes, angina may be controlled without severe complications.

2. Prinzmetal's (Variant)

   a. Pain often occurs at rest and may last up to 30 min.
   b. Pain is not usually precipitated by an increase in oxygen demand.
   c. Pain may occur in the absence of atherosclerosis.
   d. Pathology is related to spasms of the coronary arteries. Spasms are strong contractions of smooth muscle in the coronary arteries caused by an increase in intracellular calcium levels.
   e. ECG usually shows *ST segment elevation.*

3. Unstable (Pre-infarction)

   a. Chest pain lasting longer than 20–30 min
   b. Pain is more severe than with stable angina and experienced at rest or with low activity levels.
   c. Pattern of attacks usually progresses, with increased frequency, duration, and intensity.
   d. ECG may show *ST segment depression.*
   e. Nitrates are usually insufficient to relieve pain.
   f. Increased incidence of MI within 1½ years after angina begins

D. "P-Q-R-S-T" method of pain assessment[2, 7]

P = *Provocative:*	What activities elicit pain?
Q = *Quality:*	What does the pain feel like? Do other symptoms occur simultaneously?
R = *Region/Radiation:*	Where is the pain? Does the pain radiate? If so, where?
S = *Severity:*	How does the pain rate on a scale of 0–10? (Some institutions now use a 0–5 scale.)

T = *Timing/Treatment:* When did the pain begin? How long does it last? What did you do to relieve the pain? Were such measures effective?

E. Pain of angina vs. myocardial infarction[11, 24, 42]

1. Generally, anginal pain is more diffuse and vague than pain from an MI.
2. With MI, pain *may* be described as "vise-like," "crushing," substernal pressure that may or may not radiate to the jaw and/or left arm.
3. Pain from myocardial infarction *may* radiate to the jaw, back, shoulders, arms, or abdomen.
4. Approximately 15% of patients experiencing MI have no pain.
5. Generally, women experiencing angina/MI complain of more gastrointestinal-like symptoms than men. Administration of a "GI cocktail" consisting of Maalox or Mylanta, viscous lidocaine, and Donnatal should immediately relieve pain related to acute gastrointestinal causes such as esophagitis, gastritis, and gastric/duodenal ulcers. If pain is not relieved, cardiac-related causes should be thoroughly investigated.

F. Subjective/Physical examination findings of angina/MI[11]

1. Note: History and physical examination findings are very important to early dectection and diagnosis.
2. Nausea
3. Vomiting
4. Diaphoresis
5. Cool, clammy skin
6. Chest pain—usually substernal; for MI—not relieved by nitroglycerin
7. Dyspnea
8. Feeling of "impending doom."

G. Diagnostic/Laboratory findings of angina/MI[2, 11, 23, 24, 29, 38, 40, 42]

1. 12-Lead ECG changes

   a. Signs of MI progression: Heightening or peaking of T waves → ST segment elevation → Inversion of T waves → Formation of Q waves → Diminished height of R waves
   b. Note: Approximately 30% of patients experiencing MI show no immediate 12-lead ECG changes.
   c. Hallmarks of ischemia vs. injury vs. infarction
      i. *Ischemia*—T wave inversion, peaked T waves, and ST segment depression. Note: With angina, cardiac changes usually do not persist once pain is alleviated.

     ii. *Injury*—ST segment elevation of >1 mm above base line

     iii. *Infarction*—Q waves (pathologic) either >25% of the QRS complex height or >1 mm wide (0.04 s)

  d. Expected site of MI based on ECG changes

     i. *Inferior:* Leads II, III, aV_F; diaphragmatic involving the right coronary artery (80–90%) or left circumflex artery (10–20%)

     ii. *Inferolateral:* Leads II, III, aV_F, V_5 and V_6; site = left circumflex artery

     iii. *Anterior:* V_3 and V_4; site = left anterior descending artery

     iv. *Anterolateral and lateral:* Leads I, aV_L, V_5, and V_6; site = left anterior descending artery or the left circumflex artery

     v. *Anteroseptal:* V_1, V_2, and V_3; site = left anterior descending artery

     vi. *Posterior:* Reciprocal changes noted in V_1 and V_3, broad or tall R waves, and ST depression without T-wave inversion may be seen; site = right coronary artery or left circumflex artery

     vii. *Right ventricular:* V_4–V_6; elevations in all precordial leads may be seen; site = right coronary artery.

2. Serum cardiac enzymes (Table 11–1)
3. CBC with electrolytes, hemoglobin, and hematocrit levels
4. Lipid profile

H. Management of angina/Acute MI[1–4, 8, 10, 19, 37, 42, 43] (Fig. 11–1)

1. Emergency management of acute angina/MI[2, 7, 10, 26, 43]

  a. Nitroglycerin, sublingual (1 q5min × 3)

  b. Oxygen, at 2–4 L/min per NC

  c. Aspirin, 325 mg p.o.

  d. Bedside monitor—Evaluate potential life-threatening dysrhythmias.

  e. IV access—Blood for cardiac enzymes and other laboratory values may be drawn at this time.

  f. Continuous pain assessment

  g. Pulse oximetry

  h. 12-Lead ECG

  i. Consider morphine, 4–8 mg IV, or meperidine (Demerol), 50–75 mg IV, if pain not relieved; may repeat with low doses q15min until pain is relieved, unless other adverse effects occur.

  j. Consider admitting the patient to the coronary care unit to rule out acute MI, pending results of cardiac enzymes.

TABLE 11-1. SERUM CARDIAC ENZYMES

SERUM MARKER	EARLIEST INCREASE (HOURS)	PEAK (HOURS)	DURATION	OTHER CAUSES OF ELEVATION
Troponin T	4–6	10–24	14–21 days	Regenerative muscular disorders; unstable angina
Troponin I	4–6	10–24	5–7 days	100% specific for myocardial necrosis
Myoglobin	2–3	6–9	3–15 h	Regenerative muscular disorders; unstable angina
CK—MB	4–8	15–24	48–72 h	Post cardioversion, cardiac contusion, cardiac surgical procedures, myocarditis, and acute pericarditis with myocardial involvement
Total CK	3–6	24–36	18–30 h	Smooth muscle injury; nonspecific
LD1	8–12	72–144	7–12 days	Hemolytic and megaloblastic anemias, acute renal infarction, hemolysis, and testicular cancer
Total LD	10–12	48–72	10–14 days	Smooth muscle injury; nonspecific

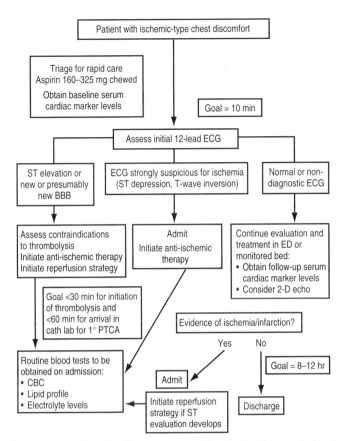

Figure 11–1. Algorithm for management of patients with suspected acute myocardial infarction in the emergency department (ED). All patients with ischemic-type chest discomfort should be evaluated rapidly and receive aspirin. The initial 12-lead electrocardiogram (ECG) is used to define the acute management strategy. Patients with ST segment elevation or new or presumably new bundle branch block (BBB) should be considered candidates for reperfusion; those without ST segment elevation but with an ECG and clinical history that are strongly suspicious for ischemia should be admitted for initiation of anti-ischemic therapy. Patients with a normal or nondiagnostic ECG should undergo further evaluation in the ED or short-term observation until results of serial serum cardiac marker levels are obtained. The following routine blood tests should be obtained in all patients admitted: a complete blood count (CBC), lipid profile, and electrolyte levels. 2-D, two-dimensional: 1°, primary; PTCA, percutaneous transluminal coronary angioplasty. (Redrawn from Goldman, L., & Braunwald, E. [1998]. *Primary cardiology* [p. 267]. Philadelphia: W.B. Saunders; modified from Antman, E. M., & Braunwald, E. [1997]. Acute myocardial infarction. In E. Braunwald [Ed.], *Heart disease* [5th ed.]. Philadelphia: W.B. Saunders; redrawn from Ryan, T.J., Anderson, J.L., Antman, E.M., et al. [1996]. ACC/AHA guidelines for the management of patients with acute myocardial infarction. *Journal of the American College of Cardiology, 28,* 1328–1428, reprinted with permission of the American College of Cardiology.)

k. *If diagnosis of unstable angina or acute MI is made or suspected, continue immediately as follows:*
l. For hemodynamically stable patients, institute beta-blocker therapy intravenously (e.g., Metoprolol [Lopressor] 5 mg IV × 3 doses, administered two minutes apart, followed by 50 mg p.o. q6h starting 15 min after the last IV dose).
m. Consider heparin continuous IV drip (e.g., 80 units/kg IV bolus followed by 18 units/kg/h continuous infusion to maintain a PTT at 1.5–2 × the patient control. Note: The emergency antagonist for heparin is protamine sulfate. The use of low molecular weight heparin (e.g., Enoxaprin [Lovenox] 1 mg/kg q12h SC for 2–8 days) is gaining clinical recognition as an alternative to the use of unfractionated heparin. Indicated in patients with non-Q–wave MI and patients with unstable angina. Monitor therapeutic co-agulation values. See section J.4.c. following.
n. Consider administration of an antiplatelet agent glycoprotein IIb/IIIa inhibitor such as Tirofiban (Aggrastat) in combination with heparin for patients with non-Q–wave MI. Initial dose 0.4 μg/kg/min IV for 30 min and then continued at 0.1 μg/kg/min. Dosing should be continued through angiography and 12–24 h after angioplasty. Monitor for bleeding. Other preparations include abciximab (ReoPro), 0.25 mg/kg bolus 10–60 min before therapy, followed by 10 μg/min continuous infusion × 12 h; or eptifibatide (Integrilin), 180 μg/kg IV (maximum 22.6 mg) over 1–2 min, then 2 μg/kg/min (maximum 15 mg/h) by continuous infusion for up to 72 h. If patient is to undergo percutaneous coronary intervention, reduce infusion to 0.5 μg/kg/min and continue for 20–24 h after the procedure, up to 96 h of therapy.
o. Consider nitroglycerin continuous IV drip (Tridil) if pain is not relieved by sublingual nitroglycerin and morphine or meperidine (Demerol). Begin at 5–10 μg/min and titrate up 5–10 μg/min q5–10 min until pain is relieved or until the patient becomes hypotensive (i.e., systolic blood pressure <90 mmHg).
p. Consider thrombolytic therapy (see section I) *OR*
q. Consider cardiac catheterization/percutaneous transluminal coronary angioplasty (PTCA) (see section J) *and then*
r. Consider coronary artery bypass graft surgery (see section K).
s. Admit to critical care unit for continuous monitoring.
t. Following emergent therapy, consider the following:

2. After an acute ischemic event, consider additional testing (Fig. 11–2).

a. *Exercise/stress test:* Use of a treadmill to monitor ECG changes for signs of ischemia, as well as heart rate and blood pressure (BP)
   i. Usually requires 10–15 min
   ii. A *maximal test* involves the patient exercising until at least 85% of predicted capacity is reached (based on age and measured by heart rate).
   iii. Excercise continues until chest pain, fatigue, or other adverse effects are experienced, including
       (1) Extreme weakness
       (2) Severe dyspnea
       (3) Syncope or dizziness
       (4) Ataxia
       (5) Claudication
       (6) Appearance of S_3 or S_4 heart sounds
       (7) ST segment elevation or depression of ≥ 1 mm
       (8) Systolic BP >250 mmHg
       (9) Decrease in systolic BP >10 mmHg
       (10) Rise in diastolic BP >90 mmHg or >20 mmHg over the patient's initial base line
       (11) "Glassy-eyed" appearance, cold sweats, or confusion.
   iv. *Submaximal tests* are usually conducted on patients who have experienced an acute MI and are ended once the patient reaches a specific, calculated target heart rate. Usually the targeted heart rate (THR) is calculated using the formula $(220 - \text{age}) \times 0.85 = \text{THR}$
   v. *Abnormal results/positive stress test:* Downsloping or flat ST segment of 1 mm or >1 mm from an originally depressed ST segment
b. *Thallium stress test:* Use of a radionuclide to detect perfusion of the myocardium.
   i. Test is conducted similarly to the treadmill test.
   ii. During the final portion of the test, a radionuclide, such as thallium 201, or other tracing preparation, such as technetium Tc 99m teboroxime (Cardiotec) or technetium Tc 99m sestamibi (Cardiolite), is intraveneously injected.
   iii. Patient is then placed on a nuclear imaging scanner, where the myocardium is scanned for distribution of the radionuclide/tracing agent.
   iv. Scan is repeated in 3–4 h.
   v. *Abnormal results:* Light distribution indicates decreased or absent perfusion on the first scan. Defects depicted

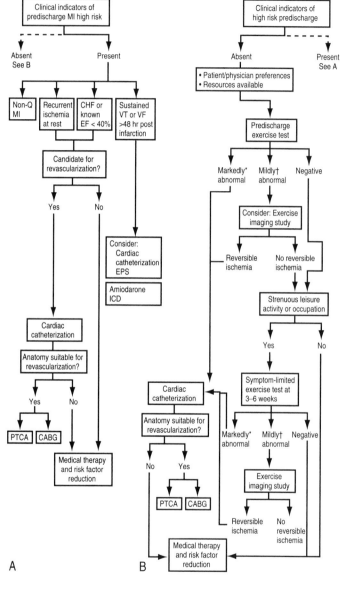

* High risk (≥2mm ST segment depression, hypotension at peak exercise, low working capacity)
† Positive, not high risk (≤1 mm ST segment depression, good working capacity)

Figure 11–2. *See legend on opposite page*

on the first scan, but not the second, indicate ischemia. Defects on both scans indicate areas of scar tissue as the result of MI.

  c. *Pharmacologic stress test:* Utilization of pharmacologic agents to increase coronary blood flow in patients who are unable to exercise to the point of reaching their target heart rates.

     i. *Drugs of choice* to increase coronary artery perfusion include dipyridamole (Persantine) and adenosine (Adenocard). Dobutamine (Dobutrex) is given primarily to increase cardiac output, rather than to increase coronary blood flow (i.e., perfusion).

     ii. *If dipyridamole (Persantine) is used,* give thallium 201 approximately 5 min after the intravenous dose, followed by a nuclear scan. Give aminophylline, 50–125 mg, to reverse the side effects of dipyridamole, which may include chest pain, nausea, dizziness, or headache. Two to three hours later, administer a second dose of thallium, and conduct a second scan.

     iii. *Abnormal results/positive test:* Downsloping or flat ST segment ≥1 mm for more than 0.08 s or >1 mm depression from an initial ST segment depression of the patient's base line

  d. Ultrasonographic testing: Consider the use of

     i. Echocardiogram

Figure 11–2. Management algorithm for risk stratification after acute myocardial infarction (MI). *A.* Patients with clinical indicators of high risk at hospital discharge, such as recurrent ischemia at rest or depressed left ventricular function, should be considered candidates for revascularization and referral to cardiac catheterization for ultimate triage to either percutaneous transluminal coronary angioplasty (PTCA); coronary artery bypass graft surgery (CABG) or medical therapy and risk factor reduction. Patients with life-threatening arrhythmias, such as sustained ventricular tachycardia (VT) or ventricular fibrillation (VF), should be considered for diagnostic cardiac catheterization, electrophysiology study (EPS), and management with either amiodarone or an implantable cardioverter-defibrillator (ICD), or both. CHF, congestive heart failure: EF., ejection fraction. *B.* Patients without indicators of high risk at hospital discharge can be evaluated either with a submaximal exercise test prior to discharge (at 5 to 7 days) or with a symptom-limited exercise test at 14 to 21 days. Patients with either a markedly abnormal exercise test or no evidence of reversible ischemia on an exercise imaging study can be managed with medical therapy and risk factor reduction. (Redrawn from Goldman, L., & Braunwald, E. [1998]. *Primary cardiology* [p. 280]. Philadelphia: W.B. Saunders; from Antman, E.M., & Braunwald, E. [1997]. Acute myocardial infarction. In E. Braunwald [Ed.], *Heart disease* [5th ed.] [p. 1262]. Philadelphia: W.B. Saunders, with permission.)

      ii. Doppler echocardiogram

      iii. Color flow Doppler imaging

      iv. Transesophageal echocardiogram (TEE)

3. Outpatient management of stable angina[3, 4, 8, 13, 37, 38] (Fig. 11–3)

  a. Nitrates—Encourage use of sublingual or buccal spray
     (0.3–0.6 mg) 5 min before exertion that may cause angina.
     Consider long-acting preparations such as

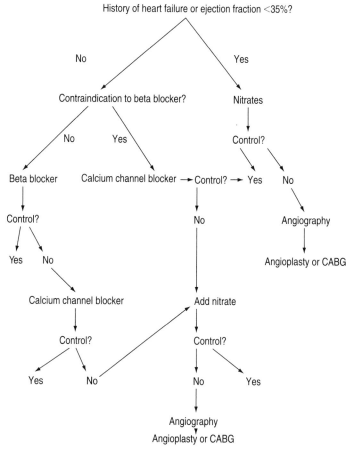

Figure 11–3. Treatment Algorithm for Stable Angina. (From Millonig,
V.L., & Miller, S.K. [1999]. *Adult nurse practitioner certification review guide*
[p. 219]. Potomac, MD: Health Leadership Associates, with permission.)

    i. Isosorbide dinitrate (Isordil), 10–40 mg p.o. t.i.d. (most commonly) *OR*

    ii. Isosorbide mononitrate (Ismo), 10–20 mg p.o. b.i.d. *OR*

    iii. Nitroglycerin sustained-release (Nitroglyn), 2.5–2.6 mg t.i.d. or q.i.d., titrating up as needed by 2.5 or 2.6 mg increments to a maximal dose of 26 mg q.i.d.

    iv. Nitroglycerin transdermal patches (Nitro-Dur; Nitro-Derm), which deliver 5–40 mg q24h; teach patient to take the patch off each morning for a nitrate-free interval of time.

b. Beta blockers: Preparation/Initial dose/(Dosage range)

    i. Propranolol (Inderal), 20 mg b.i.d./(40–320 mg in two doses)

    ii. Metoprolol (Lopressor), 50 mg in two doses/day initially and then or 100–450 mg in two or three doses for angina; Toprol XL, 50–100 mg p.o. each day in one dose

    iii. Nadolol (Corgard), 20 mg q.d./(20–160 mg q.d.)

    iv. Atenolol (Tenormin), 25 mg q.d./(25–200 mg q.d.)

    v. Major contraindications: Bradyarrhythmias, severe bronchospastic disease, heart failure

c. Calcium channel blockers—Only first indicated in patients who are unable to take beta blockers or in patients with refractory angina in which combination therapy with beta blockers is employed. Preparation/Initial dose/(Dosage range)

    i. Diltiazem (Cardizem SR), 90 mg b.i.d./(180–360 mg in two doses)

    ii. Diltiazem (Cardizem CD), 180 mg q.d./(180–360 mg q.d.)

    iii. Diltiazem (Dilacor XR), 180 or 240 mg q.d./(180–540 mg q.d.)

    iv. Diltiazem (Tiazac SA), 240 mg q.d./(180–540 mg q.d.)

    v. Verapamil (Calan SR, Isoptin SR, Verelan), 180 mg q.d./(180–480 mg in one or two doses)

    iv. Dihydropyridines (e.g., Amiodipine [Norvasc], felodipin [Plendil], nifedipine [Adalat CC, Procardia XL]) are usually not used as first line therapy because of increased side effects and reflex tachycardia.

d. If the patient is unresponsive to a single agent, use an alternative classification of agent before progressing to combination therapy.

e. If the patient remains symptomatic, use of either a beta blocker and a long-acting nitrate or a beta blocker and a calcium channel blocker (other than verapamil) is most effective.

f. Low dose aspirin therapy (162–325 mg q.d. or 325 mg every other day)

g. In patients who do not tolerate aspirin, clopidogrel (Plavix), 75 mg p.o. q.d.

h. Reduce low-density lipoproteins to ≤ 100 mg/dL as indicated.

4. Post-MI outpatient management[2, 11, 26]

a. See patient for follow-up as needed immediately after discharge.

b. Future visits after initial follow-up should be every 2–6 months.

c. Consider stress testing 3–4 weeks post-MI.

d. Repeat ECG at 3 months and every 1–2 years thereafter.

e. Continue pharmacologic therapy.

   i. Beta blocker (e.g., Propranolol [Inderal], 80–320 mg/day).

   ii. Anticoagulants (e.g., continue present warfarin [Coumadin] therapy, 2–10 mg p.o. every day for 3 months). Monitor therapeutic coagulation values—See section J.4.c. below.

   iii. Continue aspirin therapy, 325 mg q.d. indefinitely.

   iv. ACE inhibitor of choice in patients with left ventricular dysfunction and most patients with Q wave MI for remodeling (e.g., captopril, 25–50 mg t.i.d., is particularly recommended for patients with ejection fractions <40% beginning 3–16 days postinfarction).

f. Cardiac rehabilitation, as indicated.

I. Thrombolytic Therapy

1. Definition
Pharmacologic process using agents to increase oxygen supply by lysing clots that are obstructing flow to the coronary arteries

2. Indications[6, 26, 33, 34, 36]

a. Preferred mode of treatment for acute MI (see #3 and #4, Absolute and Relative contraindications, following)

b. Unrelieved chest pain of recent onset (>30 min and <6 h); variations of this indication have been used, such as administration up to 24 h after the initiation of pain, *with:*

c. ECG changes—ST segment *elevation* (in two contiguous leads, 1 mm elevation in limb leads, or 2 mm elevation in precordial leads), Q waves, or bundle branch block

d. Greatest benefit within 1–3 h of the onset of pain. Mortality may be reduced by 50%.

3. Absolute/Major contraindications[1, 6, 24, 26]

a. Active bleeding

b. Major trauma or surgery (<3 months ago)

    c. History of hemorrhagic stroke, intracranial aneurysm, or tumor

    d. Severe hypertension (systolic BP >180 mmHg, uncontrolled)

    e. Pregnancy

    f. Aortic dissection

4. Relative contraindications

    a. History of recent GI bleeding

    b. Hypertension (BP >165/95 mmHg)

    c. Prolonged/traumatic cardiopulmonary resuscitation.

    d. Cardiogenic shock—PTCA should be considered, instead.

    e. History of ischemic stroke or cerebrovascular disease

5. Major complication: Hemorrhage
6. Preparations[1, 6, 18, 24, 26]

    a. *Tissue plasminogen activator (t-PA)*—Offers less risk of bleeding because it is fibrin-specific and, therefore, will not deplete clotting factors; can be repeated later in life; see section 7, following; especially effective in

       i. Patients with large/anterior wall MIs

      ii. Patients who have undergone previous CABG surgery

     iii. Young patients

    b. *Streptokinase*—Synthetic protein derived from group C beta-hemolytic streptococci; combines with plasminogen to activate the fibrinolytic process; can only be administered once in a lifetime because of the development of antibodies; see section 7 following; especially effective in

       i. Patients with small MIs

      ii. Patients at high risk for stroke

     iii. Late treatment (>6 h following the onset of pain)

     iv. Advanced patient age (>75 years)

      v. Young patients

    c. *Reteplase (rPA)*—Agent very similar to t-PA. See #7, following.

    d. *Anisoylated plasminogen-streptokinase activator complex (anistreplase; APSAC)*—One-dose administration agent that may be used in rural hospitals where PTCA/CABG surgery is not available; similar properties to streptokinase. See section 7, following. APSAC is also useful in scenarios where cost containment may be an issue.

7. Select thrombolytic choices[6, 18, 26] (Table 11–2)
8. Considerations during administration[41]

    a. Observe for signs of tissue reperfusion.

       i. Abrupt pain relief

      ii. ECG normalization and/or appearance of Q waves

TABLE 11-2. SELECT THROMBOLYTIC CHOICES

	TISSUE PLASMINOGEN ACTIVATOR (t-PA)	STREPTOKINASE	RETEPLASE (rPA)	APSAC
Peak effect	45 min	20 min–2 h	NA	45 min
Duration	6 h–2 days	6–24 h	NA	6 h–2 days
Fibrin-specific	Yes	No	Yes	No
Dosage/Infusion	15 mg bolus followed by 50 mg over 30 min, then 35 mg over 1 h (not to exceed 100 mg)	750,000 units over 20 min, followed by 750,000 units over 40 min	10 units bolused over 2 min, repeated in 30 min	30 units over 2–5 min
Anticoagulation following administration*	Aspirin, 325 mg q.d.; heparin 5000 unit bolus followed by 1000 U/h infusion (maintain PTT 1.5–2 × control)	Aspirin, 325 mg q.d.; no evidence shown to improve outcome with use of heparin	Aspirin, 325 mg q.d.; heparin 5000 unit bolus followed by 1000 U/h infusion (maintain PTT 1.5–2 × control)	Aspirin, 325 mg q.d.
Fibrin-specific	Yes	No	Yes	No
Allergic reactions	No	Yes	No	Yes
Estimated cost	$2,750	$494	$2,750	$2,439

*Monitor therapeutic coagulation values. See Table 11–3.

iii. Reperfusion dysrhythmias, especially accelerated idio-ventricular rhythm, sinus bradycardia, ventricular tachycardia, and ventricular fibrillation
iv. Improved capillary refill, oxygen saturation, and so forth.
b. Monitor neurologic status for changes related to possible cerebrovascular accident.
c. Monitor for bleeding (e.g., gums, urine, bruising). Check therapeutic coagulation values. See section J.4.c.; following.

9. Post-thrombolytic treatment[2, 6, 26, 42]

a. Ensure adequate pain relief via the use of morphine, 4–8 mg IV, or meperidine (Demerol) 50–75 mg.
b. Consider the short-term use of IV beta blockers immediately post infarction; followed by p.o., when able.
c. Nitroglycerin for recurrent chest pain. Routine administration is not recommended.
d. Consider angiotensin-converting enzyme (ACE) inhibitors after thrombolyis and the use of beta blockers in patients with continuing ischemia in spite of the use of nitrates.

J. Percutaneous transluminal coronary angioplasty (PTCA)[6, 9, 16, 26, 30, 36]

1. Definition[46]

a. PTCA is an invasive procedure whereby a narrow catheter with an inflatable balloon tip is inserted percutaneously into the aorta and up into the coronary arteries under fluoroscopy.
b. The balloon is temporarily inflated to compress atherosclerotic plaque against the arterial wall, resulting in dilation of the lumen of the coronary artery.
c. Intracoronary arterial stents are commonly used in conjunction with PTCA.

2. Indications/Criteria for use/Incidence[6, 24, 27, 42, 46]

a. PTCA is the preferred mode of treatment for MI only when immediately available to patients (i.e., within 60 min of arrival in the emergency department) or when thrombolytics are contraindicated.
b. ECG changes
c. Evolving MI
d. Angina (stable—unresponsive to medical treatment, new-onset)
e. Adequate ventricular function and collateral circulation

    f. Relatively proximal, noncalcified lesions

    g. Lesions <10 mm in length

    h. Lesions not involving a major bifurcation

    i. It is estimated that >400,000 PTCAs are performed annually in the United States.

3. Laboratory/Diagnostics

    a. Hemoglobin and hematocrit

    b. Electrolytes

    c. Coagulation profile

    d. Type and crossmatch two units of packed red blood cells in case CABG surgery is needed.

4. Special considerations[16, 26, 28, 42, 46]

    a. Patient teaching

       i. Possibility of needing CABG surgery if complications occur

      ii. The patient will remain awake, receive local anesthesia to the groin, and must lie still.

     iii. The procedure is not painful.

     iv. NPO after midnight (unless emergency)

      v. The patient must keep the leg straight; a pressure bandage may be used following the procedure (follow hospital protocol).

     vi. The patient will be walking within 4–12 h after the procedure.

    b. Observe for signs of reperfusion

       i. ECG changes

      ii. Pain relief

     iii. Other signs of improving clinical status

    c. Monitor therapeutic coagulation values after the procedure (may vary depending on laboratory). Many institutions are solely monitoring ACT following PTCA for sheath removal (e.g., ACT <175); follow hospital protocol (Table 11–3).

    d. Observe for complications[1, 12, 35]

       i. Restenosis may occur in 30–40% of patients; evidenced by angina, ST segment elevation per 12-lead ECG, and/or dysrhythmias; emergency repeat PTCA or CABG surgery is warranted.

      ii. Contrast dye allergy (evidenced by signs of anaphylaxis; Note: Feeling warm or somewhat flushed during PTCA is normal.)

     iii. Hematoma formation at the groin site

     iv. Coronary artery perforation/rupture, embolism, spasms of coronary arteries, and MI are possible.

TABLE 11–3. THERAPEUTIC COAGULATION VALUES

TEST	NORMAL	THERAPEUTIC VALUES
International normalized ratio (INR)	<2 seconds	*MI or patients with mechanical heart valve:* 2.5–3.5 × normal *Chronic atrial fibrillation:* 2.0–3.0 × normal or <2.5 × normal if patient is >70 years old *Deep vein thrombosis or pulmonary embolus treatment:* 2.0–3.0 × normal
Activated coagulation time (ACT)	70–120 seconds	150–190 seconds or >300 seconds post PTCA/ stent application
Activated partial thromboplastin time (APTT)	28–38 seconds	1.5–2.5 × normal
Prothrombin time (PT)	11–16 seconds	1.5–2.5 × normal
Partial thromboplastin time (PTT)	60–90 seconds	1.5–2.5 × normal

K. Coronary artery bypass graft (CABG) surgery[5, 13, 15, 17, 21, 25, 37, 39, 42, 44, 45]

1. Definition
   Procedure whereby ischemic areas of the heart are revascularized using a grafting approach from the aortic root to a point distal to the ischemic lesion, using one of the following for the graft:

   a. Internal mammary artery (better for long-term patency)
   b. Saphenous vein
   c. Gastroepiploic artery
   d. Radial artery

2. Indications

   a. Refractory unstable angina
   b. MI
   c. Failure of PTCA
   d. Greater than 50% left main coronary artery occlusion
   e. Triple-vessel coronary artery disease
   f. Left ventricular failure related to either congestive heart failure or cardiogenic shock

3. Expectations in the immediate postoperative period

   a. Continous cardiac monitoring—Atrial fibrillation occurs in 20–30% of patients, warranting consideration of anticoagulation if it persists >24 h.

   b. Mechanical ventilation—Extubation within 4–6 h in most patients

   c. Pulmonary artery catheter—To measure hemodynamic profile

   d. Arterial line—For continuous BP readings and laboratory analyses

   e. Pulmonary capillary wedge pressure—Maintaining at a point slightly higher than normal (e.g., 18–20 mmHg)

   f. Hypotension—If warm cardioplegia was used, maintain BP and mean arterial pressure by volume loading with crystalloids, colloids, or packed red blood cells; autotransfusion may also be used.

   g. Serum potassium—Maintaining level in the high-normal range (e.g., 4.5–5.5 mEq/L)

   h. Serum magnesium—Maintaining level at approximately 2.0 mEq/L to assist in preventing dysrhythmias.

   i. Clotting factors—Administering fresh frozen plasma and platelets as indicated for depletion

   j. Mediastinal chest tubes ×2—If output exceeds 400 mL in 2 consecutive hours or 500 mL in one hour, re-exploratory surgery is indicated.

   k. Epicardial pacing wires ×2—May be used if heart rate drops below 80 beats/min

   l. NGT to low wall suction—for gastric decompression

   m. Foley catheter—To ensure adequate (>30 mL/h) urinary output, or per protocol

   n. Common vasoactive inotropic support agents

      i. Dopamine (Intropin)—Used for renal vascular dilation

      ii. Dobutamine (Dobutrex)—Used to increase cardiac output

      iii. Amrinone (Inocor) or Milrinone (Primacor)—Used to increase contractility and decrease preload and afterload via vasodilation

      iv. Esmolol (Brevibloc)—Beta blocker used for tachycardia

      v. Diltiazem (Cardizem)—Beta blocker used for tachycardia

      vi. Nitroprusside (Nipride)—Used for transient hypertension as a result of vasoconstriction secondary to hypothermia during surgery

      vii. Nitroglycerin (Tridil)—Used for coronary and systemic vasodilation to decrease preload and myocardial oxygen consumption

viii. Norepinephrine (Levophed)—Vasoconstrictor used for severe shock

o. Monitoring for neurologic changes—Cerebrovascular accident may occur in 5–10% of patients. Increased risk is seen with
   i. Advanced age
   ii. African American men
   iii. Hypertension
   iv. Obesity
   v. Diabetes mellitus
   vi. Atrial rhythm disorders
   vii. Cardiopulmonary bypass lasting more than 2 h

p. Monitoring for infection—Postoperative fever ≥38.5°C warrants suspicion for culture and sensitivity testing of blood, wound, urine, and sputum; provide antibiotic therapy as indicated. See Chapter 80, Infections.

L. Potential complications of MI[14, 20, 26, 42]

1. Dysrhythmias—See Chapter 18.
2. Congestive heart failure—See Chapter 15.
3. Pulmonary edema—See Chapter 25.
4. Cardiogenic shock—Most common fatal complication of MI; see Chapter 76.
5. Pericarditis—See Chapter 14.
6. Infection—Especially leg wound, sternotomy, or systemic (see Chapter 80, Infections)
7. Cardiac tamponade

   a. Definition
      Accumulation of blood and/or fluid in the pericardial space, resulting in a life-threatening decrease in cardiac output
   b. Etiology/Incidence/Predisposing factors[23, 41]
      i. Blunt/penetrating trauma to the upper chest
      ii. Postoperative cardiac surgical patients or following cardiac catheterization
      iii. Patients with pericarditis
      iv. Acute MI
      v. May be caused by viral, bacterial, or fungal infections
   c. Subjective findings—Unremarkable
   d. Physical examination findings[20, 41]
      i. Beck's triad

      • Jugular venous distention (JVD)—Rarely present with traumatic injury related to hypovolemia
      • Narrowing pulse pressure
      • Distant heart tones

    ii. Tachycardia

    iii. Pulsus paradoxus

    iv. Changes in level of consciousness (e.g., anxiety, confusion)

    v. Oliguria

    vi. Other signs of shock

  e. Diagnostic/Laboratory findings[22]

    i. Echocardiogram—Used to confirm diagnosis

    ii. Chest x-ray—May show widening mediastinum

  f. Management[2]

    i. Pericardiocentesis

    ii. Symptomatic treatment of shock (e.g., oxygen, fluid resuscitation, inotropic agents) (see Chapter 75, Management of The Patient in Shock)

References

1. Baas, L. (1996). Care of the cardiac patient. In M.R. Kinney, & D.R. Packa (Eds.), *Andreoli's comprehensive cardiac care* (8th ed.) (pp. 276–341). St. Louis: Mosby.

2. Becker, D. (1999). Coronary artery disease. In L. Bucher & S. Melander (Eds.), *Critical care nursing* (pp. 209–226). Philadelphia: W.B. Saunders.

3. Braunwald, E. (1998a). Acute myocardial infarction. In L. Goldman & E. Braunwald (Eds.), *Primary cardiology* (pp. 257–283). Philadelphia: W.B. Saunders.

4. Braunwald, E. (1998b). Unstable angina. In L. Goldman, & E. Braunwald (Eds.), *Primary cardiology* (pp. 284–295). Philadelphia: W.B. Saunders.

5. Capuano, T.A., Sullivan, K., Rothenberger, C., Meeker, C., Gallagher-Sabo, M., & Sebastian, M. (1999). A benchmark project to improve cost and quality outcomes for CABG patients. *Dimensions of Critical Care Nursing, 18,* 36–43.

6. Casey, K., Bedker, D.L., & Roussel-McElmeel, P.L. (1998). Myocardial infarction: Review of clinical trials and treatment strategies. *Critical Care Nurse, 18,* 39–51.

7. Chatterjee, K. (1998a). Ischemic heart disease. In J.H. Stein (Ed.), *Internal medicine* (4th ed.) (pp. 192–208). St. Louis: Mosby.

8. Chatterjee, K. (1998b). Stable angina pectoris. In L. Goldman & E. Braunwald (Eds.), *Primary Cardiology* (pp. 234–256). Philadelphia: W.B. Saunders.

9. Cohen, E.A., Young, W., Slaughter, P.M., Oh, P., & Naylor, C.D. (1999). Trends in clinical and economic outcomes of coronary angioplasty from 1992–1995: A population-based analysis. *American Heart Journal, 167,* 1012–1018.

10. Dracup, K.A. & Cannon, C.P. (1999). Combination treatment strategies for management of acute myocardial infarction: New directions with current therapies. *Critical Care Nurse* (Suppl.), 3–15.

11. Dunphy, L.M.K. (1999). *Management guidelines for adult nurse practitioners.* Philadelphia: F.A. Davis.

12. Fleury, J., Keller, C., & Murdaugh, C. (1996). In J.M. Clochesy, C. Breu, S. Cardin, A.A. Whittaker, & E.B. Rudy, (Eds). *Critical care nursing* (2nd ed.) (pp. 337–356). Philadelphia: W.B. Saunders.

13. Gawlinski, A., McCloy, K., Caswell, D., & Quinones-Baldrich, W.J. (1999). Cardiovascular disorders. In A. Gawlinski & D. Hamwi (Eds.), *Acute care nurse practitioner: Clinical curriculum and certification review* (pp. 136–294). Philadelphia: W.B. Saunders.

14. Goldsborough, M.A., Miller, M.H., Gibson, J., Creighton-Kelly, S., Custer, C.A., Wallop, J.M., & Greene, P.S. (1999). Prevalence of leg wound complications after coronary artery bypass grafting: Determination of risk factors. *American Journal of Critical Care, 8,* 149–153.

15. Goodwin, M.J., Bissett, L., Mason, P., Kates, R., & Weber, J. (1999). Early extubation and early activity after open heart surgery. *Critical Care Nurse, 19,* 18–26.

16. Homes, L.M., & Hollabaugh, S.K. (1997). Using the continuous quality improvement process to improve the care of patients after angioplasty. *Critical Care Nurse, 17,* 56–65.

17. Huerta-Torres, V. (1998). Preparing patients for early discharge after CABG. *American Journal of Nursing, 98,* 49–51.

18. Kline-Rogers, E., Martin, J.S., & Smith, D.D. (1999). New era of reperfusion in acute myocardial infarction. *Critical Care Nurse, 19,* 21–31.

19. Kosnik, L. (1999). Treatment protocols and pathways: Improving the process of care. *Critical Care Nurse,* (Suppl.), Oct., 3–6.

20. Lamborn, M.L., & Moseley, M.J. (1997). Cardiac alterations. In J.C. Hartshorn, M.L. Sole, & M.L. Lamborn, (Eds.), *Introduction to critical care nursing* (2nd ed.) (pp. 232–269). Philadelphia: W.B. Saunders.

21. Lindsay, M. (1998). Frequency of cerebrovascular accident after cardiac surgery. *Critical Care Nurse, 18,* 19–27.

22. Lobstein, P. (1999). In M.R. Dambro (Ed.), *Griffith's 5 minute clinical consult* (pp. 50–51). Media: Williams & Wilkins.

23. Lopez-Jiminez, F., Goldman, L., Sacks, D.B., Thomas, E.J., Johnston, P.A., Cook, E.F., & Lee, T.H. (1997). Prognostic value of cardiac troponin T after noncardiac surgery: 6 month follow-up data. *Journal of American College of Cardiology, 29,* 1241–1245.

24. Lowe, A., & Melander, S.D. (1996). PTCA and thrombolytic therapy in myocardial infarction. In S.D. Melander (Ed.), *Review of critical care nursing* (pp. 50–73). Philadelphia: W.B. Saunders.

25. Maglish, B.L., Schwartz, J.L., & Matheny, R.G. (1999). Outcomes improvement following minimally invasive direct coronary artery bypass surgery: The role of nursing in critical care and cardiovascular risk factor reduction. *Critical Care Nursing Clinics of North America, 11,* 177–188.

26. Massie, B.M. (1999). Systemic hypertension. In L.M. Tierney, S.J. McPhee, & M.A. Papadakis, (Eds.), *Current medical diagnosis & treatment* (38th ed.) (pp. 430–452). Stamford, CT: Appleton & Lange.

27. Maynard, C., Chapko, M.K., Every, N.R., Martin, D.C., & Ritchie, J.L. (1998). Coronary angioplasty outcomes in the healthcare cost and utilization project. *American Journal of Cardiology, 81,* 848–852.

28. Meluch, F., & Mitchell S.B. (1997). Preventing complication: Decreasing intracoronary stent complications. *Dimensions of Critical Care Nursing 16,* 114–121.

29. Murphy, M.J., & Berding, C.B. (1999). Use of measurements of myoglobin and cardiac troponins in the diagnosis of acute myocardial infarction. *Critical Care Nurse, 19,* 58–66.

30. Patterson, S., Citro, K., & Gillium, N. (1999). Percutaneous myocardial revascularization: New treatment option for patients with angina. *Critical Care Nurse, 19,* 27–36.

31. Pelter, M.M., Adams, M.G., Wung, S., Paul, S.M., & Drew, B.J. (1998). Peak time of occurrence of myocardial ischemia in the coronary care unit. *American Journal of Critical Care, 7,* 411–417.

32. Piatek, Y.M., & Atzori, M. (1999). PTMR: When all options are exhausted, percutaneous transmyocardial revascularization can diminish symptoms of angina. *American Journal of Nursing, 99,* 64–66.

33. Rawles, J.M. (1998). Quantification of the benefit of earlier thrombolytic therapy: Five-year results of the Grampian region early anistreplase trial (GREAT). *Journal of the American College of Cardiology, 30,* 1181–1186.

34. Rawles, J.M. (1999). Benefits of earlier thrombolytic therapy. *Cardiology Review, 16,* 22–24.

35. Ritchie, J.L., Maynard, C., Chapko, M.K., Every, N.R., & Martin, D.C. (1999). Association between percutaneous transluminal coronary angioplasty volumes and outcomes in the healthcare cost and utilization project. *American Journal of Cardiology 83,* 493–497.

36. Roberts, C. (1999). Have we reached the therapeutic ceiling in acute myocardial infarction? *Critical Care Nurse* (Suppl.), Oct., 7–11.

37. Rogers, T.B., & Vargas, G. (1999). The return of the radial artery in CABG. *American Journal of Nursing, 99,* 26–30.

38. Rogers, W.J. (1996). Disorders of the coronary arteries. In J.C. Bennett & F. Plum (Eds.). *Cecil textbook of medicine* (20th ed.) (pp. 296–301). Philadelphia: W.B. Saunders.

39. Shawgo, T., & York, N. (1999). Preoperative versus postoperative weights: Which one should be used for cardiac surgery patients' drug and hemodynamic calculations? *Critical Care Nurse, 19,* 57–67.

40. Specialty Health. (1998). *Quik ref 3: Critical care* [Brochure]. Author unknown. Blue Bell, PA.

41. Steuble, B.T. (1997). Angina pectoris. In J.H. Keen & P.L. Swearingen (Eds.), *Mosby's Critical Care Nursing Consultant* (pp. 24–25). St. Louis: Mosby.

42. Thelan, L.A., Urden, L.D., Lough, M.E., & Stacy, K.M. (1998). *Critical care nursing: Diagnosis and management* (3rd ed.). St. Louis: Mosby.

43. Whitman, G.R., & Casedonte, M. (1996). Therapeutic modalities in the treatment of the patient with cardiovascular dysfunction. In S.D. Ruppert, J.G. Kernicki, & J.T. Dolan (Eds.), *Dolan's critical care nursing* (2nd ed.) (pp 272–292). Philadelphia: F.A. Davis.

44. Zevola, D.R., Raffa, M., Brown, K., Hourihan, E., & Maier, B. (1997). Clinical pathways and coronary artery bypass surgery. *Critical Care Nursing, 17,* 20–33.

45. Zevola, D.R., & Maier, B. (1999). Improving the care of cardiothoracic surgery patients through advanced nursing skills. *Critical Care Nurse, 19,* 34–44.

46. Zygmont, D.M. (1996). Nursing management of the patient with coronary artery disease, angina pectoris, or myocardial infarction. In S.D. Ruppert, J.G. Kernicki, & J.T. Dolan, (Eds.). *Dolan's critical care nursing: Clinical management through the nursing process* (2nd ed.) (pp. 270–292). Philadelphia: F.A. Davis.

ADJUNCT EQUIPMENT/ DEVICES

12

Thomas W. Barkley, Jr., DSN, RN, CS, ACNP

I. INTRA-AORTIC BALLOON PUMP[6, 8, 12]

A. Overview

1. Introduced in late 1960s primarily for patients with cardiogenic shock
2. Classified as an assist device and designed to

    a. Increase coronary artery perfusion
    b. Decrease oxygen consumption

B. Indications

1. Preinfarction angina refractory to pharmacologic therapy
2. Acute myocardial infarction
3. Refractory ventricular dysrhythmias related to ischemia
4. Severe mitral valve regurgitation
5. Severe ventriculoseptal defect
6. Before or after heart surgery
7. Low cardiac output states, such as septic shock

C. Contraindications

1. Absolute
    a. Aortic aneurysm
    b. Bypass grafting from the aorta to peripheral vessels
    c. Aortic insufficiency

2. Relative
    a. Peripheral or central atherosclerosis
    b. Bleeding disorders
    c. History of embolic event
    d. Ethical considerations (e.g., advanced age, severe left ventricular failure, multisystem failure), weighing the benefits of intra-aortic balloon pump therapy against quality of life issues

D. Components

1. Consists of a thin, polyurethane balloon mounted on a catheter
2. The catheter is inserted into the patient's aorta either surgically or percutaneously by threading it up through the femoral artery into the descending aorta. Note that the coronary arteries originate from the aorta immediately above the aortic valve.

3. The catheter is connected to a bedside console that shuttles helium in and out of the balloon "in concert" with the cardiac cycle.

E. Therapeutic effects

1. While *inflated,* the balloon pump increases aortic pressure during diastole, which augments coronary perfusion. Thus, the patient experiences a *decrease* in *afterload.*
2. While *deflated,* the balloon pump decreases aortic pressure during systole to lessen the workload on the left ventricle. Thus, the patient experiences an *increase* in *preload.*

F. Management considerations

1. Vital signs and hemodyamics should be frequently monitored.
2. Ensure accurate timing/pump operation based on either the
   a. R wave of the ECG (Fig. 12–1)
   b. Upstroke (dicrotic notch [DN]) of the arterial line tracing
   c. Spike from a pacemaker
   d. Wave form on the balloon pump (Fig. 12–2). The following checklist may be used to ensure optimal balloon inflation/deflation:
      i. Inflated at the DN
      ii. Should see a clear V at the inflation point (IP)
      iii. Peak diastolic pressure (PDP) should be ≥ the peak systolic pressure (PSP).
      iv. Should see a clear U reflecting the balloon aortic end diastolic pressure (BAEDP)
      v. Ensure that the BAEDP is 5–15 mmHg less than the patient's aortic end-diastolic pressure (PAEDP).
      vi. Note that the assisted peak pressure is less than the peak systolic pressure (PSP).

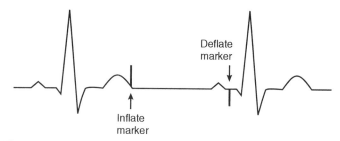

Figure 12–1. Use of timing markers as a reference on the ECG tracing. (From Mims, B.C., Toto, K.H., Leuke, L.E., & Roberts, M.K. [1996]. *Critical care skills: A clinical handbook* [p. 199]. Philadelphia: W.B. Saunders, with permission.)

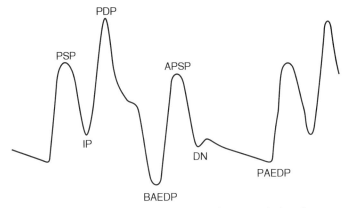

Figure 12–2. Timing the wave form to check for proper timing of counterpulsation. (From Mims, B.C., Toto, K.H., Leuke, L.E., & Roberts, M.K. [1996]. *Critical care skills: A clinical handbook* [p. 203]. Philadelphia: W.B. Saunders, with permission.)

   vii. Calculate the end-diastolic dip to reflect the decreased
        workload of the heart: BAEDP − PAEDP =
        5–15 mmHg.
3. Involved leg must be kept straight.
4. Head of the bed should be elevated only slightly.
5. Monitor for complications

   a. Lower extremity ischemia related to occlusion of the femoral artery either by the catheter or by emboli from catheter thrombus formation
   b. Displacement of the catheter related to patient movement
   c. Balloon perforation
   d. Infection

6. Weaning parameters: Hemodynamically stable vital signs including

   • Normal cardiac index (≥2.5 L/min)
   • Normal MAP (>70 mmHg)
   • Normal pulmonary capillary wedge pressure (6–12 mmHg)
   • Absence of chest pain
   • Absence of other signs of inadequate perfusion

7. Weaning methods: Either

   a. Decrease the volume in the balloon with each inflation (e.g., in periods of 25% reduction), OR
   b. Decrease the frequency of inflation (e.g., from every cardiac sequence to every other, to every third).

G. Complications

1. Balloon rupture
2. Embolus
3. Arterial occlusion
4. Destruction of red blood cells caused by the pump
5. Inability to wean the patient from the pump

II. PACEMAKERS[3, 6, 7, 11, 12]

A. Definition

1. Electronic devices that deliver stimuli (i.e., impulses) to the cardiac muscle in an effort to maintain adequate heart rate and cardiac output when the patient's intrinsic pacemaker becomes insufficient
2. May be used for single (ventricular) or dual (atrial, ventricular, or atrioventricular [AV]-sequential) chamber pacing

B. Primary indications—With symptomatic patients or those refractory to pharmacologic therapy

1. Bradyarrhythmias
2. Heart block
3. Sick sinus syndrome
4. Asystole
5. Atrial tachyarrhythmias
6. Ventricular tachyarrhythmias

C. Components

1. The pacing system consists of a power source, called the pulse generator, that senses the patient's intrinsic cardiac activity and delivers stimuli to the cardiac muscle based on the patient's intrinsic cardiac activity.
2. The pacemaker contains a unipolar or bipolar lead/electrode catheter that is placed in the right atrium or right ventricle, in contact with the endocardium.
3. The tip of the lead/electrode makes contact with the cardiac muscle and is responsible for transferring electrical stimuli from the pulse generator to the heart.
4. Temporary pacemakers usually have a pulse generator that is external to the body, while the pulse generator of permanent pacemakers is usually internal.

D. Operational definitions

1. *Capture*—The process that occurs when the pulse generator's delivered impulse/stimulus is adequate to depolarize the cardiac muscle

   a. A *single-chamber pacemaker* will depolarize either the atrium or the ventricle, resulting in a large P wave (atrial) or a large QRS complex (ventricular), following the respective pacing artifact (Fig. 12–3).

b. A *dual-chamber pacemaker* will depolarize both the right atrium and the right ventricle as needed (Fig. 12–4).

2. *Spike/artifact*—The vertical line that is seen either before the R wave or the QRS complex, indicating pacemaker firing (i.e., before the R wave [atrial pacemaker]; before the QRS complex [ventricular pacemaker])

3. *Sensing*—Activity that occurs when the pacemaker recognizes intrinsic electrical activity of the heart. The pacemaker then "resets" the timing mechanism, resulting in inhibition of the pacing stimulus. Sensing is designed to prevent potentially life-threatening competition between the artificial pacemaker and the patient's intrinsic pacemaker.

4. *Rate responsiveness*—Refers to a special modulation that enables the pacemaker to increase or decrease the rate of firing as needed.

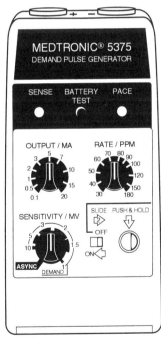

Figure 12–3. Medtronic single-chamber pacemaker. (From Mims, B.C., Toto, K.H., Leuke, L.E., & Roberts, M.K. [1996]. *Critical care skills: A clinical handbook* [p. 282]. Philadelphia: W.B. Saunders, with permission.)

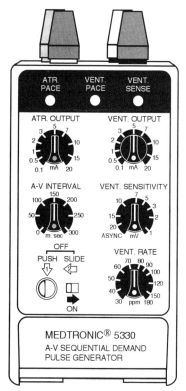

Figure 12–4. Medtronic A-V sequential demand pulse generator. (From Mims, B.C., Toto, K.H., Leuke, L.E., & Roberts, M.K. [1996]. *Critical care skills: A clinical handbook* [p. 281]. Philadelphia: W.B. Saunders, with permission.)

5. *Programmability*—The ability to painlessly and noninvasively change pacemaker settings or parameters based on the patient's needs
6. *Programmable settings/parameters*—It is possible to program three settings/parameters in all pacemakers.
   a. *Rate*—The number of times each minute that the pacemaker will fire if the patient's intrinsic rate drops to less than the set rate.
   b. *Energy output (milliamps or mA)*—Strength of electrical current needed to depolarize the myocardium; usually set at two to three times the pacemaker threshold
   c. *Sensitivity (millivolts or mV)*—Adjustment of the amplitude of myocardial electrical impulses that the pacemaker can detect; reflects the ability of the pacemaker to detect the

patient's intrinsic cardiac activity; usually set at a low
number (e.g., 2–3 mV); the lower the number, the more
sensitive the pacemaker

7. Additional settings/parameters for dual chamber pacemakers

    a. *AV interval*—Milliseconds of time between the beginning
of atrial depolarization and the beginning of ventricular
depolarization caused by the pacemaker; the usual setting
is 120–200 ms.

    b. *Maximum rate*—The upper limit of how fast the ventricle
can be paced to accompany atrial activity

    c. *Atrial refractory period*—Millisecond interval denoting
when the pacemaker will not respond to the patient's
atrial activity

E. Types of pacemakers

1. Four basic types of pacemakers are available.

    a. *Transcutaneous*—An external pacemaker used to produce
ventricular pacing; indicated in cardiac emergencies such
as severe bradycardia and asystole; temporary. An anterior
and a posterior electrode (pad) are placed on the thorax;
sedation is warranted because of painful chest wall stimulation; rate, energy output, and sensitivity are programmable.

    b. *Transthoracic*—A temporary, ventricular pacemaker used
only as a "last resort" during cardiac emergencies such as
asystole; requires a subxyphoid insertion via a long needle
into the right ventricle through which a pacing wire is
threaded to the endocardium

    c. *Transvenous*—Most common type of pacemaker used per-
manently, yet may be used temporarily; produces atrial,
ventricular, or AV-sequential pacing. The pulse generator
is implanted under the skin, usually in the upper chest;
the lead is inserted via the subclavian vein into the right
atrium and right ventricle.

    d. *Epicardial*—Commonly used after cardiac surgery. Leads
are sewn lightly to the epicardium and appear externally
on the chest through puncture sites; leads are "grounded"
using some form of rubber such as a glove or glass test
tube with a rubber cap. Use is discontinued several days
after cardiac surgery.

2. Description codes—Each type of pacemaker is programmed
using a five-position generic code, although the first three let-
ters are most commonly used. Each letter in the code has a
special meaning (Table 12–1).

TABLE 12–1. FIVE-POSITION GENERIC (NASPE/BPEG) PACEMAKER CODE

I CHAMBER PACED	II CHAMBER SENSED	III MODE OF RESPONSE	IV PROGRAMMABLE FUNCTIONS	V SPECIAL TACHYARRHYTHMIA FUNCTIONS
O—None	O—None	O—None	O—None	O—None
A—Atrium	A—Atrium	T—Triggered	P—Simple programmable	P—Pacing
V—Ventricle	V—Ventricle	I—Inhibited	M—Multiprogrammable	S—Shock
D—Dual	D—Dual	D—Dual	C—Communicating	D—Dual
			R—Rate modulation	

NASPE = North American Society of Pacing and Electrophysiology; BPEG = British Pacing and Electrophysiology Group; NBG—NASPE, BPEG Group. (From Hartshorn, J., Sole, M.L., & Lamborn, M. [1997]. *Introduction to critical care nursing* [2nd ed.], [p. 259]. Philadelphia: W.B. Saunders, with permission.)

a. I = Chamber paced
b. II = Chamber sensed
c. III = Mode of response
d. IV = Programmable functions
e. V = Special tachyarrhythmia functions
f. Examples
    i. AAI = atrial pacing, atrial sensing, and inhibited by atrial activity (i.e., P waves).
    ii. VVI = ventricular pacing, ventricular sensing, and inhibited by ventricular activity (i.e., QRS complexes).
    iii. DDD = atrial and ventricular pacing, atrial and ventricular sensing, and inhibited by responses from either the atria or the ventricles.

F. Operation and threshold measurement

1. Pacemaker settings—Table 12–2 shows settings that should be checked for each type of pulse generator or pacing mode.
2. Measuring the *pacing* threshold—To ascertain the smallest number of milliamps needed for depolarization

    a. The rate should be set on demand mode and at approximately 10 beats per minute faster than the patient's intrinsic rate.
    b. Check the ECG for 1:1 capturing (i.e., QRS complex and T wave after every pacemaker spike).
    c. Check the pace indicator on the pulse generator—it should be flashing at the set rate.
    d. Decrease the mA output slowly until a loss of capture occurs (i.e., spike occurs without a QRS complex or T wave following it).
    e. Then, slowly increase the mA output until capturing returns, and note the setting (mA) at that time.
    f. The resulting setting is indicative of the pacing threshold.
    g. Increase the mA output to two to three times the pacing threshold.
    h. Return the rate to the original setting.
    i. Repeat this process to determine the atrial pacing threshold by changing the atrial mA output setting. Capture will be seen by a P wave following the atrial pacemaker spike.

3. Measuring the *sensing* threshold—To ascertain a measurement of the smallest electrical impulse (mV) that the pacemaker can detect. The sensing threshold is measured to ensure that the pacemaker will sense intrinsic beats and not fire at the same time.

    a. Adjust the sensitivity to the lowest mV number (i.e., most sensitive setting).

TABLE 12–2. PACEMAKER SETTINGS TO BE CHECKED FOR EACH TYPE OF PULSE GENERATOR OR PACING MODE

TYPE OF PULSE GENERATOR	COMMON PACING MODE(S)	CONTROLS/RELEVANT SETTINGS
Single chamber	Ventricular demand (VVI)	Rate Output/mA Sensitivity—should be on a low number, not on asynchronous
Dual chamber	Atrial asynchronous (AOO)	AV interval Ventricular rate (will reflect atrial rate in this mode) Atrial output Ventricular output—should be set at minimum level (0.1 mA), as the ventricle is not paced in this mode Ventricular sensitivity—not relevant for this mode
	Ventricular demand (VVI)	Ventricular rate Ventricular sensitivity—should be set on a low number Ventricular output Atrial output—should be set at minimum level (0.1 mA), as the atrium is not paced in this mode AV interval—Note: should be set at minimum level (0 ms), as the atrium is not paced in this mode.
	AV-Sequential demand pacing (DVI)	Ventricular rate Ventricular output Atrial output AV interval Ventricular sensitivity

150

DDD	Atrial demand pacing (AAI)	Base pacing rate
		Atrial output
		Atrial sensitivity
		Atrial refractory (automatically set at 200 ms)
	Ventricular demand pacing (VVI)	Base pacing rate
		Ventricular output
		Ventricular sensitivity
	AV-Sequential demand (DVI)	Base pacing rate
		Atrial output
		Ventricular output
		Ventricular sensitivity
		AV interval
	Physiologic pacing (DDD)	Base pacing rate
		Maximum pacing rate
		Atrial output
		Ventricular output
		Atrial sensitivity
		Ventricular sensitivity
		Atrial refractory
		AV interval

(From Mims, B.C., Toto, K.H., Leuke, L.E., & Roberts, M.K. [1996]. *Critical care skills: A clinical handbook* [pp. 290–291]. Philadelphia: W.B. Saunders, with permission.)

151

b. Adjust the rate to 10 pulses less than the patient's intrinsic rate. Note: do not perform this procedure if the patient's intrinsic rate is unsatisfactory.

c. The pacemaker should not be firing at this time, and the patient's intrinsic activity should be visible on the monitor.

d. Ensure that the patient can tolerate the new rate.

e. Check the sense indicator on the pulse generator—it should be flashing in concert with each intrinsic beat.

f. Increase the mV slowly (i.e., decreasing the sensitivity) until a loss of sensing is indicated, evidenced by the sense indicator no longer flashing.

g. Ensure that the pace indicator flashes as the pacemaker fires asynchronously.

h. Then, increase the sensitivity slowly (i.e., decrease the mV) until flashing of the sense indicator is noted with each intrinsic beat.

i. The resulting setting is indicative of the sensing threshold.

j. Adjust the sensitivity to a setting that is less than half of the sensing threshold, or on the lowest number (most sensitive).

k. Ensure that the rate is set back at the original position.

l. Repeat this process to determine the atrial sensing threshold by changing the atrial sensitivity. Sensing of the P wave should be noted on the monitor.

G. Major complications and treatment

1. *Failure to capture*—Evidenced by pacemaker artifact's appearing without the appropriate complex following the spike (Fig. 12–5)

   a. Position the patient on the left side.
   b. Assess the chest x-ray for displacement.
   c. Reprogram to increase the pacemaker amplitude.
   d. Increase the mA output to maximum.
   e. Change the battery (temporary) or the generator (permanent).

2. *Failure to pace*—Evidenced by no pacemaker artifact appearing when firing of the pacemaker should have occurred (Fig. 12–6)

   a. Position the patient on the left side.
   b. Assess the chest x-ray for displacement.
   c. Distance the patient from possible sources of electromagnetic interference such as MRI scanners and radio towers.
   d. Warm the patient if the failure to pace is related to patient shivering.
   e. Decrease the sensitivity by *increasing* the mV.

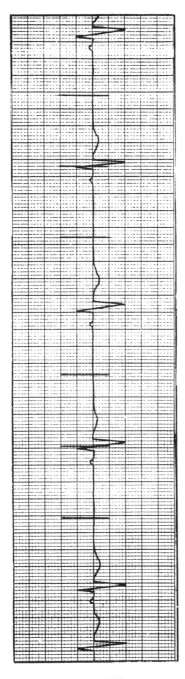

Figure 12–5. VVI mode. Rate = 71; V-V interval = 840 ms. Spikes occur at the appropriate time (the end of the V-V interval), but are not followed by a QRS complex. Pacemaker is firing appropriately, but is **failing to capture.** (From Mims, B.C., Toto, K.H., Leuke, L.E., & Roberts, M.K. [1996]. *Critical care skills: A clinical handbook* [p. 309]. Philadelphia: W.B. Saunders, with permission.)

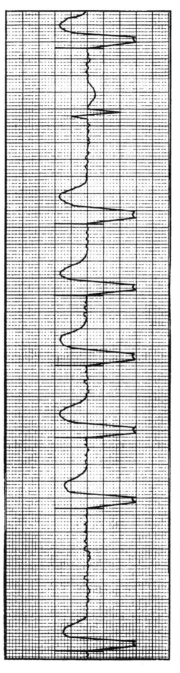

Figure 12–6. Ventricular pacemaker showing two long pauses where the pacemaker **failed to pace** as soon as it should have. (From Intermedics, Inc. [1994]. *Concepts of permanent cardiac pacing*. Angleton, TX: Intermedics, Inc., with permission of Guidant Corp.)

f. Change the battery (temporary) or the generator (permanent).

3. *Failure to sense*—Evidenced by random pacemaker spikes/artifact throughout the patient's cardiac cycle that occur in competition with the patient's intrinsic cardiac rhythm (Fig. 12–7)

a. Position the patient on the left side.
b. Assess the chest x-ray for displacement.
c. Increase the sensitivity by *decreasing* the mV.
d. Use a magnet for a minimal period of time to check pacemaker function.
e. Turn OFF the pacemaker if the patient's cardiac output is stable to prevent further competition and potentially life-threatening dysrhythmias such as ventricular tachycardia, ventricular fibrillation, and asystole.
f. Change the battery (temporary) or the generator (permanent).

III. AUTOMATIC INTERNAL CARDIOVERTER/DEFIBRILLATOR (AICD)[1, 2, 4, 5, 9, 10]

A. Definition
Electronic device implanted subcutaneously to automatically treat life-threatening dysrhythmias

B. Indications/General comments

1. Survival of sudden cardiac arrest unrelated to myocardial infarction
2. Patients with life-threatening, ventricular dysrhythmias that are refractory to pharmacologic therapy
3. Approximately 15,000 patients in the United States have AICDs.

C. Equipment

1. The AICD consists of a pulse generator and a lead system, similar to those of a pacemaker.
2. The pulse generator, designed to last more than 5 years, is usually implanted subcutaneously in the patient's abdomen or subclavian area.
3. The transvenous lead system is inserted through the left subclavian vein into the right ventricle and then tunneled and connected to the pulse generator. One ventricular patch is also connected to the pulse generator. Some models have two transvenous leads (utilizing both the right and the left subclavian veins) and two ventricular patches.

D. Programmability

1. Defibrillation
2. Cardioversion

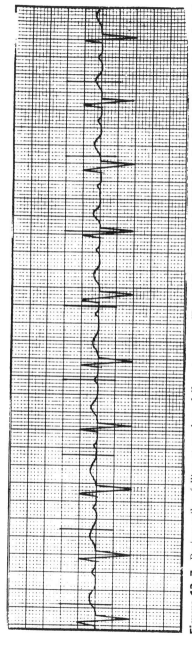

Figure 12–7. Pacing spikes falling at random; **failure to sense.** (From Mims, B.C., Toto, K.H., Leuke, L.E., & Roberts, M.K. [1996]. *Critical care skills: A clinical handbook* [p. 302]. Philadelphia: W.B. Saunders, with permission.)

TABLE 12–3. NASPE/BPEG DEFIBRILLATOR (NBO) CODE

SHOCK CHAMBER	ANTITACHYCARDIA PACING CHAMBER	TACHYCARDIA DETECTION	ANTIBRADYCARDIA PACING CHAMBER
O = None	O = None	E = Electrogram	O = None
A = Atrium	A = Atrium	H = Hemodynamic	A = Atrium
V = Ventricle	V = Ventricle		V = Ventricle
D = Dual (A + V)	D = Dual (A + V)		D = Dual (A + V)

(From Kinney, M., Packa, D., Andreoli, K., & Zipes, D. [1995]. *Andreoli's comprehensive cardiac care* [8th ed.] [p. 242]. St. Louis: Mosby; from Bernstein, A., et al. [1993]. The NASPE/BPEG defibrillator code. *PACE, 16,* 1776, with permission.)

TABLE 12–4. NASPE/BPEG DEFIBRILLATOR (NBD) CODE, SHORT FORM

ICD-S = ICD with shock capability only
ICD-B = ICD with bradycardia pacing as well as shock
ICD-T = ICD with tachycardia (and bradycardia) pacing as well as shock

---

(From Kinney, M., Packa, D., Andreoli, K., & Zipes, D. [1995]. *Andreoli's comprehensive cardiac care* [8th ed.] [p. 243]. St. Louis: Mosby; from Bernstein, A., et al. [1993]. The NASPE/BPEG defibrillator code. *PACE, 16,* 1776, with permission.)

3. Antitachycardia pacing (ATP)
4. Antibradycardia pacing (ABP)

E. Codes—Two types depict the functions of the AICD (Tables 12–3 and 12–4).
F. Patient teaching

1. Document device-related events.
2. Maintain Medicalert identification.
3. Families and significant others should be trained in CPR.
4. Magnets may either activate or deactivate the device. Monitor for tones emitted from the device signaling deactivation following exposure to external magnets.
5. Driving is usually contraindicated because of the likelihood of syncope accompanying the patient's cardiac event.

References

1. Bass, L. (1996). Care of the cardiac patient. In M.R. Kinney & D.R. Packa (Eds.), *Andreoli's comprehensive cardiac care* (8th ed.), (pp. 276–341). St. Louis: Mosby.
2. Bucher, L. (1999). Acute myocardial infarction. In L. Bucher & S. Melander (Eds.), *Critical Care Nurse* (pp. 247–250). Philadelphia: W.B. Saunders.
3. Gamrath, B., Del Monte, L., & Richards, K. (1998). Noninvasive pacing: What you should know. *Journal of Emergency Nursing, 24,* 223–233.
4. Ignatavicius, D.D., Workman, M.L., & Mishler, M.A. (1995). *Medical-surgical nursing: A nursing process approach* (2nd ed.). Philadelphia: W.B. Saunders.
5. Kruse, L., Demarco, M.K., Moyer, P., Guenther, L., Wagner, A., Torrelli, V., & Leone, D. (1998). Keeping pace with implanted defibrillators. *RN, 61,* 30–35.
6. Mims, B.C., Toto, K.H., Leucke, L.E., & Roberts, M.K. (1996). *Critical care skills: A clinical handbook*. Philadelphia: W.B. Saunders.
7. Nadim Jr., N., Pacifico, A., Doyle, T.K., Earle, N.R., Hardage, M.L., & Philip, D. (1997). Spontaneous ventricular tachycardia treated by antitachycardia pacing. *American Journal of Cardiology, 79,* 820–822.
8. Osborn, C., & Quaal, S.J. (1998). Maximizing cardiopulmonary resuscitation in patients with intra-aortic balloon pumps. *Critical Care Nurse, 18,* 25–27.

9. Pacifico, A., Johnson, J.W., Stanton, M.S., Steinhaus, D.M., Gabler, R., Church, T., & Henry, P.D. (1998). Comparison of results in two implantable defribrillators (arrhythmias and conduction disturbances). *American Journal of Cardiology, 82,* 875–880.

10. Stephenson, N., & Combs, W.J. (1996). Artificial cardiac pacemakers and implantable cardioverter defibrillator. In M.R. Kinney and D.R. Packa (Eds.), *Andreoli's comprehensive cardiac care* (8th ed.), (pp. 240–250). St. Louis: Mosby.

11. Van Orden Wallace, C.J. (1998). Dual-chamber pacemakers in the management of severe heart failure. *Critical Care Nurse, 18,* 57–67.

12. Whitman, G.R., & Casedonte, M. (1996). Therapeutic modalities in the treatment of the patient with cardiovascular dysfunction. In S.D. Ruppert, J.G. Kernicki, & J.T. Dolan (Eds.), *Dolan's critical care nursing: Clinical managment through the nursing process* (2nd ed.), (pp. 241–269). Philadelphia: F.A. Davis.

PERIPHERAL VASCULAR DISEASE

Thomas W. Barkley, Jr., DSN, RN, CS, ACNP

I. PERIPHERAL VASCULAR DISEASE: OVERVIEW

A. Definition/Incidence[2, 3, 12, 14]

1. Disorders of the peripheral arteries and veins
2. Commonly occurs in the lower extremities
3. Affects approximately one in five adults
4. Includes two categories of disease:

    a. Peripheral arterial disease (PAD)
    b. Chronic venous insufficiency (CVI)

B. Etiology/Predisposing factors

1. Same as for coronary artery disease (see Chapter 10)

C. Peripheral arterial disease (PAD)[2, 3, 9, 12, 14]

1. Subjective/Physical examination findings

    a. The "6 Ps"
        i. Pain—Intermittent claudication (i.e., pain to calf, thigh, or buttock)
        ii. Pallor
        iii. Pulse absent or diminished
        iv. Paresthesias
        v. Paralysis
        vi. Poikilothermia
    b. Loss of hair on toes or lower legs
    c. "Glossy," thin, cool, dry skin

2. Diagnostic testing

    a. Doppler ultrasound studies
    b. Arteriography

3. Management

    a. Embolectomy for emboli to extremities
    b. Thrombolytic therapy for arterial thrombosis
    c. Angioplasty, when indicated
    d. Pentoxifylline (Trental), 400 mg p.o. t.i.d., to decrease viscosity and increase RBC flexibility
    e. Control contributing factors
        i. Diabetes
        ii. Smoking
        iii. Hypertension

D. Chronic venous insufficiency (CVI)[2, 12, 14]

1. Subjective/Physical examination findings

   a. Dependent edema to the feet
   b. Leg swelling or "tightness"
   c. Shiny, taut, hyperpigmented skin
   d. Ulcerations or varicosities to legs or feet

2. Diagnostic testing

   a. Doppler plethysmographic studies to measure changes in leg size or volume
   b. Venography

3. Management

   a. Symptomatic treatment
   b. Control edema
      i. Elevation
      ii. Support hose
   c. Weight reduction, as appropriate
   d. Need for meticulous skin care
   e. Review medications for agents that may potentially cause edema (e.g., calcium channel blockers).

II. SPECIFIC DISORDERS

A. Occlusive arterial disease[3, 4, 11, 14]

1. Arteriosclerosis obliterans

   a. Definition
   Narrowing of the lumen in the arteries as a result of atherosclerosis
   b. Etiology/Incidence[4, 14]
      i. Smoking increases risk twofold.
      ii. Increased incidence in men (3:1 male to female ratio), commonly between the ages of 50 and 70
      iii. Femoropopliteal, popliteal-tibial, and aortoiliac vessels (thus mostly lower extremities) are most commonly affected.
      iv. Higher incidence among diabetics

2. Thromboangiitis obliterans (Buerger's disease)

   a. Definition
   Occlusion of the arteries as a result of thrombosis and inflammation
   b. Etiology/Incidence[4, 7]
      i. More common in young males (20–40 years of age); rarely occurs in women
      ii. Almost all patients are moderate to heavy smokers.

    iii. Higher incidence in countries other than the United States (e.g., Southeast Asia, Japan, India)
    iv. Possible genetic predisposition

3. Subjective and physical assessment findings for occlusive arterial/Buerger's disease[3, 4, 7]

   a. Intermittent claudication
   b. Pain at rest
   c. Pain relieved by dependent positioning
   d. Coldness, numbness, or pallor of the extremity or extremities
   e. Absent or diminished pulse
   f. Ulcerations of the feet or toes
   g. Usually affects the arms and legs and not just the lower extremities, as compared with arteriosclerosis

4. Diagnostic testing[6, 7, 14]

   a. Physical examination is the most accurate method for diagnosis.
   b. Doppler ultrasonography
   c. Angiography
      i. "Spider leg" appearance related to collateral circulation
      ii. Multiple, smooth, segmental, tapered occlusions
      iii. Involvement of distal small and medium-sized vessels in upper and lower extremities

5. Management[4, 6, 7]

   a. Balloon/laser angioplasty
   b. Pain relief
      i. Hyperbaric oxygen therapy
      ii. Prostaglandin vasodilators administered IV or intra-arterially
      iii. Epidural anesthesia
   c. Atherectomy
   d. Other surgical approaches, when indicated
   e. Pentoxifylline (Trental), 400 mg p.o. t.i.d., to prolong patient's ability to ambulate and exercise before claudication
   f. Appropriate foot care/hygiene
      i. Debridement of necrotic ulcers
      ii. Amputation of gangrenous digits or tissue
   g. Smoking cessation—The disease will continue to progress if patient does not stop smoking.

B. Venous disease

1. Definition[14]

   a. Condition in which there is alteration in the character of veins resulting in thrombosis or decreased venous return

    b. Manifests as either superficial thrombophlebitis or deep vein thrombosis

2. Etiology[4, 6, 7, 14]

    a. Stasis of blood (e.g., immobility)
    b. Hypercoagulability
    c. Other
    d. Deep vein thrombosis is more common in women than in men.

3. Superficial thrombophlebitis

    a. Etiology/Incidence[2, 7]
       i. Intravenous cannulation of veins—most common cause
       ii. Trauma to pre-existing varices
       iii. Infection—*Staphylococcus* most commonly
       iv. Accounts for 10% of all nosocomial infections
       v. One in five cases associated with deep vein thrombosis
    b. Subjective and physical examination findings[2, 3, 7]
       i. Palpable, cord-like, reddened vein (i.e., linear appearance of redness)
       ii. Involved area is tender and warm.
       iii. Absence of significant swelling of the extremities
       iv. Fever—in 70% of patients
    c. Management
       i. Elevation of affected limb
       ii. Warm compresses.
       iii. NSAIDs (e.g., indomethacin [Indocin SR], 75 mg a day or b.i.d.

4. Deep vein thrombosis[4, 6, 14, 15]

    a. Risk factors: Internal and acquired[1, 7, 8, 10]
       i. Internal: Virchow's triad
         (1) Stasis of blood
         (2) Vessel wall changes
         (3) Changes in blood composition
       ii. Acquired factors
         (1) Surgery
         (2) Trauma (especially to pelvis or lower extremities)
         (3) Pregnancy
         (4) Puerperium
         (5) Lupus anticoagulant
         (6) Malignant diseases
         (7) Female hormones
         (8) Obesity
         (9) Congestive heart failure

b. Subjective/Physical examination findings[1, 2, 4, 7, 14]
   i. Aching/"throbbing" pain
   ii. Tenderness to palpation
   iii. Positive Homan's sign (pain upon dorsiflexion of the foot) occurs in approximately 40% of patients.
   iv. Increased body temperature
   v. Localized edema/swelling distal to the occlusion
   vi. Other signs of inflammation (e.g., redness, swelling, fever, extremity warm to touch) may be present.
c. Laboratory/Diagnostic findings[5-7, 10]
   i. Doppler ultrasound—Usually used initially because it is noninvasive, and serial repeated studies may be easily conducted
   ii. Venography—Invasive, painful, used to evaluate the deep vein thrombosis
d. Management[2, 4, 10, 13, 14]
   i. Bed rest with elevation of involved extremity
   ii. Use of local heat to the affected area
   iii. Anticoagulation therapy
      (1) Consider the use of low molecular weight heparin SC (e.g., enoxaprin [Lovenox], 30 mg SC b.i.d. as an initial dose for 7–10 days; then 40 mg SC for up to 3 weeks may be used, as indicated). Approximately 72 h after initial administration, warfarin (Coumadin), 10–15 mg p.o. every day should be started and continued for 3 months.
      (2) Heparin IV, 5000 unit bolus, then 750–1000 units/h for 5–7 days. Adjust dosage based on PTT (1.5–2 times the control value is optimal). Approximately one day after beginning heparin, warfarin, 10–15 mg p.o. every day, should be started and continued for 3 months.
   iv. Thrombolytic therapy may be considered.
   v. Consider insertion of an inferior vena cava (IVC) filter in patients for whom anticoagulation is contraindicated to assist in preventing pulmonary embolus.
   vi. Analgesics
   vii. Walking should be resumed gradually, with the patient wearing elastic stockings.

References

1. Anand, S.S., Wells, P.S., Hunt, D., Brill-Edwards, P., Cook, D., & Ginsberg, J.S. (1998). Does this patient have deep vein thrombosis? (The rational clinical examination). *Journal of the American Medical Association, 279*, 1094–1099.
2. Dunphy, H. (1999). *Management guidelines for adult nurse practitioners.* Philadelphia: F.A. Davis.
3. Hayko, D.M. (1998). Peripheral vascular assessment: Is it venous or arterial insufficiency? *Home Health Focus, 5*, 13.

4. Kantos, H.A. (1996). Vascular diseases of the limb. In J.C. Bennett & F. Plum (Eds.), *Cecil textbook of medicine* (20th ed.) (pp. 346–357). Philadelphia: W.B. Saunders.

5. Kearon, C., Julian, J.A., Math, M., Newman, T.E., & Ginsberg, J.S. (1998). Noninvasive diagnosis of deep venous thrombosis. *Annals of Internal Medicine, 128,* 663–677.

6. Massey, B.M., & Amidon, T.M. (1999). Heart. In L.M. Tierney, S.J. McPhee, & M.A. Papadakis (Eds.), *Current medical diagnosis & treatment* (38th ed.) (pp. 339–429). Stamford, CT: Appleton & Lange.

7. Petropoulos, P. (1999). Thromboangiitis obliterans (Beurger's disease). In F.F. Ferri (Ed.), *Ferri's Clinical Advisor* (pp. 471–472). Philadelphia: Mosby.

8. Rosendaal, F. R. (1999). Venous thrombosis: A multicausal disease. *The Lancet, 353,* 1167–1173.

9. Sasaki, S., Sakuma, M., Kunihara, T., & Yasuda, K. (1999). Current trends in thromboangiitis obliterans (Buerger's disease) in women. *American Journal of Surgery, 177,* 316–320.

10. Schwartz, L.B., (1998). Conventional and alternative therapies for acute deep venous thrombosis. *Journal of Care Management: The Official Journal of the Case Management Society of America, 4,* 9–13.

11. Sims, J.R., & Hanson, E.L. (1998). Images in clinical medicine. Thromboangiitis obliterans (Buerger's disease). *New England Journal of Medicine, 339,* 672.

12. Spittell, P.C., & Spittell, J.A., Jr. (1998). Diseases of the peripheral arteries and veins. In J.H. Stein (Ed.). *Internal medicine* (4th ed.) (pp. 304–312). St. Louis: Mosby.

13. Stein, P.D., Goldhaber, S.Z., Gottschalk, A., Hull, R.D., Hyers, T.M., Leeper, K.V., Moser, K.M., Pineo, G.F., Raskob, G. Saltzman, H.A., Sostman, H.D., Tapson, V.F., & Weg, J.G. (1998). Opinions regarding the diagnosis and management of venous thromboembolic disease. *Chest: The Cardiopulmonary and Critical Care Journal, 113,* 499–504.

14. Thelan, L.A., Urden, L.D., Lough, M.E., & Stacy, K.M. (1999). *Critical care nursing: Diagnosis and management* (3rd ed) St. Louis: Mosby.

15. Thomas, S. (1999). Graduated compression and the prevention of deep vein thrombosis (Part 1). *Journal of Wound Care, 8,* 41–43.

INFLAMMATORY CARDIAC DISEASES

Thomas W. Barkley, Jr., DSN, RN, CS, ACNP

I. PERICARDITIS[4, 6, 9]

A. Definition/General comments

1. Acute, painful inflammation of the pericardium
2. May be mild or life-threatening
3. Accurate patient history is of paramount importance in making the diagnosis.

B. Etiology/Predisposing factors/Incidence[3, 4, 8, 10, 14]

1. Viruses: Most common cause, especially infections with coxsackieviruses and echoviruses, Epstein-Barr virus, influenza, hepatitis, HIV, varicella, and mumps
2. Myocardial infarction: Affects 10–15% of patients within the first week after MI
3. Higher incidence among males
4. Cardiac surgery
5. Rheumatic fever
6. Neoplasia
7. Radiation therapy
8. Uremia
9. Tuberculosis
10. Idiopathic
11. Trauma
12. Other causes, such as drug allergy or autoimmune diseases
13. Affects 2–6% of the general population acutely

C. Subjective findings[1, 4, 9, 12]

1. Complaints of precordial/retrosternal, localized, "pleuritic" chest pain; pain that usually lasts for only a few seconds; patient may complain of pain under the breast.
2. Pain reported as being intensified with coughing, swallowing, inspiration (patient may complain of shortness of breath), or recumbent positioning; relieved by sitting in a forward position
3. Fever may or may not be present (underlying cause).

D. Physical examination findings[3, 4, 8, 9, 12]

1. Pericardial friction rub: Classically heard best with the patient sitting up and leaning forward
2. Pleural friction rub may or may not be present.
3. Dyspnea

E. Laboratory/Diagnostic findings[4, 8-10, 13]

1. ST segment elevation: ST segment returns to normal in a few days, followed by possible T wave inversion.
2. Depressed PR interval: Highly diagnostic of pericarditis
3. Elevated erythrocyte sedimentation rate
4. Leukocytosis
5. Consider ordering

   a. CBC (to rule out infection/leukemia)
   b. Electrolytes
   c. Blood cultures (if bacteria/infection is suspected)
   d. Echocardiogram (to confirm pericardial fluid)

F. Management[2, 3, 9, 13]

1. Aspirin (ASA), 650 mg q4h for 2 weeks *OR*
2. NSAIDs

   a. Ibuprofen (Advil), 400–600 mg q6h for 2 weeks
   b. Indomethacin (Indocin), 25–50 mg q8h for 2 weeks

3. Corticosteroids: Indicated *only* after failure of high-dose NSAIDs (several weeks' duration) because corticosteroids may increase *viral* replication

   • Prednisone (Deltasone), 60 mg every day, then taper and discontinue

4. Antibiotics—As indicated for bacterial infections
5. Codeine, 15–60 mg p.o. q.i.d. for pain
6. Monitor closely for cardiac tamponade.

II. ENDOCARDITIS

A. Definition[5, 9, 14]

1. Inflammation/infection of the endothelial layer of the heart, usually involving the cardiac valves
2. Endocarditis should be ruled out in any patient presenting with *fever of unknown origin* and a new *heart murmur.*

B. Etiology/Incidence/Predisposing factors[2, 5, 9, 10, 14]

1. Usually caused by bacteria—most commonly

   a. *Staphylococcus aureus*
   b. *Streptococcus pyogenes*
   c. *Pneumococcus*
   d. *Neisseria* organisms

2. May also be caused by fungi and viruses, especially in immunocompromised patients
3. Increased incidence associated with congenital heart disease and in those patients with valvular disease

4. Predisposing factors include recent invasive procedures such as dental surgery, genitourinary surgery, use of invasive catheters, hemodialysis, or burns.

C. Subjective findings[2, 5, 8, 9]

1. Fever lasting for several weeks
2. Headache
3. Weight loss
4. Fatigue
5. Exertional dyspnea
6. Cough
7. General malaise

D. Physical examination findings[2, 5, 9, 14]

1. Fever—Medium- to high-grade
2. Murmur—May not be detectable in some patients, especially those with right-sided endocarditis
3. Skin changes

   a. Pallor, purpura, petechiae
   b. Osler's nodes—Painful, red nodules in distal phalanges
   c. Splinter hemorrhages—Linear, subungual, resembling splinters
   d. Janeway's lesions—Macules on palms and soles; rarely observed; smaller than Osler's nodes and not painful
   e. Roth's spots—Small retinal infarcts, white in color, encircled by areas of hemorrhage
   f. Pallor
   g. Splenomegaly

E. Diagnostic/Laboratory findings[2, 5, 7, 9]

1. Patient may have normochromic, normocytic anemia.
2. WBC count may be elevated; always a ''left shift'' in the differential with band formation
3. Erythrocyte sedimentation rate is usually elevated.
4. Microscopic hematuria and proteinuria may be present.
5. Consider ordering

   a. Blood cultures—Most important diagnostic test; perform three cultures from three different sites.
   b. Echocardiogram to assess valvular involvement

F. Management[2, 7–9]

1. Generally, antibiotic therapy is withheld until results of blood cultures are available; while results are pending, empiric therapy may be necessary if the patient is critically ill.
2. Possible pharmacologic therapy—depending on cultured organisms

a. For *most* Streptococci and particularly *S. bovis*: Penicillin G, 2 million units q4h in combination with gentamicin, 1 mg/kg IV q8h for 2 weeks *OR*

b. Ceftriaxone (Rocephin), 2 g q.d. IV or IM for 4 weeks

- For *penicillin-allergic patients:* Either cefazolin (Ancef), 1 g IV q8h for 4 weeks, OR vancomycin (Vancocin), 15 mg/kg IV q12h for 4 weeks

c. For *methicillin-resistant Staphylococcus aureus*: Nafcillin (Unipen), 1.5 g q4h for 4–6 weeks

- For *penicillin-allergic patients:* Either cefazolin, 2 g IV q8h, OR vancomycin, 15 mg/kg q12h

d. For *enterococci:* Gentamicin, 1 mg/kg q8h, in combination with either ampicillin (Omnipen), 2 g IV q4h, OR penicillin G, 3–5 million units q4h for 4 weeks

- For *penicillin-allergic patients:* Vancomycin, 15 mg/kg q12h, in combination with gentamicin, 1 mg/kg q8h

G. Endocarditis prophylaxis[5, 9, 11]

1. Procedures in which prophylaxis *IS* recommended

a. Dental procedures
   i. Extractions
   ii. Periodontal procedures including surgery, scaling and root planing, and recall maintenance
   iii. Implant replacement and reimplantation of avulsed teeth
   iv. Endodontic (root canal) instrumentation or surgery only beyond the apex
   v. Subgingival placement of antibiotic fibers or strips
   vi. Initial placement of orthodontic bands but not brackets
   vii. Intraligamentary local anesthetic injections
   viii. Prophylactic cleaning of teeth or implants in which bleeding is expected

b. Gastrointestinal tract procedures
   i. Sclerotherapy for esophageal varices
   ii. Esophageal stricture dilation
   iii. Endoscopic retrograde cholangiography with biliary obstruction
   iv. Biliary tract surgery
   v. Surgical procedures that involve intestinal mucosa

c. Respiratory tract procedures
   i. Tonsillectomy and/or adenoidectomy
   ii. Surgical procedures that include respiratory mucosa
   iii. Rigid bronchoscopy

    d. Genitourinary tract procedures
- i. Prostatic surgery
- ii. Cystoscopy
- iii. Urethal dilation

2. Procedures in which prophylaxis is generally *NOT* recommended

    a. Dental procedures
- i. Restorative dentistry (operative and prosthodontic) with or without retraction card
- ii. Local anesthetic injection (nonintraligamentary)
- iii. Intracanal endodontic treatment, after placement and buildup
- iv. Placement of rubber dams
- v. Postoperative suture removal
- vi. Placement of removable prosthodontic or orthodontic appliances
- vii. Oral impressions
- viii. Fluoride treatments
- ix. Oral radiographs
- x. Orthodontic appliance adjustment
- xi. Shedding of primary teeth

    b. Respiratory tract procedures
- i. Endotracheal intubation
- ii. Flexible bronchoscopy with or without biopsy
- iii. Tympanostomy tube insertion

    c. Gastrointestinal tract procedures
- i. Transesophageal echocardiography
- ii. Endoscopy with or without biopsy

    d. Genitourinary tract procedures
- i. Vaginal hysterectomy
- ii. Vaginal delivery
- iii. Cesarean section
- iv. Urethral catheterization (in uninfected tissue)
- v. Uterine dilation and curettage (in uninfected tissue)
- vi. Therapeutic abortion (in uninfected tissue)
- vii. Sterilization procedures (in uninfected tissue)
- viii. Insertion or removal of intrauterine devices (in uninfected tissue)

    e. Other
- i. Cardiac catheterization, including balloon angioplasty
- ii. Implanted cardiac pacemakers, implanted defibrillators, and coronary stents
- iii. Incision or biopsy of surgically scrubbed skin
- iv. Circumcision

3. Antibiotic recommendations

    a. Dental, oral, respiratory tract, or esophageal procedures
- i. Adults should receive amoxicillin (Amoxil), 2.0 g p.o., within 1 h before the procedure.

    ii. Patients unable to take oral medication: Adults should receive ampicillin, 2.0 g IM or IV, within 30 min before the procedure.

    iii. Penicillin-allergic patients: Adults should receive clindamycin (Cleocin Phosphate), 600 mg p.o., OR azithromycin (Zithromax), 50 mg/kg p.o. or 500 mg, OR clarithromycin (Biaxin), 15 mg/kg p.o., each given within 1 h before the procedure.

    iv. Penicillin-allergic and unable to take oral medications: Adults should receive clindamycin, 600 mg, within 30 min before the procedure, OR cefazolin, 1 g IM or IV.

  b. Genitourinary and gastrointestinal tract procedures

    i. High risk patients (e.g., prosthetic valves, previous endocarditis, cyanotic congenital heart disease): Adults should receive ampicillin, 20 g IM or IV, plus gentamicin, 1.5 mg/kg, within 30 min of starting the procedure, followed by ampicillin, 50 mg/kg IM or IV within 30 min of starting the procedure, followed 6 h later by ampicillin, 25 mg/kg IM or IV, OR amoxicillin, 25 mg/kg p.o.

    ii. High risk patients allergic to ampicillin or amoxicillin: Adults should receive vancomycin, 1.0 g IV, over 1–2 hours PLUS gentamicin, 1.5 mg/kg IM or IV.

    iii. Moderate risk patients (e.g., mitral valve prolapse, rheumatic heart disease, hypertrophic cardiomyopathy): Adults should receive amoxicillin, 2.0 g p.o. within 1 h before the procedure, OR ampicillin, 2.0 g IM or IV.

    iv. Moderate-risk patients allergic to ampicillin or amoxicillin: Adults should receive vancomycin, 1.0 g IV.

References

1. Baas, L.B. (1997). Pericarditis, acute. In J.H. Keen & P.L. Swearingen (Eds.), *Mosby's critical care nursing consultant* (pp. 312–313). St. Louis: Mosby.
2. De Jong, M.J. (1998). Infective endocarditis: Minor procedures may place patients at risk for developing this infection of the heart lining. *American Journal of Nursing, 5,* 34–35.
3. Ferri, F.F. (Ed.). (1999). *Ferri's clinical advisor.* St. Louis: Mosby.
4. Heiselman, D.E. (1999). Pericarditis. In M.R. Dambro (Ed.), *Griffith's 5 minute clinical consultant* (pp. 792–793). Philadelphia: Lippincott, Williams & Wilkins.
5. Levison, M.E., & Abrutyn, E. (1998). Endocarditis: Current guidelines on prophylaxis. *Consultant, 38,* 260–264.
6. Lorell, B.H. (1998). Pericardial Disease. In L. Goldman & E. Braunwald (Eds.), *Primary cardiology* (pp. 427–444). Philadelphia: W.B. Saunders.
7. Masoudi, F.A., & Sande, M.A. (1998). Infective endocarditis. In J.H. Stein (Ed.), *Internal medicine* (4th ed.) (pp. 225–234). St. Louis: Mosby.

8. Massie, B.M. (1999). Systemic hypertension. In L.M. Tierney, S.J. Mc-Phee, & M.A. Papadakis, (Eds.), *Current medical diagnosis & treatment* (38th ed.) (pp. 430–452). Stamford, CT: Appleton & Lange.

9. Pawsat, D.E., & Lee, J.Y. (1998). Inflammatory disorders of the heart: Pericarditis, myocarditis, and endocarditis. *Emergency Clinics of North America, 16*, 665–681.

10. Schkenbach, L.H. (1997). Patients with valvular disease. In J.M. Clochesy, C. Breu, S. Cardin, A.A. Whittaker, & E.B. Rudy (Eds.), *Critical care nursing* (2nd ed.) (pp. 428–457). Philadelphia: W.B. Saunders.

11. Skillings, J. (1998). Endocarditis and endocarditis prophylaxis. *Lippincott's Primary Care Practice, 2*, 529–532.

12. Thelan, L.A., Davie, J.K., Urden, L.D., & Lough, M.E. (1994). *Critical care nursing: Diagnosis and management* (2nd ed). St. Louis: Mosby.

13. Watanakunakorn, C. (1999). Endocarditis, infective (parts 1 & 2). In M.R. Dambro (Ed.), *Griffith's 5 minute clinical consultant* (pp. 358–361). Philadelphia: Lippincott, Williams & Wilkins.

14. Woolliscroft, J.O. (1996). *Handbook of current diagnosis & treatment.* Philadelphia: Mosby.

CONGESTIVE HEART FAILURE

15

Thomas W. Barkley, Jr., DSN, RN, CS, ACNP

I. CONGESTIVE HEART FAILURE (CHF)

A. Definition/General comments[1, 7, 12, 13, 15, 20]

1. CHF is a syndrome, rather than a disease, caused by a variety of pathophysiologic processes in which the heart is unable to pump an adequate amount of blood to meet the metabolic demands of tissues.
2. CHF usually develops over time and includes dysfunction of either one or both ventricles.
3. Most commonly, left-sided heart failure occurs first. After one side of the heart fails, the other may eventually fail because of increased strain and workload.

B. Incidence/Etiology/Predisposing factors[1, 3, 6, 7, 9, 11–15, 18]

1. Affects over 4.7 million persons in the United States
2. Estimated 400,000 new cases diagnosed each year
3. Most common inpatient diagnosis in patients >65 years of age
4. Single largest Medicare hospitalization expenditure
5. CHF is more common in men than in women until age 75; at that time, incidence becomes approximately equal in both genders.
6. Estimated death rates among African Americans are 50% higher than among whites.
7. Left ventricular dysfunction from coronary artery disease is the most common cause.
8. Hypertension—Risk is three times higher in patients with hypertension.
9. Other precipitating factors/disease states
   a. Infections such as pericarditis, viral or bacterial systemic infections
   b. Endocrine abnormalities such as hyperthyroidism, thyrotoxicosis, pheochromocytoma
   c. Nutritional disorders such as beriberi (thiamine deficiency), kwashiorkor (protein deficiency)
   d. Preeclampsia
   e. Alcoholic cardiomyopathy
   f. Musculoskeletal disorders such as muscular dystrophy, myasthenia gravis
   g. Autoimmune disorders such as lupus erythematosus, sarcoidosis, amyloidosis

  h. Genetic factors leading to hypertrophic cardiomyopathy
  i. Valvular heart disease
  j. Rheumatic or congenital heart disease

C. Compensatory mechanisms common with CHF[1, 7, 8, 12, 13, 15]

1. Hypertrophy: The cardiac wall thickens with increased muscle mass over time because of increased strain and workload. Wall thickening leads to higher demand for oxygenation.
2. Dilation

  a. Enlargement of the chambers develops to compensate for increased blood volume.
  b. Because of increased volume, muscle fibers are stretched to increase contractile force.

3. Sympathetic nervous system: Inadequate cardiac output activates the sympathetic nervous system to release epinephrine and norepinephrine. As a result, myocardial oxygen demands are increased.
4. Renal response (renin-angiotensin-aldosterone cascade)

  a. Blood filtration in the kidneys decreases when cardiac output decreases.
  b. The kidneys respond to a false decreased blood volume and release renin.
  c. Renin activates release of angiotensin I and II.
  d. Angiotensin causes (a) peripheral vasoconstriction and (b) the release of aldosterone.
  e. Aldosterone causes sodium retention.
  f. Sodium retention is detected by the pituitary, and antidiuretic hormone (ADH) is secreted.
  g. ADH increases water absorption in the renal tubules, and, thus, water is retained.

D. Right- vs. left-sided heart failure: Subjective and physical examination findings[1, 6–8]

1. *Right-sided heart failure:* The right ventricle is impaired, and blood backs up in the right ventricle, the right atrium, and the systemic circulation.

  a. Increased central venous pressure
  b. Jugular venous distention
  c. Peripheral edema
  d. Liver enlargement
  e. Ascites
  f. S_3 and/or S_4 heart sounds

2. *Left-sided heart failure:* The left ventricle is impaired, and blood backs up in the left ventricle, left atrium, pulmonary veins, and lungs.

  a. Increased pulmonary capillary wedge pressure
  b. Adventitious breath sounds (crackles)
  c. Dyspnea

   d. Atrial fibrillation secondary to atrial distention
   e. Pulsus alternans (every other pulse beat is diminished)
   f. S_3 and, rarely, S_4 heart sounds

E. General subjective and physical examination findings of CHF[5-7, 9]

1. *Fatigue*—May be an early sign
2. *Dyspnea*—Related to poor gas exchange secondary to fluid retention
3. *Tachycardia*—Related to the sympathetic nervous system response to decreased cardiac output
4. *Edema*

   a. Legs (peripheral)
   b. Liver (hepatomegaly)
   c. Spleen (splenomegaly)
   d. Abdominal cavity (ascites)
   e. Lungs (pulmonary edema)

5. *Nocturia*—At night, when the body is in the supine position, fluid shifts from the interstitial spaces back into the intravascular space, resulting in increased renal blood flow and diuresis.
6. *Skin Changes*—Related to increased tissue capillary oxygen extraction. Thus, skin may look dusky and may also be diaphoretic.
7. *Behavioral Changes*—Related to impaired cerebral circulation, especially in the presence of atherosclerosis (e.g., restlessness, confusion, decreased attention span, decreased memory)
8. *Chest Pain*—In the presence of atherosclerosis, chest pain is related to decreased coronary perfusion.

F. Laboratory and diagnostic testing[2, 6, 7, 9, 16, 17, 19]

1. History and physical examination are very important to diagnosis and follow-up treatment.
2. Arterial blood gases (respiratory alkalosis is common—due to compensatory hyperventilation).
3. Erythrocyte sedimentation rate (decreased)
4. Electrolyte analysis
5. Urinalysis (may show renal dysfunction)
6. Chest x-ray (may reveal an enlarged heart)
7. ECG (used to detect old myocardial infarctions)—May show small (reduced) ECG complex size
8. Echocardiogram (assesses valve and wall motion)
9. Exercise stress test (assesses base line tolerance)

G. Classification of disease[1, 7] (Table 15–1)

1. *Systolic dysfunction*—The major defect associated with this diagnosis is the inability of the heart to *contract*, leading to reduced ventricular emptying and insufficient cardiac output.

   a. Associated with eccentric hypertrophy and therefore increased size of the heart

TABLE 15–1. NEW YORK HEART ASSOCIATION FUNCTIONAL CLASSIFICATION OF HEART FAILURE

FUNCTIONAL CLASS	DEFINITION	MANIFESTATION
I	Persons with cardiac disease, but without resulting limitations of physical activity	Ordinary physical activity causing no undue fatigue, palpitations, dyspnea, or angina
II	Persons with cardiac disease resulting in slight limitation of physical activity, but comfortable at rest	Ordinary physical activity resulting in fatigue, palpitations, dyspnea, or angina
III	Persons with cardiac disease resulting in marked limitation of physical activity, but comfortable at rest	Less than ordinary physical activity causing fatigue, palpitations, dyspnea, or angina
IV	Persons with cardiac disease resulting in an inability to carry out any physical activity without discomfort	Symptoms of cardiac insufficiency or of angina often present even at rest

Data from The Criteria Committee of the New York Heart Association (1979). *Nomenclature and criteria for diagnosis of diseases of the heart and great vessels.* Boston: Little, Brown. (From L. Bucher & S. Melander [Eds.], *Critical care nursing* [p. 263]. Philadelphia: W.B. Saunders, with permission.)

  b. Left ventricular ejection fraction of <40% denotes systolic dysfunction.

2. *Diastolic dysfunction*—Impairment in the ability of the heart to *relax*, resulting in impaired filling.

  a. Leads to stiffening and thickening of the myocardial wall
  b. Associated with concentric hypertrophy, with the heart's size remaining basically normal (e.g., the cardiothoracic ratio <55% on anteroposterior chest x-ray)

H. Management[2, 4–7, 10, 12, 13, 17]

1. Treat underlying cause.
2. Sodium restriction
3. Diuretic plus ACE inhibitor should be the initial treatment for symptomatic patients. Follow the algorithm shown in Figure 15–1.
4. Mild fluid retention (thiazide or similar preparation)

  a. Hydrochlorothiazide (HCTZ) (HydroDIURIL), 25–100 mg/day in one or two doses; maximum: 200 mg/day
  b. Metolazone (Zaroxolyn), 5–10 mg p.o. every day
  c. Chlorthalidone (Hygroton), 50–100 mg p.o. per day or 100 mg every other day; maximum: 200 mg/day

5. Severe fluid retention (loop diuretics)

  a. Furosemide (Lasix), 20–80 mg/dose p.o. initially, increased in increments of 20–40 mg/dose at intervals of 6–8 h; usual maintenance dose is twice daily or every day
  b. Bumetanide (Bumex), 0.5–2 mg/dose p.o. 1–2 times/day; maximum: 10 mg/day
  c. Torsemide (Demadex), 10–20 mg p.o. or IV every day; may be titrated upward until positive diuresis occurs

6. Potassium-sparing agents may also be used in combination with loop and thiazide diuretics.

  a. Spironolactone (Aldactone), 100–200 mg/day p.o. in one or two divided doses; alternate day dosing may be effective
  b. Triamterene (Dyrenium), 100 mg p.o. b.i.d. if used alone; lower dosage should be used if other diuretics are also used
  c. Amiloride (Midamor), 5–10 mg/day p.o. up to 20 mg with careful electrolyte monitoring

7. ACE inhibitors

  a. Standard therapy with heart failure
  b. Examples with initial dosages
    i. Captopril (Capoten), 6.25 mg initially for patients with pre-existing low blood pressure and/or hyponatremia. For other patients, 12.5 mg may be given initially. If

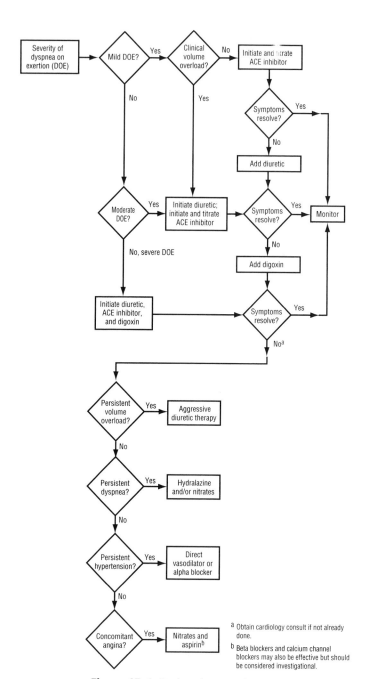

Figure 15–1. *See legend on opposite page*

178

the patient remains asymptomatic 2 h after initial administration, 12.5 mg t.i.d. may usually be safely ordered. Teach patient signs and symptoms related to hypotension. Maximal dosage = 100 mg t.i.d.

   ii. Enalapril (Vasotec), 5 mg q.d.

c. Caution: ACE inhibitors may cause profound hypotension. Diuretics and other vasodilators should be withheld or reduced for 24 h before initial administration of an ACE inhibitor. Monitor potassium levels.

d. Other adverse effects to monitor

   i. Cough—Dosage adjustment may be necessary; some coughing should be expected.

   ii. Skin rash—Dosage adjustment is usually warranted.

   iii. Renal Insufficiency—Monitor BUN and creatinine levels.

8. Digitalis (Digoxin): Positive inotropic agent used cautiously in patients with normal sinus rhythm

  a. Intravenous

    • Initial dose: 0.5 mg IV slowly over 10–20 min

    • Additional dose: 0.125 or 0.25 mg may be given 3 h later.

    • Total dose: 1.0–1.25 mg

  b. Oral

    • Initial dose: 1.0–1.25 mg divided over 24 h

    • Additional dose: 0.5 mg added in the second 24 h

    • Total dose: Best achieved by 0.5 mg q.d. for 3 days, then maintenance dosage

    • Maintenance dose: 0.125–0.5 mg q.d.

    • Monitor therapeutic level: 0.5–2.0 ng/mL

9. Vasodilators: Decrease preload, afterload, and systemic vascular resistance. Examples:

  a. Nitrates—Isosorbide dinitrate, 20–80 mg p.o. t.i.d., or nitroglycerin ointment, 12.5–50 mg (1–4 inches) q8h

  b. Oral hydralazine—Hydralazine, 200–400 mg q.d., in divided doses

   i. Not shown to be particularly effective as monotherapy, but quite effective in combination with nitrates

---

Figure 15–1. Pharmacologic management of patients with heart failure. (Redrawn from Konstam, M. Dracup, K. Baker, D., et al. [1994]. *Heart failure: Evaluation and care of patients with left-ventricular systolic dysfunction.* Clinical Practice Guideline No. 11. AHCPR Publication No. 94-0612. Rockville, MD: Agency for Health Care Policy and Research, Public Health Service, U.S. Department of Health and Human Services [pp. 50–53].)

    ii. Monitor for side effects, including gastrointestinal disturbances, hypotension, tachycardia, headache, and a lupus-like syndrome.

  c. Beta blockers—Carvedilol (Coreg) has been approved in the United States for *stable* patients. Dosage is 3.125 mg b.i.d., increased to 6.25 mg, 12.5 mg, and 25 mg b.i.d. at approximately 2-week intervals. Requires close patient monitoring.

  d. Calcium channel blockers—Contraindicated with CHF, as these agents may accelerate the progression of the disease.

References

1. Albert, N. (1999). Heart failure: The physiologic basis for current therapeutic concepts. *Critical Care Nurse, 19* (Suppl.), 2–13.
2. Davie, A.P., Francis, C.M., Caruana, L., Sutherland, G.R., & Mcmurray, J.J.V. (1997). Assessing diagnosis in heart failure: Which features are of any use. *QJM, 90*, 335–339.
3. Dunphy, L.M.H. (Ed.). (1999). *Management guidelines for adult nurse practitioners*. Philadelphia: F.A. Davis.
4. Havranek, E.P. (1999). Case report: Using ACE inhibitors to treat an elderly CHF patient. *Cardiology Review, 16*, 44.
5. Kober, L. Torp-Pederson, C., Jorgensen, S., Eliasen, P., & Camm, A.J. (1998). Changes in absolute and relative importance in the prognostic value of left ventricular systolic function and congestive heart failure after acute myocardial infarction. *American Journal of Cardiology, 81*, 1292–1297.
6. Konstam, M. Dracup, K. Baker, D., et al. (1994). *Heart failure: Evaluation and care of patients with left-ventricular systolic dysfunction.* Clinical Practice Guideline No. 11. AHCPR Publication No. 94-0612. Rockville, MD: Agency for Health Care Policy and Research, Public Health Service, U.S. Department of Health and Human Services (pp. 50–53).
7. Kotecki, C.N. (1999). Heart failure. In L. Bucher & S. Melander (Eds.), *Critical care nursing* (pp. 258–285). Philadelphia: W.B. Saunders.
8. Lamborn, M.L., & Moseley, M.J. (1997). Cardiac alterations. In J.C. Hartshorn, M.L. Sole, & M.L. Lamborn (Eds.), *Introduction to critical care nursing* (pp. 232–269). Philadelphia: W.B. Saunders.
9. Lobstein, P. (1999). Congestive heart failure. In M.R. Dambro (1999). *Griffith's 5 minute clinical consult* (pp. 256–257). Media, PA: Williams & Wilkins.
10. Mcmurray, J.J., and Stewart, S. (1998). Nurse led, multidisciplinary intervention in chronic heart failure. *Heart, 80*, 430–431.
11. Montagne, O., Le Roux, A., & Lejonc, J.L. (1999). Congestive heart failure in the aged. Causes and mechanisms of left ventricular dysfunction. *Presse Medicale, 28*, 658–660.
12. Moser, D.K., & Cardin, S. (1996). Heart failure. In J.M. Clochesy, C. Breu, S. Cardin, A.A. Whittaker, & E.B. Rudy (Eds.). *Critical care nursing* (2nd ed.) (pp. 380–412). Philadelphia: W.B. Saunders.
13. Moser, D.K., Frazier, S.K., Worster, P.L., & Clarke, J. (1999). The role of the critical care nurse in preventing heart failure after acute myocardial infarction. *Critical Care Nurse, 19* (Suppl.), 11–15.
14. Rich, M.W. (1999). Case report: Patient with chronic severe heart failure and occult shock. *Cardiology Review, 16*, 16–19.

15. Roberts, S.L. (Ed). (1996). *Critical care nursing: Assessment and intervention*. Stamford, CT: Appleton & Lange.

16. Tecce, M.A, Pennington, J.A., Segal, B.L., & Jessup, M.L. (1999). Heart failure: Clinical implications of systolic and diastolic dysfunction. *Geriatrics, 54,* 31–33.

17. Tierney, L.M., McPhee, S.J., & Papadakis, M.A. (Eds.). (1999). *Current medical diagnosis & treatment* (38th ed). Stamford, CT: Appleton & Lange.

18. Vasan, R.S., Larson, M.G., Benjamin, E.J., Evans, J.C., & Levy, D. (1997). Left ventricular dilatation and the risk of congestive heart failure in people without myocardial infarction. *New England Journal of Medicine, 336,* 1350–1355.

19. Weinberger, H.D. (1999). Diagnosis and treatment of diastolic heart failure. *Hospital Practice, 34,* 115–126.

20. Zygmont, D.M. (1996). Nursing management of the patient with coronary artery disease, angina pectoris, or myocardial infarction. In S.D. Ruppert, J.G. Kernicki, & J.T. Dolan (Eds.), *Dolan's critical care nursing: Clinical management through the nursing process* (2nd ed.) (pp. 270–291). Philadelphia: F.A. Davis.

VALVULAR DISEASE

Thomas W. Barkley, Jr., DSN, RN, CS, ACNP

16

I. VALVULAR DISEASE

A. Definition[3, 11]

1. The impairment of unidirectional flow as a result of damaged cardiac valves
2. Two types

   a. Stenosis ("narrowing"—obstructed forward blood flow)
   b. Regurgitation ("insufficiency"—backward blood flow across the valve)

3. May occur with all cardiac valves

B. Mitral stenosis

1. Definition
   Narrowing of the mitral valve resulting in obstructed forward blood flow
2. Etiology/Incidence[7]

   a. Rheumatic endocarditis from rheumatic fever is most common.
   b. Calcification of the valve with scarring
   c. Approximately two thirds of patients are female.

3. Subjective and physical examination findings[2, 5, 7, 15]

   a. Fatigue
   b. Dyspnea
   c. Orthopnea
   d. Other findings consistent with left-sided heart failure
   e. Palpitations—associated with atrial fibrillation
   f. Loud S_1 heart sound with low-pitched, mid-diastolic murmur; does not radiate
   g. Apical crescendo rumble

4. Diagnostic tests[1, 2, 5, 6, 15]

   a. Echocardiogram (two-dimensional)—Most valuable test; marked enlargement of the left atrium is the usual finding.
   b. Doppler echocardiogram—Prolonged pressure half-time across the valve
   c. Transesophageal echocardiogram (TEE)
   d. ECG—Check for atrial fibrillation, notched/broad P waves.

e. Chest x-ray—Check for the appearance of a straight left-sided heart border or large left atrium clearly indenting the esophagus.

f. Cardiac catheterization to establish severity

5. Management[1, 2, 5, 7]

a. Digoxin for atrial fibrillation

b. Diuretics for fluid mobilization

c. Anticoagulants for patients with continued atrial fibrillation

d. Percutaneous transvenous mitral valvotomy (PTMV)—Balloon approach for mechanical relief of less calcified valves.

e. Surgical valve repair or replacement for patients unresponsive to other therapy

C. Mitral regurgitation[6, 8, 12, 15, 16]

1. Definition
Backflow of blood into the left atrium as a result of deficient mitral valve closure

2. Etiology[7, 11]

a. Rheumatic disease

b. "Floppy" mitral valve

c. Papillary muscle dysfunction secondary to ischemic heart disease

d. Infective endocarditis

e. Ruptured chordae tendineae

f. Hypertrophic cardiomyopathy

g. Systemic lupus erythematosus

3. Subjective and physical examination findings[7, 11, 12, 14, 15]

a. Fatigue

b. Weakness

c. Dyspnea

d. Palpitations—Associated with atrial fibrillation

e. S_3 heart sound with systolic murmur at the 5th intercostal space-midclavicular line (apex)—May radiate to base or left axilla; blowing, musical, or high-pitched at times

f. Apical thrill may be palpable (Grade IV).

4. Diagnostic tests[12, 15, 16]

a. Echocardiogram (two-dimensional)—Thickened valve with or without flailing leaflets or vegetation

b. Doppler echocardiogram—Regurgitant flow into the left atrium

c. Transesophageal echocardiogram

d. ECG—Check for notched or broad P waves, left axis deviation.

    e. Chest x-ray—Check for enlarged left atrium and/or ventricle.

    f. Cardiac catheterization—Same as for mitral stenosis

5. Management[11, 13, 16]

    a. Vasodilators (e.g., ACE inhibitors, nitrates) to decrease afterload

    b. Digoxin for patients with atrial fibrillation

    c. Diuretics

    d. Anticoagulants for patients with atrial fibrillation

    e. Antibiotic prophylaxis for surgical or dental procedures

    f. Surgery—Reserved for severe disease refractory to other therapy

D. Mitral valve prolapse[7, 11]

1. Definition/Etiology/Incidence

    a. Protrusion of the mitral valve into the left atrium during systole as the result of damaged leaflets of the valve

    b. Usually benign

    c. Affects up to 20% of the population

    d. More prevalent in women than in men

2. Physical examination findings

    a. Often asymptomatic

    b. Fatigue

    c. Dizziness

    d. Dyspnea

    e. Chest pain or palpitations may occur.

3. Diagnostic tests
   Same as for other mitral disorders

4. Management

    a. Antibiotic prophylaxis for procedures, to prevent bacterial endocarditis

    b. Avoid stimulants in patients with palpitations.

    c. Same additional treatment as for mitral stenosis and regurgitation

    d. Monitor for complications

       i. Mitral regurgitation—Most common complication

       ii. Bacterial endocarditis—Risk is two to three times that of the general population

       iii. Supraventricular dysrhythmias

E. Aortic stenosis[7, 9]

1. Definition—Narrowing of the aortic valve resulting in obstructed forward blood flow

2. Etiology/Incidence[11]

   a. Rheumatic disease is the most common cause.
   b. Aging
   c. Idiopathic calcification of the aortic valve
   d. Congenital
   e. Most common valvular disorder in the United States

3. Subjective and physical examination findings[9, 13, 15]

   a. Dyspnea—May be marked
   b. Angina—Occurs in approximately 70% of patients
   c. Syncope—Occurs in approximately 20% of patients
   d. Murmur—Systolic, "blowing," rough, harsh at the 2nd right intercostal space, usually radiating to the neck

4. Diagnostic tests[9, 15]

   a. Same as for other mitral disorders
   b. Chest x-ray—Check for concentric hypertrophy of the left ventricle with a calcified valve.

5. Management

   a. Surgery—High mortality rate (75% of patients within 3 years of the onset of symptoms) if valve is not replaced.
   b. Symptomatic treatment (e.g., sodium restriction and diuretics if congestive heart failure is present; ACE inhibitors are contraindicated).
   c. Antibiotic prophylaxis for procedures, to prevent infective endocarditis

F. Aortic regurgitation[4, 7, 12]

1. Definition[11]
   Backflow of blood into the left ventricle as a result of deficiencies of the aortic valve leaflets or the aorta

2. Etiology[13]

   a. Rheumatic fever
   b. Rheumatoid arthritis
   c. Infectious endocarditis is the most common cause of acute presentation.
   d. Idiopathic valve calcification

3. Subjective and physical examination findings[4, 10, 12, 13, 15]

   a. Fatigue
   b. Dyspnea
   c. Syncope
   d. S_3 heart sound
   e. Murmur—Diastolic, "blowing" at the 3rd left intercostal space
   f. Signs of congestive heart failure
   g. Increased pulse pressure

4. Diagnostic tests[4, 12, 15]

    a. Same as for mitral disorders

    b. Chest x-ray—Check for moderate to severe left ventricular enlargement.

5. Management

    a. Surgery

    b. Vasodilators (e.g., ACE inhibitors)

    c. If congestive heart failure is present, symptomatic treatment, such as sodium restriction, diuretics, and digitalis

    d. Antibiotic prophylaxis against bacterial endocarditis for dental or other surgical procedures

References

1. Asorian, B. (1999). Cardiac surgery. In P. Logan (Ed.), *Principles of practice for the acute care nurse practitioner* (pp. 697–720). Stamford, CT: Appleton & Lange.
2. Bruce, C.J., & Nishimura, R.A. (1998). Newer advances in the diagnosis and treatment of mitral stenosis. *Current Problems in Cardiology, 23,* 125–192.
3. Carabello, B.A. (1998). Valvular heart disease. In L. Goldman & E. Braunwald (Eds.), *Primary cardiology* (pp. 370–389). Philadelphia: W.B. Saunders.
4. Choudhry, N.K., and Etchells, E.E. (1999). Does this patient have aortic regurgitation? *Journal of the American Medical Association, 281,* 2231–2238.
5. Fassbender, D., Schmidt, H.K., Seggewiss, H. Mannebach, H., & Bogunovic, N. (1998). Diagnosis and differential therapy of mitral stenosis. *Herz, 23,* 420–428.
6. Ferri, F.F. (Ed.). (1999). *Ferri's clinical advisor.* St. Louis: Mosby.
7. Freed, L.A., Levy, D., Levine, R.A., Larson, M.G., Evans, J.C., Fuller, D.L., Lehman, B., & Benjamin, E.J. (1999). Prevalence and clinical outcomes of mitral-valve prolapse. *New England Journal of Medicine, 341,* 1–7.
8. Kitabake, A., & Tomita, F. (1999). Mitral regurgitation associated with ischemic heart disease. *Internal Medicine, 38,* 617–618.
9. Otto, C.M. (1999). The difficulties in assessing patients with moderate aortic stenosis. *Heart, 82,* 5–6.
10. Ruppert, S.D., Kernicki, J.G., & Dolan, J.T. (Eds.) (1999). *Dolan's critical care nursing.* Philadelphia: F.A. Davis.
11. Schakenbach, L.H. (1996). Patients with valvular disease. In J.M. Clochesy, C. Breu, S. Cardin, A.A. Whittaker, & E.B. Rudy (Eds.), *Critical care nursing* (2nd ed.) (pp. 428–456). Philadelphia: W.B. Saunders.
12. Singh, J.P., Evans, J.C., Levy, D., Larson, M.G., Freed, L.A., Fuller, D.L., Lehman, B., & Benjamin, E.J. (1999). Prevalence and clinical determinants of mitral, tricuspid, and aortic regurgitation (the Framingham heart study). *American Journal of Cardiology, 83,* 897–902.
13. Steuble, B.T. (1997). Cardiac surgeries: Valvular disorders. In J.H. Keen & P.L. Swearingen (Eds.), *Mosby's critical care nursing consultant* (pp. 64–65). St. Louis: Mosby.

14. Thelan, L.A., Urden, L.D., Lough, M.E., & Stacy, K.M. (Eds.). (1998). *Critical care nursing: Diagnosis and management* (3rd ed.). St. Louis: Mosby.
15. Tierney, L.M., McPhee, S.J., & Papadakis, M.A. (Eds.). (1999). *Current medical diagnosis & treatment* (38th ed.). Stamford, CT: Appleton & Lange.
16. Tischler, M.D., Rowan, M., & LeWinter, M.M. (1998). Effect of enalapril therapy on left ventricular mass and volumes in asymptomatic chronic, severe mitral regurgitation secondary to mitral valve prolapse. *American Journal of Cardiology, 82,* 242–245.

CARDIOMYOPATHY

Thomas W. Barkley, Jr., DSN, RN, CS, ACNP

I. CARDIOMYOPATHY[3, 5, 8, 9, 12]

A. Definition

Idiopathic disorder causing cardiac muscle dysfunction resulting in heart failure

B. Types[2, 5–7, 10, 11]

1. *Dilated (Congestive)*—Characterized by abnormal systolic pump function and dilated ventricles without proportional compensatory hypertrophy; systolic heart failure
2. *Hypertrophic*—Autosomal dominant disorder characterized by a stiff left ventricle during diastole that restricts ventricular filling; ventricular hypertrophy occurs without dilation or a thickening septum; diastolic heart failure
3. *Restrictive*—Characterized by both inadequate diastolic filling and rigid ventricular walls; diastolic heart failure

C. Etiology/Incidence[1, 2, 4–7, 10]

1. Dilated (Congestive)

   a. Caused by ischemic heart disease, hypertension, alcoholism, systemic lupus erythematosus; also idiopathic causes
   b. Most common type of cardiomyopathy
   c. Approximately 1% of the general population is affected, with 10% of those older than 80 years of age.

2. Hypertrophic
   Cause is idiopathic. Chronic hypertension has been associated with increased incidence.
3. Restrictive

   a. Secondary to a variety of conditions, such as sarcoidosis, endomyocardial fibrosis (after open heart surgery); also results from radiation exposure and idiopathic causes
   b. Relatively uncommon

D. Subjective and physical examination findings[2, 4, 5, 10]

1. Dilated (Congestive)—Associated with left or biventricular congestive heart failure (CHF)

   a. Increased jugular venous distention
   b. Low pulse pressure

    c. S_3 and/or S_4 heart sounds
    d. Peripheral edema
    e. Rales
    f. Dyspnea
    g. Orthopnea
    h. Paroxysmal nocturnal dyspnea
    i. Mitral or tricuspid regurgitation (rare)
    j. Cardiomegaly

2. Hypertrophic

    a. Dyspnea
    b. Chest pain
    c. Syncope
    d. Murmur—Harsh, "diamond-shaped" (crescendo-decrescendo) systolic, at the left sternal border, that decreases with squatting and increases with the Valsalva maneuver
    e. S_4 heart sound
    f. Maximized apical pulse (double or triple)

3. Restrictive—Associated with right-sided CHF

    a. Dyspnea
    b. Fatigue
    c. Weakness
    d. Edema
    e. Jugular venous distention
    f. Ascites
    g. Murmurs (regurgitant)
    h. Kussmaul's breathing (possibly)

E. Diagnostic testing[2, 4–6, 11]

1. Dilated (Congestive)

    a. Chest x-ray
       i. Marked cardiac enlargement
      ii. Pulmonary edema (interstitial)
    b. ECG
       i. ST segment–T-wave changes with left ventricular hypertrophy
      ii. Right or left bundle branch block
     iii. Dysrhythmias common (e.g., atrial fibrillation, premature atrial contractions, premature ventricular contractions, ventricular tachycardia)
    c. Echocardiogram
      Left ventricular dilation and dysfunction with low ejection fraction
    d. Routine blood and urine chemistries

2. Hypertrophic
   a. Chest x-ray
      Mild cardiomegaly or normal heart size
   b. ECG
      i. Abnormal Q waves in anterolateral and inferior leads
      ii. Left ventricular hypertrophy
   c. Echocardiogram
      i. Left ventricular hypertrophy
      ii. Increased ejection fraction
   d. Routine blood and urine chemistries

3. Restrictive
   a. Chest x-ray
      i. Evidence of CHF, possibly including pleural effusion
      ii. Cardiomegaly is usually mild to moderate.
   b. ECG
      i. ST segment–T-wave changes
      ii. Atrial fibrillation, left axis deviation, and other dysrhythmias are possible.
   c. Echocardiogram
      i. Thickened cardiac valves
      ii. Increased wall thickness
      iii. Normal or small left ventricle size with mild to normal left ventricle function
   d. Routine blood and urine chemistries
   e. Cardiac catheterization/MRI to distinguish from constrictive pericarditis
      i. Impairment of the left ventricle is more evident than impairment of the right ventricle (e.g., pulmonary capillary wedge pressure is greater than central venous pressure) with restrictive cardiomyopathy.
      ii. MRI reveals greater thickening of the pericardium with restrictive cardiomyopathy.
      iii. With constrictive pericarditis, both ventricles are usually involved.
   f. Myocardial biopsy for definitive diagnosis

Figure 17–1. Pharmacologic management of patients with heart failure. (Redrawn from Konstam, M. Dracup, K. Baker, D., et al. [1994]. *Heart failure: Evaluation and care of patients with left-ventricular systolic dysfunction.* Clinical Practice Guideline No. 11. AHCPR Publication No. 94-0612. Rockville, MD: Agency for Health Care Policy and Research, Public Health Service, U.S. Department of Health and Human Services [pp. 50–53].)

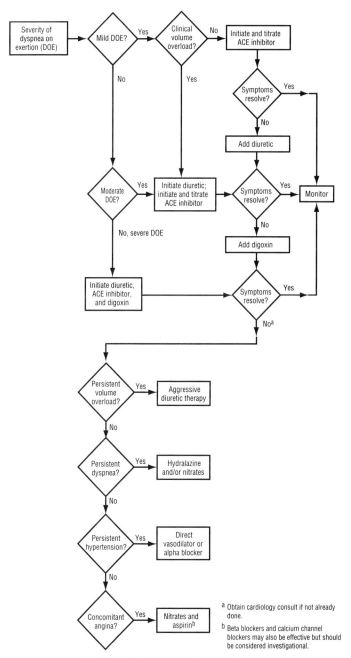

Figure 17-1. *See legend on opposite page*

F. Management[2, 5, 10, 11] (Fig. 17–1)

1. Dilated (Congestive)

   a. Treatment of the underlying condition (e.g., discontinuing use of alcohol, treating endocrine causes)
   b. For CHF (see Chapter 15)

      i. Rest
      ii. Restricted sodium
      iii. Diuretics
      iv. ACE inhibitors
      v. Digitalis

   c. Vasodilators, especially combined with ACE inhibitors and nitrates
   d. Oral anticoagulation for emboli prophylaxis
   e. Metoprolol (Lopressor; Toprol XL)—Low-dose beta blockade
   f. Diltiazem (Cardizem)—Especially effective for idiopathic causes
   g. Antidysrhythmic as needed

2. Hypertrophic

   a. Propranolol (Inderal), 160–240 mg/day, for both obstructive and nonobstructive disease
   b. Verapamil (Calan) for both obstructive and nonobstructive disease
   c. With CHF, IV normal saline in addition to propranolol or verapamil
   d. Antibiotic prophylaxis for invasive procedures
   e. Amiodarone (Cordarone) to prevent recurrence of atrial fibrillation
   f. Avoidance of alcohol
   g. Consider dual chamber pacing to prevent progression of the disease, as indicated.
   h. *ACE inhibitors, nitrates, other beta blockers, and digoxin are contraindicated with hypertrophic obstructive disease.*

3. Restrictive

   a. Control CHF—Major cause of death
      i. Restrict sodium intake.
      ii. Use diuretics as needed.
      iii. Administer antidysrhythmics as appropriate.
   b. Perform repeated phlebotomies to decrease iron deposition in the heart for patients with cardiomyopathy caused by hemachromatosis.
   c. Corticosteroids for sarcoidosis
   d. Symptomatic treatment

References

1. Bart, B.A., & O'Connor, C.M. (1999). Clinical determinants of mortality in patients with cardiomyopathy. *Cardiology Review, 16,* 8–11.
2. Borrowman, T., Love, R., & Mason, J.W. (1999). Dilated cardiomyopathy: Problems in diagnosis and management. *Chest: The Cardiopulmonary and Critical Care Journal 115,* 569–571.
3. Dec, W.G. (1998). Cardiomyopathies. In L. Goldman & E. Braunwald (Eds.), *Primary cardiology* (pp. 487–508). Philadelphia: W.B. Saunders.
4. Felker, G.M., Hu, W., Hare, J.M., Hurban, R.H., Baughman, K.L., & Kasper, E.K. (1999). The spectrum of dilated cardiomyopathy: The Johns Hopkins experience with 1,278 patients. *Medicine, 78,* 270–283.
5. Ferri, F.F. (Ed.). (1999). *Ferri's clinical advisor.* St. Louis: Mosby.
6. Kilner, P.J., Gunning, M.G., Knight, C.J., & Sigwart, U. (1997). Hypertrophic cardiomyopathy: Stress induction of subaortic stenosis and mitral regurgitation. *Circulation, 95,* 1083–1084.
7. Kotecki, C.N. (1999). Heart failure. In L. Bucher & S. Melander (Eds.), *Critical care nursing* (pp. 259–285). Philadelphia: W.B. Saunders.
8. Shah, P.M. (1998). Cardiomyopathies. In J.H. Stein (Ed.), *Internal medicine* (4th ed.) (pp. 262–271.). St. Louis: Mosby.
9. Steuble, B.T. (1997). Cardiomyopathy. In J.H. Keen & P.L. Swearingen (Eds.), *Mosby's critical care nursing consultant* (pp. 76–77). St. Louis: Mosby.
10. Tierney, L.M., McPhee, S.J., & Papadakis, M.A. (Eds.). (1999). *Current medical diagnosis & treatment* (38th ed.). Stamford, CT: Appleton & Lange.
11. Twomey, C., & Logan, P. (1999). Heart failure and cardiomyopathy. In P. Logan (Ed.), *Principles of practice for the acute care nurse practitioner* (pp. 723–739). Stamford, CT: Appleton & Lange.
12. Woolliscroft, J.O. (1996). *Handbook of current diagnosis & treatment.* Philadelphia: Mosby.

ECTOPY AND DYSRHYTHMIA EMERGENCIES

Thomas W. Barkley, Jr., DSN, RN, CS, ACNP

I. COMMON CARDIAC RHYTHMS/DYSRHYTHMIAS AND TREATMENT[1-10]

Note: Emergency cardiovascular care is an evolving science, and, as such, practitioners are strongly encouraged to attend regular advanced cardiovascular life support (ACLS) update courses, as national guidelines are periodically revised.

A. Normal sinus rhythm (NSR) (Fig. 18–1)

1. Characteristics

   a. Regular rate and rhythm
   b. PR interval and QRS complex normal
      i. PR interval ≤.20s
      ii. QRS complex ≤.12s

2. Rate = 60–100 beats per minute (bpm)

B. Sinus bradycardia (SB) (Fig. 18–2)

1. Characteristics

   a. Regular rate and rhythm
   b. PR interval and QRS complex normal

2. Rate = <60 bpm or rate less than expected relative to underlying condition or cause
3. Etiology

   a. Increased vagus nerve activity (e.g., in athletic individuals, during Valsalva maneuver)
   b. Digitalis (Digoxin)
   c. Propranolol (Inderal)
   d. Quinidine
   e. Hypoxemia

4. Clinical manifestations

   a. Decreased cardiac output
   b. Hypotension
   c. Loss of consciousness
   d. Other signs of poor perfusion

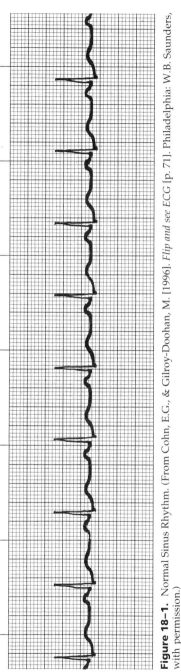

Figure 18–1. Normal Sinus Rhythm. (From Cohn, E.G., & Gilroy-Doohan, M. [1996]. *Flip and see ECG* [p. 71]. Philadelphia: W.B. Saunders, with permission.)

195

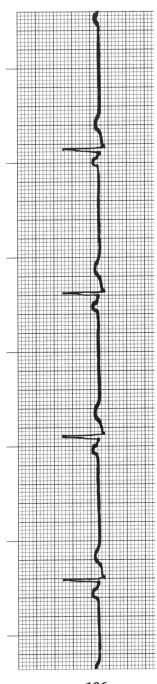

Figure 18–2. Sinus Bradycardia. (From Cohn, E.G., & Gilroy-Doohan, M. [1996]. *Flip and see ECG* [p. 75]. Philadelphia: W.B. Saunders, with permission.)

5. Treatment

   a. Primary ABCD survey: Assess ABCs, secure airway noninvasively, and ensure that monitor/defibrillator is
available.

   b. Secondary ABCD survey

- Determine if an invasive airway is needed and
administer oxygen.
- Obtain IV access, ensure rhythm per monitor, administer
fluids as needed.
- Check vital signs, oxygen saturation per pulse oximeter,
and monitor blood pressure.
- Obtain and review 12-lead ECG and portable chest
x-ray.
- Conduct a problem-focused history and physical
examination.
- Consider causes.

   c. For serious signs or symptoms related to bradycardia,
continue as follows:

- Atropine, 0.5–1 mg IV; repeated every 3–5 min as
needed, not to exceed a total dose of 0.04 mg/kg; shorter
dosing intervals (e.g., 3 min) and higher doses (e.g.,
0.04 mg/kg) should be considered with severe clinical
scenarios.
- Transcutaneous pacing—Especially indicated with
symptomatic Type II second degree AV block or third
degree AV block until transvenous pacemaker can be
inserted.
- Consider dopamine (Intropin), 5–20 μg/kg/min—lower
doses (e.g., 1–3 μg/kg/min) for renal perfusion; higher
doses for vasoconstriction; maximum dose = 20 μg/kg/
min
- Consider IV epinephrine drip at 2–10 μg/min (1 mg of
1:1000 solution mixed in 500 mL normal saline;
administered at 1–5 mL/min).

C. Sinus tachycardia (ST) (Fig. 18–3)

1. Characteristics

   a. Regular rate and rhythm
   b. PR interval and QRS complex normal

2. Rate = >100 bpm and generally <150–160 bpm
3. Etiology

   a. Pain
   b. Fever
   c. Anxiety

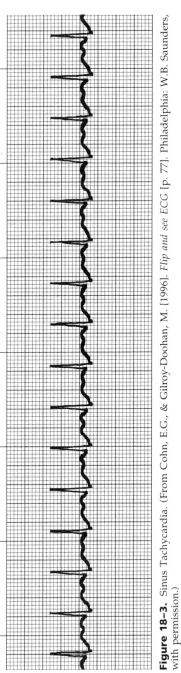

Figure 18–3. Sinus Tachycardia. (From Cohn, E.G., & Gilroy-Doohan, M. [1996]. *Flip and see ECG* [p. 77]. Philadelphia: W.B. Saunders, with permission.)

    d. Shock
    e. Hypovolemia
    f. Congestive heart failure
    g. Cocaine use

4. Clinical manifestations—If rate is greatly elevated

    a. Decreased cardiac output
    b. Hypotension
    c. Loss of consciousness
    d. Other signs of poor perfusion

5. Treatment:

    a. Treat the underlying problem or cause.
    b. Medications are not indicated.

D. Sinus arrhythmia (Fig. 18–4)

1. Characteristics

    a. Rate is variable (i.e., variable R–R interval).
    b. Normal PR interval and QRS complex
    c. Rate varies with respirations.

2. Etiology: Common in children and the elderly
3. Clinical manifestations: None
4. Treatment: None

E. Premature atrial contractions (PACs) (Fig. 18–5)

1. Characteristics

    a. Occurs when an ectopic focus in the atria fires before the next sinus node impulse. P waves usually look different (i.e., either smaller or peaked).
    b. Rate usually "resets" itself, resulting in one premature beat followed by a normal series of beats in sinus rhythm.

2. Etiology: Unknown
3. Clinical manifestations: None
4. Treatment: None

F. Atrial fibrillation (A-Fib) (Fig. 18–6) (See Fig. 18–IIB, p. 241)

1. Characteristics

    a. No discernible P waves; f (fibrillatory) are noted instead.
    b. PR interval is not measurable (wavy baseline).
    c. QRS complex is regularly irregular.
    d. Atrial rate is commonly 350–600 bpm.
    e. Ventricular rate is usually 100–160 bpm.

2. Etiology

    a. Congestive heart failure

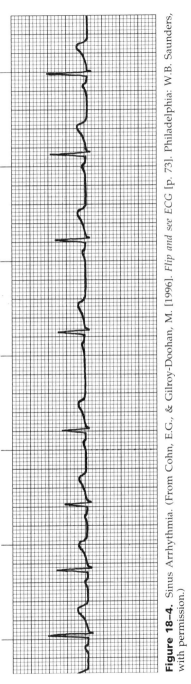

Figure 18-4. Sinus Arrhythmia. (From Cohn, E.G., & Gilroy-Doohan, M. [1996]. *Flip and see ECG* [p. 73]. Philadelphia: W.B. Saunders, with permission.)

200

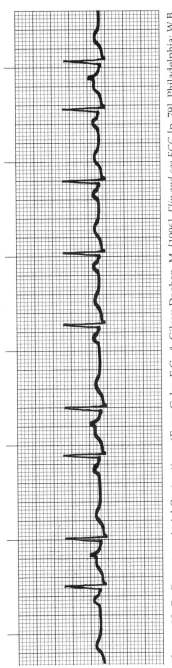

Figure 18–5. Premature Atrial Contractions. (From Cohn, E.G., & Gilroy-Doohan, M. [1996]. *Flip and see ECG* [p. 79]. Philadelphia: W.B. Saunders, with permission.)

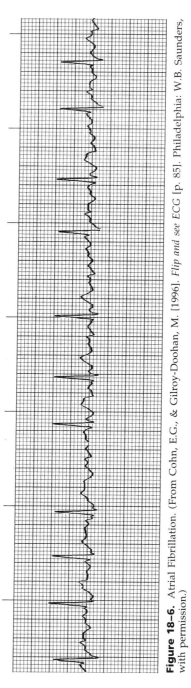

Figure 18–6. Atrial Fibrillation. (From Cohn, E.G., & Gilroy-Doohan, M. [1996]. *Flip and see ECG* [p. 85]. Philadelphia: W.B. Saunders, with permission.)

b. Hypoxemia
c. Valvular disease
d. Hyperthyroidism

3. Clinical manifestations

a. Decreased cardiac output
b. Hypotension
c. Loss of consciousness

4. Treatment

Note: Management of atrial fibrillation and/or atrial flutter is based on three parameters: (a) normal heart function, (b) whether impaired (congestive heart failure [CHF] exists or ejection fraction [EF] <40%), or (c) whether Wolff-Parkinson-White syndrome is present *and* whether the goal is either to control rate or to convert the rhythm considering the duration of onset (i.e., less than [<] or greater than [>] 48 h).

a. To control *rate* in patients with atrial fibrillation/atrial flutter AND *normal* heart function:
   i. If atrial fibrillation/flutter has persisted for longer than 48 h, converting agents should be used with extreme caution in patients not receiving adequate anticoagulation because of the possibility of embolic events.
   ii. Consider *only one* of the following choices:

      • Calcium channel blockers: e.g., diltiazem (Cardizem), 15–20 mg (0.25 mg/kg) IV over 2 min; may repeat in 15 min at 20–25 mg (0.35 mg/kg) over 2 min; maintenance infusion rate = 5–15 mg/h titrated to heart rate.
      • Beta blockers; e.g., atenolol (Tenormin), 5 mg IV slowly over 5 min; wait 10 min and then administer a second dose of 5 mg IV slowly over 5 min; in 10 additional min, if tolerated well, may begin 50 mg p.o.; then give 50 mg p.o. b.i.d.
      • Additional Class IIb agents

b. To *convert the rhythm* in a patient with atrial fibrillation/atrial flutter with *normal* heart function AND *duration* has been <*48 h:*
   i. Direct current (DC) cardioversion: consider sedation [e.g., diazepam (Valium), 5 mg, with midazolam (Versed), 2 mg, or other benzodiazepine in combination with midazolam; may also employ a low dose narcotic agent (e.g., morphine, 2–4 mg) if the patient is not severely hypotensive; cardioversion for atrial dysrhythmias begins with 50 J, then 100 J, 200 J, and so forth.

    ii. Use only *one* of the following Class IIb agents:

      (1) Amiodarone (Cordarone): maximum cumulative dose = 2.2 g/24 h IV; may cause profound vasodilation and hypotension; may be given as follows:

- *Rapid infusion:* 150 mg IV over the first 10 min (15 mg/min); may repeat rapid infusion (150 mg IV) every 10 min as needed
- *Slow infusion:* 360 mg IV over 6 h (i.e., 1 mg/min)
- *Maintenance infusion:* 540 mg IV over 18 h (i.e., 0.5 mg/min)

      (2) Ibutilide (Corvert):

- For adults ≥60 kg: Administer 1 mg (10 mL) over 10 min; a second dose may be administered at the same rate 10 min later.
- For adults <60 kg: Administer 0.01 mg/kg initially IV.

      (3) Procainamide (Pronestyl): 20 mg/min IV by infusion until one of the following occurs:

- Rate is controlled
- Hypotension
- QRS widens >50%
- Total dose of 17 mg/kg is administered

      (4) Other considerations from Class IIb

  c. To *convert the rhythm* in a patient with atrial fibrillation/atrial flutter AND *duration* has been *>48 h or unknown:*

    i. NO DC cardioversion (Note: When using pharmacologic agents or shock, embolic events may occur during the conversion of atrial fibrillation/flutter to normal sinus rhythm from atrial thrombi unless the patient has been adequately anticoagulated. Use pharmacologic agents with extreme caution if duration has been >48 h.) *or*

    ii. Delayed cardioversion

- Anticoagulation × 3 weeks, cardiovert the patient (refer to section F.4.B.i.), and then continue anticoagulation for an additional 4 weeks *or*

    iii. Early cardioversion

- Begin heparin IV immediately (e.g., heparin 80 U/kg IV bolus followed by 18 U/kg/h IV continuous infusion)
- Conduct a transesophageal echocardiogram (TEE) to rule out atrial thrombi.

- Cardiovert within 24 h following TEE (refer to section F.4.B.i.).
- Continue anticoagulation therapy for an additional 4 weeks.

d. To control *rate* in patients with atrial fibrillation/atrial flutter AND *impaired* heart function (i.e., CHF or EF <40%):

   i. If atrial fibrillation/flutter has persisted for longer than 48 h, pharmacologic converting agents should be used with extreme caution in patients not receiving adequate anticoagulation because of the possibility of embolic events.

   ii. Consider *only one* of the following Class IIb choices:

      (1) Digoxin: Loading dose = 10–15 μg/kg of lean body weight. Caution: avoid cardioversion in patients taking digoxin unless the condition is life threatening.

      (2) Diltiazem: 15–20 mg (0.25 mg/kg) IV over 2 min; may repeat in 15 min at 20–25 mg (0.35 mg/kg) over 2 min; maintenance infusion rate = 5–15 mg/h titrated to heart rate.

      (3) Amiodarone: Maximum cumulative dose = 2.2 g/ 24 h IV; may cause profound vasodilation and hypotension; may be given as follows:

         - *Rapid infusion:* 150 mg IV over the first 10 min (15 mg/min); may repeat rapid infusion (150 mg IV) every 10 min as needed
         - *Slow infusion:* 360 mg IV over 6 h (i.e., 1 mg/min)
         - *Maintenance infusion:* 540 mg IV over 18 h (i.e., 0.5 mg/min)

e. To *convert the rhythm* in a patient with atrial fibrillation/ atrial flutter with *impaired* heart function (i.e., CHF or EF <40%) AND *duration* has been *<48 h:*

   i. Consider DC cardioversion (refer to section F.4.B.i) *or*

   ii. Amiodarone: Maximum cumulative dose = 2.2 g/24 h IV; may cause profound vasodilation and hypotension; may be given as follows:

      - *Rapid infusion:* 150 mg IV over the first 10 min (15 mg/min); may repeat rapid infusion (150 mg IV) every 10 min as needed
      - *Slow infusion:* 360 mg IV over 6 h (i.e., 1 mg/min)
      - *Maintenance infusion:* 540 mg IV over 18 h (i.e., 0.5 mg/min)

f. To *convert the rhythm* in a patient with atrial fibrillation/ atrial flutter with *impaired* heart function (CHF or EF <40%) AND *duration* has been *>48 h or unknown:*

   i. Anticoagulation therapy as discussed in section 4.C.

   ii. DC cardioversion (refer to section F.4.B.i).

g. To control *rate* in patients with atrial fibrillation/atrial flutter AND *Wolff-Parkinson-White syndrome* with *preserved* heart function:

  i. If atrial fibrillation/flutter has persisted for longer than 48 h, pharmacologic converting agents should be used with extreme caution in patients not receiving adequate anticoagulation because of the possibility of embolic events.

  ii. DC cardioversion (refer to section F.4.B.i.) OR

  iii. Use *only one* of the following Class IIb agents:

   (1) Amiodarone: Maximum cumulative dose = 2.2 g/ 24 h IV; may cause profound vasodilation and hypotension; may be given as follows:

   - *Rapid infusion:* 150 mg IV over the first 10 min (15 mg/min); may repeat rapid infusion (150 mg IV) every 10 min as needed
   - *Slow infusion:* 360 mg IV over 6 h (i.e., 1 mg/min)
   - *Maintenance infusion:* 540 mg IV over 18 h (i.e., 0.5 mg/min)

   (2) Procainamide: 20 mg/min IV by infusion until one of the following occurs:

   - Rate is controlled
   - Hypotension
   - QRS widens >50%
   - Total dose of 17 mg/kg is administered OR

   (3) ONE of the following Class III agents, noting these drugs may be harmful when used in patients with Wolff-Parkinson-White syndrome:

   - Adenosine (Adenocard): The patient should be placed in mild reverse Trendelenburg postion before administration. Initially give 6 mg rapidly over 1–3 s followed by a rapid normal saline (NS) bolus of 20 mL. (Syringes containing adenosine and NS should be inserted in the same injection port nearest the patient and tubing should be clamped during administration to prevent backflow of the medication and NS; then, unclamp the tubing and elevate the extremity. Repeat a second and third dose of adenosine at 12 mg each, 1–2 min apart as needed.)
   - Beta blockers: e.g., atenolol, 5 mg IV slowly over 5 min; wait 10 min and then administer a second dose of 5 mg IV slowly over 5 min; in 10 additional min, if tolerated well, may begin 50 mg p.o.; then give 50 mg p.o. b.i.d.

- Calcium channel blockers: e.g., diltiazem, 15–20 mg (0.25 mg/kg) IV over 2 min; may repeat in 15 min at 20–25 mg (0.35 mg/kg) over 2 min; maintenance infusion rate = 5–15 mg/hour titrated to heart rate.
- Digoxin: Loading dose = 10–15 μg/kg of lean body weight. Caution: Avoid cardioversion in patients taking digoxin unless the condition is life threatening.

h. To control *rate* in patients with atrial fibrillation/atrial flutter AND *Wolff-Parkinson-White syndrome* and *impaired* (i.e., CHF or EF <40%) heart function:

   i. If atrial fibrillation/flutter has persisted for longer than 48 h, pharmacologic converting agents should be used with extreme caution in patients not receiving adequate anticoagulation because of the possibility of embolic events.

  ii. DC cardioversion (refer to section F.4.B.i.) OR

 iii. Amiodarone: Maximum cumulative dose = 2.2 g/24 h IV; may cause profound vasodilation and hypotension; may be given as follows:

- *Rapid infusion:* 150 mg IV over the first 10 min (15 mg/min); may repeat rapid infusion (150 mg IV) every 10 min as needed.
- *Slow infusion:* 360 mg IV over 6 h (i.e., 1 mg/min).
- *Maintenance infusion:* 540 mg IV over 18 h (i.e., 0.5 mg/min).

i. To *convert the rhythm* in a patient with atrial fibrillation/atrial flutter with *Wolff-Parkinson-White syndrome* AND *duration* has been >48 h:

   i. DC cardioversion (refer to section F.4.B.i) OR

  ii. Use *only one* of the following Class IIb agents:

   (1) Amiodarone: Maximum cumulative dose = 2.2 g/24 h IV; may cause profound vasodilation and hypotension; may be given as follows:

- *Rapid infusion:* 150 mg IV over the first 10 min (15 mg/min); may repeat rapid infusion (150 mg IV) every 10 min as needed.
- *Slow infusion:* 360 mg IV over 6 h (i.e., 1 mg/min).
- *Maintenance infusion:* 540 mg IV over 18 h (i.e., 0.5 mg/min).

   (2) Procainamide: 20 mg/min IV until one of the following occurs:

- Total dose of 17 mg/kg is administered
- QRS widens by >50%

- Hypotension
- Arrhythmia suppression OR

(3) ONE of the following Class III agents, noting these drugs may be harmful when used in patients with Wolff-Parkinson-White syndrome:

- Adenosine: The patient should be placed in mild reverse Trendelenburg position before administration. Initially, give 6 mg rapidly over 1–3 seconds followed by a rapid NS bolus of 20 mL. (Syringes containing adenosine and NS should be inserted in the same injection port nearest the patient and tubing should be clamped during administration to prevent backflow of the medication and NS; then, unclamp the tubing and elevate the extremity; repeat a second and third dose of adenosine at 12 mg each, 1 to 2 min apart as needed.)
- Beta blockers: e.g., atenolol, 5 mg IV slowly over 5 min; wait 10 min and then administer a second dose of 5 mg IV slowly over 5 min; in 10 additional min, if tolerated well, may begin 50 mg p.o.; then give 50 mg p.o. b.i.d.
- Calcium channel blockers: e.g., diltiazem, 15–20 mg (0.25 mg/kg) IV over 2 min; may repeat in 15 min at 20–25 mg (0.35 mg/kg) over 2 min; maintenance infusion rate = 5–15 mg/h titrated to heart rate.
- Digoxin: Loading dose = 10–15 μg/kg of lean body weight. Caution: Avoid cardioversion in patients taking digoxin unless the condition is life threatening.

j. To *convert the rhythm* in a patient with atrial fibrillation/atrial flutter with *Wolff-Parkinson-White syndrome* AND *duration* has been *>48 h or unknown:*
   i. Prescribe anticoagulation therapy as described in section F.4.C., *followed by*
   ii. DC cardioversion (refer to section F.4.B.i)

G. Atrial flutter (A-flutter) (Fig. 18–7) (See Fig. 18–IIB, p. 241)

1. Characteristics

   a. Sawtooth appearance of flutter waves (F waves), especially if the rhythm strip is turned upside down
   b. PR interval is not measurable.
   c. Atrial rate varies from 240 to 360 bpm.
   d. QRS complex is usually normal.

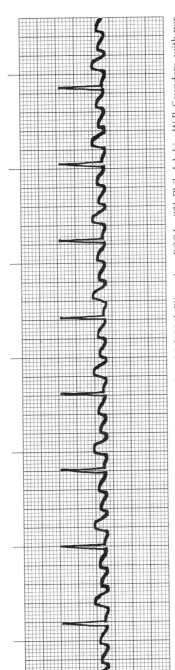

Figure 18–7. Atrial Flutter. (From Cohn, E.G., & Gilroy-Doohan, M. [1996]. *Flip and see ECG* [p. 83]. Philadelphia: W.B. Saunders, with permission.)

2. Etiology

    a. Congestive heart failure
    b. Hypoxemia
    c. Valvular disease
    d. Hyperthyroidism

3. Clinical manifestations

    a. Decreased cardiac output
    b. Hypotension
    c. Loss of consciousness

4. Treatment: Same as for atrial fibrillation—Refer to section F.4.

H. Narrow complex supraventricular tachycardia (SVT) (Fig. 18–8) (See Fig. 18–IIC, p. 243)

    • Paroxysmal supraventricular tachycardia (PSVT)
    • Junctional tachycardia
    • Ectopic or multifocal atrial tachycardia

1. Characteristics

    a. Sudden onset
    b. Rate = 160–250 bpm
    c. Regular rhythm, cannot distinguish P waves, and QRS complex is normal (<0.12 s)

2. Etiology

    a. Anxiety
    b. Stimulants
    c. Digitalis toxicity causing an ectopic impulse to originate from above the ventricles and conduct normally throughout the ventricles

3. Clinical manifestations

    a. Dizziness
    b. Decreased cardiac output
    c. Decreased blood pressure
    d. Loss of consciousness
    e. Chest pain

4. Treatment for all three types of narrow complex SVT

    a. Vagal stimulation
      i. Carotid massage—Gentle pressure, first over the right, and then over the left carotid artery for 10–20 s. Note: Contraindicated in patients with history of transient ischemic attacks or carotid bruits.
      ii. Valsalva maneuvers—Ask the patient to cough or strain as though having a bowel movement, or elicit the gag reflex in the patient.

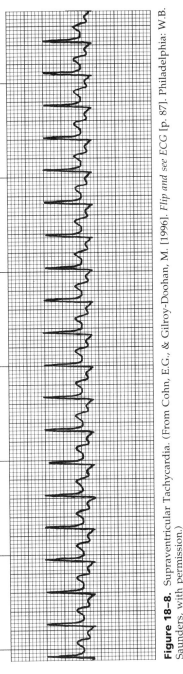

Figure 18–8. Supraventricular Tachycardia. (From Cohn, E.G., & Gilroy-Doohan, M. [1996]. *Flip and see ECG* [p. 87]. Philadelphia: W.B. Saunders, with permission.)

b. Adenosine: The patient should be placed in mild reverse Trendelenburg position before administration. Initially, give 6 mg rapidly over 1–3 s followed by a rapid NS bolus of 20 mL. (Syringes containing adenosine and NS should be inserted in the same injection port nearest the patient and tubing should be clamped during administration to prevent backflow of the medication and NS; then, unclamp the tubing and elevate the extremity; repeat a second and third dose of adenosine at 12 mg each, 1–2 min apart as needed.)

c. Other medications and therapies—Recommendations are based on whether the patient has normal (i.e., preserved) or impaired (i.e., CHF or EF <40%) heart function:

d. For patients with *paroxysmal supraventricular tachycardia* AND *preserved* (normal) heart function, the following are recommended in *priority order* after vagal maneuvers and administration of adenosine:

  i. Calcium channel blocker: For example, diltiazem, 15–20 mg (0.25 mg/kg) IV over 2 min; may repeat in 15 min at 20–25 mg (0.35 mg/kg) over 2 min; maintenance infusion rate = 5–15 mg/h titrated to heart rate.

  ii. Beta blocker: For example, atenolol, 5 mg IV slowly over 5 min; wait 10 min and then administer a second dose of 5 mg IV slowly over 5 min; in 10 additional minutes, if tolerated well, may begin 50 mg p.o.; then give 50 mg p.o. b.i.d.

  iii. Digoxin: Loading dose = 10 to 15 μg/kg of lean body weight

  iv. DC Cardioversion (refer to section F.4.B.i.)

  v. Consider the following:

     (1) Procainamide: 20 mg/min IV until one of the following occurs:

       • Total dose of 17 mg/kg is administered
       • QRS widens by >50%
       • Hypotension
       • Arrhythmia suppression

     (2) Amiodarone: Maximum cumulative dose = 2.2 g/ 24 h IV; may cause profound vasodilation and hypotension; may be given as follows:

       • *Rapid infusion:* 150 mg IV over the first 10 min (15 mg/min); may repeat rapid infusion (150 mg IV) every 10 min as needed.
       • *Slow infusion:* 360 mg IV over 6 h (i.e., 1 mg/ min).
       • *Maintenance infusion:* 540 mg IV over 18 h (i.e., 0.5 mg/min).

e. For patients with *paroxysmal supraventricular tachycardia* AND *impaired* (i.e., CHF or EF <40%) heart function, the following are recommended in *priority order* after vagal maneuvers and administration of adenosine:

   i. NO DC cardioversion

   ii. Digoxin: Loading dose = 10–15 μg/kg of lean body weight

   iii. Amiodarone (Cordarone): Maximum cumulative dose = 2.2 g/24 h IV; may cause profound vasodilation and hypotension; may be given as follows:

      • *Rapid infusion:* 150 mg IV over the first 10 min (15 mg/min); may repeat rapid infusion (150 mg IV) every 10 min as needed.

      • *Slow infusion:* 360 mg IV over 6 h (i.e., 1 mg/min).

      • *Maintenance infusion:* 540 mg IV over 18 h (i.e., 0.5 mg/min).

   iv. Diltiazem: 15–20 mg (0.25 mg/kg) IV over 2 min; may repeat in 15 min at 20–25 mg (0.35 mg/kg) over 2 min; maintenance infusion rate = 5–15 mg/h titrated to heart rate.

f. For patients with *junctional tachycardia* AND *preserved* (normal) heart function, the following are recommended after vagal maneuvers and administration of adenosine:

   i. NO DC cardioversion

   ii. Amiodarone: maximum cumulative dose = 2.2 g/24 h IV; may cause profound vasodilation and hypotension; may be given as follows:

      • *Rapid infusion:* 150 mg IV over the first 10 min (15 mg/min); may repeat rapid infusion (150 mg IV) every 10 min as needed.

      • *Slow infusion:* 360 mg IV over 6 h (i.e., 1 mg/min).

      • *Maintenance infusion:* 540 mg IV over 18 h (i.e., 0.5 mg/min).

   iii. Beta blocker: e.g.; atenolol, 5 mg IV slowly over 5 minutes; wait 10 min and then administer a second dose of 5 mg IV slowly over 5 min; in 10 additional minutes, if tolerated well, may begin 50 mg p.o.; then give 50 mg p.o. b.i.d.

   iv. Calcium channel blocker: e.g., diltiazem, 15–20 mg (0.25 mg/kg) IV over 2 min; may repeat in 15 min at 20–25 mg (0.35 mg/kg) over 2 min; maintenance infusion rate = 5–15 mg/h titrated to heart rate.

g. For patients with *junctional tachycardia* AND *impaired* (CHF or EF <40%) heart function, the following are recommended after vagal maneuvers and administration of adenosine:

   i. NO DC cardioversion

    ii. Amiodarone: Maximum cumulative dose = 2.2 g/24 h IV; may cause profound vasodilation and hypotension; may be given as follows:

- *Rapid infusion:* 150 mg IV over the first 10 min (15 mg/min); may repeat rapid infusion (150 mg IV) every 10 min as needed.
- *Slow infusion:* 360 mg IV over 6 h (i.e., 1 mg/min).
- *Maintenance infusion:* 540 mg IV over 18 h (i.e., 0.5 mg/min).

h. For patients with *ectopic or multifocal tachycardia* AND *preserved* (normal) heart function, the following are recommended after vagal maneuvers and administration of adenosine:

    i. NO DC cardioversion

    ii. Calcium channel blocker; e.g., diltiazem, 15–20 mg (0.25 mg/kg) IV over 2 min; may repeat in 15 min at 20–25 mg (0.35 mg/kg) over 2 min; maintenance infusion rate = 5–15 mg/h titrated to heart rate.

    iii. Beta blocker: e.g., atenolol, 5 mg IV slowly over 5 min; wait 10 min and then administer a second dose of 5 mg IV slowly over 5 min; in 10 additional minutes, if tolerated well, may begin 50 mg p.o.; then give 50 mg p.o. b.i.d.

    iv. Amiodarone: Maximum cumulative dose = 2.2 g/24 h IV; may cause profound vasodilation and hypotension; may be given as follows:

- *Rapid infusion:* 150 mg IV over the first 10 min (15 mg/min); may repeat rapid infusion (150 mg IV) every 10 min as needed.
- *Slow infusion:* 360 mg IV over 6 h (i.e., 1 mg/min).
- *Maintenance infusion:* 540 mg IV over 18 h (i.e., 0.5 mg/min).

i. For patients with *ectopic or multifocal atrial tachycardia* AND *impaired* (CHF or EF <40%) heart function, the following are recommended after vagal maneuvers and administration of adenosine:

    i. NO DC cardioversion

    ii. Amiodarone: Maximum cumulative dose = 2.2 g/24 h IV; may cause profound vasodilation and hypotension; may be given as follows:

- *Rapid infusion:* 150 mg IV over the first 10 min (15 mg/min); may repeat rapid infusion (150 mg IV) every 10 min as needed.
- *Slow infusion:* 360 mg IV over 6 h (i.e., 1 mg/min).
- *Maintenance infusion:* 540 mg IV over 18 h (i.e., 0.5 mg/min).

    iii. Diltiazem: 15–20 mg (0.25 mg/kg) IV over 2 min; may repeat in 15 min at 20–25 mg (0.35 mg/kg) over 2 min; maintenance infusion rate = 5–15 mg/h titrated to heart rate.

I. Junctional/Nodal (Fig. 18–9)

1. Characteristics

    a. Because the beat originates in the atrioventricular (AV) node, there are usually no P waves preceding QRS complexes.

    b. Occasionally, P waves are retrograde conducted, resulting in a downward deflection either before or after the QRS complex.

    c. Rate is usually 40–60 bpm (i.e., the intrinsic AV node rate).

    d. Accelerated junctional rhythms have the same criteria, but rates range 60–100 bpm.

2. Etiology

    a. Myocardial infarction

    b. Congestive heart failure

    c. Acidosis

    d. Hyperkalemia

3. Treatment

    a. Symptomatic treatment is rarely needed.

    b. Atropine, if patient is severely bradycardic

    c. Consider pacing if patient is severely bradycardic.

J. Pulseless electrical activity (PEA) (Fig. 18–10)

Note: While the rhythm strip in Figure 18–10 illustrates sinus tachycardia, the rhythm would be considered PEA if the patient had no pulse.

1. Characteristics

    a. Formerly called "electrical-mechanical dissociation"

    b. The heart's electrical system is still intact and working, but the heart is not mechanically functioning.

    c. PEA is simply having a rhythm without a pulse.

2. Etiology

Consider the most frequent causes of PEA: "the 5 Hs and 5 Ts":

Hypovolemia	**Tablets** (drug overdose, accidents)
Hypoxia	**Tamponade** (cardiac)
Hydrogen ion (acidosis)	**Tension** (pneumothorax)
Hyper/hypokalemia	**Thrombosis** (coronary syndromes)
Hypothermia	**Thrombosis** (pulmonary embolism)

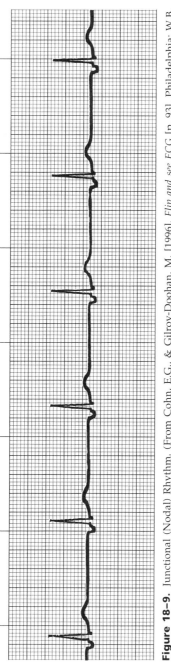

Figure 18–9. Junctional (Nodal) Rhythm. (From Cohn, E.G., & Gilroy-Doohan, M. [1996]. *Flip and see ECG* [p. 93]. Philadelphia: W.B. Saunders, with permission.)

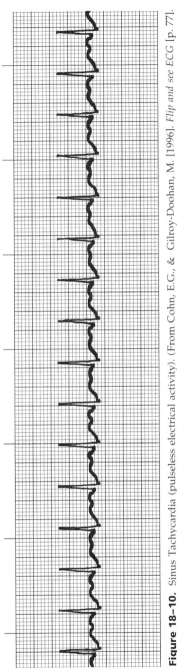

Figure 18–10. Sinus Tachycardia (pulseless electrical activity). (From Cohn, E.G., & Gilroy-Doohan, M. [1996]. *Flip and see ECG* [p. 77]. Philadelphia: W.B. Saunders, with permission.)

3. Treatment

   a. Check responsiveness, activate the emergency response system, and call for a defibrillator.

   b. A–B–Cs:

     i. A—Open airway.

     ii. B—Provide positive pressure ventilations.

     iii. C—Begin chest compressions.

     iv. D—Defibrillation: Assess and shock VF/pulseless VT.

   c. Perform rapid and ongoing secondary assessment, including:

     i. A—Airway: Place airway device as soon as possible (dual lumen airway [e.g., Combi-tube]).

     ii. B—Breathing: Confirm airway device placement by examination and confirmation device; secure airway device (preferably with purpose-made holders); confirm effective oxygenation and ventilation.

     iii. C—Circulation: Establish IV access, establish rhythm per monitor, administer appropriate medications for rhythm and condition, and assess for occult blood flow ("pseudo-EMD").

     iv. D—Differential diagnosis: Search for/treat underlying causes.

   d. Consider the most frequent causes of PEA: "the 5 Hs and 5 Ts":

Hypovolemia	Tablets (drug overdose, accidents)
Hypoxia	Tamponade (cardiac)
Hydrogen ion (acidosis)	Tension (pneumothorax)
Hyper/hypokalemia	Thrombosis (coronary syndrome)
Hypothermia	Thrombosis (pulmonary embolism)

   e. Administer epinephrine, 1 mg IV push, repeated q3–5 min.

   f. Administer atropine if PEA rate is slow, 1 mg IV, repeated q3–5 min as needed until a total dose of 0.04 mg/kg is given.

K. Premature ventricular contractions (PVCs) (Fig. 18–11)

1. Etiology

   a. Irritability of the myocardium due to

     i. Electrolyte imbalances

     ii. Hypoxia

     iii. Acidosis

     iv. Myocardial infarction

     v. Other

   b. A stimulus from the ventricle replaces the SA node as the pacemaker for one or more beats, and contraction occurs without the usual transmission from the atrium.

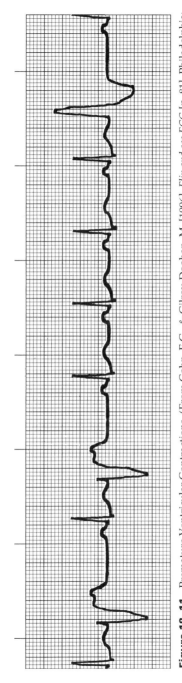

Figure 18–11. Premature Ventricular Contractions. (From Cohn, E.G., & Gilroy-Doohan, M. [1996]. *Flip and see ECG* [p. 81]. Philadelphia: W.B. Saunders, with permission.)

2. Clinical manifestations

    a. Patients may or may not be aware of PVCs.

    b. Symptoms are usually related to the number and frequency of abnormal beats.

    c. Patients may complain of ''fluttering'' or ''palpitations'' of the heart.

    d. On the monitor, PVCs exhibit a wide, bizarre configuration that is very different from that of the normal beat.

3. Implications

    a. PVCs that occur infrequently or have the same focus (i.e., have the same shape, are unifocal) have limited significance and may occur in the absence of heart disease. An increase in the frequency of these beats is more significant, especially if the PVCs occur more often than six times per minute, or if the patient has had a very recent myocardial infarction (Fig. 18–12).

    b. PVCs that are the result of more than one focus (i.e., multifocal) are more serious and may precede ventricular tachycardia or ventricular fibrillation. The risk is minimal if the beats are isolated. The danger increases if the beats are frequent (i.e., more than six per minute), or multifocal (have different shapes) (Fig. 18–13), occur with every other beat

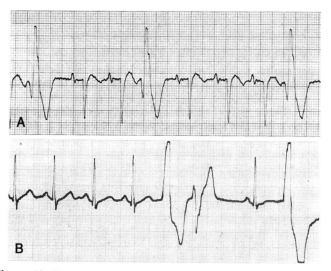

Figure 18–12. *A,* Unifocal PVCs. *B,* Multifocal PVCs. (From Thelan, L. [1997]. *Critical care nursing: Diagnosis and management* [3rd ed.], [p. 416]. St. Louis: Mosby–Year Book, with permission.)

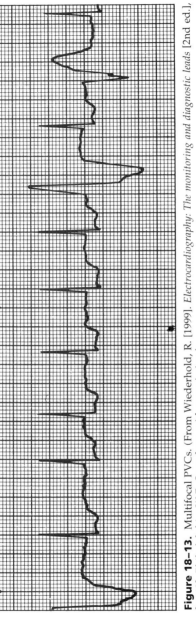

Figure 18–13. Multifocal PVCs. (From Wiederhold, R. [1999]. *Electrocardiography: The monitoring and diagnostic leads* [2nd ed.], [p. 63]. Philadelphia: W.B. Saunders, with permission.)

221

(bigeminal) (Fig. 18–14), with every third beat (trigeminal) (Fig. 18–15), or repetitively (pairs), or appear on the down-slope of the T wave (when the heart is relatively refractory and electrically unstable).

c. If a PVC lands on the downslope of the T wave, the patient may experience ventricular tachycardia and/or ventricular fibrillation.

4. Treatment

a. Drugs
   i. Oxygen
   ii. Lidocaine, 1.0–1.5 mg/kg q 5–10 min, until no ectopy or to a total of 3 mg/kg. If lidocaine resolves ectopy, use continuous lidocaine drip at 2–4 mg/min.
   iii. Consider checking potassium and digoxin levels.
   iv. Repeat lidocaine (as described in section ii.).
   v. Procainamide, 20–30 mg/min until no ectopy, 17 mg/kg reached, or side effects occur. If procainamide resolves ectopy, use continuous procainamide drip at 1–4 mg/min (check blood levels).
   vi. Bretylium (if supply is available), 5–10 mg/kg over 8–10 min. If bretylium resolves ectopy, use continuous bretylium drip at 1–2 mg/min.
   vii. Consider overdrive pacing.

b. Treat the underlying cause.

L. Ventricular tachycardia (VT) (Fig. 18–16)

1. Etiology

a. Irritability of the myocardium
b. A series of ectopic electrical impulses from the ventricles assumes control of the heart rhythm.

2. Clinical manifestations

a. The monitor pattern shows a series of beats with wide, bizarre complexes.
b. If conscious, patients may feel palpitations, be "light-headed," dizzy, or have chest pain.
c. Blood pressure usually drops significantly.
d. A weak pulse may be present.
e. If unconscious, the patient may appear clinically dead and may not have a pulse (treat as ventricular fibrillation) or demonstrate seizure-like activity.
f. Ventricular rate = 120–250 bpm.

3. Implications

a. If untreated, VT produces rapid hemodynamic decompensation due to inadequate filling and emptying of the ventricles.
b. If untreated, VT leads to ventricular fibrillation, asystole, and death.

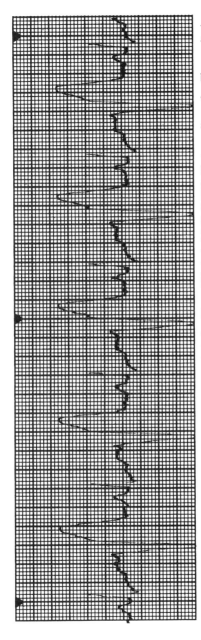

Figure 18–14. Regular Sinus Rhythm with Bigeminal PVCs. (From Wiederhold, R. [1999]. *Electrocardiography: The monitoring and diagnostic leads* [2nd ed.], [p. 65]. Philadelphia: W.B. Saunders, with permission.)

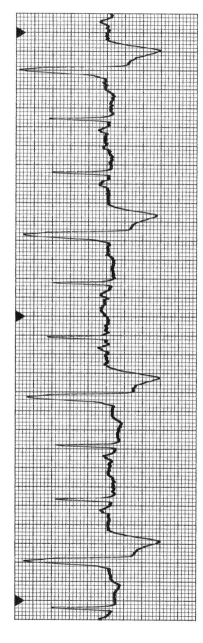

Figure 18–15. Regular Sinus Rhythm and Trigeminal PVCs. (From Wiederhold, R. [1999]. *Electrocardiography: The monitoring and diagnostic leads* [2nd ed.], [p. 66]. Philadelphia: W.B. Saunders, with permission.)

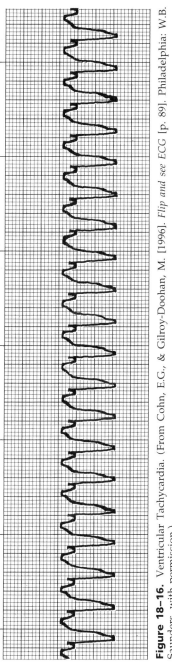

Figure 18–16. Ventricular Tachycardia. (From Cohn, E.G., & Gilroy-Doohan, M. [1996]. *Flip and see ECG* [p. 89]. Philadelphia: W.B. Saunders, with permission.)

4. Treatment of *stable* ventricular tachycardia (VT): Monomorphic or polymorphic
   Note: May go directly to cardioversion.
   a. Monomorphic VT
      i. Assess whether cardiac function is impaired
      ii. For patients with *normal function:*
         (1) Consider *one* of the following medications:
             (a) Procainamide: 20 mg/min IV infusion until one of the following criteria is met:
                 • Total dose of 17 mg/kg is administered
                 • Hypotension
                 • Arrhythmia suppression
                 • QRS widens by >50%
                 (Maintenance infusion dosage = 1–4 mg/min.)
                 OR
             (b) Amiodarone: Maximum cumulative IV dose = 2.2 g/24 h; may be administered by the following:
                 • *Rapid infusion:* 150 mg IV over the first 10 min (15 mg/min); may repeat rapid infusion (150 mg IV) every 10 min as needed.
                 • *Slow infusion:* 360 mg IV over 6 h (i.e., 1 mg/min).
                 • *Maintenance infusion:* 540 mg IV over 18 h (i.e., 0.5 mg/min). OR
             (c) Lidocaine: 1.0–1.5 mg/kg IV push; repeat 0.5–0.75 mg/kg q 5–10 min; maximum total dose = 3 mg/kg; maintenance infusion = 1–4 mg/min (30–50 μg/kg/min)
      iii. For patients with *poor ejection fractions:*
         (1) Administer either amiodarone, 150 mg IV bolus over 10 min, OR
         (2) Lidocaine, 0.5–0.75 mg/kg IV push; THEN
         (3) Employ synchronized cardioversion (refer to section F.4.B.i.), cardioversion with ventricular dysrhythmias begins at 100 J, then 200 J, and so forth.
   b. Polymorphic VT
      i. Assess whether the QT baseline interval is prolonged.
      ii. For patients with a *normal baseline QT interval:*
         (1) Treat ischemia.
         (2) Correct abnormal electrolytes.
         (3) Consider *one* of the following medications:
             (a) Beta blocker: e.g., atenolol, 5 mg IV slowly over 5 min; wait 10 min and then administer a second dose of 5 mg IV slowly over 5 min; in 10 additional minutes, if tolerated well, may begin 50 mg p.o.; then give 50 mg p.o. b.i.d.

(b) Lidocaine: 1.0–1.5 mg/kg IV push; repeat 0.5–0.75 mg/kg q 5–10 min; maximum total dose = 3 mg/kg; maintenance dose = 1–4 mg/min (30–50 μg/kg/min)

(c) Amiodarone: Maximum cumulative dose = 2.2 g/24 h IV; may cause profound vasodilation and hypotension; may be given as follows:
- *Rapid infusion:* 150 mg IV over the first 10 min (15 mg/min); may repeat rapid infusion (150 mg IV) every 10 min as needed.
- *Slow infusion:* 360 mg IV over 6 h (i.e., 1 mg/min).
- *Maintenance infusion:* 540 mg IV over 18 h (i.e., 0.5 mg/min).

(d) Procainamide: 20 mg/min IV infusion until one of the following criteria is met:
- Total dose of 17 mg/kg is administered
- Hypotension
- Arrhythmia suppression
- QRS widens by >50%

(Maintenance infusion dosage = 1–4 mg/min.)

iii. For patients with *prolonged baseline QT intervals* (suggestive of torsades de pointes):

(1) Correct abnormal electrolytes.

(2) Consider one of the following medications/therapies:

(a) Magnesium: Loading dose of 1–2 g mixed in 50–100 mL D5W given over 5–60 min IV; follow with 0.5–1.0 g/h IV (titrate dose to control torsades de pointes).

(b) Overdrive pacing

(c) Isoproterenol (Isuprel): Administer 2–10 μg/min; titrate to adequate heart rate (i.e., VT is suppressed).

(d) Phenytoin (Dilantin): 10–15 mg/kg slowly IV; do not exceed 50 mg/min; maintenance dose = 100 mg IV q 6–8 h; follow each administration by an injection of sterile NS to avoid local venous irritation.

(e) Lidocaine: 1.0–1.5 mg/kg IV push; repeat 0.5–0.75 mg/kg q 5–10 min; maximum total dose = 3 mg/kg; maintenance infusion 1–4 mg/min (30–50 μg/kg/min).

5. Treatment of *unstable* VT (*with* a pulse but with *any* signs of hemodynamic compromise)

a. Consider sedation, e.g., diazepam (Valium), 5 mg, with midazolam (Versed), 2 mg, or other benzodiazepine with midazolam; may also employ a low-dose narcotic (e.g.,

morphine, 2–4 mg) if the patient is not severely hypotensive.
  b. DC Cardioversion at 100 J
  c. DC Cardioversion at 200 J
  d. DC Cardioversion at 300 J
  e. DC Cardioversion at 360 J
  f. Consider lidocaine, 1.5 mg/kg IV; then 0.5–0.75 mg IV q5–10 min until VT resolves or up to 3 mg/kg is given; follow with a continuous drip of 2–4 mg/min.
6. Treatment of *pulseless* VT (See Fig. 18–IIA, p. 240.)
  a. Check responsiveness, activate the emergency response system, and call for a defibrillator.
  b. A–B–Cs:
    i. Open airway.
    ii. Provide positive pressure ventilations.
    iii. Begin chest compressions (CPR for approximately 1 min).
  c. Defibrillate up to 3 times (e.g., 200 J, 300 J, 360 J).
  d. Check rhythm—If persistent or recurrent, continue with the following:
  e. Perform rapid and ongoing secondary assessment, including:
    i. A—Airway: Place airway device as soon as possible (i.e., dual lumen airway [e.g., Combi-tube]).
    ii. B—Breathing: Confirm airway device placement by examination and confirmation device, secure airway device (preferably with purpose-made holders), confirm effective oxygenation and ventilation.
    iii. C—Circulation: Establish IV access, establish rhythm per monitor, and administer appropriate medications for rhythm and condition.
    iv. D—Differential diagnosis: Search for/treat underlying causes.
  f. Administer epinephrine, 1 mg IV push, repeated q3–5 min, OR
  g. Vasopressin, 40 units IV, single dose, one time only; THEN
  h. Defibrillate with 360 J (within 30–60 s).
  i. Following defibrillation, consider the following antiarrhythmics options:
    i. Amiodarone for cardiac arrest states: 300 mg IV push; consider repeating 150 mg IV push in 3–5 min; maximum cumulative dose 2.2 g/24 h. OR
    ii. Lidocaine (indeterminate) for cardiac arrest states from VT/VF: Administer 1.0–1.5 mg/kg IV initially; for refractory VF, may administer another 0.5–0.75 mg/kg IV push, and repeat in 5–10 min; maximal total dose = 3 mg/kg. Note: a single dose of 1.5 mg/kg IV is

also acceptable; endotracheal administration dosage = 2–4 mg/kg; maintenance infusion dosage = 1–4 mg/min (30–50 μg/kg/min).

iii. Magnesium if hypomagnesemia is present or torsades de pointes resulting in cardiac arrest: 1–2 g (2–4 mL of 50% solution) diluted in 10 mL of D_5W given by IV push.

iv. Procainamide for intermittent/recurrent VT/VF: 100 mg IV push given q 5 min; maximum dose = 17 mg/kg; maintenance infusion dosage = 1–4 mg/min.

v. Consider buffers.

j. Defibrillate at 360 J: Defibrillation with 360 J should continue following the administration of each agent above (i.e., "drug, shock, drug, shock," and so forth)

M. Ventricular fibrillation (V-fib) (Fig. 18–17)

1. Etiology

   a. Caused by irritable ventricles due to
      i. Ischemia
      ii. Acidosis
      iii. Electrolyte imbalances
   b. The coordinated contractions of the ventricles are replaced by rapid irregular contractions and twitching of the ventricles.
   c. Electrical activity is not unified.

2. Clinical manifestations

   a. Sudden loss of consciousness and/or seizure-like activity
   b. Absence of pulse or respirations
   c. Cyanosis
   d. Dilated pupils

3. Implications

   a. V-fib results in sudden death unless the dysrhythmia is immediately terminated.
   b. Although V-fib may be reversed, irreversible brain damage may result from lack of perfusion.

4. Treatment: Same as for pulseless ventricular tachycardia—Refer to section L.6.

N. Asystole (Fig. 18–18)

1. Etiology

   a. The electrical force within the heart becomes inadequate to stimulate it, and the ventricles cease to contract.

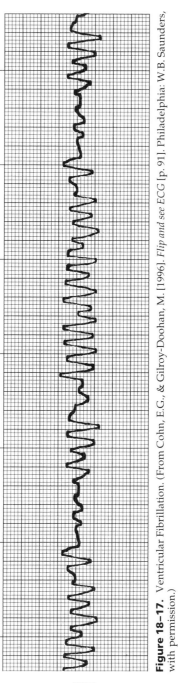

Figure 18–17. Ventricular Fibrillation. (From Cohn, E.G., & Gilroy-Doohan, M. [1996]. *Flip and see ECG* [p. 91]. Philadelphia: W.B. Saunders, with permission.)

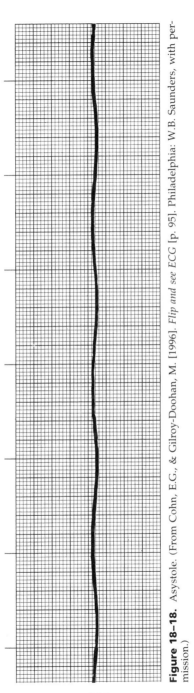

Figure 18–18. Asystole. (From Cohn, E.G., & Gilroy-Doohan, M. [1996]. *Flip and see ECG* [p. 95]. Philadelphia: W.B. Saunders, with permission.)

  b. The end result is a "straight line" on the monitor.
  c. Asystole is often seen with drug overdoses, electrolyte imbalances, and myocardial infarction.

2. Clinical manifestations: Same as V-fib
3. Implications: Same as V-fib

4. Treatment

  a. Check responsiveness, activate the emergency response system, and call for a defibrillator.
  b. A–B–Cs:
    i. A—Open airway.
    ii. B—Provide positive pressure ventilations.
    iii. C—Begin chest compressions and confirm true asystole (check two leads).
    iv. D—Defibrillation: Assess and shock VF/pulseless VT; note: defibrillation is not indicated for asystole.
  c. Perform rapid and ongoing secondary assessment including
    i. A—Airway: Place airway device as soon as possible (i.e., dual lumen airway [e.g., Combi-tube]).
    ii. B—Breathing: Confirm airway device placement by examination and confirmation device, secure airway device (preferably with purpose-made holders), confirm effective oxygenation and ventilation.
    iii. C—Circulation: Confirm true asystole, establish IV access, identify rhythm per monitor, and administer appropriate medications for rhythm and condition
    iv. D—Differential diagnosis: Search for/treat underlying causes.
  d. Transcutaneous pacing—If considered, should be performed immediately.
  e. Administer epinephrine, 1 mg IV push, repeated q 3–5 min.
  f. Administer atropine, 1 mg IV, repeated q 3–5 min as needed until a total dose of 0.04 mg/kg is given.
  g. If asystole persists, consider quality of resuscitation, whether atypical clinical features may be present, and whether to withhold or cease resuscitative efforts.

O. Idioventricular rhythm (Fig. 18–19)

1. Characteristics

  a. A regular, slow rhythm with wide ventricular complexes without P waves
  b. The rate is <40 bpm.

2. Clinical manifestations: Same as for asystole
3. Treatment: Same as for asystole

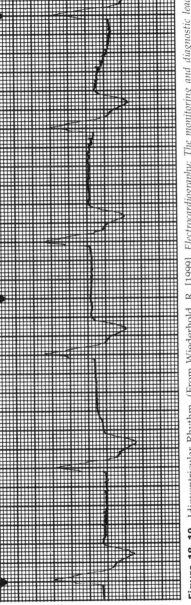

Figure 18–19. Idioventricular Rhythm. (From Wiederhold, R. [1999]. *Electrocardiography: The monitoring and diagnostic leads* [2nd ed.]. [p. 100]. Philadelphia: W.B. Saunders, with permission.)

P. Agonal rhythm (Fig. 18–20)

1. Characteristics

   a. Dying heart beat—Extremely slow, irregular, and becomes slower to the point of asystole
   b. Usually of ventricular nature, but may also have sinus or junctional qualities

2. Clinical manifestations: Same as for asystole
3. Treatment: Same as for asystole

Q. First degree (AV) block (Fig. 18–21)

1. Characteristics

   a. A delay in the impulse from the atria to the ventricles characterized by a PR interval of >0.20 s
   b. Rhythm is regular, and the QRS complex is not affected.

2. Etiology

   a. Occurs in all ages in both normal and diseased hearts
   b. Drugs
      i. Digitalis
      ii. Quinidine
      iii. Procainamide
      iv. Damage to the junction

3. Clinical manifestations: Usually asymptomatic
4. Treatment

   a. Rarely, if ever, needs treatment. *Untreated if asymptomatic.*
   b. Atropine, 0.5–1 mg IV if symptomatic, followed by transcutaneous pacing and preparation for a transvenous pacemaker

R. Second degree block (Mobitz type I) (Wenckebach) (Fig. 18–22)

1. Characteristics

   a. Usually transient and occurs at the AV node
   b. Progressive prolongation of the PR interval until an impulse is completely blocked (dropped)
   c. Then, the pattern usually repeats.
   d. There is also a decreasing R–R interval prior to the blocked beat.
   e. Atrial rhythm is usually regular, and the ventricular rhythm is usually irregular, with progressive shortening of the R–R interval before the blocked impulse.
   f. QRS complex is not affected.

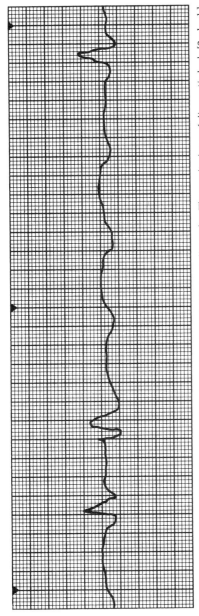

Figure 18–20. Agonal Rhythm. (From Wiederhold, R. [1999]. *Electrocardiography: The monitoring and diagnostic leads* [2nd ed.], [p. 102]. Philadelphia: W.B. Saunders, with permission.)

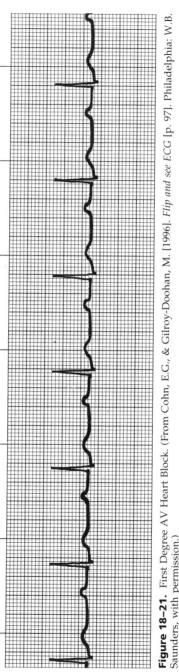

Figure 18–21. First Degree AV Heart Block. (From Cohn, E.G., & Gilroy-Doohan, M. [1996]. *Flip and see ECG* [p. 97]. Philadelphia: W.B. Saunders, with permission.)

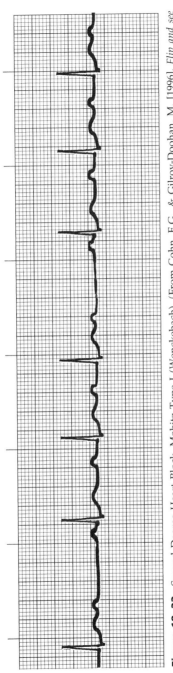

Figure 18–22. Second Degree Heart Block, Mobitz Type I (Wenckebach). (From Cohn, E.G., & Gilroy-Doohan, M. [1996]. *Flip and see ECG* [p. 99]. Philadelphia: W.B. Saunders, with permission.)

2. Etiology
   a. Usually from drug effects (e.g., digitalis, verapamil, propranolol) OR
   b. Myocardial infarction
3. Clinical manifestations
   a. Often asymptomatic
   b. If symptomatic, may see:
      i. Decreased cardiac output
      ii. Hypotension
      iii. Loss of consciousness
4. Treatment
   a. Atropine, 0.5–1 mg IV if symptomatic, followed by transcutaneous pacing and preparation for a transvenous pacemaker
   b. Consider the use of dopamine, 5–20 μg/kg/min, if the patient is severely hypotensive.
   c. Consider epinephrine, 2–10 μg/min, as appropriate.
   d. Obtain serum drug levels of agents prescribed to patient (e.g., digoxin).

S. Second degree block (Mobitz type II) (Fig. 18–23)

1. Characteristics
   a. Usually occurs below the level of the AV node
   b. Associated commonly with an organic lesion in the conduction pathway
   c. Associated with poorer prognosis than Mobitz type I
   d. PR interval does not lengthen prior to a dropped beat.
   e. More than one dropped beat may occur in succession.
   f. Sometimes associated with widened QRS complex
   g. Overall, the atrial rate is unaffected, but the ventricular rate is less than the atrial rate.
2. Etiology
   a. Usually anterior myocardial infarction
   b. Digitalis toxicity is not a cause.
3. Clinical manifestations: Same as second degree type I
4. Treatment
   a. Atropine, 0.5–1 mg IV if symptomatic, followed by transcutaneous pacing and preparation for a transvenous pacemaker
   b. Consider the use of dopamine, 5–20 μg/kg/min, if the patient is severely hypotensive.
   c. Consider epinephrine, 2–10 μg/min, as appropriate.

T. Third degree AV block (complete heart block) (Fig. 18–24)

1. Characteristics
   a. Complete absence of conduction between the atria and the ventricles

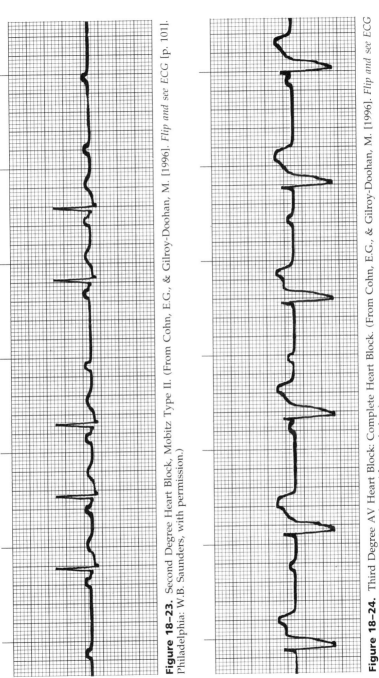

Figure 18–23. Second Degree Heart Block, Mobitz Type II. (From Cohn, E.G., & Gilroy-Doohan, M. [1996]. *Flip and see ECG* [p. 101]. Philadelphia: W.B. Saunders, with permission.)

Figure 18–24. Third Degree AV Heart Block: Complete Heart Block. (From Cohn, E.G., & Gilroy-Doohan, M. [1996]. *Flip and see ECG* [p. 103]. Philadelphia: W.B. Saunders, with permission.)

239

   b. Atrial rate is unaffected, and the ventricular rate is slower than the atrial rate.

   c. Ventricular rate is usually 40–60 bpm.

   d. PR interval will vary, since the atria and ventricles are depolarized from different pacemakers.

2. Etiology

   a. Myocardial infarction is the most common cause.

   b. May also be caused by digitalis toxicity or any other degeneration of the conduction system

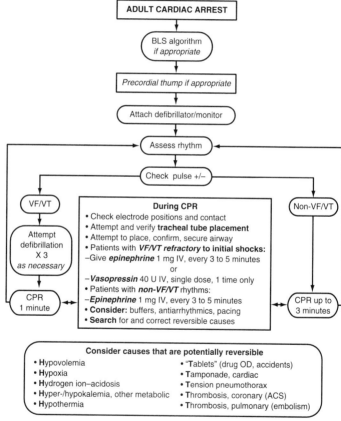

Figure 18–IIA. Universal algorithm for adult advanced cardiovascular life support cardiac care. (Redrawn from Hazinski, M.F., Cummins, R.O., & Field, J.M. [Eds.] [2000]. *2000 Handbook of emergency cardiovascular care for healthcare providers* [p. 8]. Dallas, TX: American Heart Association, with permission.)

Control of Rate and Rhythm

Atrial fibrillation/ atrial flutter with • Normal heart • Impaired heart • WPW	1. Control Rate		2. Convert Rhythm	
	Heart Function Preserved	**Impaired Heart EF <40% or CHF**	**Duration <48 Hours**	**Duration >48 Hours or Unknown**
Normal cardiac function	**Note:** If AF >48 hours' duration, use agents to convert rhythm with extreme caution in patients not receiving adequate anticoagulation because of possible embolic complications. Use only 1 of the following agents (see note below): • Calcium channel blockers (Class I) • β-blockers (Class I) • For additional drugs that are Class IIb recommendations, see Guidelines or ACLS text	(Does not apply)	**Consider:** • DC cardioversion Use only 1 of the following agents (see note below): • Amiodarone (Class IIa) • Ibutilide (Class IIa) • Flecainide (Class IIa) • Propafenone (Class IIa) • Procainamide (Class IIa) • For additional drugs that are Class IIb recommendations, see Guidelines or ACLS text	• **NO DC cardioversion!** • **Note:** Conversion of AF to NSR with drugs or shock may cause embolization of atrial thrombi unless patient has adequate anticoagulation. • Use antiarrhythmic agents with extreme caution if AF >48 hours' duration (see note above) *or* ***Delayed cardioversion*** **Anticoagulation X 3 weeks at proper levels** • Cardioversion, *then* • Anticoagulation X 4 weeks more *or* ***Early cardioversion*** • Begin IV heparin at once • TEE to exclude atrial clot ***then*** • Cardioversion within 24 hours ***then*** • Anticoagulation X 4 more weeks
Impaired heart (EF <40% or CHF)	(Does not apply)	Note: If AF >48 hours' duration, use agents to convert rhythm with extreme caution in patients not receiving adequate anticoagulation because of possible embolic complications. Use only 1 of the following agents (see note below): • Digoxin (Class IIb) • Diltiazem (Class IIb) • Amiodarone (Class IIb)	**Consider:** • DC cardioversion *or* • Amiodarone (Class IIb)	**Consider:** • Anticoagulation as described above, followed by • **DC cardioversion**

WPW indicates Wolff-Parkinson-White syndrome; AF, Atrial fibrillation; NSR, normal sinus rhythm; TEE, transesophageal echocardiogram; and EF, ejection fraction.

Note: Occasionally 2 of the named antiarrhythmic agents may be used, but use of these agents in combination may have proarrythmic potential. The classes listed represent the Class of Recommendation rather than the Vaughn-Williams classification of antiarrhythmics.

Figure 18–IIB. Tachycardia: Atrial fibrillation and flutter. (Redrawn from Hazinski, M.F., Cummins, R.O., & Field, J.M. [Eds.] [2000]. *2000 Handbook of emergency cardiovascular care for healthcare providers* [pp. 16–17]. Dallas, TX: American Heart Association, with permission.)

Figure continues on next page.

Control of Rate and Rhythm

Atrial fibrillation/ atrial flutter with • Normal heart • Impaired heart • WPW	1. Control Rate		2. Convert Rhythm	
	Heart Function Preserved	**Impaired Heart EF <40% or CHF**	**Duration <48 Hours**	**Duration >48 Hours or Unknown**
WPW	**Note:** If AF >48 hours' duration, use agents to convert rhythm with extreme caution in patients not receiving adequate anticoagulation because of possible embolic complications. • DC cardioversion *or* • **Primary anti-arrythmic agents** Use only 1 of the following agents (see note below): • Amiodarone (Class IIb) • Flecainide (Class IIb) • Procainamide (Class IIb) • Propafenone (Class IIb) • Sotalol (Class IIb) **Class III** **(Can be harmful)** • Adenosine • β-blockers • Calcium blockers • Digoxin	**Note:** If AF >48 hours' duration, use agents to convert rhythm with extreme caution in patients not receiving adequate anticoagulation because of possible embolic complications. • DC cardioversion *or* • Amiodarone (Class IIb)	• DC cardioversion *or* • **Primary anti-arrythmic agents** Use only 1 of the following agents (see note below**): • Amiodarone (Class IIb) • Flecainide (Class IIb) • Procainamide (Class IIb) • Propafenone (Class IIb) • Sotalol (Class IIb) **Class III** **(Can be harmful)** • Adenosine • β-blockers • Calcium blockers • Digoxin	• **Anticoagulation** as described above, followed by • **DC cardioversion**

Note: Occasionally 2 of the named antiarrhythmic agents may be used, but use of these agents in combination may have proarrhythmic potential. The classes listed represent the Class of Recommendation rather than the Vaughn-Williams classification of antiarrhythmics.

Figure 18–IIB *Continued*

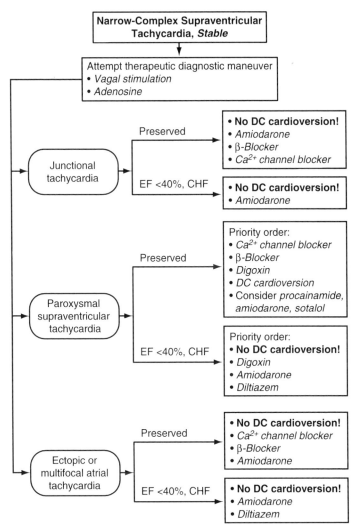

Figure 18–IIC. Narrow-complex tachycardia. (Redrawn from Hazinski, M.F., Cummins, R.O., & Field, J.M. [Eds.] [2000]. *2000 Handbook of emergency cardiovascular care for healthcare providers* [p. 18]. Dallas, TX: American Heart Association, with permission.)

3. Clinical manifestations

    a. Asymptomatic if the ventricular rate is adequate

    b. Otherwise, progressive decrease in cardiac output, loss of consciousness

4. Treatment

    a. Atropine, 0.5–1 mg IV if symptomatic, followed by transcutaneous pacing and preparation for a transvenous pacemaker

    b. Consider the use of dopamine, 5–20 μg/kg/min, if the patient is severely hypotensive.

    c. Consider epinephrine, 2–10 μg/min, as appropriate.

    d. Obtain serum drug levels of agents prescribed to patient.

II. ALGORITHMS FOR CARDIAC EMERGENCIES[2, 8, 9]

A. Universal algorithm for adult advanced cardiovascular life support cardiac care (Fig. 18–IIA)

B. Tachycardia: Atrial fibrillation and flutter (Fig. 18–IIB)

C. Narrow-complex tachycardia (Fig. 18–IIC)

References

1. Cohn, E.G., & Gilory-Doohan, M. (1996). *Flip and see ECG.* Philadelphia: W.B. Saunders.

2. Cummins, R.O. (Ed.) (1997). *Advanced cardiac life support 1997–1999.* American Heart Association.

3. DiGregorio, G.J., & Barbieri, E.J. (1998). *Handbook of commonly prescribed drugs* (13th ed.). West Chester, PA: Medical Surveillance, Inc.

4. Gwinnutt, C.L. (1998). Advanced life support in adults. *Pre-Hospital Immediate Care, 2,* 27–34.

5. Hazinski, M.F., Cummins, R.O., & Field, J.M. (Eds.) (2000). *2000 Handbook of Emergency Cardiovascular Care for Healthcare Providers.* Dallas, TX: American Heart Association.

6. Karch, A.M. (Ed.) (2000). *Lippincott's nursing drug guide 2000.* Philadelphia: J.B. Lippincott.

7. Mancini, M.E., & Kaye, W. (1999). AEDs changing the way you respond to cardiac arrest. *American Journal of Nursing, 99,* 26–30.

8. Saver, C.L. (1994). Decoding the ACLS algorithms. *American Journal of Nursing, 94,* 27–36.

9. Thelan, L.A., Urden, L.D., Lough, M.E., & Stacy, K.M. (1998). *Critical care nursing: Diagnosis and management* (3rd ed.). St. Louis: Mosby.

10. Wiederhold, R. (1998). *Electrocardiography: The monitoring lead* (2nd ed.). Philadelphia: W.B. Saunders.

Management of Patients with Pulmonary Disorders

DIAGNOSTIC CONCEPTS OF OXYGENATION AND VENTILATION

Judith Azok, MSN, RN, ARNP, GNP-C

I. PULMONARY PERFUSION[2, 6, 7, 9, 14]

A. Definition

Movement of mixed venous blood through the pulmonary capillary bed for the purpose of gas exchange between the blood and alveolar air

B. The pulmonary vascular system is a high-volume system with low capillary resistance.

1. Pulmonary blood flow is about 6 L/min.
2. The mean pulmonary arterial pressure is 15 mmHg.

C. Regional differences in blood flow in the lungs

1. Lung bases receive a greater percentage of blood flow than do the apices.
2. Factors that affect distribution of pulmonary blood flow

   a. Gravity and hydrostatic pressure differences within the blood vessels: Blood must flow against gravity to the apices when a person is in the upright position.
   b. Effect of alveolar pressure: Alveolar pressure may be greater than pulmonary capillary pressure in the apical and middle regions of lungs because of
      i. Positive pressure ventilation
      ii. Decreased right ventricular preload (decreased hydrostatic pressure), dehydration, hemorrhage
      iii. Air trapping: chronic obstructive pulmonary disease
   c. Effect of decreased P_{AO_2} (alveolar gas): Local reflex that causes vasoconstriction of pulmonary arterioles supplying hypoxic alveoli

II. VENTILATION[1, 2, 6, 8, 10–12]

A. Definition

1. The mechanical movement of air into and out of the alveoli for the purpose of gas exchange between the atmosphere and capillary blood
2. Gas flows from higher atmospheric to lower intrapulmonary pressure during inhalation.

B. Regulation of ventilation

1. CNS control

   a. Brain stem centers (medulla and pons): Cells fire automatically to trigger inhalation; others fire to halt inhalation; exhalation occurs passively.

   b. Cerebral cortex: Allows voluntary control to override brain stem centers in response to chemical stimuli and lung inflation changes

2. Chemical regulation

   a. *Central* chemoreceptors in medulla respond to ↑ $Paco_2$ (hypercapnia) and decreased pH (acidosis) through medullary stimuli by increasing ventilatory depth and rate; hypercapnia is the major stimulus to alter ventilation.

   b. *Peripheral* chemoreceptors in aortic and carotid bodies respond to ↓ Pao_2 (hypoxemia) by stimulating medullary centers to increase ventilation.

   c. Patients with chronically high $Paco_2$: Hypercapnic ventilatory drive is lost; these patients respond only to changes in Pao_2 by stimulation of peripheral receptors in order to adjust ventilation (hypoxemic respiratory drive).

      i. Supplemental O_2: Administer low liter flows very carefully to prevent apnea (e.g., begin 1–2 L/min and assess).

      ii. Do not withhold O_2 if needed; be prepared to assist with mechanical ventilation if respiratory drive is depressed.

C. Work of breathing (WOB)

1. Definition: The amount of effort required to overcome the elastic and resistive properties of the lungs and chest wall

2. Elasticity (elastic recoil): The tendency of the lungs to return to their original shape

   a. Lungs try to collapse because of tension between the interstitial elastic fibers and the surface of the alveoli.

   b. Chest wall attempts to resist inward-moving recoil.

3. Compliance: Measure of distensibility or how easily the lungs and thorax can be stretched; describes resistance as a result of elastic properties

   Note: ↑ Compliance: Less pressure needed to stretch lungs and/or thorax

   a. High compliance: Easier to expand lung tissue (e.g., chronic obstructive pulmonary disease)

   b. Low compliance: Stiff lungs; chest wall less distensible (e.g., pneumonia, acute respiratory distress syndrome)

4. Resistance is determined by the radius of the airway through which air is flowing.

   Note: ↑ Resistance: ↑ Effort for ventilation → ↑ WOB

D. Alveolar ventilation (V_a): Amount of air that reaches alveoli and participates in gas exchange

1. Pa_{CO_2}: Best indicator of V_a
2. Normal: Pa_{CO_2} = 35–45 mmHg

III. ALVEOLAR DIFFUSION[1, 2, 4, 7, 11, 13, 14]

A. Definition

Exchange of O_2 and CO_2 across the alveolocapillary membrane

1. Oxygen diffuses down the concentration gradient from higher alveolar pressure (Pa_{O_2}) to lower pulmonary capillary pressure (Pa_{O_2}).
2. CO_2 diffuses at a *rate* 20 times greater than that of O_2 from capillary to alveolus.

B. A-a gradient: Alveolar-to-arterial oxygen gradient

Aa_{DO_2}: Alveolar-to-arterial oxygen difference

1. A *calculation* to aid in diagnosing the degree of a patient's hypoxemia
2. *Formula:* Difference between partial pressure of O_2 in the alveoli (Pa_{O_2}) and partial pressure of O_2 in arterial blood (Pa_{O_2})
   Pa_{O_2}: calculated
   Pa_{O_2}: from arterial blood gases

   Note: A-a gradient OR Aa_{DO_2} = Pa_{O_2} − Pa_{O_2}

   a. Formula to calculate Pa_{O_2}

   Pa_{O_2} = [Fi_{O_2} × (Pb − PH_2O)] − Pa_{CO_2}/0.8 (Resp. Quotient)
   Fi_{O_2} = Fraction of inspired oxygen: 21–100%
   Pb = Barometric pressure: 760 mmHg (at sea level)
   PH_2O = Water vapor pressure: 47 mmHg

   $$Pa_{O_2} = [0.21 \times (760 - 47)] - 40/0.8$$
   $$Pa_{O_2} = 0.21 \times 713 - 50$$
   $$Pa_{O_2} = 100 \text{ mmHg}$$
   $$\text{Normal } Pa_{O_2} = 60\text{--}100 \text{ mmHg}$$

3. Normal values: Difference between alveolar and arterial oxygen

   a. Young adult breathing room air (Fi_{O_2} = 21%): <10 mmHg difference
   b. Adult >60 years of age on room air: <20 mmHg difference
   c. Breathing Fi_{O_2} 100 % = <50 mmHg difference

IV. OXYGEN TRANSPORT IN THE CIRCULATION[2–5, 7, 8, 11–13]

A. O_2 carried in the blood

1. O_2 dissolved in plasma (3% of total) = Pa_{O_2}; normal = 80–100 mmHg.

2. O_2 bound to hemoglobin (Hgb) (97% of total) = Sao_2; normal = 95–100%.

> Note: Reserve for times of increased demand.

Note: Assess Hgb level for oxygen-carrying capacity. If Hgb level is decreased yet adequately saturated, the patient is *not* adequately oxygenated.

B. Pao_2 and Sao_2: Indirect measurement of O_2 *available* to tissues

C. O_2 that stays bound to Hgb is useless to body cells.

1. Affinity: Ability of Hgb to release O_2

   a. Weak affinity: Easily releases O_2 to tissues
   b. Strong affinity: Easily accepts and retains O_2

D. Oxyhemoglobin dissociation curve: Demonstrates affinity of Hgb for O_2

1. Flat part of curve: *Binding* portion in lungs.

   a. Increased affinity; binds easily: Pao_2 is 60–100 mmHg, with $Sao_2 > 90\%$.

2. Steep part of curve: *Dissociation* portion at the tissue level

   a. Weaker affinity: Hgb readily dissociates O_2 when Pao_2 falls <60 mmHg.

E. Shifts in oxyhemoglobin dissociation curve: Other patient variables affect affinity of Hgb for O_2.

1. Shift to the *left*: Greater affinity

   a. Binds easily in lung; less unloading to tissues
   b. Increased affinity → possible tissue hypoxia due to strong bond between Hgb and O_2; need for O_2 may have decreased
   c. Causes
      i. Alkalosis
      ii. Hypothermia
      iii. Decreased 2,3-diphosphoglycerate

2. Shift to the *right*: Decreased affinity

   a. Hgb unloads more O_2 to tissues.
   b. Delivery of O_2 to tissues improves as long as loading of O_2 in lungs is adequate.
   c. Causes
      i. Acidosis
      ii. Increased tissue metabolism, anaerobic metabolism, hyperthermia
      iii. Increased 2,3-diphosphoglycerate

F. Continuous Svo_2 monitoring: Monitoring O_2 transport and extraction

1. Measure of mixed venous O_2 saturation by the pulmonary artery catheter

   a. Continuous measure and display of mixed venous oxygen saturation
   b. Hgb reflects light, which can be measured according to its saturation.

2. Normal Svo_2: 75%; Hgb unloads 25% of its O_2 before returning to the heart.

   a. Normal ratio of supply of O_2 to demand: 4 : 1
   b. Acceptable Svo_2 range: *60–80%*

Venous blood gases	Arterial blood gases
pH = 7.36	pH = 7.4
$Pvco_2$ = 47 mmHg	$Paco_2$ = 40 mmHg
Hco_3 = 24 mEq/L	Hco_3 = 24 mEq/L
Pvo_2 = 40 mmHg	Pao_2 = 100 mmHg
Svo_2 = 75%	Sao_2 = 99%
Hgb = 15 g	Hgb = 15 g

3. Trends in *changes* in Svo_2: Assesses the effectiveness of peripheral oxygen delivery; may signal need to assess cardiac profile

   a. Svo_2 <60% or trend downward: Patient has tapped the venous reserve of O_2
      i. Implies increased tissue extraction of O_2

         Note: Greater risk for anaerobic metabolism

      ii. Causes
         (1) ↓ O_2 supply (e.g., ↓ Fio_2, anemia, ↓ CO)
         (2) ↑ O_2 demand (e.g., fever, ↑ WOB, shivering)
      iii. Svo_2 <40% = anaerobic metabolism → organ dysfunction
   b. Svo_2 >80%: Implies decreased tissue extraction of oxygen
      i. High return of O_2 is often an earlier indicator of change in patient status than change in hemodynamic parameters.
      ii. Causes
         (1) ↑ O_2 supply (e.g., Fio_2 > need, polycythemia)
         (2) ↓ O_2 demand (e.g., sleep, hypothermia)
         (3) ↓ effective O_2 delivery and uptake by cells (e.g., sepsis, cyanide toxicity, shift of O_2/Hgb curve to left)

G. Oxygen supply/demand balance: Calculations

ROI_2 = Venous O_2 return to heart	DOI_2 = Arterial O_2 delivery to tissues

$$= \text{Cardiac Index} \times (\text{venous } O_2 \text{ content}) \times 10$$
$$= CI \times (1.34 \times Hgb \times Svo_2) \times 10$$
$$= 3 \times (1.34 \times 15 \times .75) \times 10$$
$$= 3 \times (15) \times 10$$
$$= 450 \text{ mL/min/m}^2$$

$$= \text{Cardiac Index} \times (\text{arterial } O_2 \text{ content}) \times 10$$
$$= CI \times (1.34 \times Hgb \times Sao_2) \times 10$$
$$= 3 \times (1.34 \times 15 \times .98) \times 10$$
$$= 3 \times (20) \times 10$$
$$= 600 \text{ mL/min/m}^2$$

$$\dot{V}o_2 = \text{Tissue } O_2 \text{ demand}$$
$$DOI_2 - ROI_2 = VO_2$$
$$600 \text{ mL} - 450 \text{ mL} = 150 \text{ mL/min/m}^2$$
$$\text{Prolonged} \downarrow Svo_2 \text{ and/or prolonged} \downarrow Vo_2 \rightarrow \text{poor prognosis}$$

References

1. Bucher, L., & Melander, S. (1999). *Critical care nursing.* Philadelphia: W.B. Saunders.
2. Chuly, M., Guzzetta, C., & Dossey, B. (1997). *AACN handbook of critical care nursing.* Stamford, CT: Appleton & Lange.
3. Dickson, S. (1995). Understanding the oxyhemoglobin dissociation curve. *Critical Care Nurse, 15,* 54–58.
4. Goodfellow, T. (1997). Application of pulse oximetry and the oxyhemoglobin dissociation curve respiratory management. *Critical Care Nurse Quarterly, 10,* 22–27.
5. Gopinath, S., Valadka, A., Uzura, M., & Robertson, C. (1999). Comparison of jugular venous oxygen saturation and brain tissue PO_2 as monitors of cerebral ischemia after head injury. *Critical Care Medicine, 27,* 2337–2345.
6. Hudak, C., Gallo, B., & Marten, P. (1998). *Critical care nursing: A holistic approach* (7th ed.). Philadelphia: J.B. Lippincott.
7. Misasi, R., & Keyes, J. (1996). Matching and mismatching ventilation and perfusion in the lung. *Critical Care Nurse, 16,* 23–38.
8. Palmer, C., & Grave, S. (1996). Developing the nursing diagnosis of impaired oxygenation: Abnormally low SVO_2 value. *Critical Care Nurse, 16,* 69–76.
9. Roberts, S.L. (1996). *Critical care nursing: Assessment and intervention.* Stamford, CT: Appleton & Lange.
10. Rupport, S., Kernicki, J., & Dolan, T. (1996). *Dolan's critical care nursing: Clinical management through the nursing process* (2nd ed.). Philadelphia: F.A. Davis.
11. Schallom, L., & Ahrens, T. (1999). Using oxygenation profiles to manage patients. *Critical Care Clinics of North America, 11,* 437–446.
12. Schumacker, P. (1998). Oxygen supply dependency in critical illness: An evolving understanding. *Intensive Care Medicine, 24,* 97–99.
13. Tasatar-Erhard, M. (1995). The effect of patient position on arterial oxygen saturation. *Critical Care Nurse, 15,* 31–36.
14. Thelan, L.A., Davie, J.K., Urden, L.D., & Taugh, M.E. (1998). *Critical care nursing: Diagnosis and management* (3rd ed.). St. Louis: Mosby.

MEASURES OF OXYGENATION AND VENTILATION

John P. McGuinness, MD

I. OXYGENATION AND VENTILATION[7, 10, 13]

A. Definition

1. Closely related terms but *not identical* in meaning
2. The term *oxygenation* refers to the content of oxygen in blood and the adequacy of oxygen transport and is determined by the partial pressure of oxygen present in the alveoli, condition of the alveolar capillary membrane, amount of hemoglobin, and cardiac output.
3. *Ventilation* refers to the exchange of oxygen and carbon dioxide at the alveolar capillary membrane. As a rough approximation, oxygenation is best measured by Pao_2 (or, by extension, the peripheral oxygen saturation, Spo_2), and ventilation is measured by $Paco_2$. There are a number of measurement techniques for these terms.

B. Clinical measurements

1. Exercise tolerance: The ability to perform a normal exercise load (e.g., climb a flight of stairs without stopping) suggests adequate oxygenation and ventilation.
2. Air hunger: Ask the patient, "Are you getting enough air?"
3. Cyanosis: A bluish tint due to the presence of excessive amounts of deoxygenated hemoglobin; the more central the cyanosis, the greater its severity. For example, cyanosis evident on the face and chest is more severe than cyanosis limited to the fingertips.
4. Arterial blood gases (ABGs): Measurement of ABGs allows determination of the partial pressure of oxygen and carbon dioxide as well as pH.

   a. Normal values for arterial blood gas
      i. pH = 7.35–7.45
      ii. Pao_2 = 80–97 mmHg
      iii. $Paco_2$ = 35–45 mmHg
      iv. HCO_3 = 22–26 mEq/L
      v. Base excess −3 to +3 mEq/L
      vi. Arterial oxygen saturation >98%
   b. The partial pressures of arterial oxygen and carbon dioxide, and arterial oxygen saturation will decline as altitude above sea level increases.

   c. Interpret Pa_{O_2} in light of F_{IO_2}. As a general rule, the Pa_{O_2} should be five times the F_{IO_2} (e.g., the F_{IO_2} of room air is 21%, and an acceptable Pa_{O_2} is 95–100 mmHg).

   d. Interpret pH in light of Pa_{CO_2}. For every 10 mmHg shift in Pa_{CO_2}, a pure respiratory acidosis will cause a reciprocal change in pH of 0.08 (e.g., if the measured Pa_{CO_2} is 50 mmHg, the pH due to purely respiratory causes should be 7.32). A lower or higher value of the measured pH would be attributed to a metabolic acidosis or metabolic alkalosis, respectively.

C. Limitations

1. Invasiveness

   a. Drawing blood for an ABG measurement is often painful for the patient, even at the hands of an experienced technician.

   b. If frequent measurements are required, as in a critically ill or mechanically ventilated patient, an indwelling arterial catheter should be placed.

2. An ABG is not a continuous measurement.

   a. ABG is accurate only at the time it is obtained.

   b. A more continuous measurement would be peripheral oxygen saturation, measured by a pulse oximeter or an end-tidal CO_2 measurement device.

3. The ABG sample must be handled with care.

   a. The sample must not be allowed to clot and must be heparinized.

   b. Excessive amounts of heparin in a small blood sample will alter the pH.

   c. Any air bubbles must be expelled from the syringe because the oxygen and carbon dioxide in the sample will equilibrate with the air bubble.

   d. If more than a few minutes may pass before the sample is measured, it must be chilled to limit the ongoing metabolism of the cellular components.

II. PULSE OXIMETRY[10–12]

A. Definition

1. Pulse oximetry is a noninvasive, continuous, and relatively inexpensive method to measure the percentage of oxyhemoglobin during pulsatile blood flow

2. Inexpensive devices are available to measure oxygen saturation, and the measurement may become as ubiquitous as determinations of blood pressure.

B. Mechanism

1. Pulse oximetry utilizes a light-emitting diode to transmit light in the trans-red and near-infrared wavelengths; this light is variably absorbed by oxygenated and deoxygenated blood.
2. Blood is measured during pulsatile and nonpulsatile blood flow, and the higher blood saturation level is displayed as the SpO_2.
3. The pulse oximetry probe is typically placed on a digit but can be placed on an earlobe, cheek, nose, or toe.
4. It is not always necessary to remove nail polish to obtain an accurate reading; often, an accurate reading can be obtained across the pad of the finger or at another site.
5. The pulse oximetry probe may be applied continuously.
6. The accuracy of the reading is affected by hemoglobin concentration; ideally, hemoglobin should be >10 mg/dL.

C. The normal values are variable and must be interpreted in light of altitude, the patient's age, and cardiopulmonary function.

1. The pulse oximetry reading is a percentage of saturation of the available hemoglobin and not a partial pressure.

   a. The number must be interpreted in light of the oxyhemoglobin saturation curve.
   b. Factors that influence the dissociation curve, such as pH, must be considered as well.

2. Remember that the relationship between oxygen saturation and partial pressure of oxygen is nonlinear. It is prudent to commit to memory that

   a. SpO_2 of 90% represents a PaO_2 of 60 mmHg
   b. SpO_2 of 75% is a PaO_2 of 40 mmHg
   c. SpO_2 50% is a PaO_2 of 27 mmHg

D. Limitations of pulse oximetry

1. Pulse oximetry does not provide information regarding pH, $PaCO_2$, or respiratory rate.
2. Pulse oximetry is confounded by the presence of carbon monoxide.

   a. The device will misinterpret carboxyhemoglobin as oxyhemoglobin and thereby provide a falsely elevated reading.
   b. When carbon monoxide poisoning is suspected, an ABG analysis is a more reliable measurement of oxygenation.

3. Pulse oximetry is confounded by the presence of certain intravascular dyes.

a. Methylene blue dye will be misinterpreted by the oximeter as deoxygenated hemoglobin, thus indicating a falsely lowered oxygen saturation.
b. Similarly, methemoglobinemia will confound pulse oximetry sensors.

4. Pulse oximetry is most valuable as a reading of *central* oxygenation.

a. Occasionally, a peripherally placed oximeter sensor will not be indicative of central oxygenation.
b. Circumstances in which a peripherally placed oximeter will not be indicative of central oxygenation include hypothermia and severe peripheral vascular disease.

5. Pulse oximetry is also influenced by hemoglobin concentration.

a. However, it is important to remember that pulse oximetry measures oxygen saturation, not oxygen content.
b. For example, an anemic patient may have a high oxygen saturation but a low oxygen content.

III. PULMONARY ARTERY CATHETERIZATION[1-3, 5, 6]

A. Definition
Technique in which a balloon-tipped catheter is placed through a large vein into the vena cava, and then through the right side of the heart and into the pulmonary artery

B. General description

1. The pulmonary artery catheter is typically 70 cm in overall length and is inserted up to 50 cm. The catheter contains three lumina.

a. One for a proximal port
b. One for a distal port located at the tip of the catheter
c. One for an inflatable balloon that is located a few centimeters proximal to the distal end

2. Most pulmonary artery catheters have a temperature sensor at the tip that not only provides an accurate core temperature, but also permits calculation of cardiac output via a thermodilution technique.
3. Newer versions of the catheter are antibiotic-impregnated and may include an oxygen sensor.
4. The optimal position of the pulmonary artery catheter is in zone III of the lung.

a. Zone III is characterized by a continuous flow of blood.
b. The pulmonary artery pressure in zone III exceeds the pulmonary venous pressure.

   c. The pulmonary venous pressure in zone III in turn exceeds the intra-alveolar pressure.

C. Indications for placement

1. Pulmonary artery catheterization is especially useful in determining a patient's volume status.

   a. A hypotensive patient with a high pulmonary wedge pressure would not benefit from additional volume loading.
   b. A hypotensive patient with a low wedge pressure would benefit from a fluid bolus.

2. Pulmonary catheters are valuable in determining a patient's cardiac output and cardiac index.

D. Contraindications to the placement of a pulmonary artery catheter

1. No absolute contraindications
2. Relative contraindications include

   a. Latex allergy
   b. Thrombocytopenia
   c. Coagulopathies
   d. Left bundle branch blocks (for fear of damaging the functioning right bundle branch during catheter placement)

E. Information provided by the pulmonary catheter is extensive; however, pulmonary artery catheterization requires skill both in using pressure transducers and in interpreting analog tracings.

1. The proximal port indicates pressure in the central venous space. This port is also useful for administering vasoactive medications.
2. The distal port, when the balloon is deflated, measures pulmonary artery pressures.
3. When the balloon is inflated, the pressure at the distal port at the end of expiration reflects the pulmonary capillary wedge pressure (PCWP), which serves as an approximation of the left ventricular end-diastolic pressure or preload.
4. The temperature probe accurately measures core temperature.
5. Cardiac output can be determined using a thermodilution technique via the proximal port. Knowledge of cardiac output allows computation of the systemic vascular resistance.

F. Complications

1. Thrombocytopenia—May be associated with prolonged catheter placement
2. Pulmonary hemorrhage—May occur with balloon hyperinflation or inflation in a hypothermic patient. Pulmonary hemorrhage is usually heralded by hematemesis.

3. Cardiac rhythm disturbances may occur, especially during catheter placement as the tip of the catheter impinges on the ventricular wall.

4. Sepsis—Always a risk with intravascular foreign bodies

IV. FLUID RESUSCITATION[4, 8, 9]

A. Definition

Process in which intravascular volume is replaced to ensure optimal cardiac output, thereby providing adequate perfusion to vital organs

B. Indicators of inadequate intravascular volume

1. Decreased urine output—less than 0.5 mL/kg/h
2. Capillary refill time >3 s
3. Obvious massive blood loss, as may result from trauma or obstetric hemorrhage
4. Evidence of significant preload reduction, such as hypotension and tachycardia.

   a. It is important to remember that not all hypotension is due to hypovolemia.
   b. Careful consideration must be given to other common causes, such as cardiac dysfunction and neurogenic shock.

C. Fluid resuscitation in a seriously ill patient should be managed in a critical care setting.

1. Consideration should be given to the placement of adequate monitoring devices, including

   a. An arterial catheter for monitoring and sampling purposes
   b. A urinary bladder catheter to provide an accurate measurement of urine production.

2. In addition, the patient's body temperature must be monitored during large volume resuscitations.

   a. Substantial amounts of room-temperature fluids or chilled blood products can rapidly chill a patient.
   b. Ideally, fluids should be warmed before administration.

3. At least one, preferably two, 16-gauge intravenous catheters in antecubital vessels may be lifesaving.

   a. Concerns about the limitation of the patient's ability to flex an arm should be deferred until the patient's condition is stabilized.
   b. Generally, a longer catheter is better tolerated by the patient than a shorter catheter.

D. Choices for fluid resuscitation

1. Packed red blood cells (RBCs)

   a. Have largely taken the place of fresh whole blood
   b. Fluid of choice for major hemorrhage
   c. Each unit of red cells typically increases the hematocrit of a 70-kg person by 3%.

2. Fresh frozen plasma (FFP)

   a. Should *not* be used in fluid resuscitation
   b. Should be used instead for coagulopathies

3. Crystalloid solutions

   a. Normal saline is a good choice for routine fluid resuscitation.
   b. Lactated Ringer's solution has a wider variety of elemental constituents than normal saline and is commonly employed in the operating suite.
   c. Dextrose-containing solutions come in a wide variety of concentrations.
      i. They should be used only after considering the patient's need for dextrose.
      ii. Dextrose-containing solutions are not first-line agents for volume expansion.

4. Colloid solutions, such as albumin, may be thought of as intravascular sponges that absorb volume from the extravascular space and hold it in the intravascular space.

   a. Unfortunately, this holding effect is transient and does little to correct the primary problem of decreased intravascular volume.
   b. Colloid solutions should be reserved for specific indications.

E. Adequacy of fluid resuscitation may be judged by clinical indicators such as

1. Urine output
2. Improved capillary refill time
3. Vital signs
4. Specific hemodynamic parameters such as PCWP

References

1. Cowley, C.G., & Lloyd, R. (1999). Interventional cardiac catheterization advances in nonsurgical approaches to congenital heart disease *Current Opinions in Pediatrics, 11,* 425–432.
2. Findlay, J.Y., Harrison, B.A., Plevak, D.J., & Krowka, M.J. (1999). Inhaled nitric oxide reduces pulmonary artery pressures in portopulmonary hypertension. *Liver Transplant Surgery, 5,* 381–387.

3. Fontes, M.L., Bellows, W., Ngo, L., & Mangano, D.T. (1999). Assessment of ventricular function in critically ill patients: Limitations of pulmonary artery catheterization. Institutions of the McSPI Research Group. *Journal of Cardiothoracic and Vascular Anesthesia, 13*, 521–527.

4. Glupczynski, Y., & Sibille, Y. (1999). Nosocomial pneumonia: Diagnosis, epidemiology and treatment. *Acta Clinica Belgium, 54*, 178–190.

5. Koobi, T., Kaukinen, S., & Turjanmaa, V.M. (1999). Cardiac output can be reliably measured noninvasively after coronary artery bypass grafting operation [see comments]. *Critical Care Medicine, 27*, 2206–2211.

6. Marik, P.E. (1999). Pulmonary artery catheterization and esophageal Doppler monitoring in the ICU. *Chest, 116*, 1085–1091.

7. McCarthy, M.C., Cline, A.L., Lemmon, G.W., & Peoples, J.B. (1999). Pressure control inverse ratio ventilation in the treatment of adult respiratory distress syndrome in patients with blunt chest trauma. *American Surgeon, 65*, 1027–1030.

8. Murphy, J.T., Horton, J.W., Purdue, G.F., & Hunt, J.L. (1999). Cardiovascular effect of 7.5% sodium chloride-dextran infusion after thermal injury. *Archives of Surgery, 134*, 1091–1097.

9. Novak, L., Shackford, S.R., Bourguignon, P., Nichols, P., Buckingham, S., Osler, T., & Sartorelli, K. (1999). Comparison of standard and alternative prehospital resuscitation in uncontrolled hemorrhagic shock and head injury. *Journal of Trauma, 47*, 834–844.

10. Robertson, P.W., & Hart, B.B. (1999). Assessment of tissue oxygenation. *Respiratory Care Clinics of North America, 5*, 221–263.

11. Shoemaker, W.C., Thangathurai, D., Wo, C.C., Kuchta, K., Canas, M., Sullivan, M.J., Farlo, J., Roffey, P., Zellman, V., & Katz, R.L. (1999). Intraoperative evaluation of tissue perfusion in high-risk patients by invasive and noninvasive hemodynamic monitoring. *Critical Care Medicine, 27*, 2147–2152.

12. Smith, R.P., Argod, J., Pepin, J.L., & Levy, P.A. (1999). Pulse transit time: An appraisal of potential clinical applications. *Thorax, 54*, 452–457.

13. Valta, P., Uusaro, A., Nunes, S., Ruokonen, E., & Takala, J. (1999). Acute respiratory distress syndrome: Frequency, clinical course, and costs of care [In Process Citation]. *Critical Care Medicine, 27*, 2367–2374.

THE CHEST X-RAY

John P. McGuinness, MD, and
David A. Miller, MD, FCCP

I. GENERAL PRINCIPLES[1, 2]

A. Anteroposterior (AP) films are usually obtained with a portable x-ray machine in the case of critically ill patients.

B. Posteroanterior (PA) films

1. These films are usually obtained in the x-ray suite.
2. Because the patient's heart is closer to the film in the PA position, these studies depict the heart size more accurately than do AP films.

C. Heart size, or, more accurately, the cardiac shadow, is a major component of the chest x-ray. The size of the cardiac shadow is contingent on several factors.

1. Because of the spatial relationships between the x-ray beam source, the patient's heart, and the film cassette, the heart may appear artificially enlarged.
2. The cardiac shadow appears larger on inspiration than on expiration.
3. The cardiac shadow is larger in a supine patient than in a standing patient.

D. Lateral films are usually obtained in the x-ray suite.

1. The lateral view is particularly useful in evaluating structures in the posterior mediastinal and retrocardiac spaces.
2. This view is also useful in evaluating the thoracic vertebrae.

E. Adequacy of the film

1. X-ray beam penetration may be judged by the clarity of the vertebrae viewed when the beam is passed through the sternum. The vertebral bodies should be visible.

   a. An overpenetrated film, i.e., one in which the x-ray beam is too intense, will have lost evidence of subtle pathology; the earliest pathologic changes will have been ''burned through'' and rendered invisible.
   b. An underpenetrated film will be uninterpretable; an insufficiently intense x-ray beam will not reveal adequate detail.

2. The symmetry of the clavicles is an indicator of chest rotation.

   a. The clavicles should be approximately equal in length.

b. The clavicular heads should be in the center of the film.
c. Excessive rotation will distort anatomic relationships and heart size.

II. READING A CHEST X-RAY[5, 8]

A. A systematic approach is helpful in reading a chest x-ray.

1. To ensure that you are looking at the proper film

a. Identify the patient.
b. Verify the date and time of the film.

2. When multiple chest x-rays have been obtained, it is useful to look at the films in sequential order.

B. Examine the bony structures visible in the film.

1. Look for evidence of both old and new fractures (particularly in children).
2. Evaluate bone density in older patients.
3. Examine

a. Clavicles
b. Ribs
c. Vertebrae—Best seen in the lateral view

C. Examine the pulmonary parenchyma.

1. Always look for evidence of pneumothorax.

a. Ensure that the pulmonary markings extend throughout the lung fields and especially up to the apices.
b. Be especially vigilant for indications of pneumothorax
   i. In mechanically-ventilated patients
   ii. In patients who have sustained blunt or penetrating chest trauma

2. Because much of the parenchyma consists of air-filled structures, pay particular attention to evidence of fluid-filled alveoli.

a. Fluid-filled alveoli appear as radiodensities.
b. They may be suggestive of heart failure or pneumonia.

3. The lines visible in the medial pulmonary parenchyma are indicators of intravascular volume status and are caused by vascular structures rather than bronchi.

a. Lines in the periphery are called Kerley's lines; exaggeration of these lines is often caused by interstitial edema from congestive heart failure.
b. The specific Kerley lines are named as follows:
   i. Kerley A lines are several inches long and extend from the hilum.

    ii. Kerley B lines begin at the lung bases and radiate from the pleura.

    iii. Kerley C lines extend throughout the lungs.

4. Look for atelectasis.

   a. Typically found in a lobar or segmental pattern

   b. Suggestive of collapsed or fluid-filled alveoli from which air has been displaced

D. Examine the cardiac shadow.

1. Heart size is influenced by

   a. The patient's body habitus; thinner people typically have thinner hearts than heavier people.

   b. Degree of inspiration can be judged by the number of visible ribs.

   c. When the film is obtained in diastole, it will show a larger cardiac silhouette than a film taken in systole.

2. Specific features of cardiac anatomy

   a. On the shadow from the right side of the heart, the ascending aorta and right atrium can be identified.

   b. On the shadow from the left side of the heart, prominent structures include

     i. The aortic knob

     ii. The left pulmonary artery

     iii. The left atrial appendage

     iv. The left atrium

     v. The left ventricle

E. Examine the diaphragm and visible abdominal structures.

1. The diaphragm separates the thoracic cavity from the abdominal cavity.

2. Ensure that there is not a layer of air outlining the diaphragm; the presence of such a layer suggests a perforated abdominal viscus.

3. Look for evidence of the presence of abdominal structures in the thoracic cavity (e.g., a diaphragmatic hernia).

4. The chest x-ray often includes a portion of the abdominal viscera. Look at the included portions of bowel for evidence of obstruction, such as distended loops of bowel or multiple air-fluid levels.

5. Always evaluate the area immediately inferior to the diaphragm for evidence of free air. The presence of subdiaphragmatic free air suggests a perforated hollow viscus.

F. Examine the chest x-ray for the correct placement of lines and tubes.

1. Endotracheal tubes should be in the trachea, with the tip of the tube above the carina.
2. Gastric tubes should extend beneath the diaphragm and into the gastric air bubble.
3. Pulmonary artery catheters should be seen to extend into the pulmonary vasculature without curling or looping in the heart chambers.
4. Duodenal tubes should be seen below the diaphragm, extending across the left side and into the right side of the abdomen, suggesting that the tube has traversed the pylorus.

III. HELPFUL SIGNS[4, 6]

A. Silhouette sign

1. Conceptually, a silhouette that is ordinarily present is obliterated by an abnormal density, i.e., tissues of different organs that have similar densities will obliterate the margins between the organs.
2. An infiltrate in the lingular portion of the left upper lobe or the right middle lobe of the lung obliterates a normally visible portion of the cardiac border.

B. Consolidation

1. An air bronchogram is formed when the alveoli adjacent to a bronchiole are consolidated, thus outlining the air remaining in the bronchiole.
2. Usually, airways beyond the main stem are not visible, but if adjacent lung tissue is consolidated or collapsed, the airway will be outlined.

IV. SPECIFIC DISEASE ENTITIES[3, 7]

A. Congestive heart failure—Often manifested by an enlarged cardiac shadow and increased pulmonary vascular markings
B. Pericardial effusions

1. Chest x-ray is not sensitive enough to detect pericardial effusions.

    a. Changes in the size of the cardiac silhouette seen in serial films may, however, be suggestive of an effusion.
    b. Previous films should be reviewed to recognize and note subtle changes.

2. Cardiac echocardiography is more reliable than chest x-ray to detect pericardial effusions.

C. Emphysema

1. Pulmonary parenchyma tends to be more lucent than normal, reflecting the loss of tissue and hyperinflation.

2. Cardiac silhouette is often narrow.
3. Diaphragmatic domes are often flattened.

D. Pneumonia

1. A chest x-ray is an essential part of the initial workup of a suspected pneumonia.
2. Pneumonia is suspected when an infiltrate is seen in a specific segment of the lung. The diagnosis of pneumonia requires clinical and laboratory findings as well.
3. Improvement in the appearance of a chest film often lags behind clinical improvement by a factor of weeks.

E. Pulmonary nodules (also called coin lesions)

1. A nodule is defined as a lesion <6 cm in size. Larger lesions are referred to as "masses."
2. Solitary nodules should always be evaluated.
3. The most valuable method for evaluation of a pulmonary nodule is comparison with earlier films.

    a. Benign nodules are more often found in nonsmokers under age 35 years.
    b. Benign nodules tend to be calcified.
    c. Calcifications in benign nodules are typically described as central, laminar, diffuse, or popcorn.
    d. Nodules described as eccentric or stippled may be either benign or malignant.
    e. Benign nodules tend to remain unchanged over time.

4. Computerized tomography is useful in evaluating questionable nodules.
5. Nodules may be followed with serial chest x-rays.

    a. Repeat the chest x-ray in 1 month.
    b. Then repeat every 6 months for 2 years.

6. If the nodule has not changed in 2 years, it is likely to be benign.
7. Cytologic examination of sputum has only limited value in the evaluation of pulmonary nodules.

References

1. Chapman, W.W., & Haug, P.J. (1999). Comparing expert systems for identifying chest x-ray reports that support pneumonia. *Proceedings of the AMIA Symposium*, 216–20.
2. Fiszman, M., Chapman, W.W., Evans, S.R., & Haug, P.J. (1999). Automatic identification of pneumonia related concepts on chest x-ray reports. *Proceedings of the AMIA Symposium*, 67–71.
3. Katz, D.S., & Leung, A.N. (1999). Radiology of pneumonia. *Clinical Chest Medicine, 20*, 549–562.
4. Knisely, B.L., Mastey, L.A., Collins, J., & Kuhlman, J.E. (1999). Imaging of cardiac transplantation complications. *Radiographics, 19*, 321–39.

5. Krupinski, E.A., Evanoff, M., Ovitt, T., Standen, J.R., Chu, T.X., & Johnson, J. (1998). Influence of image processing on chest radiograph interpretation and decision changes. *Academic Radiology, 5*, 79–85.
6. Kurihara, Y., Yakushiji, Y.K., Nakajima, Y., Niimi, H., Arakawa, H., & Ishikawa, T. (1999). The vertical displacement sign: A technique for differentiating between left and right ribs on the lateral chest radiograph. *Clinical Radiology, 54*, 367–369.
7. Ng, C.S., Wells, A.U., & Padley, S.P. (1999). A CT sign of chronic pulmonary arterial hypertension: the ratio of main pulmonary artery to aortic diameter. *Journal of Thoracic Imaging, 14*, 270–278.
8. Obayashi, Y., Fujita, J., Suemitsu, I., Kamei, T., Nii, M., & Takahara, J. (1999). Successive follow-up of chest computed tomography in patients with Mycobacterium avium-intracellulare complex. *Respiratory Medicine, 93*, 11–15.

DIFFERENTIAL DIAGNOSIS OF PULMONARY DISORDERS

22

David A. Miller, MD, FCCP

I. SYMPTOM POSSIBILITIES AND ORIGINS[1-5]

A. Major symptoms suggesting a pulmonary disorder

1. Dyspnea

    a. Air flow obstruction and/or altered ventilation/perfusion relationship

    b. Altered pulmonary compliance

    c. Respiratory muscle weakness

2. Cough

    a. Mucus

    b. Foreign body

    c. Exposure to noxious stimuli

    d. Bronchospasm

3. Production of sputum or blood—Hemoptysis: below the vocal cords

4. Chest pain

    a. Cardiac

    b. Pleural

    c. Pericardial

    d. Esophageal

    e. Vascular

5. "Noisy" breathing

    a. Wheezing

    b. Retained secretions

    c. Snoring with obstruction to air flow

6. Altered mental status or daytime functioning

B. Potential origins of symptoms (pathophysiologic alterations) in the thorax

1. Pulmonary parenchyma—Altered ventilation and/or perfusion

2. Pulmonary vasculature—Altered perfusion

3. Trachea and bronchi—Altered secretion and/or air flow

4. Chest wall, pleura, and pericardium

    a. Altered perfusion and/or ventilation

    b. Altered sense of comfort in breathing

5. Great vessels—Altered comfort
6. Esophagus—Altered comfort
7. Hemoglobin

   a. Altered perfusion
   b. Altered systemic oxygen distribution

8. Heart and cardiac valves—Altered sense of comfort in breathing
9. Constitutional changes

   a. Altered body temperature
   b. Altered appetite and/or weight
   c. Altered sweating/chills

C. Special considerations

1. The lung parenchyma—Absent pain fibers below the glottis
2. The chest wall and pleura—Pain with ventilation and/or with movement of the chest
3. Changes in sputum

   a. Color
   b. Amount
   c. Production
   d. Expectoration

4. Hemoptysis

   a. Lung infection
   b. Tumor
   c. Anticoagulation
      i. Medical therapy
      ii. Severe intrinsic liver disease
      iii. Thrombocytopenia
   d. A source of bleeding above the vocal cords is not considered hemoptysis but, rather, is believed to be related to the upper airway or gastrointestinal tract.

5. Circadian variation in symptoms

   a. Usual increase in airway resistance between 2 AM and 6 AM
   b. Aggravation of symptoms during periods of recumbency

6. Chest pain during the night—Usually of cardiac and/or esophageal origin
7. Chest pain 3 to 4 h after rising—Usually cardiac in origin
8. Chest pain after meals—Usually of esophageal and/or cardiac origin

D. Detailing symptoms referable to breathing in differential diagnosis of breathing problems

1. About what is the patient complaining?
2. When did the apparent problem actually begin?

3. To what does the patient attribute the problem?
4. Does the review of symptoms suggest systemic rather than localized disease?
5. Are risk factors known?
6. Are comorbidities present?

II. RISK FACTORS AND COMORBIDITIES[1, 3, 4]

A. Risk factors for respiratory problems other than work-related causes

1. Lighted tobacco

    a. Cigarettes
    b. Pipes
    c. Cigars

2. "Recreational" drug use

    a. Marijuana
    b. Cocaine

3. Particulate matter

    a. Dust with or without household mites
    b. Pollens
    c. Molds
    d. Pollution

4. Household chemicals

    a. Cleaning materials
        i. Ammonia
        ii. Bleach
    b. Insecticides

5. Reaction to airborne allergens
6. Known or suspected autoimmune disorder
7. Exposure to pets (including animal dander) and exotic birds

B. Comorbidities

1. Heart disease
2. Esophageal disease
3. Chest trauma/surgery
4. Other surgery (especially pelvic and orthopedic)
5. Venous insufficiency/edema
6. Recent travel
7. Malignancy
8. Immobility
9. Diabetes mellitus

III. EXPOSURE TO ENVIRONMENTAL RISKS: WORK AND MEDICATIONS[1-4]

A. Work-related exposure to substances that create risk

1. Chemical toxins (examples)

   a. Toluene diisocyanate
   b. Chlorine
   c. Fluorine
   d. Insecticides

2. Particulate matter (examples)

   a. Asbestos
   b. Fiberglass
   c. Smoke
   d. Moldy agricultural material

B. Medication-induced respiratory problems

1. Dry cough

   a. ACE inhibitors
   b. Certain chemotherapeutic agents

2. Dyspnea

   a. Amiodarone
   b. Beta blockers

3. Hemoptysis

   a. Aspirin
   b. Coumadin
   c. Heparin
   d. Platelet-activation inhibitors

4. Wheezing—Beta blockers
5. Pulmonary infiltrates

   a. Methotrexate
   b. Amiodarone
   c. Others

IV. EXPOSURE TO INFECTIOUS AGENTS[1, 3, 4]

A. Traditional seasonal respiratory pathogens

1. Winter

   a. Influenza
   b. Pneumococcal pneumonia

2. Spring

   a. *Mycoplasma pneumoniae*
   b. *Chlamydia pneumoniae*

3. Summer: *Legionella pneumophila*

B. Additional pathogens that exacerbate chronic respiratory problems

1. Gram-positive: *Streptococcus pneumoniae*
2. Gram-negative

   a. *Moraxella catarrhalis*
   b. *Haemophilus influenzae*
   c. Others (especially in chronic pulmonary disorders)
      i. *Klebsiella pneumoniae*
      ii. *Pseudomonas aeruginosa*

C. Exposure to mycobacterial infections

1. *Mycobacterium tuberculosis*—Increased risk with affected family member or close significant other
2. Atypical mycobacteria—*Mycobacterium avium-intracellulare* (Mycobacterium-avium complex)

D. Geographic-based fungal infections

1. Histoplasmosis

   a. Upper Midwest
   b. Mississippi River

2. Coccidioidomycosis

   a. Desert Southwest
   b. San Joaquin Valley

E. Immunodeficiency-based pulmonary infections associated with HIV infection, chemotherapy, congenital conditions, and transplant-related immunosuppression

1. Mycobacteria (see C. Exposure to mycobacterial infections)
2. Protozoa

   a. *Pneumocystis carinii*
   b. *Toxoplasma gondii*

3. Bacteria
4. Viral

   a. Cytomegalovirus
   b. Varicella zoster

5. Fungal infections, including aspergillosis

References
1. Albert, R., Spiro, S., & Jett, J. (Eds.). (1999). *Comprehensive respiratory medicine*. London: Mosby.
2. Barker, L.R., Burton, J.R., & Zieve, P.D. (Eds.). (1999). *Principles of ambulatory medicine* (5th ed.). Baltimore: Williams & Wilkins.

3. Fauci, A.S., Braun E., Isselbacher, K.J., Wilson, J.D., Martin, J.B., Kasper, D.L., Hauser, S.L., & Longo, D.L. (Eds). (1998). *Harrison's principles of internal medicine* (14th ed.). New York: McGraw-Hill.
4. Goldman, L., & Bennett, J.C. (Eds.). (2000). *Cecil textbook of medicine* (21st ed.). Philadelphia: W.B. Saunders.
5. Tierney, L.M., McPhee, S.J., & Papadakis, M.A. (Eds.). (1999). *Current medical diagnosis & treatment* (38th ed.). Stamford, CT: Appleton & Lange.

PULMONARY FUNCTION TESTING

David A. Miller, MD, FCCP

I. PULMONARY FUNCTION TESTING

A. Purpose of a pulmonary function test (PFT)[1, 2]

1. To determine the existence of a ventilatory defect that may then be used to

   a. Assign a potential diagnosis to explain a patient's symptoms
   b. Differentiate between obstruction of airways and decreased pulmonary parenchymal compliance as the source of a patient's symptoms
   c. Evaluate the response to treatment of a pulmonary disease process

2. Indications for a PFT

   a. Evaluate unexplained dyspnea and cough
   b. Assess severity of pulmonary pathology
   c. Determine potential reversibility of airway obstruction

3. Limitations of the PFT

   a. The patient must be able to cooperate with the testing; inadequate cooperation negates the value of the testing.
   b. The patient should be relatively stable with respect to symptoms. Temporary worsening of symptoms may invalidate the determination of severity of dysfunction present.

B. Types of PFT

1. Spirometry

   a. Determines the forced vital capacity and forced expiratory flow rates
   b. If expiratory air flow obstruction is defined, the response to an aerosolized bronchodilator should be measured.
      i. An increase of 15–20% or more is often accepted as a reason to use a bronchodilator.
      ii. However, a smaller improvement in flow rate in the presence of more severe obstruction is a reason to consider using a bronchodilator.

2. Spirometry with bronchodilator challenge (evaluation for bronchospasm)

   a. Determines the vital capacity and expiratory flow rates before and after aerosolized bronchodilator challenge

b. Degree of responsiveness may be useful in determining the need for bronchodilator therapy.

3. Body plethysmography
   a. Useful in determining all lung volumes, including
      i. Vital capacity (measured during spirometry)
      ii. Residual volume in the chest after expiration
      iii. Total lung capacity
   b. More completely differentiates between a restrictive ventilatory defect (lowered lung volumes) and an obstructive ventilatory defect (increased total lung volume and residual volume)

C. Understanding "normal" values or "predicted" values

1. PFT laboratories use a comparison of the patient being studied with a larger population of persons of similar age, gender, height, and weight.
2. The nomograms used vary among laboratories and may prevent absolute comparison when testing is done in different locations.

D. Lung volume measurements and the meaning of lung "capacities" (Tables 23–1 and 23–2)

1. Lung volume is reported as a single value.
2. Lung capacity refers to the combination of one or more lung volumes.

TABLE 23–1. LUNG VOLUMES AND LUNG CAPACITIES

LUNG VOLUME	LUNG CAPACITY	
Inspiratory reserve volume (IRV) The amount of air that can be inhaled following a full inspiration	**Vital Capacity (Forced; FVC)**	**Total Lung Capacity (TLC)**
Tidal volume (VT) The amount of air inhaled or exhaled during a normal breath		
Expiratory reserve volume (ERV) The amount of air that can be forced out of the lungs following a full expiration		
Residual volume (from plethysmography) **(RV)** The amount of air remaining in the lungs following a forced expiration		

TABLE 23–2. EXPIRATORY FLOW RATES

FLOW RATE MEASUREMENT	PARAMETER ASSESSED Comment on Effort Dependency
FEV_1: Forced expiratory volume in 1 second	Central and smaller airways Effort-dependent
FEV_1% (FEV_1/FVC): FEV_1 as a percentage of the vital capacity	How much of the vital capacity can be exhaled forcibly in one second Effort-dependent
FEF25–75: Expiratory flow rate over the midportion of expiration	Small airways Relatively effort-independent

E. Determination of the presence of obstructive and restrictive ventilatory defects

1. Obstructive ventilatory defects

   a. Flow rate is reduced compared with normal values for similar persons.
   b. Lung volumes generally are within normal range or are larger than normal because of air trapping and hyperinflation (with increased reserve volume and total lung capacity).

2. Restrictive ventilatory defects

   a. Flow rates may be normal.
   b. Lung volumes and expiratory flow rates are proportionally reduced.

F. Determining severity of defects (lung volumes and flow rates)

1. Values over 70% of predicted volumes/flow rates are considered within normal limits.
2. Values 60–70% of predicted volumes/flow rates are mildly reduced.
3. Values 50–60% of predicted volumes/flow rates are moderately reduced.
4. Values lower than 50% of predicted volumes/flow rates are severely reduced.
5. When the values for the residual volume and total lung capacity exceed 120% of predicted, air trapping and hyperinflation are present.
6. If air flow obstruction is present, bronchodilator responsiveness is considered significant if the expiratory air flow measurements improve at least 15% over baseline values.

a. The absence of such a response is, by itself, not justification for withholding these medications.
b. Bronchodilators may improve other parameters of lung function, including secretion clearance.

G. The peak expiratory flow meter and asthma[3]

1. A simple and inexpensive device (indeed, usually provided by pharmaceutical companies that manufacture bronchodilators) intended for home use by asthmatics and those with other forms of potentially reversible airway obstruction
2. Ideally, the patient will measure his or her peak expiratory flow rate (PEFR) at least once daily initially, at the same time each day, to provide a measure of functional air flow limitation over time.

   a. Values are recorded in a diary provided with the device.
   b. The patient's "best" flow rate, typical flow rates, and altered flow rates may then be used to determine the need for additional medication.
      i. PEFR 80–100% of baseline, the "green" zone: No change in therapy is necessary.
      ii. PEFR 50–80% of baseline, the "yellow" zone: Temporary increase in intensity of therapy, or additional therapy, should be considered.
      iii. PEFR below 50% of baseline, the "red" zone: Urgent/emergency care is advised.

References

1. Albert, R., Spiro, S., & Jett, J. (Eds.). (1999). *Comprehensive respiratory medicine*. London: Mosby.
2. Goldman, L., & Bennett, J.C. (Eds.). (2000). *Cecil textbook of medicine* (21st ed.). Philadelphia: W.B. Saunders.
3. National Asthma Education and Prevention Program. (1997). Expert Panel Report 2: Guidelines for the Diagnosis and Management of Asthma. National Institutes of Health Pub No. 97-4051. Bethesda: NIH.

OBSTRUCTIVE (VENTILATORY) LUNG DISEASES

David A. Miller, MD, FCCP

I. CHRONIC OBSTRUCTIVE PULMONARY DISEASE (COPD)[1-7, 10]

A. Definition

1. COPD is a mixture of diseases, including emphysema, chronic bronchitis, and bronchospastic airway disease, all characterized by limitation of expiratory air flow.
2. Acute exacerbations are superimposed upon chronic symptoms.

B. Etiologies/Incidence

1. Tobacco smoking (cigarettes, cigars, pipes) is the most common cause.

   a. Most persons who smoke a pack of cigarettes per day for over 40 years will have manifestations of COPD.
   b. Note: One pack of cigarettes per day multiplied by the number of years smoked equals the number of pack-years of cigarettes smoked.

2. Inhalation of environmental pollutants (e.g., oxides of sulfur and nitrogen): The incidence depends on exposure in heavily polluted areas.
3. Occupational exposure to inorganic chemicals (chlorine, fluorine) and organic chemicals (toluene, for example) may result in airway obstruction.

C. Subjective findings

1. Cough, dry and occasionally productive, especially in the early morning
2. Sputum production

   a. Usually clear in color, but may be discolored (e.g., yellow, purulent, or green)
   b. A change in the amount produced or the color of the sputum is important in management decisions.

3. Exertional dyspnea
4. Weight loss with progressive disease owing to early satiety and difficulty breathing after food is consumed
5. Fatigue

6. Complaints of chest tightness, owing either to

   a. Alterations that are slowly occurring in the chest wall (e.g., increase in anteroposterior chest diameter), or to
   b. Acute air retention within the thorax

D. Physical examination findings

1. General

   a. Respiratory rate is normal or increased.
   b. Mental status should be alert and oriented.
   c. Note sitting position for presence of classic "emphysema stance."
      i. The patient sits with the chest forward and the arms straightened.
      ii. The upper body is lifted to allow for greater expansion of the chest as gravity pulls the abdominal contents downward and away from the diaphragm.
   d. Inspect for clubbing of the nail beds (chronic bronchitis, bronchiectasis) and for pursed-lip breathing.

2. Chest inspection

   a. Increase in the anteroposterior diameter of the chest
      i. Giving rise to a "barrel" configuration
      ii. Normally, the diameter of the chest from axilla to axilla is about twice the anteroposterior diameter.
   b. Use of accessory muscles of respiration
      i. Sternocleidomastoids
      ii. Intercostals

3. Chest percussion

   a. Hyper-resonance
   b. Low diaphragm

4. Chest auscultation

   a. Diminished breath sounds throughout the chest
   b. Prolonged forced expiratory time (Auscultation while asking the patient to forcibly exhale shows that the effort to exhale the air requires over 3 s.)
   c. Rhonchi on inspiration and/or expiration, especially when secretions are increased
   d. Occasional wheezing on expiration
      i. Asthma
      ii. Chronic bronchitis

E. Laboratory/Diagnostic findings

1. Pulmonary function testing

   a. Expiratory flow rates are reduced.
      i. Early disease: Reduction in small airway flow rates

    ii. Late disease: Reduction in FEV_1 (forced expiratory volume in 1 s, a measure of the potential for severe complications of COPD)

  b. Lung volume changes

    i. Air trapping indicated by increased residual volume

    ii. Hyperinflation indicated by increased total lung capacity

    iii. Forced vital capacity may be reduced by air trapping.

    iv. Related to the reduction in air flow, the reduction in the forced vital capacity is, on a percentage of normal basis, less than the percentage reduction in predicted expiratory air flow.

2. Arterial blood gases and pulse oximetry

  a. Earlier in the course of disease, and often during the later stages, both studies show normal oxygenation and ABGs show no evidence of chronic respiratory acidosis.

  b. Seen more frequently later in the course of disease, or during exacerbations of moderately severe disease

    i. Hypoxemia (Pao_2 <55 mmHg)

    ii. Hypercarbia (chronic respiratory acidosis)

  c. During acute exacerbations of COPD, hypoxemia and acute hypercarbia may be seen.

    i. Assessment requires at least one arterial blood gas analysis.

    ii. Increasing respiratory distress and changes in mental status (confusion; stupor) require more frequent checks of arterial blood gases.

  d. Pulse oximetry

    i. Used frequently to assess for adequacy of oxygen transport within the blood at rest and during exertion

    ii. Adequate oxygenation is implied when Sao_2 >88% when the hemoglobin level is above 10 g/dL.

3. Other laboratory values

  a. Hemoglobin and hematocrit

    i. Hemoglobin <10 g/dL may be suboptimal for oxygen transport.

    ii. Hematocrit >55 mL/dL is evidence for secondary polycythemia due to chronic hypoxemia.

  b. Serum bicarbonate is elevated with chronic hypercarbia.

4. Chest x-ray

  a. Air trapping

  b. Blebs and bullae (dilated air spaces within the pulmonary parenchyma)

  c. Flattened diaphragm

F. Nonpharmacologic management

1. Nonpharmacologic therapy using heated or cooled aerosols of water may help thin airway secretions in combination with chest physiotherapy.
2. The value of chest physiotherapy (percussion and postural drainage) in COPD is controversial, but it may be worthwhile when patients perceive a benefit from it.

G. Pharmacologic management[7, 8]

1. Anticholinergic agents

   a. Decrease airway secretions and airway smooth muscle tone
   b. Agent of choice in COPD: Ipratropium bromide (Atrovent), 2 puffs q.i.d.; also premixed in saline for use in hand-held nebulizer
      i. Mainstay of therapy for COPD
      ii. Side effects: Dry mouth and dry, hacky cough

2. Bronchodilators

   a. Beta-2 adrenergic receptor agonists
      i. Reduce airway smooth muscle tone
      ii. Stimulate ciliary motion to promote secretion mobilization
   b. Short-acting inhaled agents: Metered dose inhaler, 2 puffs q.i.d. and as needed, or premixed (unit dose) solution
      i. Albuterol (Proventil, Ventolin); also premixed in saline for use in hand-held nebulizer
      ii. Metaproterenol (Alupent), premixed for use in hand-held nebulizer
      iii. Pirbuterol (Maxair)
      iv. Terbutaline (Brethine), 2 puffs t.i.d.

3. Long-acting inhaled agent

   a. Metered dose inhaler, 2 puffs q12h
   b. Salmeterol (Serevent)—Prolonged receptor binding requires patient education about proper use to avoid induction of cardiac arrhythmias.

4. Short-acting agents: Oral preparations

   a. Albuterol (Volmax), 2–4 mg t.i.d.
   b. Albuterol extended release (Proventil Repetab), 4 mg q12h

5. Corticosteroids

   a. Used to decrease inflammatory effects
   b. Patients taking oral and parenteral corticosteroids need to be warned against abrupt withdrawal from these agents.[9]

   c. Metered-dose inhalers
- i. Triamcinolone acetonide (Azmacort), 2 puffs q.i.d. or 4 puffs b.i.d.
- ii. Fluticasone propionate (Flovent 44 [0.11 mg/inhalation], 110 [0.22 mg/inhalation], 220 [0.44 mg/inhalation]), 2 puffs b.i.d.
- iii. Budesonide (Pulmicort), 2 puffs b.i.d.
- iv. Beclomethasone dipropionate (Beclovent, Vanceril), 2 puffs q.i.d.

   d. Oral tablets
- i. Prednisone (Deltasone), 60 mg/day tapered quickly to less than 20 mg/day
- ii. Methylprednisolone (Medrol), 64 mg/day tapered to less than 16 mg/day

   e. Intravenous preparations: Methylprednisolone sodium succinate (Solu-Medrol), 20–40 mg IV q6–8h for severe exacerbations of COPD, tapered as the patient's condition allows

   f. Intramuscular preparations
- i. Methylprednisolone (Depo-Medrol), 80–240 mg IM in divided IM dosage to decrease discomfort
- ii. Triamcinolone acetonide (Kenalog), 60 mg IM

6. Drugs for respiratory muscles (i.e., diaphragm and intercostals) and bronchodilator activity

   a. Theophylline timed release
- i. Theo-Dur, 300 mg b.i.d.; may also be given intravenously
- ii. Uni-Dur, 400–600 mg in the evening
- iii. Theophylline timed release (Uniphyl), 400–600 mg in the evening
  Note: Evening dosages acknowledge the circadian increase in airway smooth muscle tone.

7. Comments

   a. Maintenance therapy for COPD should incorporate as many different classes of pharmacologic agents as needed to maintain the patient's usual performance status.

   b. During exacerbations, inhaled bronchodilators may be needed more frequently than every 4 h.

   c. Parenteral steroids should be added and rapidly tapered over several days until it is clear whether or not the preparations have contributed to improving the patient's general condition.

8. Antimicrobial agents

   a. Indications

      i. Changes in sputum quantity and color are considered important.

         (1) A Gram's stain may be helpful.

         (2) Sputum culture is usually not indicated.

         (3) In most instances both sputum and blood cultures should be obtained prior to beginning antimicrobial therapy if pneumonia is suspected.

      ii. A recent upper respiratory infection has led to an exacerbation of COPD.

      iii. Radiographic evidence compatible with pneumonia is present.

      iv. Bacteremia is suspected.

   b. Agent chosen should cover usually expected respiratory pathogens (see Chapter 31), without being unnecessarily broader in spectrum than is required.

9. Agents to thin sputum

   a. Glyceryl guaiacolate (Hytuss, Robitussin) may be of help in thinning respiratory secretions, although adequate total body hydration is clearly more important. These agents should therefore be combined with adequate hydration.

   b. Acetylcysteine (Mucomyst 10% or 20%)

      i. Reduces sputum viscosity

      ii. One to ten milliliters of either 10% or 20% solution are inhaled q6–8h, generally after an inhaled beta-2 agonist (see previously, under Bronchodilators).

      iii. This solution can provoke bronchospasm.

      iv. "Tastes like rotten eggs" because of sulfur content

10. Supplemental oxygen (see Chapter 33)

II. EMPHYSEMA[8]

A. Definition

1. A clinical disorder characterized by exertional dyspnea
2. Defined anatomically as a loss of lung support tissue with air trapping, creating large air spaces (e.g., blebs, bullae) deficient in vascular tissue (increased residual volume and total lung capacity, reduced flow rates)

B. Etiology

1. Usually caused by cigarette use
2. May be genetic (alpha$_1$-antitrypsin deficiency)

C. Physical examination findings

1. Reduced air entry sounds
2. Prolonged forced expiratory time
3. Increase in the anteroposterior diameter of the chest (i.e., "barrel chest")

D. Diagnosis/Therapy (see I. COPD, G. Pharmacologic management)[8]

III. CHRONIC BRONCHITIS[8]

A. Definition

1. A clinical disorder characterized by cough with sputum production
2. Sputum production must occur daily for 2 or more consecutive months for 2 or more consecutive years.
3. Daily sputum is usually most prominent in the morning or upon arising.
4. Dyspnea may be present.

B. Physical examination findings

1. Reduced air entry sounds with rhonchi
2. Prolonged expiration that may include wheezing
3. Cyanosis, either acutely or chronically, is more common than in "pure" emphysema.

C. Diagnosis/Therapy (see I. COPD, G. Pharmacologic management)

IV. ASTHMA[11]

A. Definition

1. A clinical disorder characterized by periodic cough with episodic wheezing
2. Sputum is usually described as "plugs" of sputum.
3. When the disorder is exacerbated, the patient may complain of "tightness" in the chest and dyspnea.
4. Patient often has a family history of asthma.

B. Physical examination findings

1. Reduced air entry sounds
2. Prolonged expiration with expiratory wheezing

C. Diagnosis/Therapy

Current standards of care are based on the report of the Expert Panel, Report 2: Guidelines for the Diagnosis and Management of Asthma, 1997.

1. Step 1: Mild intermittent asthma
   a. No daily therapy
   b. Periodic inhaled beta-2 agonists

2. Step 2: Mild persistent asthma
    a. Anti-inflammatory therapy (inhaled corticosteroid; see COPD therapy) OR leukotriene receptor antagonist
        i. Zafirlukast (Accolate), 20 mg p.o. b.i.d.
        ii. Montelukast (Singulair), 10 mg p.o. daily
    b. Periodic inhaled beta-2 agonists

3. Step 3: Moderate persistent asthma
    a. Medications in Step 2 plus
    b. An oral theophylline (sustained release) or a long-acting oral beta-2 agonist

4. Step 4: Severe persistent asthma
    a. Medications in Step 3 plus
    b. Oral or parenteral systemic corticosteroids that are tapered as rapidly as possible

V. BRONCHIECTASIS[12]

A. Definition

1. A clinical disorder characterized by periodic cough with production of copious sputum
2. Copious sputum means one or more cups per day that is occasionally bloody.
3. Often postinflammatory
    a. After severe pneumonia or obstruction of a bronchus by a foreign body
    b. Following healing of tuberculosis

B. Physical examination findings

1. Inspiratory rhonchi during acute exacerbations
2. Noisy expiration

C. Diagnostic findings

1. Chest x-ray may show fibrotic changes.
2. Chest computed tomography will usually document dilation of airways and thickening of bronchial walls.

D. Management

1. See I. COPD, G. Pharmacologic management.
2. Emphasis is on antibiotics (even prophylactically).

VI. OBSTRUCTIVE AIRWAY LESIONS

A. Endobronchial lesions (e.g., tumors, foreign bodies)— Seen on chest x-ray or suspected because of atelectasis

1. Subjective findings
    a. Cough
    b. Dyspnea

   c. Hemoptysis

   d. Weight loss

   e. May include findings outside the chest in other regions of the body when metastatic from another organ

2. Diagnostics

   a. Computed tomographic scan showing a solid mass or irregularly shaped cavity within one lung

   b. Chest x-ray demonstrating a mass

   c. Fiberoptic bronchoscopy with biopsy

3. Treatment: Based on discovered pathology; may include

   a. Surgical removal

   b. Chemotherapy

   c. Radiation therapy

   d. Combination of the preceding

References

1. Tierney, L.M., McPhee, S.J., & Papadakis, M.A. (Eds.). (1999). *Current medical diagnosis & treatment* (38th ed.). Stamford, CT: Appleton & Lange.

2. Barker, L.R., Burton, J.R., & Zieve, P.D. (Eds.). (1999). *Principles of ambulatory medicine* (5th ed.). Baltimore: Williams & Wilkins.

3. Fauci, A.S., Braun E., Isselbacher, K.J., Wilson, J.D., Martin, J.B., Kasper, D.L., Hauser, S.L., & Longo, D.L. (Eds). (1998). *Harrison's principles of internal medicine* (14th ed.). New York: McGraw-Hill.

4. Goldman, L., & Bennett, J.C. (Eds.). (2000). *Cecil textbook of medicine* (21st ed.). Philadelphia: W.B. Saunders.

5. Albert, R., Spiro, S., & Jett, J. (Eds.). (1999). *Comprehensive respiratory medicine*. London: Mosby.

6. Mihalas, L.S. (1999). An approach to the diagnosis of occupational asthma. *Annals of Allergy, Asthma, & Immunology, 83,* 577–582.

7. Thoonen, B.P., van Schayck, C.P., van Weel, C., Levy, M.L., Spelman, R., Price, D., Ryan, M., Bellamy, D., van Grunsven, P., Cloosterman, S., van den Boom, G., Gorgels, W., & Schonberger, H. (1999). Present and future management of asthma and COPD: Proceedings from WONCA 1998. *Family Practice, 16,* 313–315.

8. American Thoracic Society. (1995). Standards for the diagnosis and care of patients with chronic obstructive pulmonary disease. *American Journal of Respiratory and Critical Care Medicine, 152,* 78–121.

9. Davies, L., Nisar, M., Pearson, M., Pearson, M.G., Costello, W., Earis, J.E., & Calverley, P.M. (1999). Oral corticosteroid trials in the management of stable chronic obstructive pulmonary disease. *Quarterly Journal of Medicine, 92,* 395–400.

10. Sethi, S. (1999). Infectious exacerbations of chronic bronchitis: Diagnosis and management. *Journal of Antimicrobial Agents and Chemotherapy, 43* (Suppl. A), 97–105.

11. National Asthma Education and Prevention Program. (1997). Expert Panel Report 2: Guidelines for the Diagnosis and Management of Asthma. National Institutes of Health Pub No. 97-4051. Bethesda: NIH.

12. Tasker, A.D., Flower, C.D. (1999). Imaging the airways. Hemoptysis, bronchiectasis, and small airway disease. *Clinics in Chest Medicine, 20,* 761–773.

RESTRICTIVE (INFLAMMATORY) LUNG DISEASES AND CONGESTIVE HEART FAILURE/ PULMONARY EDEMA

David A. Miller, MD, FCCP

I. PNEUMONIA[1-7]

A. Definition of pneumonia

1. An acute febrile inflammatory disorder of the lung(s), associated with cough and exertional dyspnea
2. Infiltrate is present on chest x-ray. The appearance of the infiltrate may lag behind the appearance of symptoms by 24–48 h, justifying a repeat chest x-ray at that time.
3. Leukocytosis may be present.

B. Incidence/Etiology

1. Pneumonia is one of the most common of all serious lung conditions and a frequent cause of acute care hospitalization and mortality.
2. Organisms that are potential causes of community-acquired pneumonia:

   a. Bacteria
      i. *Streptococcus pneumoniae* (most common bacterial cause in adults)
      ii. *Klebsiella pneumoniae*
      iii. *Haemophilus pneumoniae*
      iv. Gram-negative organisms
   b. "Atypical" pathogens
      i. *Chlamydia pneumoniae*
      ii. *Mycoplasma pneumoniae*
      iii. *Mycobacterium tuberculosis*
   c. Viruses
      i. Respiratory syncytial virus
      ii. Adenovirus
      iii. Rhinovirus

3. Overzealous treatment of mild respiratory infections in the past has contributed to the development of antimicrobial drug resistance, especially to *Streptococcus pneumoniae*.

4. Comorbidity from the following conditions contributes to high mortality from pneumonia:

   a. Congestive heart failure
   b. Diabetes mellitus
   c. Chronic liver and renal disease
   d. Chronic obstructive pulmonary disease

5. The very young and the very old are at increased risk of death from pneumonia, despite the remarkable array of anti-microbial agents available to treat this disorder.

C. Classification of pneumonia

1. "Typical" pneumonias manifest with the "classic" findings.

   a. Fever
   b. Chills
   c. Leukocytosis
   d. Cough
   e. Sputum production

2. "Atypical" pneumonias vary in their presentation.

   a. Fever may be high.
   b. Leukocytosis
      i. May be absent
      ii. May be associated with a "left shift" in the differential white blood cell count to include a high number of "band" forms
   c. Cough is often dry.

3. Both forms demonstrate an infiltrate on chest x-ray.

   a. Atypical pneumonias are more often diffuse.
   b. Atypical pneumonias may involve more than one lung segment or both lungs.

4. Occurrence information may assist in defining the type of pneumonia present.

   a. Time of year
   b. Known epidemic disease
   c. Presence of comorbid conditions

5. Community-acquired pneumonias are those acquired within the community setting.
6. Nosocomial pneumonias are the result of exposure to infection while staying in a health care facility.

   a. Hospital
   b. Nursing home
   c. Rehabilitation facility

7. Pneumonias are often categorized by risk factors present that predispose the patient to the pneumonia.

    a. Aspiration pneumonias (related to altered mental status)
    b. Obstructive lesions of the airway
       i. Tumor
       ii. Retained bronchopulmonary secretions
    c. Inhalation injury–related pneumonia
       i. Hypersensitivity pneumonia
       ii. Near-drowning

D. Evaluation for possible pneumonia

1. Historical information
2. Physical examination

    a. Tachypnea
    b. Tachycardia
    c. Fever
    d. Discomfort
    e. Rales (or "crackles") on auscultation over the affected area(s)

3. Chest x-ray, looking for new pulmonary infiltrates
4. Laboratory studies

    a. CBC, including differential WBC
    b. Blood cultures
    c. Gram's stain and culture of sputum
    d. Arterial blood gases and/or pulse oximetry

E. Treatment[8]

1. Antimicrobial therapy with cultures pending (see Chapter 31). If the patient is

    a. Less than 40 years old, without comorbidity: Macrolide
    b. Over 40 years old, or with comorbidity: Macrolide plus third-generation cephalosporin
    c. Over 60 years old: Macrolide plus third-generation cephalosporin plus additional gram-negative organism coverage

2. Antimicrobial therapy should be revised as culture information becomes available and as improvement occurs. In general, the narrowest spectrum antimicrobial to which known organisms are expected to respond should be used.
3. Simultaneous treatment of coexisting illnesses is needed.

    a. Chronic obstructive pulmonary disease
    b. Congestive heart failure
    c. Diabetes
    d. Dehydration

4. Not all patients, especially young adults, need hospitalization for pneumonia.

   a. The decision to hospitalize a patient with pneumonia should be guided by
      i. The possibility of rapidly progressive disease
      ii. The overall status of the patient (coexisting problems)
      iii. The patient's ability to reliably self-administer medication for this illness
   b. If in doubt, it is reasonable to observe the patient in hospital during initial therapy, and to reassess the early response to treatment.

F. Prevention of pneumonia

1. Vaccination against influenza: Fluvax

   a. Repeated annually
   b. Some revaccinate within a season if the patient
      i. Is immunocompromised
      ii. Has severe underlying chronic obstructive pulmonary disease or heart disease

2. Vaccination against *Streptococcus pneumoniae:* Pneumovax

   a. Repeated every 7–10 years or as recommended by the Centers for Disease Control
   b. Only covers the 23 most virulent strains of *S. pneumoniae*

II. TUBERCULOSIS (TB)[1-5, 9]

A. Etiology: *Mycobacterium tuberculosis*
B. Incidence

1. The rates of new infections by *M. tuberculosis* are increasing, especially among the homeless and among those living in crowded conditions in larger metropolitan areas.
2. Alarmingly, the incidence of multidrug-resistant TB (defined as resistant to isoniazid and to rifampin) also appears to be rising, especially along the east and west coasts of the United States.
3. This rise has coincided with the increased numbers of patients with HIV and AIDS.

C. Clinical findings

1. Symptoms

   a. Fever
   b. Cough, generally productive of purulent sputum that may contain blood
   c. Weight loss
   d. Night sweats that may require changing of bed linen

2. Physical examination findings
   a. Body temperature elevation
   b. Cachexia may be noted.
   c. Rales over the affected areas: Apical post-tussive rales for apical disease

3. Laboratory/Diagnostic findings
   a. Normal complete CBC
   b. Low serum cortisol level if disseminated disease to the adrenal glands has destroyed the adrenal cortices
   c. Sputum
      i. Acid-fast smears are often positive, but therapy may need to be started empirically if other findings are suggestive of TB in the absence of positive smears.
      ii. Cultures for *M. tuberculosis* are usually positive within 6 weeks.
   d. TB skin testing (intradermal purified protein derivative [PPD])
      i. 0.1 mL PPD injected intradermally; read 48 hours later
      ii. Interpretation based on measurement of the largest diameter of the indurated area (not including flat but erythematous area):
         (a) <5 mm: Negative test
         (b) 5 mm: Positive test in an HIV-infected patient
         (c) 10 mm: Positive test in health care worker
         (d) 15 mm: Positive test in the general population

4. Chest x-ray
   a. Infiltrate
      i. Especially present in the upper lobes of the lungs, or in the superior segments of the lower lobes
      ii. Can be present in any portion of the lungs
   b. Cavity within the lungs

D. Treatment

1. Patient isolation during initial evaluation and treatment, according to Occupational Safety and Health Administration (OSHA) standards, is mandatory.
2. Suspected disease, or smear-positive disease, pending the return of sputum cultures
   a. Four-drug therapy
      i. Isoniazid/INH, 300 mg p.o. each day, with pyridoxine, 50 mg p.o., to prevent INH-induced peripheral neuropathy
      ii. Rifampin/rifampicin, 600 mg p.o. each day
      iii. Ethambutol (Myambutol), 15 mg/kg p.o. each day, preceded by screening of color vision. Note: Ethambutol

may cause red/green color blindness as an adverse effect.

    iv. Pyrazinamide, 15–30 mg/kg in three divided doses daily

  b. Revision of therapy when drug sensitivities are known, usually to INH with rifampin

  c. Therapy is continued for 9 months.

  d. For nonadherent patients, directly observed therapy (DOT) may begin three times per week, usually after 2 weeks of observed therapy, often in hospital.

3. Prophylaxis

  a. Patients

    i. Asymptomatic, with a positive PPD and a normal chest x-ray

    ii. Exposed to active TB who have a negative PPD

    iii. Undergoing immunosuppressive therapy for other reasons

    iv. Who have HIV infections

  b. Treatment

    i. INH, 300 mg p.o. daily for 1 year

    ii. Pyridoxine, 50 mg p.o. daily during INH therapy

III. ACUTE RESPIRATORY DISTRESS SYNDROME (ARDS)/ ACUTE LUNG INJURY[1-5, 10, 11]

A. Etiologies: Any of the numerous causes of acute systemic inflammation

1. Bacteremia or other severe systemic infections
2. Massive trauma or injury, including burns and smoke inhalation
3. Pancreatitis
4. Shock (any cause)
5. Cardiopulmonary bypass
6. Increased intracranial pressure, especially after trauma or intracranial bleeding
7. Aspiration of fluid, including gastrointestinal contents and near-drowning

B. Incidence

1. The annual incidence is unknown, largely owing to lack of required reporting and misunderstanding about when and how the diagnosis is made.
2. Overall incidence in any locale will be proportional to the incidence of the known causes of the syndrome itself.

C. Clinical findings

1. Severe respiratory distress occurring during the course of one of the inciting events

2. Respiratory distress often requires the early institution of mechanical ventilatory assistance.
3. Symptoms

   a. Breathlessness
   b. Agitation
   c. Confusion
   d. Obtundation as oxygen delivery and uptake by tissues falls

4. Other manifestations include failure of other organ systems.

   a. Kidneys
   b. Liver
   c. Bone marrow (reduced platelet count)
   d. Multisystem organ failure

5. Physical findings depend on the presentation of the condition placing the patient at risk for ARDS. Lungs often sound clearer than the chest x-ray would suggest.
6. Laboratory testing

   a. CBC with differential white count and platelet count
   b. Coagulation studies
      i. Prothrombin time
      ii. Partial thromboplastin time
      iii. Fibrinogen level
      iv. Fibrin degradation products
   c. Renal and liver function
   d. Urinalysis
   e. Blood and urine cultures
   f. Sputum culture and Gram's stain

7. X-rays

   a. Chest x-ray—Often shows evolving bilateral infiltrates
   b. Other x-rays—As indicated by the patient's presenting problems (e.g., trauma)

D. Treatment

1. Airway

   a. Assess adequacy of ventilation and the degree of work used during spontaneous ventilation.
   b. Intubate if ventilation is significantly compromised, especially if altered mentation is noted.

2. Breathing: Institute mechanical ventilation

   a. If work of breathing is not being met, evidenced by
      i. Patient fatigue
      ii. Elevated Pa_{CO_2}
   b. If measured hypoxemia is not correctable by an FiO_2 of 0.5

3. Circulation: Vigorous fluid resuscitation should be started if hypotension is present
   a. Regulated by hemodynamic parameters
   b. Best monitored by an indwelling pulmonary artery catheter
4. Correct the underlying etiology of the ARDS.
5. Support needed
   a. Mechanical ventilatory assistance often requires the institution of positive end-expiratory pressure.
   b. Ventilatory pressures over 45 cm H_2O may require the use of
      i. Reduced tidal volumes
      ii. Pressure-cycled ventilation
   c. The patient should be sedated for comfort.
   d. Nutritional support should be started early.
      i. Use the enteral route, if possible, or total parenteral nutrition.
      ii. Most patients require nearly twice their usual daily caloric requirements to counteract the tremendous energy expenditure used in combating ARDS.

E. Despite refinements in the provision of care for ARDS patients, the mortality overall remains nearly 40%.
F. Special considerations

1. The risk of pulmonary barotrauma, including pneumothorax or pneumomediastinum, is high with this disorder.
2. Sudden increases in ventilating pressures with desaturations in arterial oxygen tension indicate the need for an immediate repeat chest x-ray and for possible chest tube insertion.
3. Repeated physical and radiographic assessments of the lungs may be needed to rule out barotrauma in the mechanically ventilated patient with ARDS.

IV. IDIOPATHIC PULMONARY FIBROSIS (IPF)[1–5, 12, 13]
A. Etiology/General concepts

1. Etiology is unknown.
2. Prior to treatment, rule out
   a. Inhalation exposure
   b. Autoimmune disorders
   c. Chronic lung infections
      i. Tuberculosis
      ii. Deep fungal infections
         (1) Histoplasmosis
         (2) Coccidioidomycosis
3. In patients with prior malignancy, lymphangitic spread of tumor to the lungs should be excluded.

B. Incidence

1. Unknown; IPF is the most common cause of interstitial lung disease among elderly patients.
2. More common in men than in women

C. Clinical findings

1. Symptoms
   a. Progressive (slow or rapid) dyspnea
   b. Cough (nonproductive)
   c. Specific questioning of the patient about prior exposure to the following:
      i. Inorganic dusts
         (1) Silica
         (2) Asbestos
      ii. Organic dusts (e.g., in silos, where hypersensitivity pneumonia may be acquired)
      iii. Fumes
         (1) Chlorine
         (2) Sulfur dioxide
      iv. Drugs
         (1) Chemotherapeutic agents (e.g., bleomycin)
         (2) Antibiotics (e.g., nitrofurantoin and sulfas)
         (3) Gold salts (during the course of therapy for rheumatoid arthritis)
         (4) Amiodarone (for cardiac arrhythmias)
      v. Radiation to lung parenchyma
      vi. Risk factors for *Pneumocystis carinii* pneumonia
         (1) Immunosuppression from HIV infection
         (2) Chemotherapy for lymphoma or lymphocytic leukemia and other malignancies
         (3) Immunosuppression for organ transplantation
      vii. Known chronic congestive heart failure

2. Physical examination findings
   a. Rales ("Velcro crackles") may be heard on auscultation.

3. Laboratory/Diagnostic findings
   a. Changes within the lung parenchyma, especially in the lower lobes, demonstrated by chest x-ray and high resolution CT scanning
      i. Interstitial infiltrates
      ii. Nodules
      iii. Cystic (or "honey-combing") changes
   b. Pulmonary function testing typically demonstrates a restrictive ventilatory defect.
      i. Some patients may show a coexisting bronchoconstriction in small airways.

    ii. The diffusing capacity of lung for carbon monoxide (D_{LCO}) is commonly reduced, a manifestation of altered ventilation and perfusion relationships within the lungs.

  c. Arterial blood gas analysis and pulse oximetry

    i. May demonstrate hypoxemia, typically as the disease progresses

    ii. Carbon dioxide retention indicates severe disease.

  d. Laboratory findings generally are not helpful.

    i. PPD testing should be done.

    ii. Prior exposure to deep fungi including *Histoplasma capsulatum* (chicken coops, in the Midwest) and *Coccidioides immitis* (dust, desert Southwest and Central Valleys of California), may be assessed with complement fixation serologic studies for deep fungi, although prior exposure does not necessarily equate with active disease.

      (1) Histoplasmosis

      (2) Coccidioidomycosis

      (3) Blastomycosis

  e. Obtaining tissue for diagnosis

    i. Fiberoptic bronchoscopy with transbronchial biopsy of the lung parenchyma is safe and should be done first.

    ii. Bronchoalveolar lavage to assess for inflammation and to obtain secretions for culture (e.g., acid-fast bacilli [AFB] and fungi, and for *Nocardia*) may be performed at the same time.

    iii. Since biopsies obtained at bronchoscopy may be inadequate for diagnosis and are subject to sampling error, patients deemed healthy enough to undergo open-lung biopsy should be considered for thoracoscopic lung biopsy if further assurance is required that the diagnosis of idiopathic pulmonary fibrosis is correct.

4. Therapy

  a. Corticosteroids (prednisone, 1 mg/kg/day for 12 weeks)

    i. Many patients report subjective improvement.

    ii. Far fewer demonstrate objective improvement radiographically or by pulmonary function testing.

  b. Alternative treatments that may be considered in selected patients include cycylophosphamide (Cytoxan), 1 mg/kg/day, or azathioprine (Imuran), 3 mg/kg/day.

  c. Noninvasive use of positive airway pressure (by mask) may be beneficial in selected patients.

5. Prognosis: IPF is usually a progressive illness, and the prognosis is often poor over time.

V. SARCOIDOSIS[1–5, 14, 15]

A. Definition

1. Characterized pathologically by the presence of noncaseating granulomas and interstitial lung disease
2. Systemic manifestations

   a. Lymphadenopathy
   b. Cardiac involvement
   c. Iritis
   d. Cutaneous lesions
   e. Arthritis
   f. Gastrointestinal involvement
   g. Other organs may be involved.

B. Incidence

1. Unknown
2. More common among females, North American African Americans, and northern European whites.
3. May be seen in all races.
4. Typically, onset of symptoms is between the ages of 20 and 40.

C. Clinical findings

1. Symptoms

   a. Progressive dyspnea (slow or rapid)
   b. Nonproductive cough

2. Physical examination findings

   a. Depends on specific organ involvement
   b. The lung examination may be normal.
   c. Rales ("Velcro crackles") may be heard on auscultation when interstitial disease, including fibrosis, is present.

3. Laboratory/Diagnostic findings

   a. The chest x-ray may demonstrate the following; the stages shown are useful in staging pulmonary involvement by sarcoidosis.[15]
      i. Stage 0: Normal chest x-ray
      ii. Stage I: Bilateral hilar lymphadenopathy (BHL)
      iii. Stage II: BHL plus pulmonary infiltrates
      iv. Stage III: Pulmonary infiltrates without BHL
      v. Stage IV: Pulmonary fibrosis
   b. Pulmonary function testing typically demonstrates a restrictive ventilatory defect.
      i. Some patients may show a coexisting bronchoconstriction in small airways.

    ii. The D$_{LCO}$ is commonly reduced, a manifestation of altered ventilation and perfusion relationships within the lungs.

  c. Arterial blood gas analysis and pulse oximetry

    i. May demonstrate hypoxemia, typically as the disease progresses

    ii. Carbon dioxide retention indicates severe disease.

  d. Laboratory findings generally are not helpful.

    i. PPD testing should be done.

    ii. Prior exposure to deep fungi may be assessed with complement fixation serologic studies for deep fungi, although prior exposure does not necessarily equate with active disease.

      (1) Histoplasmosis

      (2) Coccidioidomycosis

      (3) Blastomycosis

  e. Obtaining tissue for diagnosis of pulmonary sarcoidosis

    i. Fiberoptic bronchoscopy with transbronchial biopsy of the lung parenchyma is safe and should be done first.

    ii. Bronchoalveolar lavage to assess for inflammation and to obtain secretions for culture (e.g., AFB and fungi, and for *Nocardia*) may be performed at the same time.

    iii. Since biopsies obtained at bronchoscopy may be inadequate for diagnosis and are subject to sampling error, patients deemed healthy enough to undergo open lung biopsy should be considered for thoracoscopic lung biopsy if further assurance is required that the diagnosis of idiopathic pulmonary fibrosis is correct.

    iv. If other organs are involved, biopsy of one of those sites may be beneficial in establishing the diagnosis.

    v. If BHL is present, cervical mediastinal exploration with biopsy of a node is reasonable.

  f. Blood tests

    i. CBC

    ii. Calcium (Sarcoidosis is associated with hypercalcemia.)

    iii. Liver function tests

    iv. BUN

    v. Creatinine

  g. ECG

  h. Urinalysis

  i. PPD

  j. Ophthalmologic examination

4. Therapy

  a. Corticosteroids (prednisone, 1 mg/kg/day for 12 weeks)

    i. Many patients report subjective improvement.

    ii. Far fewer demonstrate objective improvement radiographically or by pulmonary function testing.

   b. Alternative treatments that may be considered in selected patients include cyclophosphamide (Cytoxan), 1 mg/kg/day, or azathioprine (Imuran), 3 mg/kg/day.

   c. Methotrexate and hydroxychloroquine also have been used alternatively in sarcoidosis.

VI. CONGESTIVE HEART FAILURE (CHF)/CARDIOGENIC PULMONARY EDEMA[1–5, 16]

A. Etiology: Numerous causes are known.

1. Coronary artery disease with myocardial ischemia and infarction, aggravated by

   a. Obesity
   b. Limited exercise
   c. Dyslipidemia
   d. Cigarette smoking

2. Cardiac arrhythmias

   a. Tachycardia (especially)
   b. Bradycardia

3. Hypertension
4. Valvular dysfunction of the heart
5. Thyroid dysfunction, including

   a. Hyperthyroidism
   b. Hypothyroidism
   c. Diabetes mellitus

6. Viral myocarditis
7. Idiopathic cardiomyopathy
8. Renal failure
9. Drug therapy, especially with

   a. Calcium channel blockers
   b. Beta adrenergic antagonists

B. Incidence

1. CHF is a common disorder that leads to frequent outpatient visits and inpatient hospitalizations, despite the availability of modern therapeutic interventions.
2. In general, CHF

   a. Is progressive
   b. Eventuates in frequent hospitalizations
   c. Carries a guarded prognosis over time

C. Clinical manifestations are related to the development of restrictive ventilatory defects within the lung parenchyma that are initially mild and later severe.

1. Symptoms

   a. Progression from exertional dyspnea to orthopnea and paroxysmal nocturnal dyspnea
   b. Frank respiratory failure may be noted.
   c. A dry cough is commonly seen.
   d. The time course of this progression may be slow or abrupt.

2. Physical examination findings: Secondary responses lead to detectable signs of fluid retention.

   a. Edema and jugular venous distention
   b. Rales
   c. Tachycardia or bradycardia
   d. Inability to tolerate lying flat in the supine position
   e. Tachypnea
   f. Ascites (when CHF is advanced)

3. Diagnosis

   a. ECG
      i. Assess for ischemia or infarction.
      ii. Determine cardiac rhythm.
   b. Chest x-ray, looking for
      i. Vascular redistribution to the upper lung fields
      ii. Presence of
         (1) Interstitial edema
         (2) Kerley's B lines
      iii. Pleural effusions (usually bilateral or on the right)
      iv. Cardiomegaly
   c. Assessment of oxygenation to ensure adequate oxygenation of blood and to assess for carbon dioxide retention
      i. Arterial blood gas analysis
      ii. Pulse oximetry
   d. CBC to rule out anemia
   e. Chemistries
      i. Thyroid function
         (1) Triiodothyronine (T_3)
         (2) Levorotatory thyroxine (T_4)
         (3) Thyroid-stimulating hormone (TSH)
      ii. Renal function
         (1) BUN
         (2) Creatinine
      iii. Liver function
      iv. Electrolytes (including magnesium levels)
   f. Cardiac enzyme evaluation, especially if recent myocardial infarction or unstable angina pectoris is suspected

    g. Echocardiography to assess
      i. Systolic function of the heart
      ii. Valvular function
      iii. Dyskinesis
        (1) Global
        (2) Segmental
    h. Pulmonary function studies are not useful during acute pulmonary edema, but, when the patient is stable:
      i. May help to demonstrate the presence of a restrictive ventilatory defect in early CHF (reduced VC)
      ii. May help to evaluate for coexisting chronic obstructive pulmonary disease, especially among smokers
    i. Occasionally, patients in CHF will require pulmonary artery catheterization to document the severity of the problem, especially when hypotension is present or when needed.
      i. Aggressive fluid therapy could further aggravate CHF.
      ii. If needed, determination can be made of
        (1) Cardiac output
        (2) Cardiac index
        (3) Systemic vascular resistance
        (4) Pulmonary capillary wedge pressure
    j. In general, insertion of a pulmonary artery catheter is not necessary in treating CHF.

4. Treatment

    a. Correct the cause of the CHF, if known (especially ischemia). Nitrates may be indicated clinically.
      i. Sublingual nitroglycerine
      ii. Nitroglycerine patches such as Nitro-Dur, 0.4 mg, applied daily
    b. Emphasize long-term priorities of improved diet, weight control, and exercise.
    c. Control dyslipidemia with diet, exercise, and pharmacologic therapy.
    d. Supplement oxygen, usually via nasal cannula at low flow rates (e.g., 2 L/min).
      i. In frank pulmonary edema, oxygen should be supplied in higher amounts.
      ii. Use mask delivery as needed to adequately oxygenate the blood.
    e. If the patient is unable to sustain the work of breathing during an acute episode of CHF, intubation and mechanical ventilatory assistance are often required.
    f. Improve contractility of the myocardium.
      i. Eliminate cardiac depressants
        (1) Calcium channel blockers
        (2) Beta adrenergic antagonists

ii. Supplying additional inotropic force (e.g., digitalis)
iii. Decrease afterload with an ACE inhibitor.
iv. Decrease preload with morphine and diuresis.
v. These measures will reduce the interstitial edema and ventilatory restriction, improving respiratory symptoms.
vi. Aggressiveness of these measures needs to be proportional to the severity of the interstitial edema and the degree of respiratory distress present.

References

1. Tierney, L.M., McPhee, S.J., & Papadakis, M.A. (Eds.). (1999). *Current medical diagnosis & treatment* (38th ed.). Stamford, CT: Appleton & Lange.
2. Barker, L.R., Burton, J.R., & Zieve, P.D. (Eds.). (1999). *Principles of ambulatory medicine* (5th ed.). Baltimore: Williams & Wilkins.
3. Fauci, A.S., Braun E., Isselbacher, K.J., Wilson, J.D., Martin, J.B., Kasper, D.L., Hauser, S.L., & Longo, D.L. (Eds.). (1998). *Harrison's principles of internal medicine* (14th ed.). New York: McGraw-Hill.
4. Goldman, L., & Bennett, J.C. (Eds.). (2000). *Cecil textbook of medicine* (21st ed.). Philadelphia: W.B. Saunders.
5. Albert, R., Spiro, S., & Jett, J. (Eds.). (1999). *Comprehensive respiratory medicine*. London: Mosby.
6. Boersman, W.G. (1999). Assessment of severity of community-acquired pneumonia. *Seminars in Respiratory Infections, 14*, 103–114.
7. Ewig, S. (1999). Community acquired pneumonia: Definition, epidemiology and outcome. *Seminars in Respiratory Infections, 14*, 94–102.
8. Halm, E.A., Atlas, S.J., Borowsky, L.H., Benzer, T.I., Metlay, J.P., Chang, Y.C., & Singer, D.E. (2000). Understanding physician adherence with a pneumonia practice guideline: Effects of patient, system, and physician factors. *Archives of Internal Medicine, 160*, 98–104.
9. King, M.A., & Tomasic, D.M. (1999). Treating TB today. *RN, 62*, 26–31.
10. Goodman, L.R., Fumagalli, R., Tagliabue, R., Tagliabue, M., Ferraro, M., Gattinoni, L., & Pesenti, A. (1999). Adult respiratory distress syndrome due to pulmonary and extrapulmonary causes: CT, clinical and functional correlations. *Radiology, 213*, 545–552.
11. Kramer, B. (1999). Ventilator-associated pneumonia in critically ill patients. *Annals of Internal Medicine, 130*, 1027–1028.
12. Consensus Report. (1999). Clinical indications for noninvasive positive pressure ventilation in chronic respiratory failure due to restrictive lung disease, COPD, and nocturnal hypoventilation: A consensus conference report. *Chest, 116*, 521–524.
13. Gay, S.E., Kazerooni, E.A., Toews, G.B., Lynch, J.P., Gross, B.H., Cascade, P.N., Spizarny, D.L., Flint, A., Schork, M.A., Whyte, R.I., Popovich, J., Hyzy, R., & Martinez, F.J. (1998). Idiopathic pulmonary fibrosis: Predicting response to therapy and survival. *American Journal of Respiratory and Critical Care Medicine, 157*, 1063–1072.
14. Lynch, J.P., Kazerooni, E.A., & Gay, S.E. (1997). Pulmonary sarcoidosis. *Clinics in Chest Medicine, 18*, 755–785.
15. American Thoracic Society. (1999). Statement on sarcoidosis. *American Journal of Respiratory and Critical Care Medicine, 160*, 736–755.
16. LeConte, P., Coutant, V., N'Guyen, J.M., Baron, D., Touze, M.D., & Potel, G. (1999). Prognostic factors in acute cardiogenic pulmonary edema. *American Journal of Emergency Medicine, 17*, 329–332.

PATHOPHYSIOLOGICALLY DERIVED THERAPY FOR RESPIRATORY DYSFUNCTION

David A. Miller, MD, FCCP

I. RATIONALE[1]

A. Therapy of lung and respiratory dysfunction relies on an understanding of the pathophysiologic basis of the underlying condition.

1. Asthma is believed to result from episodic inflammatory changes within the airways due to inhaled pollen, dusts, and other irritants.

   a. Hence, anti-inflammatory agents are the first-line drugs of choice.
      i. Corticosteroids
      ii. Leukotriene-receptor antagonists
   b. Other medications targeted at controlling infection, bronchospasm, and mucus plugging are used as needed.

2. Chronic obstructive pulmonary disease (COPD) is also the result of more persistent inflammatory changes, usually due to inhalation of tobacco smoke.

   a. The resulting increase in cholinergic effects results in an increase in airway mucus and in bronchial smooth muscle tone.
   b. Hence, anticholinergic therapy is indicated first.
   c. Bronchodilators and corticosteroids are indicated periodically as well.
   d. An improvement in skeletal muscle endurance, specifically of the diaphragm and the chest wall, may be the primary effect of theophylline.
   e. Note that a polypharmacotherapeutic approach is often employed.
   f. In addition, antimicrobial agents are used when infection is also present.

3. The acute respiratory distress syndrome (ARDS) may result from any severe inflammatory injury, including bacteremia, burns, pancreatitis, and trauma.

   a. As a restrictive ventilatory defect, ARDS results in a reduction in pulmonary compliance.

    b. The primary therapy for the condition remains the treatment of its cause. This primary treatment may involve
       i. Antimicrobials
      ii. Surgery
      iii. Correction of additional dysfunction
         (1) Hyperglycemia
         (2) Azotemia
         (3) Encephalopathy
    c. Supportive care often involves the use of mechanical ventilatory assistance, it is hoped temporarily, to sustain the patient during the treatment of the underlying condition.

4. Similarly, other restrictive ventilatory defects (e.g., interstitial pulmonary fibrosis [IPF], sarcoidosis, vasculitis) require treatment of the underlying cause of the defect if any possible reduction in the degree of restriction is to be achieved.

B. Respiratory dysfunction requires an integrated approach to sustain both the supply of oxygen to the client and the removal of carbon dioxide.

1. It is equally important to consider nutrition as a primary treatment modality.
2. Respiratory disease causes the consumption of energy to sustain the work of breathing.
3. Extra nutritional resources must be available to provide the substrate that, with oxygen, will restore energy stores.

II. GOOD AND BAD MEDICINE FOR THE LUNGS[2, 3]

A. Medications can induce respiratory symptoms. The careful practitioner always reviews current medications as possible causes of patient problems.

1. Classically, the angiotensin-converting enzyme (ACE) inhibitors can induce a dry cough.
2. Beta-2 adrenergic blocking agents can induce wheezing.
3. Many chemotherapeutic agents can induce pulmonary infiltrates, for example:

    a. Busulfan
    b. Methotrexate

4. Discontinuing these medications often helps to relieve the patient's symptoms.

B. Sometimes medications that can induce side effects in the lungs or in other organs must be used despite concern for patient safety and symptoms.

1. Patients with COPD may develop rapid heart rhythms or myocardial ischemia.

    a. The use of ACE inhibitors or beta adrenergic blocking agents may be required.
    b. Judicious explanation of the clinical situation to the patient and family members is prudent in these situations.

2. Pharmacologic agents evolve over time.

    a. Beta-2 adrenergic agonists often cause tremors and can induce cardiac arrhythmias.
    b. The drug albuterol has been altered by purifying it as a specific isomer of the active agent.
        i. Patients who previously have had problems with albuterol may tolerate the more specific agent.
        ii. This agent is the levo-optical isomer of levalbuterol, available as Xopenex (0.63–1.25 mg/3 mL, as a unit dose)
            (1) Reduces the incidence of aggravating tremors
            (2) Permits the treatment of patients with COPD with a form of the drug that may be less likely to aggravate cardiac arrhythmias (given that it is used only every 8 h)

C. Respiratory infections require appropriate treatment.

1. Antimicrobial agents should be used when it is reasonably certain that an acute infection is present.

    a. Treatment with antimicrobial agents for any reason will potentially change the flora within the respiratory tract.
    b. Flora may change from "normal" to organisms not ordinarily found in the respiratory tract, including gram-negative organisms and potentially drug-resistant strains.

2. Treatment with antimicrobials should be targeted as specifically as possible to expected pathogens.

    a. Antimicrobial agents should be as narrow-spectrum as possible as long as the expected pathogens are "covered."
    b. In the event that a drug-resistant organism is cultured (e.g., methicillin-resistant *Staphylococcus aureus*), the decision to treat must be based on the probability that the organism is a true pathogen.
    c. Simply culturing an organism (colonization without clinical infection) does not mean that treatment is required.
    d. The treatment decision should be based on clinical findings:
        i. Increased quantities of sputum
        ii. Fever
        iii. Pulmonary infiltrates

References

1. Albert, R., Spiro, S., & Jett, J. (Eds.) (1999). *Comprehensive respiratory medicine*. Philadelphia: Mosby.
2. Reese, R.E., & Betts, R.F. (1996). *A practical approach to infectious diseases* (4th ed.). Boston: Little, Brown and Company.
3. Xopenex information. March 25, 1999. www.fda.gov/cder/consumer info/druginfo/xopenex.htm.

PULMONARY HYPERTENSION AND PULMONARY VASCULAR DISORDERS

David A. Miller, MD, FCCP

I. PULMONARY HYPERTENSION[1-5]

A. Etiology

1. Increased pulmonary vascular resistance

   a. Vasoconstriction (e.g., due to hypoxemia, acidosis)
   b. Loss of vasculature (e.g., due to emphysema, lung resection)
   c. Occlusion of the pulmonary vasculature (e.g., due to pulmonary embolism)
   d. Relative stenosis of the pulmonary vasculature (vasculitis)

2. Increased pulmonary venous pressure

   a. Left ventricular failure or hypertrophy
   b. Valvular heart disease (e.g., mitral valve stenosis, aortic valve stenosis)
   c. Constrictive pericarditis

3. Increased pulmonary blood flow (left-to-right shunt)
4. Polycythemia (primary or secondary, e.g., from hypoxemia)
5. Primary (idiopathic) pulmonary hypertension, seen most often in young women

B. Incidence

The incidence of secondary pulmonary hypertension is related to the incidence of the cause of pulmonary hypertension.

C. Clinical

1. Symptoms[6]

   a. Dyspnea with exertion and later at rest
   b. Those related to the cause of the pulmonary hypertension
   c. Substernal discomfort
   d. Fatigue
   e. Syncope

2. Physical examination findings

   a. Splitting of the second cardiac sound; pulmonic valve component of the second heart sound (P_2) is increased in intensity.

b. Peripheral edema related to right ventricular failure
c. Ascites

3. Laboratory

a. CBC: Increase in the hemoglobin and hematocrit if hypoxemia is present
b. ECG: Right-axis deviation

4. Chest x-ray

a. Increased size of the pulmonary arteries
b. Visible narrowing of the pulmonary arteries in the medial third of the lung (typically seen in emphysema)

5. Echocardiogram to rule out valvular heart disease and left atrial myxoma
6. Pulmonary function testing

a. To assess for obstructive and restrictive ventilatory defects
b. Primary pulmonary hypertension is a diagnosis of exclusion.

D. Treatment[7, 8]

1. Treatment of underlying disorders that contribute to hypoxemia, including

a. Chronic obstructive pulmonary disease (COPD)
b. Congestive heart failure (CHF)
c. Obstructive sleep apnea (OSA)

2. Supplemental oxygen during the night
3. Consider anticoagulation if there is a risk of small recurrent pulmonary emboli.
4. If polycythemia is severe, with hematocrit >60%, therapeutic phlebotomy should be considered to result in a hematocrit of about 55%.
5. Primary pulmonary hypertension is treated with calcium channel blockers and anticoagulation.

II. PULMONARY VASCULAR DISORDERS[1–5, 9, 10]

A. Pulmonary embolism (PE)

1. Definition

a. A clot (thromboembolus) or other undissolved solid, liquid, or gaseous material that has traveled to the lung via the venous system, lodged in the pulmonary arterial circulation, and interrupted blood flow
b. The extent of lung tissue injury is determined by the size of the embolus, which is considered massive if over 50% of flow is obstructed.
c. Accurate diagnosis is the key to reducing associated mortality.

2. Etiology/Incidence/Predisposing factors

   a. Predisposing factors for thrombotic emboli (Virchow's triad):

      i. Venous stasis: Deep venous thrombosis in lower extremities and pelvis leads to 90–95% of pulmonary emboli.

        (1) Prolonged immobility or surgery involving general anesthesia longer than 30 min

        (2) CHF

        (3) Dehydration

        (4) Obesity

        (5) Advanced age

      ii. Vessel wall injury (surgery; fractured hip and/or pelvis)

      iii. Hypercoagulability (e.g., increased owing to estrogen supplies, malignancy)

   b. Other etiologies

      i. Fat embolism: Orthopedic trauma (especially through marrow-containing bone) and surgery

      ii. Air embolism (e.g., from a central line)

      iii. Tumor fragments

      iv. Amniotic fluid embolism

      v. Septic debris (e.g., indwelling venous access device)

3. Subjective findings[10]

   a. Dyspnea, either insidious or sudden in onset, is the most common symptom.

   b. Apprehension, anxiety, perception of "impending doom"

   c. Substernal discomfort

   d. Pleuritic pain with pulmonary embolism with infarction

   e. Hemoptysis with pulmonary infarction

   f. Syncope

4. Physical examination findings (may range from none to frank cardiovascular collapse)

   a. Tachycardia

   b. Tachypnea and dyspnea

   c. Initially elevated blood pressure

   d. Diaphoresis

   e. Chest pain (dull central, pleuritic with pulmonary infarction)

   f. Decreased cardiac output

   g. Hypotension and shock

   h. Signs of right ventricular overload

      i. jugular venous distention

      ii. increased intensity, second heart sound

   i. Peripheral phlebitis

j. Signs of fat embolization
   i. Sudden, marked dyspnea in a susceptible patient
   ii. Altered consciousness
   iii. Body temperature elevation over 102°F
   iv. Petechiae over the thorax, shoulders, and axillae

5. Laboratory/Diagnostic findings

   a. Arterial blood gas analysis
      i. Acute respiratory alkalosis
      ii. Variable degrees of hypoxemia
   b. ECG: Nonspecific changes (Atrial fibrillation is not uncommon.)
   c. Chest x-ray: Normal, or with small infiltrates and/or effusion
   d. Ventilation/Perfusion lung scan
      i. If read as high probability for pulmonary embolism, treat with anticoagulants.
      ii. If read as indeterminate or low probability for pulmonary embolism, consider pulmonary angiography if clinical suspicion remains high.
      iii. If the chest x-ray is abnormal, or if COPD is present, lung scanning may lead to an erroneous interpretation. Consider pulmonary angiography.
   e. Pulmonary angiography remains the accepted diagnostic standard for detecting the presence of pulmonary emboli.
   f. Venous Doppler studies of the lower extremities may reveal the presence of deep venous thrombosis, which requires anticoagulation, in part obviating the need for angiography.
   g. Some authorities believe that spiral-cut, high-resolution CT scanning of the chest reliably shows central pulmonary emboli.

6. Management

   a. Anticoagulation for venous thromboembolism
      i. Heparin may be started while confirmatory tests are being conducted.
         (1) IV bolus of 5000–10,000 units, followed by a continuous infusion of 25,000–40,000 units q24h
         (2) Dosage sufficient to maintain the partial thromboplastin time (PTT) at 2–2.5 times control
         (3) Some hospitals use a heparin protocol, with PTT checks every 6 h, to guide heparin therapy.
      ii. Low molecular weight heparin (e.g., enoxaparin [Lovenox]) at 1 mg/kg subcutaneously q12h is currently an acceptable alternative to heparin. It also carries a lower risk of bleeding and of heparin-induced thrombocytopenia. No monitoring of coagulation parameters is needed.

    iii. Warfarin (Coumadin)

        (1) Begun at the time diagnosis of PE is confirmed; usual first dose: 5–10 mg p.o.

        (2) Heparin is continued until therapeutic anticoagulant levels are achieved with warfarin.

        (3) Monitor the International Normalized Ratio (INR) following initial daily doses of Coumadin. Adequate oral anticoagulant effect is achieved when the INR is 2–2.5.

        (4) Length of treatment: 3–6 months for the initial episode of PE. For recurrent episodes, treat for 6–12 months or longer, or consider placement of an indwelling vena cava filter to protect against massive embolization in patients with ongoing risk factors.

  b. Thrombolytic treatment: Note contraindications prior to instituting this therapy (see Thrombolytic Therapy for Myocardial Infarction in Chapter 11, Angina/Myocardial Infarction).

  c. May be appropriate for massive proximal PE associated with persistent systemic hypotension, and in patients with very little cardiopulmonary reserve

  d. Recombinant tissue plasminogen activator (r-TPA; Alteplase): 100 mg as a continuous infusion over 2 h

  e. Streptokinase: 250,000 units over 30 min, then 100,000 units/h for 24 h

  f. After thrombolytic therapy is completed, begin heparin or enoxaparin when the PTT is less than two times control.

  g. Hemodynamic support may be needed for massive emboli with hypotension.

  h. Surgical embolectomy: Reserved for those patients with massive emboli in central pulmonary arteries in whom the clot is creating hypotension and shock

  i. Inferior vena caval interruption ("umbrella" device; Greenfield filter)

    i. Indicated when the risk of further emboli is perceived to be high

    ii. Indicated when there is an absolute risk to anticoagulation

  j. Supplemental oxygen is indicated to keep oxygen saturation above 90%.

B. Pulmonary Vasculitis[2–5]

1. Wegener's granulomatosis

  a. Necrotizing granulomas of the respiratory tract (upper and lower), pulmonary microangiitis, and glomerulonephritis

   b. Associated with
      i. hemoptysis
      ii. dyspnea
      iii. cough
      iv. pulmonary infiltrates
   c. Antineutrophilic cytoplasmic antibodies are often positive.
   d. Treatment includes prednisone, 1 mg/kg per day, or cyclo-
      phosphamide (Cytoxan, 2 mg/kg per day, with reasonable
      chance of remission within one year.

2. Lymphomatoid granulomatosis

   a. A systemic granulomatous angiitis involving
      i. Lung
      ii. Brain
      iii. Skin (especially)
      iv. Upper respiratory tract (rarely)
      v. Kidneys (rarely)
   b. Associated with the eventual development of lymphoma
      in many cases
   c. Treatment is similar to that for Wegener's granulomatosis.

References

1. Tierney, L.M., McPhee, S.J., & Papadakis, M.A. (Eds.). (1999). *Current medical diagnosis & treatment* (38th ed.). Stamford, CT: Appleton & Lange.
2. Barker, L.R., Burton, J.R., & Zieve, P.D. (Eds.). (1999). *Principles of ambulatory medicine* (5th ed.). Baltimore: Williams & Wilkins.
3. Fauci, A.S., Braun E., Isselbacher, K.J., Wilson, J.D., Martin, J.B., Kasper, D.L., Hauser, S.L., & Longo, D.L. (Eds.). (1998). *Harrison's principles of internal medicine* (14th ed.). New York: McGraw-Hill.
4. Goldman, L., Bennett, J.C. (Eds.). (2000). *Cecil textbook of medicine* (21st ed.). Philadelphia: W.B. Saunders.
5. Albert, R., Spiro, S., & Jett, J. (Eds.). (1999). *Comprehensive respiratory medicine.* London: Mosby.
6. Butler, J., Chomsky, D.B., & Wilson, J.R. (1999). Pulmonary hypertension and exercise intolerance in patients. *Journal of the American College of Cardiology, 34,* 1802–1806.
7. Albert, N.M. (1999). Optimizing care of patients with pulmonary hypertension. *Dimensions of Critical Care Nursing, 18,* 2–11.
8. Frazier, S.K. (1999). Diagnosing and treating primary pulmonary hypertension. *Nurse Practitioner, 24,* 21–26.
9. Slipman, C.W., Lipetz, J.S., Jackson, H.B., & Vresilovic, E.J. (2000). Deep venous thrombosis and pulmonary embolism as a complication of bed rest for low back pain. *Archives of Physical Medicine and Rehabilitation, 81,* 127–129.
10. Koutkia, P., & Wachtel, T.J. (1999). Pulmonary embolism presenting as syncope. Case report and review of the literature. *Heart and Lung: The Journal of Acute and Critical Care, 28,* 342–347.

CHEST WALL
AND SECONDARY
PLEURAL DISORDERS

David A. Miller, MD, FCCP

I. DISORDERS OF THE CHEST WALL[1-5]

A. Components of the chest that can contribute to respiratory dysfunction

1. Spine
2. Rib cage
3. Costosternal margins
4. Pleura

B. Disorders of the spine

1. Congenital scoliosis

   a. The spine assumes an S-shaped curvature
   b. May induce a restrictive ventilatory defect
   c. Most often scoliosis remains an insignificant variable unless
      i. The curvature is severe.
      ii. Superimposed chest disease makes the work of breathing difficult.
   d. In these instances, the risk of respiratory failure may increase.

2. Kyphosis of the spine

   a. The spine has an accentuated dorsal curve.
   b. May induce a restrictive ventilatory defect
   c. Can coexist with scoliosis
   d. Can increase the risk of breathing problems in the presence of other chest diseases
   e. Acquired kyphosis
      i. Results from osteoporosis
      ii. A common clinical problem resulting from vertebral collapse with pain
      iii. Treatment of the pain potentially can also create additional risk of ventilatory compromise.

C. Rib and sternal fracture and sternal dehiscence following cardiac surgery

1. Fracture of the ribs, or even of the sternum, can occur either spontaneously or as the result of trauma or surgery.
2. Instability of the chest wall, with flailing of the wall outward during inspiration and the associated chest pain resulting

from fractures, limits chest wall movement, especially if multiple fractures are present.
3. Abnormal movement of the chest wall can result in hypoventilation and in poor secretion clearance.
4. Pain medication may facilitate breathing, but it can also lead to hypoventilation and ventilatory failure.
5. Milder problems can theoretically be helped with chest wall binders; however, with significant impairment of ventilation, positive pressure ventilation to stabilize the chest wall may be necessary.
6. Sternal dehiscence following open heart surgery or surgical procedures involving the mediastinum similarly can result in respiratory embarrassment.

D. Costochondral junctions

1. The costosternal junctions may become inflamed due to

   a. Arthritis (e.g., autoimmune in origin)
      i. Rheumatoid disease
      ii. Systemic lupus erythematosus
   b. Costochondritis (Tietze's syndrome)

2. While generally not serious, costochondritis may be confused with other, more serious, conditions within the chest.
3. Costochondritis is more common in young women.
4. Tenderness over the affected area is also common.
5. Nonsteroidal anti-inflammatory agents (NSAIDs; e.g., naproxen sodium [Aleve], 200–400 mg p.o. q8h) and heat are helpful in relieving the pain.

II. PLEURAL DISORDERS[1-6]

A. Pleurisy

1. Pleural pain is typically associated only with inspiration and expiration.
2. Pleurisy, painful breathing, usually is the result of inflammation of the parietal or of the visceral pleura, or of both.
3. The causes of pleurisy are the same as those of pleural effusion, listed in B.1.

B. Pleural effusion

1. Etiology of fluid accumulation within the pleural space

   a. Respiratory infection, especially viral
   b. Pulmonary embolism, with infarction extending to the visceral pleura
   c. Empyema
      i. Infection within the pleural fluid and space
      ii. Often extending from infection of the adjacent pulmonary parenchyma

    d. Malignancy, with spread to the pleural surfaces
    e. Autoimmune disorders, including
       i. Vasculitis
       ii. Systemic lupus erythematosus
       iii. Rheumatoid arthritis

2. Symptoms

    a. Dyspnea
    b. Pleuritic chest pain

3. Physical examination findings

    a. Tachypnea
    b. Dullness on percussion, with diminished or absent breath sounds over the affected area
    c. Pleural friction rub
    d. Fever, especially if the fluid is infected

4. Chest x-ray

    a. Pleural fluid between the lung and the chest wall
    b. Layering out of the fluid on decubitus chest x-rays
    c. Loculation of fluid along the lateral chest wall (may be confirmed by ultrasonography over the affected area)

5. Management

    a. Observation with or without diuresis. If the risk of infection is small and it is likely that the effusion is due to congestive heart failure, then the response may be assessed by
       i. Following the effusion
       ii. Looking for a decrease in the amount of fluid over time during diuresis
    b. Thoracentesis is indicated if
       i. The cause of the effusion must be evaluated for
         (1) Risk of infection
         (2) Malignancy
       ii. The patient is dyspneic
         (1) Procedure is therapeutic.
         (2) Procedure is theoretically also diagnostic.
    c. Laboratory evaluation of pleural fluid
       i. Cell count and differential white blood cell count
       ii. Chemistries
         (1) Total protein
         (2) Glucose (accompanied by a random blood glucose level)
         (3) Lactate dehydrogenase (LDH) levels
         (4) Amylase levels
       iii. Gram's stain and fluid cultures, as indicated by the patient's clinical status
         (1) Bacteria (aerobic and anaerobic)

   (2) Acid-fast bacilli
   (3) Fungi
   iv. Special serologic tests may be considered.
      (1) Carcinoembryonic antigen (CEA) in a patient with known colon cancer
      (2) CA125 in a woman with known ovarian cancer
   v. Determination of fluid pH, which tends to be low in
      (1) Empyema due to tuberculosis or anaerobic bacterial pathogens
      (2) Rheumatoid involvement of the pleura
   vi. Pleural fluid cytologic examination to assess for metastatic cancer to the pleura
 d. Further management issues
   i. If the fluid is bloody, insertion of a chest tube is often required.
   ii. Empyema requires chest tube insertion.
      (1) Antimicrobials alone are rarely, if ever, curative when empyema is present.
      (2) All antimicrobials used should be selected based on smear and culture results, including antimicrobial sensitivity data.
   iii. Repeated thoracentesis is an acceptable method of draining reaccumulations of malignant effusions, especially when the procedure is needed infrequently.
   iv. Malignant effusions treated with chest tube drainage may also be sclerosed (scarred down, in hopes of preventing recurrence).
      (1) A sclerosing agent, e.g., doxycycline, 100 mg, is introduced through the chest tube after drainage of the effusion is completed.
      (2) This sclerosing process is called pleurodesis.

References

1. Tierney, L.M., McPhee, S.J., & Papadakis, M.A. (Eds.). (1999). *Current medical diagnosis & treatment* (38th ed.). Stamford, CT: Appleton & Lange.
2. Barker, L.R., Burton, J.R., & Zieve, P.D. (Eds.). (1999). *Principles of ambulatory medicine* (5th ed.). Baltimore: Williams & Wilkins.
3. Fauci, A.S., Braun E., Isselbacher, K.J., Wilson, J.D., Martin, J.B., Kasper, D.L., Hauser, S.L., & Longo, D.L. (Eds). (1998). *Harrison's principles of internal medicine* (14th ed.). New York: McGraw-Hill.
4. Goldman, L., & Bennett, J.C. (Eds.). (2000). *Cecil textbook of medicine* (21st ed.). Philadelphia: W.B. Saunders.
5. Albert, R., Spiro, S., & Jett, J. (Eds.). (1999). *Comprehensive respiratory medicine*. London: Mosby.
6. Augusti, A.G., Cardus, J., Roca, J., Grau, J.M., Xaubert, A., & Rodriguez-Roisin, R. (1997). Ventilation-perfusion mismatch in patients with pleural effusion: Effects of thoracentesis. *American Journal of Respiratory & Critical Care Medicine, 156*, 1205–1209.

RESPIRATORY FAILURE

David A. Miller, MD, FCCP

I. DEFINITIONS AND CONCEPTS[2]

A. Breathing

1. A lay term, breathing is understood as the movement of air into and out of the lungs.
2. Physiologically, breathing is controlled by the metabolic needs of the body (i.e., oxygen and carbon dioxide levels in the blood) as perceived by the central nervous system (chemoreceptor input).
3. Breathing is also under voluntary control in conscious, alert individuals.

B. Ventilation

1. Ventilation is the aspect of breathing that refers to the actual movement of air into and out of the lungs.
2. Ventilation is determined by the volume of air moved (tidal volume) and by the ventilatory rate.
3. Individuals who are alert and spontaneously breathing vary the amount of air inhaled and exhaled with each breath, and in respiratory rate, responding to the central nervous system's control over the ventilatory act.
4. Yawning and sighing are normal variations seen during the act of ventilation.

C. Respiration

1. Respiration refers to

    a. Actual use of oxygen at the cellular level, and
    b. Removal from the cellular environment of
       i. Carbon dioxide
       ii. Metabolic wastes, especially metabolic acids
          (1) Lactic acid
          (2) Ketoacids

2. Cellular respiration is dependent on two variables:

    a. Perfusion of capillaries with oxygen and nutrient-laden blood in adequate amounts (Cellular uptake and use of oxygen normally are independent of oxygen delivery.)

  b. Venous blood flow removing cellular metabolic wastes to the heart, lungs, and kidneys
    i. For distribution to other cells, especially
      (1) Alveoli
      (2) Liver
      (3) Kidneys
    ii. For further metabolism as needed and eventual removal from the body via
      (1) Expiration
      (2) Stool
      (3) Urine

II. VENTILATORY FAILURE[1, 2]

A. Ventilatory failure refers to absent or inadequate movement of oxygen into the lungs and/or of carbon dioxide out of the lungs.

1. Apnea—Absence of movement
2. Hypopnea—Inadequate movement

B. Ventilatory failure is best assessed by measurement of the $Paco_2$ and/or the end-tidal CO_2 levels.
C. Causes of ventilatory failure

1. Ventilatory failure may be induced by overdose of medications (e.g., sedatives, hypnotics, and narcotics), relative to the body's ability to continue to respond to metabolic and cellular respiratory needs while influenced by these drugs.

  a. Unintentional overdose (e.g., iatrogenic oversedation in the presence of COPD)
  b. Intentional overdose, e.g.,
    i. Iatrogenic sedation with the intent to control ventilation
    ii. Drug overdose with suicidal intent

2. The ability to get oxygen into, and carbon dioxide out of, the lungs is impaired by acquired acute pathology secondary to

  a. Infections of the lungs (e.g., in patients with COPD)
  b. Neuromuscular disease
    i. Myasthenia gravis in crisis
    ii. Guillain-Barré syndrome
    iii. Traumatic head or spinal cord injury
  c. Pulmonary edema of either cardiogenic or noncardiogenic cause

III. RESPIRATORY FAILURE[1, 2]

A. Definition

1. Failure of adequate oxygen delivery to cells (during hypotension)
2. Failure of the cell's ability to use oxygen (e.g., cyanide poisoning, carbon monoxide poisoning)

B. The term *shock* is best reserved for situations in which respiratory failure is generalized throughout the body.

1. The sepsis syndrome with hypotension poses risk not only to the lungs but also to critically important organs, including the kidneys, heart, liver, gut, and central nervous system.
2. In sepsis syndrome, oxygen delivery to cells becomes pathophysiologically supply-dependent. Hence,

   a. Ventilation must ensure adequate supply of oxygen to the body.
   b. Circulation needs adequate volume support and systemic vascular resistance to ensure delivery of oxygen and nutrients to cells without overloading the ability of the heart to pump blood into the circulation.
   c. Pulmonary artery catheter monitoring becomes essential to determine cardiac status and systemic vascular resistance.
   d. Measuring the amount of oxygen returning to the heart reflects the overall distribution of oxygen and nutrients to cells (Svo_2 monitoring).

C. The goal of treating respiratory failure is prevention of cellular ischemia and death while the cause of the respiratory failure is corrected.

1. Control of ventilation, oxygen supply, and nutrient supply are all critical.
2. Also critical is the prevention of problems associated with mechanical ventilation.

   a. Pneumothorax
   b. Nosocomial pneumonia
   c. Indwelling catheter–related sepsis
   d. Malnutrition during the course of respiratory failure

References

1. Albert, R., Spiro, S., & Jett, J. (Eds.). (1999). *Comprehensive respiratory medicine.* London: Mosby.
2. Goldman, L., & Bennett, J.C. (Eds.). (2000). *Cecil textbook of medicine* (21st ed.). Philadelphia: W.B. Saunders.

PNEUMOTHORAX

Judith Azok, MSN, RN, ARNP, GNP-C

I. PNEUMOTHORAX

A. DEFINITION

1. A presence of air in the pleural space resulting from a perforation through the chest wall or pleura causing collapse of the lung
2. Types[1, 2, 7, 9, 11]

   a. Spontaneous: Disruption of the visceral pleura; air enters the pleural space from the lung; occurs in individuals with or without underlying lung disease.
   b. Traumatic
      i. Open: Penetrating chest trauma; parietal pleura disrupted, allowing air to enter the pleural space from the atmosphere
      ii. Closed: Blunt chest trauma; the visceral pleural is disrupted, allowing air to enter the pleural space from the lung
      iii. Iatrogenic: Disruption of the visceral pleura as a complication of an invasive thoracic procedure; may also follow procedures involving the neck or the abdomen
   c. Tension: Air enters the pleural space as a result of a spontaneous or traumatic pneumothorax, but is unable to exit; as pressure rises in the pleural space, the lung collapses and mediastinum shifts to the other side; tension pneumothorax is a medical emergency.

B. Etiology/Incidence/Predisposing factors[1, 3, 7, 8, 10]

1. Penetrating or blunt chest trauma
2. Rupture of a subpleural bleb or invasian of visceral pleura by disease (e.g., necrotizing pneumonia)
3. Intrinsic lung disease

   i. Chronic obstructive pulmonary disease
   ii. Tuberculosis
   iii. Sarcoidosis
   iv. Pulmonary fibrosis
   v. Bronchogenic carcinoma

4. Barotrauma resulting from mechanical ventilation with increased positive end-expiratory pressure

5. Complication of invasive thoracic, neck, or abdominal diagnostic or therapeutic procedures

    i. Insertion of intravenous access device
    ii. Needle biopsy of liver or lung
    iii. Thoracentesis

C. Subjective findings: Dependent on degree of lung collapse and mechanism involved[4, 8, 11]

1. Possible sudden onset of dyspnea
2. Pleuritic chest pain, at times sharp and severe
3. Apprehension, agitation

D. Physical examination findings: Manifestations depend on degree of lung collapse and mechanism involved.[2, 3, 5, 6, 8, 10]

1. Splinting and decreased inspiratory expansion of involved hemithorax
2. Bulging of intercostal spaces on affected side during exhalation
3. Decreased breath sounds and fremitus, and a hyper-resonant percussion note over affected area
4. Tracheal deviation toward unaffected side
5. Subcutaneous emphysema
6. Possible Hamman's sign (mediastinal crepitus on auscultation)
7. In the mechanically ventilated patient with positive end-expiratory pressure: Development of high peak inspiratory pressure with decreased compliance
8. Tension pneumothorax: Signs of decreased cardiac output

E. Laboratory and diagnostic findings[2, 10]

1. Arterial blood gases: Mild to moderate hypoxemia; hypercapnia with severe embolus
2. Chest x-ray: Confirms degree of lung collapse

F. Management[2, 5, 6, 8, 10]

1. Tension pneumothorax

    a. Immediate decompression with 14- to 16-gauge needle into the 2nd intercostal space, midclavicular line
    b. Insertion of chest tube at the 4th or 5th intercostal space midaxillary line to closed water-seal drainage

2. Spontaneous pneumothorax: Depends on size

    a. If small, give supplemental oxygen and observe
    b. Collapse >20%: Insert chest tube to water-seal drainage

3. Traumatic pneumothorax

    a. Prompt chest tube insertion, 4th or 5th intercostal space midaxillary line with closed chest drainage

4. Negative pressure (application of suction to chest drainage apparatus)

 a. Use when underwater seal fails to re-expand lung after 24–48 h, or
 b. When persistent pneumothorax perpetuates hypoxemia and/or hypercapnia

References

1. Bardow, R., & Mose, K. (1996). *Manual of clinical problems in pulmonary medicine* (4th ed.). Boston: Little, Brown & Co.
2. Bucher, L., & Melander, S. (1999). *Critical care nursing*. Philadelphia: W.B. Saunders.
3. Chulay, M., Gizzetta, C., & Dossey, B. (1997). *AACN handbook of critical care nursing*. Stamford CT: Appleton & Lange.
4. Hudak, C., Gallo, B., & Marten, P. (1998). *Critical care nursing: A holistic approach* (7th ed.). Philadelphia: J.B. Lippincott.
5. Rakel, R. (1999). *Conn's current therapy*. Philadelphia: W.B. Saunders.
6. Roberts, S.L. (1996). *Critical care nursing: Assessment and intervention*. Stamford, CT: Appleton & Langue.
7. Ruppert, S., Kernicki, J., & Dolan, T. (1996). *Dolan's critical care nursing: Clinical management through the nursing process* (2nd ed.). Philadelphia: F.A. Davis.
8. Stein, J.H. (1998). *Internal medicine* (4th ed.). St. Louis: Mosby.
9. Thelan, L.A., Davie, J.K., Urden, L.D., & Zough, M.E. (1998). *Critical care nursing: Diagnosis and management* (3rd ed.). St. Louis: Mosby.
10. Tierney, L.M., McPhee, S.J., & Papadakis, M.A. (2000). *Current medical diagnosis and treatment*. (39th ed.). Samford, CT: Appleton & Lange.
11. Ureden, L.D., Tough, M.E., & Stacey, K.M. (1996). *Priorities in critical care nursing* (2nd ed.). St. Louis: Mosby.

LOWER RESPIRATORY TRACT PATHOGENS

David A. Miller, MD, FCCP

I. LOWER RESPIRATORY TRACT PATHOGENS

A. Defined as those pathogens found below the larynx

1. Note that the pathogens are the same in all parts of the lower respiratory tract.
2. Recommended pharmacologic treatment may require revision after the results of sputum and blood cultures are complete (Table 31–1).[1, 2, 3]

B. Milder disease requires only narrow-spectrum antimicrobials, if any.
C. Severe disease requires a combination of antimicrobials while cultures are pending.
D. The suggestions in Table 31–1 are for empirically chosen therapy while sputum and blood cultures are completed.

1. When culture data are available, antimicrobials used should be reviewed and changed if necessary.
2. The narrowest spectrum antimicrobial that is reasonably expected to effectively treat the patient's lower respiratory tract infection should be used.

E. Recall that antimicrobial therapy is intended to help clear the pulmonary infection.

1. Other pharmacologic and nonpharmacologic therapy should be considered as well.
2. Examples

   a. Supplemental oxygen
   b. Treatment of underlying chronic obstructive pulmonary disease
   c. Nutritional support

TABLE 31-1. LOWER RESPIRATORY TRACT PATHOGENS AND TREATMENTS

LOWER RESPIRATORY TRACT INFECTION	ORGANISM	RECOMMENDED PHARMACOLOGIC TREATMENT
Acute tracheobronchitis	Viral *Mycoplasma pneumoniae* *Chlamydia pneumoniae* *Bordetella pertussis*	No therapy indicated.
Acute bacterial exacerbation of COPD	Viral, with secondary bacterial infection *Streptococcus pneumoniae* *Haemophilus pneumoniae* *Moraxella catarrhalis*	Therapy may be unnecessary. Consider trimethoprim-sulfamethoxazole DS (Bactrim DS; Septra DS), one pill b.i.d. for 7–10 days. *OR* doxycycline (Vibramycin), 100 mg b.i.d. for 7–10 days. Clarithromycin (Biaxin), 500 mg b.i.d. for 7 days. Azithromycin (Zithromax), 500 mg, then 250 mg, q.d. for 4 more days.
Pneumonia: Community-acquired	Influenza (winter months)	Amantadine (Symmetrel), 100 mg b.i.d. for 10 days. *OR* rimantadine (Flumadine), 100 mg b.i.d. for 10 days.
	Other viral	Supportive therapy. May check for respiratory syncytial virus in elderly or immunocompromised patients, although ribavirin (Virazole) effectiveness in this setting is unknown.

Table continued on following page

LOWER RESPIRATORY TRACT INFECTION	ORGANISM	RECOMMENDED PHARMACOLOGIC TREATMENT
	Streptococcus pneumoniae *Mycoplasma pneumoniae* *Chlamydia pneumoniae* *Legionella pneumophila* (summer)	Erythromycin (ERYC), 500 mg q.i.d. for 7–10 days, OR Clarithromycin (Biaxin), 500 mg b.i.d. for 7–10 days, OR Azithromycin (Zithromax), 500 mg, then 250 mg, q.d. for 5 days (given IV as 500 mg daily if unable to take by mouth).
	Streptococcus pneumoniae *Haemophilus pneumoniae* *Mycoplasma pneumoniae* *Chlamydia pneumoniae*	Erythromycin (ERYC), 500 mg q.i.d. for 7–10 days, OR Clarithromycin (Biaxin), 500 mg b.i.d. for 7–10 days, OR Azithromycin (Zithromax), 500 mg, then 250 mg, q.d. for 5 days.
Pneumonia: Community-acquired with comorbidity and over age 60 years, or admitted to ICU (*Note: Initial therapy may dictate broad-spectrum coverage, including gram-positive, and gram-negative bacteria, pending culture results.*)	Anaerobes (aspiration pneumonia) *S. pneumoniae* covered by penicillin.	Aqueous penicillin G, 2 million units IV q4h, OR Clindamycin (Cleocin), 600–900 mg IV q8h.

	Gram-positive organisms and some Gram-negative organisms.* Note that many clinicians choose to treat with two antipseudomonal antibiotics when *Pseudomonas* infection is suspected.	Cefotaxime (Claforan), 1–2 g IV q8h, *OR* Ceftazidime (Fortaz), 1 g IV q8h. Levofloxacin (Levaquin), 500 mg IV q24h.
Pneumonia: Causing respiratory failure without neutropenia	*Staphylococcus aureus*	Methicillin-resistant: Vancomycin (Vancocin), 1 g IV q8–12h.
	Gram-negative organisms*	Cefotaxime (Claforan), 1–2 g IV q8h, *OR* Ceftazidime (Fortaz), 2 g IV q8h, *OR* Imipenem/cilastatin (Primaxin), 500 mg IV q6h.
	Legionella pneumophila	Erythromycin (ERYC), 1 g IV q6h for 7–10 days, *OR* Azithromycin (Zithromax), 500 mg, then 250 mg IV, q.d. for 5 days.
Pneumonia: Causing respiratory failure with neutropenia	Gram-negative organisms*	Cefotaxime (Claforan), 1–2 g IV q8h, *OR* Ceftazidime (Fortaz), 1 g IV q8h, *OR* Imipenem/cilastatin (Primaxin), 500 mg IV q6h.
	Staphylococcus aureus	Vancomycin (Vancocin), 1 g IV q8h *if sputum Gram stain suggests staphylococcus.*
	Fungi (*Candida* spp.; *Aspergillus*)	Amphotericin B (Fungizone), IV in titrated doses.

*Gram-negative bacteria: *Klebsiella pneumoniae, Haemophilus pneumoniae, Escherichia coli, Pseudomonas* spp., *Acinetobacter* spp., *Enterobacter cloacae,* and others.

References

1. Albert, R., Spiro, S., & Jett, J. (Eds.). (1999). *Comprehensive respiratory medicine*. London: Mosby.
2. Gilbert, D.N., Moellering, R.C., & Sande, M.A. (1999). *The Sanford guide to antimicrobial therapy, 1999* (29th ed.). Vienna, VA: Antimicrobial Therapy.
3. Goldman, L., & Bennett, J.C. (Eds.). (2000). *Cecil textbook of medicine* (21st ed.). Philadelphia: W.B. Saunders.

OBSTRUCTIVE SLEEP APNEA

David A. Miller, MD, FCCP

I. CHARACTERISTICS OF BREATHING AND SLEEP[1, 3]

A. Tidal volume and respiratory rate decline as a person becomes more deeply asleep. Skeletal muscle tone decreases progressively in deeper stages of sleep, with frank atony during rapid eye movement (REM) sleep.

B. Peak airway resistance tends to be highest during the period from 2 AM to 6 AM and lowest during the period from 2 PM to 6 PM.

C. Symptoms of cough and shortness of breath may be aggravated during the normal sleeping period at night.

D. Normal pauses in respiration are infrequent and brief, lasting 5–10 s. These pauses are central in origin and are not associated with physical obstruction of the oropharynx or hypopharynx.

II. OBSTRUCTIVE SLEEP APNEA (OSA)[3]

A. Etiology

1. Obstruction of the upper airway by collapse of the soft tissues (muscle, fat) during sleep
2. Obstruction causes arousals and awakenings from sleep, and effective sleep time is reduced.

B. Incidence

1. The incidence is unknown. However, obstructive sleep apnea and hypopnea are often under-recognized in clinical practice.
2. OSA is more commonly noted among obese individuals, but the absence of obesity does not rule out the possible existence of OSA.

C. Clinical manifestations[4]

1. The classic manifestation of significant OSA is excessive daytime sleepiness (EDS).
2. Snoring is commonly heard, although severe sleep apnea may be accompanied by quiet snoring.
3. Severe daytime sleepiness interferes with normal daytime functioning.

   a. Additional attempts to "catch up" on sleep fail.
   b. Driving a vehicle or operating heavy machinery may become dangerous.

4. Hypoxemia during the apneic and hypopneic episodes may lead to adverse health consequences, including

   a. Myocardial ischemia, infarction, arrhythmias, and congestive heart failure

   b. Cerebral ischemia and stroke

   c. Sudden death

   d. Cardiorespiratory arrest following surgery or administration of sedatives, hypnotics, and narcotics

D. Physical findings

1. Mental status demonstrates less than optimal alertness.
2. Obesity, with fatty infiltration of the soft palate and pharyngeal wall and a decrease in the posterior pharyngeal space. Tonsillar enlargement, if present, aggravates the obstruction, as does enlargement of the adenoids.
3. Right-sided heart failure, with peripheral edema, may be seen.

E. Diagnosis[2]

1. Polysomnography (PSG), or an overnight sleep study measuring air flow, muscle tone, and brain wave activity, is required.
2. The finding of more than 10 obstructive apneas/hypopneas (respiratory effort in the absence of, or significant reduction in, air flow during sleep) per hour is abnormal and justifies treatment, especially if oxygen desaturations below 88% are documented.
3. Oxygen desaturations below 88% during sleep may require supplemental oxygen if they do not improve with therapy.

F. Treatment

1. General

   a. Avoidance of alcohol, sedatives, hypnotics, and narcotics until effective therapy is begun

   b. Weight loss and maintenance, if indicated

   c. Avoidance of driving and operation of heavy machinery until effectively treated, and there is a significant reduction in daytime sleepiness

2. Specific

   a. Institution of nasal continuous positive airway pressure (nCPAP) or bilevel, inspiratory and expiratory, positive airway pressure (nbiPAP) to stent the posterior pharynx.

      i. The pressure is delivered by a mechanically driven device and applied through a snugly and appropriately fitted mask over the nose or a pair of fitted nasal "pillows."

    ii. A chin strap may be required to avoid pressure leaks through the mouth.

    iii. Humidification added to the mechanical circuitry may help avoid mucosal dryness.

  b. The pressure needed to treat the OSA may be empirically chosen (e.g., 10 cm water pressure); however, the optimal therapy is best determined by repeat PSG and titration of the pressure to the level that fully alleviates the obstructive events and oxygen desaturations.

  c. Follow-up to determine adherence to the recommended therapies is crucial. The patient should use the nCPAP during all sleeping periods.

3. Other therapies

  a. Surgical removal of excessive tissue in the posterior pharynx, if nCPAP/nbiPAP fail to alleviate EDS and to reduce the frequency of apneas and hypopneas and oxygen desaturation as determined by follow-up PSG

    i. Uvulopalatopharyngoplasty

    ii. Tonsillectomy and/or adenoidectomy

  b. Mandibular advancement to pull the tongue forward to create additional posterior pharyngeal space

  c. Oral devices to increase the posterior pharyngeal space tend to be uncomfortable and therefore ineffective in treating OSA.

  d. Tracheostomy relieves OSA promptly and was the definitive therapy before nCPAP. It is now reserved for those individuals with severe disease who are unable to use nCPAP or nbiPAP, or who are not candidates for surgical resection of redundant tissue.

References

1. Albert, R., Spiro, S., & Jett, J. (Eds.) (1999). *Comprehensive respiratory medicine*. Philadelphia: Mosby.
2. Herer, B., Roche, N., Carton, M., Roig, C., Poujol, V., & Huchon, G. (1999). Value of clinical, functional, and oximetric data for the prediction of obstructive sleep apnea in obese patients. *Chest, 116*, 1537–1544.
3. Kryger, M.H., Roth, T., & Dement, W.L. (2000). *Principles and practice of sleep medicine* (3rd ed.). Philadelphia: W.B. Saunders.
4. Strohl, K.P., & Redline, S. (1996). Recognition of obstructive sleep apnea. *American Journal of Respiratory and Critical Care Medicine, 154*, 279–292.

OXYGEN SUPPLEMENTATION

John P. McGuinness, MD

I. BASIC PRINCIPLES OF OXYGEN SUPPLEMENTATION[6-8]

A. Hospital oxygen supplies typically originate at a wall source or from a portable oxygen cylinder.

1. Wall source oxygen comes from a bulk supply and originates from a large tank outside the hospital. The pressure at the wall source is 50 lb per square inch (psi).
2. Oxygen cylinders are uniformly green in color; all full oxygen cylinders have a pressure of 2000 to 2200 lb psi.

   a. The cylinder pressure varies directly with the volume of oxygen in the cylinder; a cylinder with a pressure of 1100 lb psi is half full.
   b. Oxygen cylinders require pressure reduction valves to deliver oxygen to a patient.

3. Oxygen delivered from either the wall source or the cylinder is dehumidified and is very drying to mucous membranes unless humidified.
4. Patients are typically transported with supplemental oxygen in D cylinders.

   a. A D cylinder contains 400 L oxygen (at 2200 lb psi).
   b. A D cylinder will provide 80 min of flow at 5 L/min. Plan accordingly.

B. Indications for oxygen supplementation

1. All patients with chest pain should be provided oxygen supplementation until evaluation for cardiac injury is completed.
2. Patients with a history of carbon dioxide retention (e.g., chronic obstructive pulmonary disease) should receive oxygen supplementation with caution.

   a. Overzealous oxygenation will suppress hypoxic respiratory drive and lead to apnea.
   b. Those who require oxygen supplementation may benefit from assisted ventilation.

3. Each time oxygen supplementation is initiated, the effects of the intervention must be measured.

   a. In most circumstances, determination of peripheral oxygen saturation (SpO_2) with a pulse oximeter will suffice.
   b. A reasonable goal is to maintain the SpO_2 at 92–75%.

4. The need for oxygen supplementation in a hospitalized patient should be regularly reassessed on at least a daily basis.

   a. Periodic pulse oximetry is very useful in documenting the benefits and continued need for supplemental oxygen.
   b. Oximetry should be performed both at rest and after exertion.

II. OXYGENATION WITH FACILITATION OF VENTILATION[1, 5]

A. Occasionally patients are unable to maintain spontaneous ventilation.

1. Example of such patients are victims of trauma, cardiac arrest, or drug overdose.
2. These patients require both oxygen supplementation and ventilatory assistance.

B. Airway maintenance and mouth-to-mouth ventilation are the first lines of ventilatory assistance.

1. Airway maintenance focuses on proper head position and jaw thrust maneuver and is well covered in basic and advanced life support courses.
2. Even well-administered mouth-to-mouth breathing delivers a fraction of inspired oxygen (FIO_2) of only 16–17%, compared with 21% oxygen in room air.

C. A pocket mask device allows mouth-to-mouth ventilation without personal contact.

1. Some pocket masks have a port allowing the administration of supplemental oxygen.
2. Pocket mask devices are eminently portable.

D. Bag valve mask devices

1. Bag valve mask devices allow administration of supplemental oxygen via a face mask and reservoir bag.
2. Depending on oxygen flow and operator skill, it is possible to administer high concentrations of oxygen.
3. Self inflating bags are

   a. Versatile
   b. Can be used with or without supplemental oxygen
   c. Available in various sizes appropriate for infants, children, and adults

4. The major complication of a bag valve mask device is inflation of the stomach resulting from poor airway maintenance or high ventilation pressures.

   a. Be alert for the development of gastric distention.
   b. Relieve the distention through placement of a nasogastric tube.

    c. Do not compress the distended stomach manually; emesis may result.

5. The mask is an essential component of the device and should be sized to the patient.

    a. A well fitting mask with a seal that encompasses the nose and the mouth is important in ensuring adequate ventilation.

    b. The mask should be clear to allow visualization of emesis.

6. The airway in an unconscious patient is more easily maintained with an oropharyngeal airway.

    a. The device will lift the tongue from the posterior pharynx.

    b. Oropharyngeal airways are not tolerated by patients with intact gag reflexes.

    c. The oropharyngeal airway requires a small degree of skill for placement.

       i. Inept placement may traumatize the soft tissues of the oropharynx or occlude the airway.

      ii. To safely place the airway

        (1) Open the patient's mouth.

        (2) Move the tongue aside with a tongue blade.

        (3) Insert the oropharyngeal airway.

7. A nasopharyngeal airway is a soft plastic device placed through the nares that provides a passage through the posterior pharynx.

    a. Lubrication with lidocaine jelly facilitates placement and enhances patient tolerance.

    b. A nasopharyngeal airway is usually tolerated by a conscious patient.

    c. Nasopharyngeal airways are especially useful in patients

       i. With orofacial trauma

      ii. In whom the oropharynx is not accessible

E. Suction devices are an important adjunct to ventilation.

1. Sudden cessation of ventilation may be due to airway occlusion by emesis or a mucus plug.

2. Accumulation of saliva and airway secretions can also cause occlusion.

3. A rigid suction device (e.g., Yankauer suction) is generally more useful than a flexible catheter for airway maintenance in the posterior pharynx because the rigid device can be operated with one hand.

III. DEVICES FOR OXYGEN SUPPLEMENTATION[2-4]

A. Nasal prongs are the simplest means of delivering supplemental oxygen.

1. As a general rule, each liter of oxygen flow increases FIO_2 by 4% up to 6 L/min.
2. Use of nasal prongs assumes the patient is a nose breather and has a near-normal tidal volume.

   a. The device relies on the anatomic reservoir in the nasopharynx to store oxygen between inhalations.
   b. The oxygen stored in the nasopharynx is mixed with room air during inhalation.

3. Patients may find nasal prongs uncomfortable with prolonged use. High flows of nasal oxygen will dry the mucous membranes even when the oxygen is humidified.

B. Face masks provide a higher FIO_2 than nasal prongs; most patients can tolerate the mask well.

1. A properly functioning face mask can provide an FIO_2 of 40–60%, depending on the oxygen flow.
2. Because exhaled gas may accumulate in the mask, the oxygen flow must be sufficient to expel exhaled gases. A flow of 6 L/min prevents rebreathing.
3. Some face masks have one-way flap valves on the flange of the mask.

   a. These valves often become sticky with moisture and fail to allow exhaled gas to escape.

   b. The flap valve should be removed if not functional and the mask replaced if a high FIO_2 is required.

C. A face mask with a reservoir bag can provide a higher FIO_2 than a plain face mask.

1. A face mask with a reservoir bag and a high oxygen flow rate can deliver an FIO_2 of nearly 100%.
2. To obtain a high FIO_2 the mask must fit snugly and must not be removed.
3. The reservoir bag serves to store oxygen delivered from the source between inspirations.
4. A one-way valve between the mask and the reservoir bag prevents accumulation of exhaled gas in the reservoir bag.

D. A Venturi mask is a refinement in oxygen delivery systems that allows the delivery of a known FIO_2.

1. Most mask systems deliver an approximate FIO_2, and the flow must be titrated to effect.
2. The heart of the Venturi mask is a nozzle with an aperture of known diameter.

   a. As the oxygen flow passes through the aperture, the gas flow entrains a fixed amount of room air.

b. The amount of air entrained depends on the velocity of oxygen through the aperture and the pressure gradient.

3. To change the FIO_2 delivered, the Venturi valve must be changed.

4. The Venturi mask offers little advantage over other masks except that the FIO_2 is more accurately determined. This feature may be useful in patients in whom a high FIO_2 may be harmful.

5. Differing colors of valves in Venturi masks provide varying percentages of oxygen; the amount of oxygen delivered is visible on the valve.

References

1. Charters, P., & O'Sullivan, E. (1999). The 'dedicated airway': A review of the concept and an update of current practice. *Anaesthesia, 54,* 778–786.

2. Holm, C., Christensen, M., Schulze, S., & Rosenberg, J. (1999). Effect of oxygen on tachycardia and arterial oxygen saturation during colonoscopy. *European Journal of Surgery, 165,* 755–758.

3. Orme, R.M., & Williams, M. (1999). Supplementary oxygen and the laryngeal mask airway—Evaluation of a heat-and-moisture exchanger. *Anaesthesia and Intensive Care, 27,* 509–511.

4. Poh, J., & Brimacombe, J. (1998). A comparison of the T-piece, Venturi T-piece, and T-bag for emergence with the laryngeal mask. *Anaesthesia and Intensive Care, 26,* 526–528.

5. St. John, R.E. (1999). Advances in artificial airway management. *Critical Care Nursing Clinics of North America, 11,* 7–17.

6. Waldau, T., Larsen, V.H., & Bonde, J. (1998). Evaluation of five oxygen delivery devices in spontaneously breathing subjects by oxygraphy. *Anaesthesia, 53,* 256–263.

7. Wilkes, A.R., & Vaughan, R.S. (1999). The use of breathing system filters as oxygen-delivery devices. *Anaesthesia, 54,* 552–558.

8. Zielinski, J. (1999). Indications for long-term oxygen therapy: a reappraisal. *Archive of Chest Diseases, 54,* 178–182.

MECHANICAL VENTILATORY SUPPORT

John P. McGuinness, MD

I. INDICATIONS FOR MECHANICAL VENTILATION[2, 3, 5, 14]

A. Indicated when a patient is unable to maintain a ventilatory effort adequate to prevent hypoxemia or has insufficient ventilation for adequate gas exchange, thus causing hypercarbia

B. Hypoxic patients: Those who are extremely sedated may lack sufficient ventilatory drive.

C. Hypercarbic patients

1. These patients typically have a $Paco_2$ >45 mmHg.
2. A common scenario is hypercarbia in an asthmatic patient who has become exhausted by the effort to ventilate against increased airway resistance.
3. In these patients, hypoxemia is an early and common finding.
4. However, hypercarbia is far more ominous and signals the possibility of respiratory failure due to impending exhaustion.

D. Apneic patients require mechanical ventilation.

II. GENERAL PRINCIPLES OF VENTILATION[4, 15–17]

A. Normal human ventilation is based on a negative pressure created when the contraction of the diaphragm causes the volume of the thoracic cavity to expand, leading to inspiration of ambient air.

B. Mechanical ventilation relies on an external positive pressure generated by a device to force air into the lungs. Along with this fundamental change in the method of ventilation, mechanical ventilation requires the determination of certain ventilatory parameters.

C. Mechanical ventilators allow many rate settings, depending on the respiratory condition of the patient. A typical initial ventilator rate setting is 10 breaths per minute; however, the actual rate will vary with the patient's condition.

D. Tidal volume (V_T) is the size of an individual breath.

1. A typical initial setting for tidal volume for mechanical ventilation is 7–10 mL/kg.
2. However, this volume represents a starting point and may go as high as 15 mL/kg.

E. The fraction of inspired oxygen (F_{IO_2}) is the percentage of oxygen in the inspired gas mixture.

1. Room air has an F_{IO_2} of 21%.
2. The initial setting of F_{IO_2} for a ventilated patient is contingent on the patient's condition and usually ranges from 60 to 100%.
3. An F_{IO_2} >50% is associated with the risk of pulmonary oxygen toxicity.
4. Over time, efforts should be made to decrease an elevated F_{IO_2} as quickly as the patient can tolerate it.

F. Positive end-expiratory pressure (PEEP) may be thought of as a "back pressure" at the end of expiration intended to maintain the expanded volume of peripheral alveoli.

1. In a normally breathing person, the occasional cough or yawn may be thought of as a sort of physiologic PEEP.
2. Manipulation of PEEP during mechanical ventilation is useful in allowing a decrease of F_{IO_2} by recruiting peripheral alveoli to take part in gas exchange.
3. A typical initial setting of PEEP is 5 cm H_2O.
4. PEEP may range as high as 40 cm H_2O in conditions such as adult respiratory distress syndrome (ARDS).

G. An important principle of mechanical ventilator management is that each time V_T, F_{IO_2}, or PEEP is adjusted, the effect of the alteration should be evaluated within 20–30 min with

1. Arterial blood gas analysis
2. Peripheral arterial oxygenation saturation measurement
3. End-tidal carbon dioxide reading

H. Chest x-rays

1. A patient requiring mechanical ventilation usually requires a daily chest x-ray to evaluate

    a. Endotracheal tube placement
    b. Status of pulmonary infiltrates
    c. Presence of a pneumothorax
    d. Atelectasis
    e. Heart size

2. A stable patient undergoing a prolonged course of mechanical ventilation may be managed with a chest x-ray on alternate days.

I. Nutritional needs

1. Although it is not directly related to ventilation, adequate nutrition must be ensured during periods of ventilation.

2. As a general rule, a patient who is ventilated for >48 h should be considered for nutritional supplementation, either by tube feeding or by total parenteral nutrition.

III. MODES OF VENTILATION[5, 13]

A. Continuous mechanical ventilation (CMV)

1. Provides mechanical ventilation in the absence of spontaneous patient effort
2. Delivers a defined volume per minute at a fixed rate and tidal volume

B. Intermittent mandatory ventilation (IMV)

1. Permits a patient breathing spontaneously but inadequately to breathe without assistance above a set rate provided the preset minimal parameters are achieved. For example:

   a. A minimal ventilation rate might be 6 breaths per minute.
   b. A patient with a spontaneous respiratory rate <6 breaths per minute will be ventilated by the device.

2. Allows a gradual reduction in the amount of ventilatory support provided
3. Aids in the transition from mechanical to spontaneous ventilation
4. Allows a reduction in mean airway pressure, thus decreasing the potential for barotrauma

C. Assist control ventilation (ACV)

1. ACV detects a patient's inspiratory effort and delivers a set tidal volume.
2. In the absence of patient effort, this mode provides continuous mechanical ventilation.

D. Pressure support ventilation (PSV)

1. Senses a spontaneous ventilatory effort
2. Provides additional pressure as needed
3. Useful in weaning a ventilator-dependent patient
4. Greatly decreases the work associated with ventilation

E. Pressure cycled ventilation

1. Unlike the other modes, which deliver a set *volume* to an apneic patient, pressure cycled ventilation delivers a set *pressure* to the patient.
2. Implicit in delivering a set pressure is that an adequate volume will be achieved.

   a. Typically used in infants and small children
   b. Gaining popularity for use among critically ill adults

F. Continuous positive airway pressure (CPAP)

1. Uses a positive pressure generator to augment the normal variation in airway pressure

   a. A spontaneously ventilating patient will initiate inspiration by generating a negative intrathoracic pressure.
   b. CPAP maintains a positive pressure during inspiration.

2. The artificially generated positive pressure may be visualized as making the physiologic negative pressure a little less negative, thus limiting airway collapse with negative inspiratory pressures.
3. CPAP is important in the treatment of sleep apnea.

   a. Prevents airway collapse
   b. Mitigates snoring

IV. SPECIAL ISSUES IN MANAGEMENT OF MECHANICAL VENTILATION[6, 7, 19]

A. Positive end-expiratory pressure (PEEP)

1. "Back pressure" intended to maintain inflation of peripheral alveoli; by aiding in maintaining alveolar patency, protects functional reserve capacity
2. May decrease ventilation-perfusion $\dot{V}/\dot{Q}$ mismatch (i.e., PEEP helps ensure adequate alveolar surface area to permit sufficient pulmonary gas exchange)
3. Indications for PEEP

   a. Need for a high FIO_2 to maintain an adequate PaO_2
   b. Circumstances in which alveoli have collapsed
      i. Pulmonary consolidation
      ii. ARDS
      iii. Generalized infiltrates

4. Limitations

   a. May increase intrathoracic pressure and can result in a decrease in cardiac preload and thus in cardiac output
   b. High levels of PEEP can shift the cardiac intraventricular septum.
   c. May cause barotrauma leading to pneumothorax
   d. May increase central venous pressure, leading to an increase in intracranial pressure

B. Patient positioning can improve oxygenation.

1. Pulmonary blood flow is governed largely by gravity. Thus, when one lung is better ventilated than the other, the *good* side should be *down,* as in a decubitus position.
2. Positioning the patient in a semi-sitting position relieves the pressure of the abdominal contents on the diaphragm and allows greater functional reserve capacity.

3. Lateral rotational beds allow the patient's position to be altered, thereby assisting in positioning and employing the favorable effects of gravity on lung function.

C. Suctioning

1. Frequency of suctioning should be minimized. Each attempt removes not only pulmonary secretions but also oxygen in the lungs.
2. Each episode of suctioning should be preceded by ventilation with a 100% FIO_2 to maximize the volume of oxygen in the lungs.

D. Sedation

1. Patients may be made comfortable with small amounts of benzodiazepines (e.g., midazolam [Versed], 0.5 mg IV titrated to effect, or morphine in 2 mg boluses titrated to effect).
2. Note: Neuromuscular blocking agents such as pancuronium or vecuronium have no sedative effects.

V. WEANING[5, 9, 18]

A. Definition: Process by which a patient is transitioned from mechanical ventilation to spontaneous ventilation

B. The FIO_2 is gradually decreased to maintain a PaO_2 between 60 and 100 mmHg, or a SpO_2 >90%.

1. Decrease the FIO_2 in 10–20% decrements as tolerated. Recall that PEEP is useful in recruiting peripheral alveoli, thereby

   a. Increasing arterial oxygen content
   b. Allowing downward titration of the FIO_2

2. There is no benefit obtained by decreasing the FIO_2 > 40%; prolonged use of higher FIO_2 may lead to pulmonary oxygen toxicity.

C. The ventilatory rate is gradually decreased by 1–2 breaths per minute and titrated against the $PaCO_2$, with the goal of a $PaCO_2$ of 35–45 mmHg.

1. There is little benefit to decreasing the rate below 4 breaths per minute.
2. Certain patients are chronically hypercarbic.

   a. In these patients it is quite difficult to obtain a $PaCO_2$ of less than 45 mmHg.
   b. The premorbid $PaCO_2$, if known, is a reasonable target value.

D. A patient's potential for extubation may be tested by a period of spontaneous ventilation while he or she is still intubated.

1. Remember that the presence of an endotracheal tube prevents physiologic PEEP.
2. Thus, 5 cm H_2O PEEP may be required.

VI. EXTUBATION CRITERIA[1, 5, 8]

A. General policies

1. Best performed in the morning when the normal sleep-rest cycle favors alertness. Hospitals are usually better prepared to deal with ventilatory problems during the daytime hours.
2. Avoid sedation in the hours before extubation.
3. The equipment for reintubation should be readily available.
4. Once extubated, the patient should be observed in a critical care setting to ensure the adequacy of sustained ventilation.

   a. Generally, respiratory failure occurs sooner rather than later.
   b. An observation period of 1 h should suffice.

B. Specific criteria

1. The patient should be alert enough to respond to simple instructions.
2. All neuromuscular blockade must be reversed.
3. FIO_2 should be ≤40%.
4. Measured vital capacity should be ≥15 mL/kg.
5. Measured maximum inspiratory force should be ≥20 cm H_2O.
6. The patient's ventilatory status should be evaluated 15–20 min after extubation, with continuing assessments for 6–12 h.

VII. PROLONGED VENTILATION REQUIRING TRACHEOSTOMY[10–12]

A. Generally, a tracheostomy

1. Decreases airway dead space
2. Decreases the work of breathing
3. Has the disadvantage of circumventing the small amount of positive end-expiratory pressure provided by an intact glottis.

B. Indications

1. Prolonged mechanical ventilation or ventilatory assistance
2. Need for simplification of pulmonary toilet

References

1. Afessa, B., Hogans, L., & Murphy, R. (1999). Predicting 3-day and 7-day outcomes of weaning from mechanical ventilation. *Chest, 116*, 456–461.
2. Babb, T.G. (1999). Mechanical ventilatory constraints in aging, lung disease, and obesity: Perspectives and brief review. *Medical Science, Sports, & Exercise, 31* (Suppl), S12–S22.

3. Brochard, L. (1998). Breathing: Does regular mean normal? *Critical Care Medicine, 26,* 1773–1774.

4. Calderini, E., Confalonieri, M., Puccio, P.G., Francavilla, N., Stella, L., & Gregoretti, C. (1999). Patient-ventilator asynchrony during noninvasive ventilation: The role of expiratory trigger. *Intensive Care Medicine, 25,* 662–667.

5. Charters, P., & O'Sullivan, E. (1999). The 'dedicated airway': A review of the concept and an update of current practice. *Anaesthesia, 54,* 778–786.

6. Christensen, B.V., & Thunedborg, L.P. (1999). Use of sedatives, analgesics and neuromuscular blocking agents in Danish ICUs 1996/97. A national survey. *Intensive Care Medicine, 25,* 186–191.

7. Devlin, J.W., Boleski, G., Mlynarek, M., Nerenz, D.R., Peterson, E., Jankowski, M., Horst, H.M., & Zarowitz, B.J. (1999). Motor Activity Assessment Scale: A valid and reliable sedation scale for use with mechanically ventilated patients in an adult surgical intensive care unit. *Critical Care Medicine, 27,* 1271–1275.

8. Dumas, A., Dupuis, G.H., Searle, N., & Cartier, R. (1999). Early versus late extubation after coronary artery bypass grafting: Effects on cognitive function. *Journal of Cardiothoracic & Vascular Anesthesia, 13,* 130–135.

9. Ely, E.W., Baker, A.M., Evans, G.W., & Haponik, E.F. (1999). The prognostic significance of passing a daily screen of weaning parameters. *Intensive Care Medicine, 25,* 581–587.

10. Haberthur, C., Fabry, B., Stocker, R., Ritz, R., & Guttmann, J. (1999). Additional inspiratory work of breathing imposed by tracheostomy tubes and non-ideal ventilator properties in critically ill patients. *Intensive Care Medicine, 25,* 514–519.

11. Kollef, M.H., Ahrens, T.S., & Shannon, W. (1999). Clinical predictors and outcomes for patients requiring tracheostomy in the intensive care unit [see comments]. *Critical Care Medicine, 27,* 1714–1720.

12. Lawn, N.D., & Wijdicks, E.F. (1999). Tracheostomy in Guillain-Barré syndrome. *Muscle & Nerve, 22,* 1058–1062.

13. Marquette, C.H., Wermert, D., Wallet, F., Copin, M.C., & Tonnel, A.B. (1999). Characterization of an animal model of ventilator-acquired pneumonia. *Chest, 115,* 200–209.

14. Poponick, J.M., Renston, J.P., Bennett, R.P., & Emerman, C.L. (1999). Use of a ventilatory support system (BiPAP) for acute respiratory failure in the emergency department. *Chest, 116,* 166–171.

15. Powell, F.L., Milsom, W.K., & Mitchell, G.S. (1998). Time domains of the hypoxic ventilatory response. *Respiration Physiology, 112,* 123–134.

16. Putensen, C., Mutz, N.J., Putensen-Himmer, G., & Zinserling, J. (1999). Spontaneous breathing during ventilatory support improves ventilation-perfusion distributions in patients with acute respiratory distress syndrome. *American Journal of Respiratory & Critical Care Medicine, 159,* 1241–1248.

17. Ren, X., & Robbins, P.A. (1999). Ventilatory responses to hypercapnia and hypoxia after 6 h passive hyperventilation in humans. *Journal of Physiology, 514,* 885–894.

18. Rumbak, M.J., Walsh, F.W., Anderson, W.M., Rolfe, M.W., & Solomon, D.A. (1999). Significant tracheal obstruction causing failure to wean in patients requiring prolonged mechanical ventilation: A forgotten complication of long-term mechanical ventilation. *Chest, 115,* 1092–1095.

19. Swart, E.L., van Schijndel, R.J., van Loenen, A.C., & Thijs, L.G. (1999). Continuous infusion of lorazepam versus medazolam in patients in the intensive care unit: Sedation with lorazepam is easier to manage and is more cost-effective. *Critical Care Medicine, 27,* 1461–1465.

Management of Patients with Gastrointestinal Disorders

PEPTIC ULCER DISEASE

Charlene M. Myers, MSN, RN, CS,
ACNP, CCRN

I. PEPTIC ULCER DISEASE (PUD)

A. Definition[2, 6, 7]

1. A gastrointestinal ulcer is a loss of enteric surface epithelium that extends deeply enough to penetrate the muscularis mucosae.
2. PUD refers to a chronic disorder in which there is a life-long underlying tendency to develop mucosal ulcers at sites that are exposed to peptic juice (i.e., acid and pepsin).

   a. Most common locations are the duodenum and stomach.
   b. Ulcers may also occur in the esophagus, jejunum, and ileum, and at gastroenteric anastomoses.

B. Etiology[2, 4, 8, 13]

1. *Helicobacter pylori* (*H. pylori*) is present in >90% of duodenal ulcers and >75% of gastric ulcers.
2. There is an imbalance between mucosal defense mechanisms (protective factors) and mucosal damaging mechanisms (aggressive factors).

   a. Protective factors
      i. Mucosal barrier (bicarbonate and gastric mucus)
      ii. Sufficient blood supply to the gastric mucosa and submucosa
      iii. Competent sphincters (pyloric and lower esophageal sphincter [LES]), which prevent bile salt reflux into the stomach and esophagus
      iv. Certain medications
         (1) H_2 blockers
         (2) Antacids
         (3) Sucralfate (Carafate)
         (4) Colloidal bismuth suspension
         (5) Anticholinergics
         (6) Misoprostol (Cytotec)
         (7) Omeprazole (Prilosec)
   b. Aggressive factors
      i. Gastric acid
      ii. Pepsin
      iii. Bile acids
      iv. Decreased blood flow to gastric mucosa
      v. Incompetent sphincters

      vi. Various medications
- (1) Aspirin
- (2) NSAIDs
- (3) Glucocorticoids

    vii. Cigarette smoking

   viii. Gastrinoma

     ix. Stress (especially post-traumatic)

      x. Alcohol

     xi. Impaired proximal duodenal bicarbonate secretion

    xii. *H. pylori* infection

C. Risk factors[2, 3, 5, 6]

1. Highly associated

   a. Smoking more than than ½ pack of cigarettes per day
   b. Drugs (NSAIDs)
   c. Family history
   d. Zollinger-Ellison syndrome (condition caused by non-insulin–secreting tumors of the pancreas, which secretes excess amounts of gastrin)

2. Possibly associated

   a. Corticosteroids
   b. Stress

3. Low or not associated

   a. Spices
   b. Alcohol
   c. Caffeine
   d. Acetaminophen

D. Types of peptic ulcers[3, 4, 7, 13, 14]

1. Duodenal ulcers

   a. Ninety to ninety-five percent occur in the first portion of the duodenum.
   b. Four times more common than gastric ulcers
   c. Ten percent lifetime prevalence for men and 5% for women
   d. New cases annually: 200,000–400,000
   e. The most common age range is 25–75 years.

2. Gastric ulcers

   a. Most commonly seen in the lesser curvature of the stomach near the incisura angularis
   b. New cases annually: 87,500
   c. Three to four times more prevalent than duodenal ulcers in NSAID users
   d. Peak age of incidence: 55–65 (rare before age 40)

E. Subjective findings[2, 4, 6, 7, 9, 10, 12, 14]

1. Duodenal ulcers

    a. Epigastric pain (''gnawing,'' ''aching,'' ''hunger-like'') occurring 1–3 h after eating. The pain is rhythmic and periodic.
    b. Nocturnal pain that awakens a patient from sleep
    c. Usually relieved by antacid or food ingestion
    d. Heartburn (suggesting reflux disease)
    e. Epigastric tenderness: Usually midline or right of midline

2. Gastric ulcers

    a. Epigastric pain similar to that associated with duodenal ulcers and also rhythmic and periodic
    b. Pain is not usually relieved by food.
    c. Food may precipitate the symptoms.
    d. Nausea and anorexia

F. Physical findings[2, 4, 6, 7, 9, 10, 12, 14]

1. Often unremarkable
2. Patient may have epigastric tenderness.

    a. At or to the left of the midline with gastric ulcer
    b. One inch or more to the right of the midline with duodenal ulcer

3. Signs and symptoms of shock from acute or chronic blood loss
4. Nausea and vomiting if the pyloric channel is obstructed
5. Board-like abdomen and rebound tenderness in the event of perforation
6. Hematemesis or melena if the ulcer is bleeding

G. Laboratory studies[3, 4, 6–8, 12, 13]

1. Laboratory findings do not play a major role in diagnosing PUD, but may assist in defining an underlying disorder or complication.
2. Laboratory studies are generally normal in uncomplicated disease.
3. For detection of *H. pylori*

    a. Histopathology
    b. Culture
    c. Urea breath test
    d. Serum *H. pylori* antibody test

4. CBC: May indicate anemia owing to acute or possibly chronic blood loss
5. Leukocytosis suggests ulcer penetration or perforation.

6. An elevated serum amylase level with severe epigastric pain suggests possible ulcer penetration into the pancreas.
7. Fasting serum gastrin levels to identify Zollinger-Ellison syndrome

H. Diagnostics[3, 4, 7, 14]

1. Upper GI barium studies

   a. For uncomplicated dyspepsia
   b. Those diagnosed with gastric ulcers should have an endoscopy performed after 8–12 weeks of treatment to distinguish benign from malignant ulcers.

2. Endoscopy

   a. Highest accuracy rate (90–95%)
   b. Identifies superficial and very small ulcers
   c. Biopsy can be performed.
   d. Electrocautery of any bleeding ulcers can be carried out.
   e. Gastric pH can be measured in suspected gastrinoma.
   f. Esophagitis, gastritis, or duodenitis can be diagnosed.
   g. *H. pylori* can be detected.
   h. Higher cost than barium studies

I. Complications of PUD[3, 4, 14]

1. GI bleeding (20% of cases)

   a. Clinical manifestations
      i. Hematemesis
      ii. Melena
      iii. Hematochezia
      iv. "Coffee-ground" emesis
   b. Physical examination
      i. Pallor
      ii. Tachycardia
      iii. Hypotension
      iv. Diaphoresis
   c. Laboratory findings
      i. Decreased hematocrit owing to bleeding or hemodilution from IV fluids
      ii. BUN may rise owing to absorption of blood nitrogen from the small intestine and from prerenal azotemia.
   d. Diagnostics: Endoscopy after the patient has stabilized
   e. Management
      i. In approximately 80% of cases, bleeding stops spontaneously within a few hours after admission to the hospital.
      ii. IV hydration with normal saline
      iii. Blood transfusion as required

iv. Continuous IV infusion of H_2 blockers at a dose adequate to maintain gastric pH >4

v. Vasopressin (Pitressin) and IV octreotide (Sandostatin) should not be used for bleeding ulcers.

f. Surgery if bleeding persists

2. Perforation (5–10% of cases)

a. Subjective data
   i. Severe abdominal pain
   ii. Epigastric pain that radiates to back or right upper quadrant

b. Physical examination
   i. Ill appearance
   ii. Board-like abdomen
   iii. Severe epigastric tenderness
   iv. Absent bowel sounds
   v. Knee-to-chest position
   vi. Patient may have symptoms of hypovolemia, fever.

c. Laboratory findings
   i. Leukocytosis is almost always present.
   ii. Mildly elevated amylase levels may be present.

d. Diagnostics
   i. Abdominal x-rays may reveal free air in the peritoneal cavity.
   ii. UGI radiography with water-soluble contrast may be useful.
   iii. Barium studies are contraindicated

e. Therapy
   i. Surgery
   ii. Patients who are considered poor candidates for surgery or who present >24 h after perforation and are stable may be followed closely on IV fluids, nasogastric suction, and broad-spectrum antibiotics.
   iii. If their condition deteriorates, they should be taken to surgery.

3. Gastric outlet obstruction (2% of cases)

a. Caused by edema or narrowing of the pylorus or duodenal bulb

b. Subjective findings
   i. Early satiety
   ii. Nausea
   iii. Vomiting of undigested food
   iv. Epigastric pain unrelieved by food or antacids
   v. Weight loss

c. Physical examination
   i. "Succussion splash" may be audible on physical examination, secondary to large amounts of air and fluid in the stomach.

     ii. Nasogastric aspiration may return a large amount (>200 mL) of foul-smelling fluid.

  d. Diagnostics

     i. Upper GI endoscopy should be performed after 24–72 h to determine the source of obstruction.

     ii. At 72 h, all patients should have the saline-load test by instilling 750 mL of normal saline into the stomach and checking the residual in 30 min.

     iii. A residual volume of more than 400 mL is considered positive.

     iv. That patient should remain on nasogastric suction for 5–7 more days.

  e. Laboratory: Metabolic alkalosis and hypokalemia may be present.

  f. Therapy:

     i. Normal saline IV infusion with potassium chloride if patient has an electrolyte imbalance due to vomiting and poor digestion (i.e., 1 L normal saline with 40 mEq potassium chloride/L at 100 mL/h—titrate up or down based on patient's condition)

       (1) For example, someone who is dehydrated with an increased heart rate, decreased urinary output, and decreased central venous pressure/pulmonary capillary wedge pressure may require more fluids.

       (2) By comparison, those with a history of congestive heart failure or who have signs and symptoms of cardiac overload (e.g., crackles, jugular venous distention, edema) may require less fluid.

     ii. IV H_2 blockers, e.g.

       (1) Ranitidine (Zantac), 50 mg q6–8h up to 150 mg/day

       (2) Cimetidine (Tagamet), 400 mg at bedtime or b.i.d.

       (3) Famotidine (Pepcid), 20 mg at bedtime or b.i.d.

     iii. Nasogastric decompression

     iv. Total parenteral nutrition for the severely malnourished

  g. Surgery: Traditional

  h. Upper GI endoscopy with dilation of the obstruction has proven successful.

J. Medical therapy for PUD[2–4, 7, 13, 14]

1. Acid-antisecretory agents

  a. Proton pump inhibitors

     i. Suppresses gastric acid secretion by inhibition of the H^+,K^+-ATPase enzyme system at the secretory surface of the gastric parietal cell.

     ii. Indications: Treatment of
        (1) Duodenal ulcers
        (2) Severe erosive esophagitis
        (3) Poorly responsive gastroesophageal reflux disease
           (GERD)
    iii. Agents: Omeprazole and lansoprazole (Prevacid)
    iv. Duodenal ulcers: Omeprazole, 20 mg/day, lansoprazole, 15 mg/day, result in 90% ulcer healing in 4 weeks.
     v. Gastric ulcers: Omeprazole, 40 mg/day, lansoprazole, 30–60 mg/day, heal 90% of gastric ulcers after 8 weeks.
    vi. Should be administered 30 min before meals
   vii. Serum gastrin levels may rise >500 pg/mL; therefore, serum gastrin levels should be checked after 6 months of therapy and treatment terminated or decreased if levels rise over 500 pg/mL.
  b. Acid-antisecretory agent (H_2 receptor antagonists)
     i. Decrease gastric acid secretion by blocking histamine H_2 receptors on parietal cells
    ii. Agents
        (1) Cimetidine
        (2) Ranitidine
        (3) Famotidine
        (4) Nizatidine (Axid)
    iii. Dosages: Twice daily or once at bedtime. Recommended:
        (1) Cimetidine, 800 mg at bedtime
        (2) Ranitidine and nizatidine, 300 mg at bedtime
        (3) Famotidine, 40 mg at bedtime
    iv. Symptom relief usually occurs within 2 weeks.
     v. Healing of duodenal ulcers is usually obtained within 8 weeks of beginning therapy.
    vi. Gastric ulcer healing is delayed by 2–4 weeks compared with duodenal ulcers, but 8 weeks' duration of therapy is sufficient.
2. Agents enhancing mucosal defenses

  a. Sucralfate
     i. Forms a protective barrier against acid, bile, and pepsin
    ii. May cause constipation
    iii. May bind some medications; therefore, doses should be administered at least 2 h apart
    iv. Associated with decreased incidence of nosocomial pneumonia in some studies
     v. Requires an acidic environment; therefore, antacids and H_2 blockers should be avoided.

    vi. One gram q.i.d. has the same efficacy as H_2 blockers in the treatment of duodenal ulcers (6–8 weeks' duration).

    vii. Efficacy against gastric ulcers is less established.

    viii. Maintenance dose: 1 g b.i.d.

b. Bismuth subsalicylate (Pepto-Bismol)

    i. Used to treat dyspepsia, PUD, and diarrhea

    ii. Promotes ulcer healing through stimulation of mucosal bicarbonate and prostaglandin production

    iii. Has direct antibacterial action against *H. pylori*

c. Prostaglandin analog (misoprostol [Cytotec])

    i. Promotes ulcer healing by stimulating mucus and bicarbonate secretion and modest inhibition of acid secretion

    ii. Used solely as a prophylactic agent in prevention of NSAID-induced ulcers rather than for treatment of active ulcers

    iii. High incidence of diarrhea

    iv. May stimulate contractions in pregnant patients and induce abortion

    v. Initial dose: 100 μg q.i.d. with food, increased to 200 μg q.i.d. if well tolerated

d. Antacids

    i. No longer used as first line agents; commonly used as required to supplement other antiulcer therapies owing to the rapid relief of symptoms

    ii. Low-dose aluminum- and magnesium-containing antacids promote ulcer healing by stimulating gastric mucosal defenses, not by neutralizing gastric acidity.

    iii. Dosage: 30 mL 1–3 h after meals and at bedtime

    iv. High dosages are associated with diarrhea, hypermagnesemia, and hypophosphatemia.

3. *H. pylori* eradication therapy

a. Combination drug therapy is necessary to achieve adequate rates of eradication and to decrease failures due to antibiotic resistance.

b. Combination therapy consists of two antibiotics plus either a proton pump inhibitor or bismuth.

c. Regimens using proton pump inhibitors

    i. MOC

        (1) Metronidazole (Flagyl), 500 mg b.i.d. with meals, omeprazole, 20 mg b.i.d. before meals, and clarithromycin (Biaxin), 500 mg b.i.d. with meals, for 7 days

        (2) Instruct patient that Flagyl should not be taken with alcohol or vinegar.

      ii. AOC
         (1) Amoxicillin (Amoxil), 1 g b.i.d. with meals, ome-
            prazole, 20 mg b.i.d. before meals, and clarithro-
            mycin (Biaxin), 500 mg b.i.d. with meals, for
            7 days
         (2) Preferred for those whose disease is resistant to
            metronidazole
      iii. MOA
         (1) Metronidazole, 500 mg b.i.d. with meals, omepra-
            zole, 20 mg b.i.d. before meals, amoxicillin, 1 g
            b.i.d. with meals, for 7 to 14 days
   d. Regimens using bismuth compounds
      i. Require q.i.d. dosing and have more side effects than
        the proton pump regimens
      ii. BMT: Bismuth subsalicylate, 2 tabs q.i.d., metronida-
        zole, 250 mg q.i.d., and tetracycline (Tetracyn) 500 mg
        q.i.d. All pills are taken with meals and at bedtime.
      iii. BMT + omeprazole: The above regimen plus omepra-
        zole, 20 mg b.i.d., before meals for 7 days.
   e. Antiulcer therapy is recommended for 3 to 7 weeks follow-
     ing the preceding treatment regimens to ensure symptom
     relief and ulcer healing.
      i. Duodenal ulcers: Omeprazole, 40 mg/day, or lanso-
        prazole, 30 mg/day, should be continued for 7 addi-
        tional weeks.
      ii. H_2 blockers or sucralfate can be given for 6–8 weeks.

F. Suggested follow-up[3, 4, 7, 10, 14]

1. Duodenal ulcer: No further evaluation is necessary if the patient is symptom-free after 8 weeks of therapy.
2. Gastric ulcer: Repeat endoscopy should be performed 4–6
weeks after therapy.

   a. Completely healed ulcers will require no follow-up.
   b. Partially healed ulcers
      i. If more than 50% healing and negative for carcinoma,
        requires 6 more weeks of therapy followed by
        re-evaluation
      ii. If more than 59% healing but positive for carcinoma,
        requires surgical intervention.
      iii. Less than 50% healing requires surgery.

II. GASTROESOPHAGEAL REFLUX DISEASE (GERD)

A. Definition[1, 2, 4]

1. A chronic condition in which gastric contents enter and remain in the lower esophagus owing to impaired esophageal
function

2. GERD is a symptomatic clinical condition or histologic alteration resulting from episodes of gastroesophageal reflux that may result in inflammation of the esophagus (reflux esophagitis).

B. Etiology[1–3, 14]

1. Anatomic factors

   a. Hypotensive lower esophageal sphincter (LES) pressures
   b. Hiatal hernias

2. Decreased esophageal clearance of gastric contents: Severity will depend on length of contact time between the gastric contents and the esophagus.
3. Composition and volume of refluxate: The combination of acid, pepsin, and bile produces a potent refluxate that may cause damage to the esophagus.
4. Delayed gastric emptying may contribute to gastroesophageal reflux owing to an increase in gastric volume that may increase the frequency and amount of fluid that is refluxed.

B. Contributing factors[1, 2, 4, 12, 13]

1. Dietary factors

   a. Caffeinated food and/or drinks
      i. Coffee
      ii. Tea
      iii. Cola
      iv. Chocolate
   b. Esophageal irritants
      i. Citrus fruits
      ii. Vinegar
      iii. Spicy foods
      iv. Tomatoes
   c. Excessive fluids with meals
   d. Large meals
   e. Fatty meals
   f. Meals within 2–3 h of bedtime
   g. LES relaxants
      i. Onions
      ii. Garlic
      iii. Mint
      iv. Alcoholic beverages
   h. Lying down immediately after eating

2. Nondietary features

   a. Anxiety
   b. Obesity
   c. Pregnancy

    d. Tight-fitting clothing
    e. Smoking

3. Pharmacologic agents

    a. Alpha-adrenergic antagonists
    b. Anticholinergics
    c. Antihistamines
    d. Aspirin
    e. Benzodiazepines
    f. Calcium channnel blockers
    g. Beta adrenergic agonists
    h. Cholecystokinin
    i. Levodopa
    j. Narcotics
    k. Nitrates
    l. NSAIDs
    m. Progestins
    n. Prostaglandins
    o. Secretin
    p. Somatostatin
    q. Theophylline
    r. Tricyclic antidepressants
    s. Transdermal nicotine

C. Clinical manifestations[1-4, 7, 11, 12]

1. Hallmark symptom: Heartburn (pyrosis)

    a. Described as substantial sensation of warmth or burning that may radiate to the neck, throat, and/or back
    b. Generally associated with large meals and occurs 30–60 min after eating
    c. Often aggravated by the supine position and bending over

2. Regurgitation
3. Water brash (hypersalivation)
4. Dysphagia (difficulty swallowing)
5. Odynophagia (pain on swallowing)
6. Hemorrhage
7. Belching
8. Early satiety
9. Atypical symptoms

    a. Pulmonary symptoms
        i. Recurrent pneumonia
        ii. Bronchospasm
    b. Chest pain
    c. Cough
    d. Hoarseness

   e. Hiccups
   f. Sore throat
   g. Nighttime choking
   h. Halitosis

D. Diagnosis[1–4, 10, 11, 13, 14]

1. Clinical history, including presenting symptoms and associated risk factors, is the most useful tool in the diagnosis of GERD.
2. Barium swallow is the simplest, least expensive test, but also the least sensitive. Useful as a screening tool to

   a. Rule out complications
      i. Inflammation
      ii. Ulcers
      iii. Strictures
   b. Evaluate
      i. Dysphagia
      ii. Odynophagia
      iii. Significant weight loss
      iv. Occult blood loss

3. Endoscopy is an excellent study for the diagnosis and evaluation of reflux esophagitis and other complications of GERD (strictures, Barrett's esophagus). During endoscospy

   a. Biopsy specimens can be obtained.
   b. Strictures can be dilated.

4. The Bernstein test is an intraesophageal acid perfusion study that can be used to confirm that the patient's symptoms are acid-related.

   a. The test requires an alternating infusion of 0.1 N hydrochloric acid and normal saline into the esophagus.
   b. With reflux esophagitis, there are symptoms of heartburn with the infusion of acid but not with the infusion of saline.

5. The most specific and sensitive diagnostic test for the presence of abnormal acid reflux is 24-h ambulatory pH monitoring.

   a. This test remains the gold standard for many practitioners.
   b. It is performed by passing a small electrode pH probe intranasally and placing it about 5 cm above the LES.
   c. Determination of the frequency and severity of reflux can be made by this study.

E. Management[1, 2, 4, 13, 14]

1. Phase I treatment modalities

   a. Elevate the head of the bed 4–6 in (increases esophageal clearance).

   b. Avoid large, high-fat meals and eating 2–3 h before bedtime (decreases gastric volume).

   c. Avoid foods that may decrease LES pressure.
      i. Fats
      ii. Chocolate
      iii. Alcohol
      iv. Peppermint
      v. Spearmint

   d. Avoid foods that have an irritant effect directly on the esophageal mucosa.
      i. Spicy foods
      ii. Citrus juice
      iii. Tomato juice
      iv. Coffee

   e. Add protein-rich meals to diet (augments LES pressure).

   f. Reduce weight (reduces symptoms).

   g. Eliminate smoking, if applicable (decreases spontaneous esophageal sphincter relaxation).

   h. Avoid alcohol (increases amplitude of the LES and peristaltic waves, and frequency of contraction).

   i. Avoid tight-fitting clothes.

   j. Eliminate exacerbating medications (see contributing factors).

   k. Use antacids and alginic acid as needed.
      i. 80–100 mEq of neutralizing activity (usually 30 mL/ 8–10 tabs) after meals and at bedtime. For example:
         (1) Chooz
         (2) Gaviscon
         (3) Gelusil
         (4) Gelusil II
         (5) Maalox Plus
         (6) Maalox TC
         (7) Mylanta
         (8) Mylanta II
         (9) Riopan
         (10) Tums
      ii. Prefer liquid to tablet form.

   l. Try over-the-counter H_2 blockers
      i. Famotidine, 10 mg up to twice a day.
      ii. Cimetidine, 200 mg up to twice a day
      iii. Ranitidine, 50–100 mg up to twice a day

2. Phase II treatment modalities

   a. Continue phase I management and add one of the following:

b. H_2 blocker at prescription dose
   i. Cimetidine, 400–800 mg p.o. b.i.d for 12 weeks max. (High dose: 800 mg t.i.d.)
   ii. Ranitidine, 150 mg p.o. b.i.d–t.i.d (No high dose)
   iii. Famotidine, 20–40 mg p.o. b.i.d (High dose: 160 mg q6h max)
   iv. Nizatidine, 150 mg p.o. b.i.d. or 300 mg p.o. at bedtime for 12 weeks max. (No high dose)
   v. Start on standard doses. If the patient does not respond, or has severe disease, higher doses may be recommended. OR
c. Prokinetic agents
   i. Cisapride (Propulsid), 10 mg p.o. t.i.d.–20 mg p.o. q.i.d
   ii. Metoclopramide (Reglan), 10–15 mg p.o. t.i.d. or 20 mg p.o. prn (12 weeks max). OR
d. Mucosal protectants
   i. Sucralfate, 1 g p.o. q.i.d.

3. Phase III treatment modalities

a. An inadequate response after 2–4 weeks of phase II management necessitates progression to phase III.
b. Increase the dose of the initial drug, OR
c. Add a second drug, OR
d. Add a Proton pump inhibitor.
   i. Omeprazole, 20 mg p.o. q.d. (4–8 weeks max. [High dose: 120 mg t.i.d.])
   ii. Lansoprazole, 15–30 mg p.o. q.d. (8 week max. [High dose: 90 mg p.o. b.i.d.])

4. Phase IV treatment modalities

a. Surgical Intervention.
   i. Reserved for those in whom medical management has failed or complications have developed
   ii. Indications include
      (1) Reflux-related pulmonary disease
      (2) Persistent ulcerative esophagitis
      (3) Recurrent esophageal strictures
      (4) Large hiatal hernia
   iii. The Nissen fundoplication procedure has a cure rate of approximately 90%.

References

1. Claussen, J.R. (1999). Gastrointestinal reflux disease: A rational approach to management. *Clinical Review, 9,* 69–82.
2. DiPiro, J.T. (1998). Gastrointestinal Disorders. In B.G. Wells, J.T. Dipiro, T.L. Schwinghammer, & C.W. Hamilton (Eds.), *Pharmacotherapy handbook.* Stamford, CT: Appleton & Lange.

3. Ferri, F.F. (1995). *Practical guide to the care of the medical patient* (3rd ed.). St. Louis: Mosby.

4. Grendell, J.H., McQuaid, K.R., & Friedman, S.L. (1996). *Current diagnosis and treatment in gastroenterology.* Stamford, CT: Appleton and Lange.

5. Hawkey, C.J., Karrasch, J.A., Szczepanski, L., Walker, D.G., Barkun, A., Swannell, A.J., & Yeomans, N.D. Omeprazole compared with misoprostol for ulcers associated with nonsteroidal antiinflammatory drugs. *New England Journal of Medicine, 338,* 727–734.

6. Hector Dunphy, L.M. (1999). *Management guidelines for adult nurse practitioners.* Philadelphia: F.A. Davis.

7. Hirsch, C.G. & Caswell, D. (1999). Gastrointestinal disorders. In A. Gawlinski & D. Hamwi (Eds.), *Acute care nurse practitioner: Clinical curriculum and certification review.* Philadelphia: W.B. Saunders.

8. Hood, H.M., Wark, C., Burgess, P.A., Nicewander, D., & Scott, M.W. (1999). Screening for Helicobacter pylori and nonsteroidal antiinflammatory drug use in medicare patients hospitalized with peptic ulcer disease. *Archives of Internal Medicine, 159,* 149–154.

9. Lindsetmo, R., Johnson, R., & Revhaug, A. (1998). Abdominal and dyspeptic symptoms in patients with peptic ulcer treated medically or surgically. *British Journal of Surgery, 85,* 845–849.

10. McColl, K.E.L., El-Nujumi, A., Murray, L.S., El-Omar, E.M., Dickso, A.W., & Hilditch, T.E. (1998). Assessment of symptomatic response as predictor of Helicobacter pylori status following eradication therapy in patients with ulcer. *Gut, 42,* 618–622.

11. Peters, S. (1998). Is it heart attack, or is it GERD? *Advance for Nurse Practitioners, 6,* 57–62.

12. Rakel, R.E. (1996). *Saunders manual of medical practice.* Philadelphia: W.B. Saunders.

13. Salerno, Sr. M. (1999). Gastrointestinal disorders. In V.L. Millonig & S.L. Miller (Eds.), *Adult nurse practitioner certification review guide.* (3rd ed.). Potomac, MD: Health Leadership Associates, Inc.

14. Tierney, L.M., McPhee, S.J., & Papadakis, M.A. (1999). *Current medical diagnosis & treatment* (38th ed.). Stamford, CT: Appleton & Lange.

LIVER DISEASE

*Charlene M. Myers, MSN, RN, CS,
ACNP, CCRN*

I. HEPATITIS

A. Definition[4-6, 9, 14, 15]

1. Hepatitis refers to an inflammation of the liver that can be caused by many drugs and toxic agents as well as by viruses.
2. The common forms of viral hepatitis are

   - Hepatitis A virus (HAV)
   - Hepatitis B virus (HBV)
   - Hepatitis C virus (HCV/non-A non-B virus)
   - Hepatitis D virus (delta agent)
   - Hepatitis E virus (HEV/enterically transmitted or epidemic non-A non-B virus)
   - Hepatitis G virus (HGV)

B. Etiology[4-9, 13-15]

1. HAV: Usually spread by fecal-oral route, including contaminated food sources, water, and shellfish; the parenteral route is rare.

   a. Spread is enhanced by crowding and poor sanitation.
   b. Maximum infectivity is 2 weeks prior to clinical illness.
   c. Blood and stools are infectious during a 2–6 week incubation period.
   d. Mortality rate is low, and fulminant hepatitis A is uncommon.

2. HBV: A blood-borne virus that is present in saliva, semen, and vaginal secretions

   a. It is transmitted
      i. Sexually
      ii. Through contaminated blood and blood products
      iii. Through parenteral drug abuse
      iv. Perinatally
   b. There are approximately 500 million chronic carriers worldwide.
   c. This chronic carrier state is responsible for much of the world's liver cirrhosis.
   d. Coinfection, superinfection, or chronic infection with HDV markedly increases mortality and morbidity of HBV.

3. HCV: A blood-borne virus

  a. In many patients the source of infection is uncertain.

  b. Approximately 50% of cases are related to IV drug abuse.

  c. Although HCV causes approximately 90% of post-transfusion hepatitis, only 4% of HCV cases are related to blood transfusions.

  d. Forty to sixty percent of patients with post-transfusion hepatitis develop chronic hepatitis C that, in turn, leads to cirrhosis in 20–40% of the cases.

  e. The risk of sexual and perinatal transmission is small.

4. HDV: A defective RNA virus that causes hepatitis only when accompanied by hepatitis B infection (as shown by HbsAg)

  a. Combined infection has a worse prognosis than HBV alone, with an increased incidence of fulminant hepatitis.

5. HEV: Fecal/oral route primarily seen in less developed countries (e.g., India, Mexico, Burma, Algeria, Afghanistan)

  a. Incubation period is 2–9 weeks (mean of 6 weeks).

  b. Clinical disease is similar to HAV except more severe.

  c. Mortality rate is 1–2% in general population and 10–20% in pregnant women—significantly higher than HAV.

6. HGV: Recently identified virus that is transmitted percutaneously and may cause mild acute hepatitis and chronic viremia lasting as long as 9 years.

  a. HGV has been detected in 50% of IV drug abusers and in 20% of hemophiliacs.

  b. Diagnostic tests are not currently available.

C. Risk factors[6]

1. Health care providers/other occupational risks; positive needle stick
2. Hemodialysis patients
3. Recipients of blood and/or blood products
4. IV drug users
5. Sexually active homosexual males or multiple heterosexual partners
6. Household exposure
7. Intimate exposure
8. Persons in underdeveloped countries

D. Subjective findings (Extremely variable)[4–6, 9, 14, 15]

1. Prodromal phase

  a. Malaise, myalgia, arthralgia, easily fatigued

  b. Upper respiratory symptoms (nasal discharge, pharyngitis)

   c. Anorexia, nausea, and vomiting are frequent.
   d. Diarrhea or constipation may occur.
   e. Aversion to smoking (HBV)
   f. Skin rashes, arthritis, or serum sickness may be seen early in HBV.
   g. Fever usually less than 39.5°C (more common in HAV)
   h. Mild, constant abdominal pain in the right upper quadrant or epigastrium that is often aggravated by exertion

2. Icteric phase

   a. Clinical jaundice occurs after 5–10 days, but may occur at the same time as the initial symptoms.
   b. Most patients never develop clinical icterus.
   c. There is usually an intensification of the prodromal symptoms with the onset of jaundice, followed by progressive improvement.
   d. Dark urine/clay colored stools
   e. The patient may be asymptomatic.

E. Physical findings[5–8]

1. Jaundice
2. Tender hepatomegaly
3. Splenomegaly
4. Posterior cervical lymphadenopathy (rare)
5. Rash (HBV)
6. Arthritis (rare)
7. Examination may be normal.

F. Laboratory findings[5–7, 9]

1. WBC count is normal or may be low.
2. Urinalysis—Proteinuria is common; bilirubinuria may occur prior to jaundice.
3. Greatly increased alanine transaminase (ALT) and aspartate transaminase (AST) levels (>500 IU/L) (Normal: 0–35 IU/L)
4. Increased bilirubin and alkaline phosphatase levels; may remain elevated after ALT and AST have normalized.
5. Prothrombin time (PT) and glucose level are usually normal; an increased PT or decreased glucose level indicates severe liver damage.

G. Diagnosis[5–7, 9, 17]

1. Hepatitis A

   a. IgM anti-HAV: Excellent diagnostic test
      i. Immunoglobulin M occurs during the first week of clinical disease.
      ii. IgM disappears after 3–6 months.
   b. IgG anti-HAV
      i. Immunoglobulin G peaks after one month and may persist for years.

      ii. Presence of IgG
        (1) Indicates previous exposure and noninfectivity
        (2) Confers lifelong immunity

2. Hepatitis B

   a. Detection of HbsAG or Anti-HBc-IgM
   b. Anti-HBc is very useful as a serologic marker of acute hepatitis during a gap when patients have cleared HbsAg but anti-HBs cannot be detected.
   c. Anti-HBs
      i. Appears
        (1) After the clearance of HbsAg
        (2) After successful hepatitis vaccination
      ii. Appearance of Anti-Hbs and disappearance of HbsAg indicates
        (1) Recovery from HBV
        (2) Noninfectivity
        (3) Protection from recurrent infection

3. Hepatitis C

   a. Anti-HCV[17]
      i. First-line test when diagnosis is suspected
      ii. Highly sensitive—If negative, infection is unlikely.
      iii. Specificity depends on situation—If positive in a person with risk factors and elevated liver enzymes, specificity is high.
      iv. A positive anti-HCV—Hepatitis C infection is present until proven otherwise.
   b. With the standard ELISA assay, there is an inability to isolate the virus, and there are problems with false-positive results. Sensitivity and specificity are low.
   c. A second-generation recombinant immunoblot assay (RIBA II) avoids these problems.
      i. "Confirmatory" test for hepatitis C
      ii. Rarely needed in clinical practice
      iii. A positive anti-HCV *no longer needs* to be confirmed by RIBA.
   d. Most RIBA-positive patients are infectious, and a polymerase chain reaction (PCR) can be used to identify HCV RNA chains.
      i. Gold standard to confirm infection
      ii. Detects actual virus, not the antibodies
      iii. Differentiates prior exposure from current viremia

4. Hepatitis D

   a. Diagnosis is made by detection of anti-HDV.
   b. Remember that HDV can occur as a coinfection or superinfection with HBV.

5. Hepatitis E: Diagnosis is made by detection of anti-HEV in the serum.
6. Hepatitis G: Diagnostic tests are not commercially available.

H. Medical management[1-4, 6, 7, 10-13, 16]

1. Supportive

   a. Consists of bed rest until jaundice resolves
   b. No heavy lifting, straining, or activity

2. A high-calorie diet

   a. Small, frequent meals with supplements
   b. High carbohydrates
   c. Low proteins
   d. No fatty foods

3. Avoidance of potentially hepatotoxic medications
4. Restriction of alcohol
5. Most patients do not require hospitalization.
6. If patients show signs of encephalopathy or severe coagulopathy, fulminant hepatic failure should be suspected, and hospitalization is necessary.
7. Administer antiemetics to decrease nausea and vomiting.
8. The goal for treatment of chronic hepatitis is aimed at decreasing inflammation, symptoms, and infectivity.
9. Alpha interferon therapy is used in chronic active cases. Today, combination therapy is preferred. Interferon monotherapy remains a viable option only for patients with contraindications to combination therapy.

   a. Five million units/day or 10 million units three times a week for 16 weeks (20 weeks in HBV)
   b. Three million units three times a week for 24 weeks in HCV
   c. Ten million units three times a week for HDV. Treatment for a year or longer may be necessary.
   d. A positive HbeAg (which indicates viral replication and infectivity as well as chronic hepatitis, if present, longer than 3 months) and a positive liver biopsy proving chronic hepatitis should be obtained prior to initiation of therapy.
   e. May cause prominent flu-like side affects, making it difficult to tolerate for many patients.
      i. Hyperexia
      ii. Myalgias
      iii. Weakness
      iv. Fatigue
      v. Anorexia
      vi. Leukopenia

vii. Depression

viii. Hair loss

   f. Higher ALT levels result in a better response rate to therapy.

10. Lamivudine (Epivir), also known as 3TC, has been approved for the treatment of hepatitis B.

   a. One hundred mg p.o./day for 1 year has shown regression in the severity of the disease as measured by improvements in liver histologic studies and decreases in the levels of transaminases.

   b. Some patients have also undergone seroconversion to a less active state.

11. In patients with chronic hepatitis C, initial therapy with interferon in combination with ribavirin (1000 or 1200 mg p.o./day, depending on body weight, for 24 weeks) has been shown to be more effective than treatment with interferon alone in inducing virologic and histologic improvement.

II. HEPATIC FAILURE[4–6, 9]

A. Definition

Acute liver failure is a rare but catastrophic illness resulting from sudden, marked impairment of liver cell function.

B. Etiology

1. Viral hepatitis
2. Hepatitis caused by other viruses
3. Drug-induced injury
4. Toxins
5. Metabolic disorders
6. Vascular events
7. Miscellaneous disorders

C. Clinical manifestations

1. Initial signs are vague and include

   a. Weakness

   b. Fatigue

   c. Loss of appetite

   d. Weight loss

   e. Abdominal discomfort

   f. Nausea and vomiting

   g. Change in bowel pattern

2. As liver destruction progresses, liver function becomes impaired, resulting in loss of the normal vascular, secretory, and metabolic functions of the liver.

3. When severe, the sequelae of liver disease can be characterized by

   a. Multiorgan failure, especially
      i. Cardiac
      ii. Renal
   b. Reduced liver metabolic processes
   c. Impaired bile formation and flow
   d. Increased incidence of infection

4. Cardiac

   a. Hyperdynamic circulation
   b. Portal hypertension
   c. Dysrhythmias
   d. Edema
   e. Activity intolerance

5. Dermatologic

   a. Jaundice
   b. Spider angiomas
   c. Pruritus

6. Fluid and electrolytes

   a. Ascites
   b. Water retention
   c. Decreased vascular volume
   d. Hypokalemia
   e. Hyponatremia (hemodilution)
   f. Hypernatremia
   g. Hypoglycemia
   h. Hypoalbuminemia

7. Gastrointestinal

   a. Abdominal discomfort
   b. Decreased appetite
   c. Diarrhea
   d. GI bleeding
   e. Varices
   f. Malnutrition
   g. Nausea and vomiting

8. Hematologic

   a. Anemia
   b. Impaired coagulation
   c. Disseminated intravascular coagulopathy

9. Immune system

   a. Increased risk for infection

10. Neurologic
    a. Hepatic encephalopathy

11. Respiratory
    a. Dyspnea
    b. Hyperventilation
    c. Hypoxemia

12. Renal
    a. Renal failure (hepatorenal syndrome): Patients in end-stage liver disease may develop
       i. Azotemia
       ii. Oliguria
       iii. Hyponatremia
       iv. Low urinary sodium levels
       v. Hypotension.
    b. The cause is unknown.
    c. Death may occur as a result of infection or hemorrhage.

D. Laboratory findings/Diagnostics

1. Bilirubin—Elevated (normal = 1.0 mg/dL)
2. Albumin—Decreased (normal = 3.5–5.5 g/dL)
3. PT—Prolonged; high prognostic value in acute liver injury (normal = 10–12 s)
4. Partial thromboplastin time—Prolonged (normal = 25–41 s).
5. Liver enzyme levels are not liver function tests!

    a. These tests provide information about liver dysfunction but do not actually assess liver function.
    b. Liver enzymes can be classified into two major types:
    c. Aminotransaminases
       i. AST (formerly SGOT)—Elevated (normal = 0–40 U/L)
       ii. ALT (formerly SGPT) has a greater specificity for liver disease.
       iii. In most liver diseases, AST increase is < than that of ALT (AST/ALT ratio <1) (normal ALT = 0–35 U/L).
    d. Phosphatases
       i. Alkaline phosphatase (ALP)—Normal = 30–120 U/L.
       ii. Gamma-glutamyl transpeptidase (GGT)—Normal = 0–30 U/L.
          (1) These liver enzymes are released during cellular injury and stop being released when hepatocytes begin to heal.
          (2) If injury is severe enough to cause necrosis, the enzymes will initially be very high and then will decline because there are no further enzymes to be released.

6. Ammonia—Elevated (normal = 10–80 μg/dL)

E. Management

1. Hepatic encephalopathy

   a. Protein restriction: 20–30 g/day
   b. Administer lactulose (Cephulac), 15–30 mL q3–4h until the patient produces 3–4 loose stools/day.
   c. Enteral neomycin, 1 g b.i.d.
   d. Metronidazole (Flagyl), 250 mg t.i.d.
   e. Bromocriptine (Parlodel), 2.5 mg t.i.d.
      i. May be added to those who are receiving lactulose and continue to demonstrate encephalopathic symptoms.
      ii. Initiated when the serum ammonia level is low.

2. Monitor for hypoglycemia.

   a. Ten percent glucose IV infusion
      i. Rate depends on blood glucose level.
      ii. May start at 50–100 mL/h and titrate depending on glucose levels
   b. 50% glucose IV push if needed

3. Coagulopathy

   a. Vitamin K, 10 mg SC q.d. for 3 days, if PT is >14 s, INR >2, or platelets <75,000
   b. Fresh frozen plasma

4. Hyponatremia

   a. Free water restriction
   b. Less than 1500 mL of water per day for those with a serum sodium level <125 mEq/L

5. Hypokalemia: Potassium chloride replacement
6. Variceal bleeding: Refer to Chapter 40, Gastrointestinal Bleeding.
7. Ascites

   a. Low sodium diet—2–4 g/day
   b. Fluid restriction—1500 mL/day for those with a serum sodium level <125 mEq/L
   c. Diuretic therapy
      i. Spironolactone, 100 mg/day in divided doses to 400 mg maximum
      ii. Furosemide (Lasix), 20–40 mg/day
         (1) The goal is to reduce weight by 1 lb/day in those with ascites and by 2 lb/day in those with ascites and edema.
         (2) Dose may need to be increased to achieve this weight loss.

iii. For those with tense ascites, paracentesis may be necessary to drain 3–6 L for comfort and to decrease the risk for respiratory complications.

    (1) Administer albumin, 6–8 g for each liter removed, to protect intravascular volume.

    (2) Dextran may be used as well.

8. IV bicarbonate may be necessary for severe acidosis.
9. Monitor BUN/CR for elevation—Dialysis may be necessary.
10. Monitor respiratory and hemodynamic status closely— Vasopressors and intubation may be necessary.
11. Avoid hepatotoxic substances.
12. Cholestyramine, 4 g, or colestipol, 5 g, in water or juice may be helpful for those with pruritus.

References

1. Barbaro, G., Di Lorenzo, G., Belloni, G., Ferrari, L., Paiano, A., Del Poggio, P., Bacca, D., Fruttaldo, L., Mongio, F., Francavilla, R., Scotto, G., Grisorio, B., Calleri, G., Annese, M., Barelli, A., Rocchetto, P., Rizzo, G., Gualandi, G., Poltronieri, I., & Barbarini, G. (1999). Interferon alpha-2B and ribavirin in combination for patients with chronic hepatitis C who failed to respond to, or relapsed after, interferon alpha therapy: A randomized trial. *American Journal of Medicine, 107,* 112–118.

2. Balfour, H.H. (1999). Drug therapy: Antiviral drugs. *New England Journal of Medicine, 340,* 1255–1268.

3. Davis, G.L., Esteban-Mur, R., Rustgi, V., Hoefs, J., Gordon, S.C., Trepo, C., Shiffman, M.L., Zeuzem, S., Craxi, A., Ling, M.H., & Albrecht, J. (1998). Interferon alpha-2b alone or in combination with ribavirin for the treatment of relapse of chronic hepatitis C. *New England Journal of Medicine, 339,* 1493–1499.

4. DiPiro, J.T. (1998). Gastrointestinal disorders. In B.G. Wells, J.T. Dipiro, T.L. Schwinghammer, & C.W. Hamilton (Eds.), *Pharmacotherapy handbook* (pp. 271–288). Stamford, CT: Appleton & Lange.

5. Ferri, F.F. (1995). *Practical guide to the care of the medical patient* (3rd ed.). St. Louis: Mosby.

6. Grendell, J.H., McQuaid, K.R., & Friedman, S.L. (1996). *Current diagnosis and treatment in gastroenterology.* Stamford, CT: Appleton & Lange.

7. Gross, J.B. (1998). Clinician's guide to hepatitis C. *Mayo Clinic Proceedings, 74,* 355–361.

8. Hector Dunphy, L.M. (1999). *Management guidelines for adult nurse practitioners.* Philadelphia: F.A. Davis.

9. Hirsch, C.G., & Caswell, D. (1999). Gastrointestinal disorders. In A. Gawlinski & D. Hamwi (Eds.), *Acute care nurse practitioner: Clinical curriculum and certification review* (pp. 652–660). Philadelphia: W.B. Saunders.

10. Josefson, D. (1998). Oral treatment for hepatitis B gets approval in United States. *British Medical Journal, 317,* 1034.

11. Koff, R.S. (1999). Advances in the treatment of chronic viral hepatitis. *Journal of the American Medical Association, 282,* 511–512.

12. Lam, N.P. (1999). Hepatitis C: Natural history, diagnosis, and management (Clinical review). *American Journal of Health-System Pharmacy, 56,* 961–973.

13. Lindsetmo, R., Johnson, R., & Revhaug, A. (1998). Abdominal and dyspeptic symptoms in patients with peptic ulcer treated medically or surgically. *British Journal of Surgery, 85*, 845–849.
14. Rakel, R.E. (1996). *Saunders manual of medical practice.* Philadelphia: W.B. Saunders.
15. Salerno, Sr. M. (1999). Gastrointestinal disorders. In V.L. Millonig & S.L. Miller (Eds.), *Adult nurse practitioner certification review guide* (3rd ed.) (pp. 278–327). Potomac, MD: Health Leadership Associates, Inc.
16. Tierney, L.M., McPhee, S.J., & Papadakis, M.A. (1999). *Current medical diagnosis & treatment* (38th ed.). Stamford, CT: Appleton & Lange.
17. Herrera, J.L., & Roveda, K.P. (1999). Hepatitis C: What recent advances in therapy mean for your patients. *Consultant, 32*, 436–447.

BILIARY DYSFUNCTION

CHAPTER 37

Charlene M. Myers, MSN, RN, CS, ACNP, CCRN

I. CHOLECYSTITIS[1-7, 11-13]

A. Definition

Inflammation of the gallbladder occurring acutely or chronically, associated with gallstones (cholelithiasis) in more than 90% of cases

B. Etiology/Contributing factors/Risk factors

1. Gallstones

   a. Become impacted in the cystic duct
   b. Inflammation occurs behind the obstruction.

2. Acalculous cholecystitis

   a. Five percent of cases
   b. Should be considered when there is unexplained fever 2–4 weeks after surgery or any stressful situation
      i. Multiple trauma
      ii. Critical illness with a prolonged period of poor oral intake

3. Bacteria
4. Neoplasms
5. Strictures of the common bile duct
6. Ischemia
7. Torsion (twisting of cystic duct)
8. Possible contributing factors

   a. Obesity
   b. Pregnancy
   c. Sedentary lifestyle
   d. Low fiber diets

9. Risk factors

   a. Female
   b. Advanced age
   c. Rapid weight loss
   d. Fad diets

C. Clinical manifestations

1. Biliary colic

   a. Sudden onset

    b. Intense epigastric or right upper quadrant pain that may radiate to the shoulder or back

    c. Often associated with a full or fatty meal

2. Nausea and vomiting

    a. Occurs in approximately 70% of cases

    b. Vomiting offers some relief to many patients.

3. Feeling of abdominal fullness
4. Anorexia (inability to finish an average-sized meal)
5. Dyspepsia
6. Recurrent episodes of biliary colic lasting >12 h

D. Physical findings

1. Elevated body temperature
2. Local tenderness that is almost always accompanied by muscle guarding and rebound pain
3. Positive Murphy's sign (deep pain on inspiration while fingers are placed under the right rib cage)
4. Palpable gallbladder in 5% of cases
5. Jaundice in 20% of cases
6. Right upper quadrant pain, tenderness, guarding, fever, and leukocytosis that continues or progresses after 2–3 days indicate severe inflammation and possible gangrene, empyema, or perforation.

E. Laboratory/Diagnostics

1. Mild leukocytosis: WBCs 12,000–15,000/μL
2. Serum bilirubin mildly increased (1–4 mg/dL)
3. Increased levels of

    a. Alanine transaminase (ALT)

    b. Aspartate transaminase (AST)

    c. Lactate dehydrogenase (LDH)

    d. Alkaline phosphatase

4. Amylase level

    a. Elevated

    b. If >1000 units, concomitant pancreatitis should be suspected.

5. ECG

    a. Normal

    b. ECG is important to rule out myocardial infarction as cause of symptoms.

6. Chest x-ray to rule out pneumonia
7. Flat plat of the abdomen may show radiopaque gallstones (20% of cases).

8. Hepato-iminodiacetic acid (HIDA) scan to visualize cystic duct obstruction
9. Ultrasound: Best study to diagnose gallstones, thickened gallbladder wall
10. Endoscopic retrograde cholangiopancreatography (ERCP)

   a. Can diagnose stones in the gallbladder if noninvasive studies have been found negative
   b. Gives information on the status of biliary and pancreatic ducts

F. Treatment

1. NPO or low fat, low volume meals
2. If NPO, nasogastric tube to low wall suction
3. IV fluids

   a. To maintain intravascular volume and electrolytes: 5% dextrose in ½ NS, 125 mL/h
   b. Note signs of dehydration, and increase fluids as needed.
      i. Tachycardia
      ii. Hypotension
      iii. Decreased urinary output

4. Analgesics: Meperidine (Demerol), 75–100 mg IM/IV q4h as needed, is preferred to morphine.
5. Broad-spectrum IV antibiotics such as piperacillin (Pipracil)
6. Antispasmodics and antiemetics
7. Surgery consultation: Open cholecystectomy is recommended for symptomatic cholecystitis rather than a laparoscopic procedure, owing to the higher risk of future complications.
8. Extracorporeal shock wave lithotripsy (ESWL)

   a. May be used to remove gallstones instead of excision of the gallbladder
   b. Best in patients who have a solitary radiolucent stone <2 cm in diameter

9. Gallstones that are primarily composed of cholesterol and are <2 cm in diameter can be treated by pharmacologic dissolution.

   a. Ursodiol/ursodeoxycholic acid (10–15 mg/kg/day) for 12–24 months
      i. Monitor every 6 months with an ultrasound scan of the gallbladder.
      ii. Recurrence rate has been found to be high after discontinuation of the medication.
   b. Nonoverweight patients who have stones that are radiolucent, small, lacking in calcification, few in number, and floating may benefit from chenodeoxycholic acid (CDCA)/chenodiol, which blocks hepatic synthesis of cholesterol,

and ursodeoxycholic acid (UDCA)/ursodiol, which blocks intestinal uptake.

c. Contact dissolution by instillation of methyl *tert*-butyl ether (MTBE) percutaneously into the gallbladder

II. ACUTE PANCREATITIS[1-3, 5, 8-13]

A. Definition

An acute, inflammatory, autodigestive process of the pancreas

B. Etiology

1. Biliary tract disease (e.g., gallstones)
2. Alcoholism and acute intoxication
3. Medications

   a. Azathioprine (Imuran)
   b. Sulfonamides
   c. Thiazide diuretics
   d. Estrogen
   e. Furosemide (Lasix)

4. Hyperlipidemia
5. Hypercalcemia
6. Abdominal trauma/surgery
7. ERCP
8. Viral infections
9. Ischemia
10. Vasculitis
11. Peptic ulcer disease (PUD [rare])

C. Clinical manifestations

1. Epigastric abdominal pain

   a. May radiate to the back or to the right or left
   b. Usually
      i. Has an abrupt onset
      ii. Is steady and severe
      iii. Is worsened by walking or lying supine
   c. May be alleviated by
      i. Knee-to-chest position
      ii. Leaning forward
      iii. Sitting

2. Nausea and vomiting
3. In severe attacks

   a. Weakness
   b. Sweating
   c. Anxiety

4. Epigastric tenderness and guarding

5. Absent or hypoactive bowel sounds, distention (secondary to ileus)
6. Fever
7. Tachycardia, hypotension, cool/pale skin (due to decreased intravascular volume)
8. Tachypnea, decreased breath sounds (secondary to pleural effusion)
9. Jaundice
10. Steatorrhea
11. If hypocalcemic

    a. Chvostek's sign and/or
    b. Trousseau's sign

12. Ascites
13. Crackles if pleural effusion is present
14. A right upper quadrant mass may be palpated.
15. If intra-abdominal bleeding is present (hemorrhagic pancreatitis)

    a. Flank discoloration (Grey Turner's sign) and/or
    b. Umbilical discoloration (Cullen's sign)

D. Laboratory/Diagnostic findings

1. Elevated serum amylase and lipase levels. Serum lipase remains elevated longer than does serum amylase and is more specific.
2. Elevated urine amylase level
3. Leukocytosis (10,000–30,000/μL)
4. Hematocrit may be elevated initially, owing to hemoconcentration; a decreased hematocrit may suggest hemorrhage or disseminated intravascular coagulopathy.
5. Hyperglycemia (in severe disease)
6. Elevated BUN concentration (usually secondary to dehydration)
7. AST and LDH levels may be elevated secondary to tissue necrosis.
8. Bilirubin and alkaline phosphatase levels may be increased as a result of common bile duct obstruction.
9. Hypocalcemia (<7 mg/dL) in severe disease (due to saponification of fat)
10. Abdominal plain film may show

    a. A sentinel loop (ileus)
    b. Pancreatic calcifications
    c. Gallstones

11. Contrast-enhanced CT scan is superior to ultrasound in defining the extent of pancreatitis and in diagnosing pseudocysts, necrosis, and fistulas.

12. ERCP may be indicated for some patients, but should not be performed during the acute stage of the disease.

E. Management

1. Pain control: Meperidine is preferred (75–150 mg IM q3–4h).
2. IV hydration to maintain intravascular volume

   a. Lactated Ringer's or normal saline with 20 mEq KCl/L at 75–100 mL/h
   b. Increase as needed to maintain adequate blood pressure, urinary output, and pulmonary capillary wedge pressure/central venous pressure.

3. NPO until clinical improvement, then
   a. Supplements
   b. Small, frequent meals
      i. High cholesterol
      ii. High protein
      iii. Low fat
      iv. Bland

4. Nasogastric tube for ileus or vomiting
5. Monitor calcium levels and replace as needed.
6. Monitor pulmonary function.
7. Antibiotics

   a. For patients who have evidence of
      i. Septicemia
      ii. Pancreatic abscess
      iii. Inflammation secondary to biliary stones
   b. Example: Piperacillin, tazobactam (Zosyn), 3.375 g IV q6h

8. Current experimental evidence supports the use of prophylactic antibiotics in the initial management of patients with acute pancreatitis.
9. Total parenteral nutrition may be necessary.
10. Insulin may be needed in cases of hyperglycemia.
11. Surgery in selected cases

    a. Gallstones
    b. Perforated peptic ulcer
    c. Need for excision or drainage

12. If pancreatitis is secondary to biliary obstruction, stent placement via ERCP may be used to decrease recurrent episodes.

F. Prognosis (Ranson's criteria)[6]

1. Ranson has identified criteria for predicting the prognosis of patients with acute pancreatitis. The number of prognostic signs present within the first 48 h of admission help identify the patient's chance of morbidity and mortality.

   a. Less than 3 risk factors: Approximately 1% mortality rate

b. 3–4 risk factors: 15% mortality
c. 5–6 risk factors: 40% mortality
d. >7 risk factors: Close to 100% mortality

2. Prognostic signs at admission or diagnosis

a. More than 55 years of age (more than age 70 for gall-stones)
b. WBCs > 16,000/μL
c. Blood glucose >200 mg/dL
d. LDH > 350 IU/L
e. AST > 250 IU

3. Prognostic signs during initial 48 hours

a. Hematocrit drops >10 mL/dL.
b. BUN increases >5 mg/dL.
c. Calcium level <8 mg/dL
d. Arterial oxygen pressure <60 mmHg
e. Base deficit >4 mEq/L
f. Estimated fluid sequestration >6000 mL

References

1. Ferri, F.F. (1995). *Practical guide to the care of the medical patient* (3rd ed.). St. Louis: Mosby.
2. Greenberger, N.J. (1998). Update in gastroenterology. *Annals of Internal Medicine, 124,* 309–316.
3. Grendell, J.H., McQuaid, K.R., & Friedman, S.L. (1996). *Current diagnosis and treatment in gastroenterology.* Stamford, CT: Appleton & Lange.
4. Hector Dunphy, L.M. (1999). *Management guidelines for adult nurse practitioners.* Philadelphia: F.A. Davis.
5. Hirsch, C.G., & Caswell, D. (1999). Gastrointestinal disorders. In A. Gawlinski & D. Hamwi (Eds.). *Acute care nurse practitioner: Clinical curriculum and certification review* (pp. 677–680). Philadelphia: W.B. Saunders.
6. Krumberger, J.M., & Hammer, B. (1997). Gastrointestinal alterations. In J.C. Hartshorn, M.L. Sole, & M.L. Lamborn (Eds.). *Introduction to critical care nursing* (pp. 425–472). Philadelphia: W.B. Saunders.
7. Lujan, J.A., Parrilla, P., Robles, R., Marin, P., Torralba, J.A., & Garcia-Ayllon, J. (1998). Laparoscopic cholecystectomy vs open cholecystectomy in the treatment of acute cholecystitis: A prospective study. *Archives of Surgery, 133,* 173–175.
8. Mergener, K., & Baillic, J. (1998). Fortnightly review: Acute pancreatitis. *British Medical Journal, 316,* 44–48.
9. Mergener, K., & Baillic, J. (1997). Chronic pancreatitis. *The Lancet, 350,* 1379–1385.
10. Powell, J.J., Miles, R., & Siriwardena, A.K. (1998). Antibiotic prophylaxis in the initial management of severe acute pancreatitis. *British Journal of Surgery, 85,* 582–587.
11. Rakel, R.E. (1996). *Saunders manual of medical practice.* Philadelphia: W.B. Saunders.
12. Tierney, L.M., McPhee, S.J., & Papadakis, M.A. (1999). *Current medical diagnosis & treatment* (38th ed.). Stamford, CT: Appleton & Lange.
13. Wright, J.A. (1997). Seven abdominal assessment signs every emergency nurse should know. *Journal of Emergency Nursing, 23,* 446–450.

INFLAMMATORY GASTROINTESTINAL DISORDERS

Charlene M. Myers, MSN, RN, CS, ACNP, CCRN

I. DIVERTICULITIS[2, 3, 5, 8, 9]

A. Definition

1. Inflammation or localized perforation of diverticulum with abscess formation
2. Occurs in approximately 5% of patients with diverticulosis annually

B. Etiology

1. Not clearly proven
2. Low stool weight, leading to high colonic pressure
3. Low fiber diet
4. Abnormal colonic motility leading to increased colonic pressure
5. Weakness and defects in the colon wall

C. Clinical manifestations

1. Lower left quadrant pain (mild to moderate) and fever are the main clinical features.
2. Constipation is common and may alternate with diarrhea.
3. Fever and abdominal tenderness, guarding, palpable mass, spasms, and rebound tenderness indicate inflammation due to abscess.
4. Nausea and vomiting
5. Bowel sounds are usually hypoactive.
6. Abdominal distention and exaggerated bowel sounds if obstruction occurs
7. Dysuria and frequency may be present, owing to colonic inflammatory process, which causes irritation to the bladder.

D. Laboratory/Diagnostic findings

1. Leukocytosis is common, although those with mild diverticulitis may have a normal WBC count.
2. Elevated erythrocyte sedimentation rate owing to inflammation
3. Barium enema may reveal strictures, obstruction, masses, or fistulas, but it should not be used in the acute stage because it may cause free perforation.
4. Flexible sigmoidoscopy may show inflamed mucosa, but should also be avoided during the acute phase.

5. CT scan may reveal abscess cavity.
6. ALL patients should have plain abdominal radiography to look for free air (perforation) and ileus.

E. Management

1. Patients with mild symptoms can be managed conservatively at home.

    a. Rest the bowel.
        i. Clear liquids, then low residue for 24–48 h
        ii. Progress to a high fiber diet as normal bowel function returns.
    b. Bed rest during acute phase
    c. Antibiotic therapy may consist of
        i. Metronidazole (Flagyl), 500 mg t.i.d., plus
        ii. Ciprofloxacin (Cipro), 500 mg b.i.d., OR
        iii. Trimethoprim-sulfamethoxazole (Bactrim DS), 160/800 mg b.i.d. for 14 days
    d. Instruct patient to avoid laxatives and enemas.

2. More severe cases—Hospitalization is necessary.

    a. NPO, NGT
    b. IV fluids
    c. IV antibiotics to cover both aerobic and anaerobic intestinal flora
        i. Ampicillin (Ampicin). 1–2 g per day in divided doses q4–6h
        ii. Cefoxitin (Mefoxin), 1–2 g IV q6–8h, OR
        iii. An aminoglycoside (amikacin) plus clindamycin (Cleocin) or metronidazole
    d. Morphine is contraindicated as an analgesic because it may increase colonic pressure. Pentazocine (Talwin) or meperidine (Demerol) is preferred.
    e. Severe disease or failure to respond to treatment within 72 h requires surgical consultation.
    f. Emergency surgical consultation is necessary for those patients who have an abscess, obstruction, free air, or peritonitis, which will require surgery.

II. ULCERATIVE COLITIS[2, 3, 5, 6, 9]

A. Definition

1. Inflammatory bowel disease of unknown etiology that is characterized by bouts of inflammation of part or all of the colon
2. In most patients, the disease is intermittent, with episodes of flare-ups and remission.

B. Clinical manifestations

1. Bloody diarrhea is the cardinal sign.

2. Fever
3. Abdominal pain
4. Weight loss
5. Extracolonic complications

   a. Arthralgias and arthritis (15–20% of patients)
   b. Ocular complications
   c. Skin disorders
      i. Erythema nodosum
      ii. Pyoderma gangrenosum
      iii. Mouth ulcers
   d. Liver disorders
      i. Cirrhosis
      ii. Fatty liver
      iii. Bile duct cancer
   e. Spondylitis
   f. Thromboembolic disease

6. Patient may exhibit signs and symptoms of hypovolemic shock in severe disease. Symptoms may range from mild to systemic toxicity, depending on the severity of the bleeding and inflammation.
7. Assessment of disease activity (Table 38–1)

C. Laboratory/Diagnostic findings

1. See Table 38–1.
2. Leukocytosis during inflammation
3. Anemia
4. Electrolyte abnormalities (hypokalemia)
5. Causes elevated values on liver function tests (if hepatobiliary disease is present)
6. Stool cultures for infectious disease are negative.
7. Sigmoidoscopy/colonoscopy with biopsy determines the extent of the disease and provides histologic confirmation.

TABLE 38–1. ASSESSMENT OF DISEASE ACTIVITY IN ULCERATIVE COLITIS

	MILD	MODERATE	SEVERE
Stool, #/day	<4	4–6	>6 (bloody)
Heart rate (beats/min)	<90	90–100	>100
Hematocrit	Normal	30–40 mL/dL	<30 mL/dL
Weight loss	None	1–10%	>10%
Temperature	Normal	99°–100°F	>100°F
Erythrocyte sedimentation rate	<20 mm/h or normal	20–30 mm/h	>30 mm/h
Albumin	Normal	3–3.5 g/dL	<3.0 g/dL

8. Plain abdominal x-rays exclude dilation and guide in the determination of disease state (bowel containing feces is most likely not severely inflamed).
9. Barium enema is used less frequently.
10. Colonoscopy and barium enema should not be performed in an acute attack because they could cause exacerbation.

D. Management

1. Sulfasalazine (Azulfidine) is the cornerstone of drug therapy for mild to moderate cases of ulcerative colitis.

   a. Four grams per day for active disease and 2 g/day for maintaining remission
   b. Should be initiated at 500 mg/day and increased every few days up to 4 g/day or the maximum tolerated (up to 8 g/day)

2. There are reported problems of hypersensitivity and intolerance with sulfasalazine.

   a. New forms have been developed (e.g., mesalamine [Asacol] and olsalazine [Dipentum]).
   b. These may be better tolerated, but are no more effective than sulfasalazine and cost significantly more.

3. Mesalamine suppositories, 500 mg b.i.d. for 3–12 weeks, are beneficial for ulcerative proctitis.
4. Patients with disease beyond the rectum but not beyond the descending colon may benefit from mesalamine enemas (4 g/d).
5. Corticosteroids, such as prednisone, 1 mg/kg/day, may prove to be beneficial in moderate to severe cases and for those who do not respond to mesalamine in 2–4 weeks. Taper off gradually after remission is induced (over 3–4 weeks).
6. Azathioprine (Imuran) has been shown to be effective in preventing relapse of ulcerative colitis for periods of up to 2 years.
7. For severe cases of ulcerative colitis, hospitalization is required because patients may deteriorate rapidly.

   a. NPO—Total parenteral nutrition may be necessary for those with poor nutritional status.
   b. Avoid opiates and anticholinergics.
   c. Administer IV resuscitation and blood products as needed.
   d. Monitor and correct electrolyte imbalances.
   e. Plain abdominal x-ray (to detect toxic megacolon)
   f. Stool samples (to detect infectious disease)
   g. Surgery consultation
   h. Methylprednisolone (Solu-Medrol), 48–60 mg IV daily

    i. Add IV cyclosporine for patients who have not improved after 7–10 days on corticosteroid therapy (as an alternative to a surgical intervention).

   j. Surgical indications include

      i. Toxic megacolon

      ii. Fulminant colitis

      iii. Perforation

      iv. Hemorrhage

      v. High-grade dysplasia

      vi. Carcinoma

      vii. Refractory disease requiring high-dose steroids

   k. If toxic megacolon is identified

      i. Administer broad-spectrum antibiotics, such as piperacillin (Pipracil), 2–4 g q4–6h, to cover gram-negative bacteria and anaerobes.

      ii. Insert a nasogastric tube.

      iii. Instruct the patient to roll from side to side and to lie prone to decompress the distended colon.

      iv. Serial plain abdominal x-rays

III. PERITONITIS[1–4, 8–10]

A. Definition

An acute inflammation of the visceral and parietal peritoneum

B. Etiology

1. Primary—Spontaneous bacterial peritonitis as a complication of cirrhotic ascites

   a. Low total protein in ascitic fluid (<1.5 g/dL)—Higher risk

   b. *Escherichia coli* is the most frequent causative organism.

   c. *Klebsiella, pneumococci,* and *enterococcus* are common as well.

2. Secondary

   a. Following abdominal trauma

   b. Following penetrating wounds

   c. Continuous ambulatory peritoneal dialysis (CAPD)

   d. Perforation resulting from

      i. Appendicitis

      ii. Colitis

      iii. Peptic ulcer disease

      iv. Diverticulitis

      v. Pancreatitis

      vi. Cholecystitis

   e. Postoperative

   f. Gangrene of the bowel

   g. Tuberculosis

   h. Familial Mediterranean fever

C. Clinical manifestations

1. Acute abdominal pain

   a. Exacerbated by motion
   b. Can be localized, generalized, or referred to shoulder or thorax

2. High fever
3. Nausea and vomiting
4. Constipation
5. Abdominal examination

   a. Distention
   b. Rebound tenderness
   c. Generalized rigidity
   d. Decreased bowel sounds
   e. Hyper-resonance to percussion

6. Ascites
7. Dyspnea, tachypnea
8. Dehydration (hypotension, tachycardia)

D. Laboratory/Diagnostic findings

1. Peritoneal aspirate: WBC counts $>500/\mu L$ with more than 50% neutrocytic ascites (>250 PMNs/μL)
2. Blood cultures—Positive in 25% of patients
3. Leukocytosis
4. Elevated BUN levels
5. Hemoconcentration (increased hematocrit)
6. Metabolic and respiratory acidosis
7. Elevated amylase levels
8. Abdominal x-ray

   a. Free air in peritoneal cavity
   b. Dilation of large or small bowel

9. Chest x-ray—Elevated diaphragm
10. CT and ultrasound

    a. Ascites
    b. Intra-abdominal mass

E. Management

1. Surgical consultation
2. Antibiotic therapy—3rd generation cephalosporin

   a. Cefotaxime (Claforan), 1–2 g IV q4–6h
   b. or Ceftriaxone (Rocephin), 1–2 g IV q24h
   c. Ampicillin, 1–2 g q6h, or ampicillin/sulbactam (Unasyn), 1.5–3 g q6–8h, may be added if enterococcal infection is suspected.

   d. Aminoglycoside such as gentamicin (Garamycin), 1 mg/ kg q8h, plus anaerobic coverage with metronidazole, 500 mg q6h, is needed for severe cases.

   e. Aminoglycosides (gentamicin, tobramycin) and vancomycin should not be used in patients with chronic liver failure because of the high risk of nephrotoxicity. Use a 3rd generation cephalosporin such as ceftazidime (Fortaz), 1–2 g IV q8h.

   f. Traditionally 10 days of therapy is recommended, although recent studies suggest 5 days is sufficient.

   g. Fluid resuscitation
     i. IV fluids
       (1) Lactated Ringer's solution
       (2) Normal saline
     ii. Monitor
       (1) Heart rate
       (2) Blood pressure
       (3) Mean arterial pressure
       (4) Urinary output
       (5) Pulmonary capillary wedge pressure/central venous pressure
     iii. Titrate fluid rates as needed.

   h. NPO, NGT

   i. Monitor for respiratory support.

   j. Colchicine, 0.6 mg b.i.d. or t.i.d., has been used prophylactically in patients with a history of familial Mediterranean fever (rare).

   k. Continuous ambulatory peritoneal dialysis (CAPD)
     i. Intraperitoneal vancomycin, 20 mg/L dialysate + 1 g IV load, plus gentamicin, 6–8 mg/L dialysate
     ii. Intraperitoneal cefazolin (Ancef)

IV. APPENDICITIS[2, 3, 5, 7–10]

A. Definition

1. Acute inflammation of the vermiform appendix caused by obstruction of the appendiceal lumen by

   a. Fecaliths (most common)
   b. Inflammation
   c. Foreign body
   d. Intestinal worms
   e. Strictures
   f. Tumors

2. Gangrene and perforation can develop if appendicitis is not treated within 36 h.

B. Clinical manifestations

1. Abdominal pain (100% of patients)

   a. Periumbilical pain initially, then right lower quadrant pain

b. Flexion of the thigh lessens the pain.
c. Movement usually worsens the pain.

2. Anorexia
3. Nausea with or without vomiting
4. Constipation—Urge to defecate, although some report diarrhea
5. Low-grade fever (High fever suggests possible perforation or another diagnosis.)
6. Motionless, with right thigh drawn up
7. Point tenderness (McBurney's point)
8. Guarding of the right lower quadrant
9. Positive Rovsing's sign—Right lower quadrant pain when pressure is applied to the left lower quadrant
10. Positive psoas sign—Pain with right thigh extension
11. Positive obturator sign—Pain with internal rotation of flexed right thigh

C. Laboratory/Diagnostic findings

1. Moderate leukocytosis—10,000–20,000/μL in 75% of cases
2. Urinalysis

   a. Elevated specific gravity
   b. Hematuria
   c. Pyuria
   d. Albuminuria

3. For patients who fit the picture of typical appendicitis, no imaging is necessary.
4. Ultrasound is 85% accurate in diagnosing appendicitis.
5. CT scan to detect

   a. Perforation
   b. Periappendiceal abscess

6. History and clinical findings are the cornerstones of diagnosis.

D. Management

1. Surgical consultation—Appendectomy (open or closed)
2. IV fluids; correct fluid and electrolyte imbalances as indicated
3. Broad-spectrum antibiotic (cefoxitin, 1–2 g q6–8h IV, cefotetan [Cefotan])
4. Gangrenous or perforated appendicitis

   a. Antibiotic coverage for aerobic and anaerobic enteric pathogens (all IV)
      i. Ampicillin (150–200 mg/kg/day in divided doses q3–4 h)
      ii. Gentamicin (1 mg/kg q8h [up to 5 mg/kg/day in 3–4 divided doses])

    iii. Clindamycin (300–600 mg q6–8h or 900 mg q8h [up to 4.8 g/day])

  b. Continue antibiotics for 7 days after surgery.

5. Pain management after diagnosis is made and surgery is scheduled.

  a. Meperidine, 25–50 mg IM, or

  b. Morphine sulfate, 1–2 mg IV push

References

1. Dalaman, G., Haklar, G., Sipahiu, A., Ozener, C., Akoglu, E., & Yalcin, A.S. (1998). Early detection of peritonitis in continuous ambulatory peritoneal dialysis patients by use of chemiluminescence: Evaluation of diagnostic accuracy by receiver-operating characteristic curve analysis. *Clinical Chemistry, 44,* 1680–1684.

2. Ferri, F.F. (1995). *Practical guide to the care of the medical patient* (3rd ed.). St. Louis: Mosby.

3. Grendell, J.H., McQuaid, K.R., & Friedman, S.L. (1996). *Current diagnosis and treatment in gastroenterology.* Stamford, CT: Appleton & Lange.

4. Hector Dunphy, L.M. (1999). *Management guidelines for adult nurse practitioners.* Philadelphia: F.A. Davis.

5. Hirsch, C.G., & Caswell, D. (1999). Gastrointestinal disorders. In A. Gawlinski & D. Hamwi (Eds.), *Acute care nurse practitioner: Clinical curriculum and certification review* (pp. 618–722). Philadelphia: W.B. Saunders.

6. Martin, F.L. (1997). Ulcerative colitis: How to manage this chronic inflammatory disease and prevent systemic complications. *American Journal of Nursing, 97,* 38–39.

7. Pisarra, V.H. (1999). Recognizing the various presentations of appendicitis. *Nurse Practitioner, 24,* 42–53.

8. Rakel, R.E. (1996). *Saunders manual of medical practice.* Philadelphia: W.B. Saunders.

9. Tierney, L.M., McPhee, S.J., & Papadakis, M.A. (1999). *Current medical diagnosis & treatment* (38th ed.). Stamford, CT: Appleton & Lange.

10. Wright, J.A. (1997). Seven abdominal assessment signs every emergency nurse should know. *Journal of Emergency Nursing, 23,* 446–450.

ANATOMIC INTESTINAL DISORDERS

Charlene M. Myers, MSN, RN, CS, ACNP, CCRN

I. SMALL BOWEL OBSTRUCTION[3-8, 11]

A. Definition

1. Blockage of the lumen of the intestine that prevents normal functioning and results in distention and tremendous losses of fluid into the gut
2. Necrosis with toxicity and possible perforation may occur if there is strangulation.

B. Etiology

1. Adhesions—Most common
2. Hernias—External and internal
3. Volvulus—A twisting of the bowel on itself, causing obstruction
4. Strictures—Due to

   a. Crohn's disease
   b. Radiation
   c. Ischemia

5. Hematomas—Related to

   a. Trauma
   b. Anticoagulants

6. Intussusception—Slipping of one part of an intestine into another part just below it
7. Feces (impaction)
8. Tumors
9. Foreign bodies

C. Clinical manifestations

1. Cramping periumbilical pain initially occurs sporadically, lasting seconds to minutes.
2. The pain becomes constant and diffuse as distention develops.
3. High or proximal bowel obstruction

   a. Variable upper abdominal pain
   b. Profuse vomiting

4. Middle or distal small bowel obstruction

   a. Cramping, colicky, periumbilical, or diffuse pain

    b. Distention
    c. Episodic vomiting

5. The more distal the obstruction, the greater the distention.

    a. More vomiting of feculent contents
    b. Increase in the nasogastric output

6. Obstipation (extreme constipation) develops in complete obstruction.
7. Partial obstruction—Watery, possibly mucus diarrhea
8. Mild tenderness
9. High-pitched "tinkling" bowel sounds and peristaltic rushes are noted early on auscultation; these sounds may become absent later.
10. Visible peristalsis may be present.
11. Signs and symptoms of dehydration

D. Laboratory/Diagnostic findings

1. Leukocytosis may be present.
2. Hemoconcentration and electrolyte imbalances
3. Supine and upright abdominal x-rays

    a. Ladder-like pattern of dilated bowel with air-fluid levels
    b. In complete obstruction there is little or no air in the colon or rectum.
    c. With strangulation there is thickening or "thumbprinting" of the intestinal wall.

4. Transabdominal ultrasonography

    a. Noninvasive, radiation-free method
    b. Well tolerated by patients with acute abdominal symptoms
    c. Accurate and highly specific in the diagnosis of small bowel obstruction

5. Barium radiography confirms the diagnosis if there is uncertainty.

E. Management

1. IV fluids and electrolyte replacement as indicated
2. Nasogastric tube to low wall suction
3. Initiate broad-spectrum antibiotics if strangulation is suspected (e.g., cefoxitin [Mefoxin] 1–2 g q6–8h IV piggyback, cefotetan [Cefotan]).
4. Partial obstructions usually resolve spontaneously within a few days.
5. Surgical consultation is indicated for complete obstruction, or for partial obstructions that fail to improve with traditional treatment.

II. MESENTERIC ISCHEMIA[1-4, 6, 9-11]

A. Definition

1. Mesenteric ischemia results when the bloodstream fails to carry sufficient amounts of oxygen and other nutrients to meet intestinal needs.
2. Ischemia may be related to an artery occluded by an embolus or thrombus, or there may be no physical occlusion.

B. Etiology

1. Embolism—From the left atrium, mitral valve, arterial thrombus, or elsewhere
2. Thrombus—Thrombus formation. A link has been found between prothrombin gene 20210G/A mutation and thrombosis of digestive vessels.
3. Arterial thrombus—May occur

    a. On atheromatous plaque
    b. Spontaneously (in women on oral contraceptives)

4. Surgical accidents
5. Abdominal trauma
6. Tumors
7. Occlusion of the arteriole occurs with systemic diseases.

    a. Thrombotic thrombocytopenic purpura.
    b. Disseminated intravascular coagulopathy
    c. Polyarteritis nodosa
    d. Systemic lupus erythematosus

8. Nonocclusive mesenteric vascular disease is more common than the preceding and is related to low flow conditions and mesenteric vasoconstrictive states.

    a. Congestive heart failure
    b. Aortic stenosis
    c. Shock
    d. Cardiac arrhythmias
    e. Vasoconstrictor drugs

C. Clinical manifestations

1. Severe, cramping, generalized, or periumbilical abdominal pain
2. Early in the course of the disorder, no abnormalities are found on examination. Diagnosis requires a high index of suspicion.
3. Possible rectal bleeding with colonic ischemia
4. Hypotension and abdominal distention suggest infarction.

D. Laboratory/Diagnostic findings

1. Leukocytosis

2. Lactic acidosis—Suggests infarction
3. Mesenteric arteriography (digital subtraction angiography [DSA])—Useful in locating a vascular occlusion
4. Barium contrast radiography—"Thumbprinting" or thickening of the intestinal wall
5. Contrast-enhanced MR angiography has sensitivity and specificity approaching those of DSA in the detection of mesenteric ischemia.
6. Noninvasive techniques, such as superconducting quantum interference devices (SQUIDs)

   a. Under investigation for early detection of mesenteric ischemia
   b. Can detect basic electrical rhythm by measuring the magnetic fields generated by the electrical activity of the smooth muscle of the small bowel

E. Management

1. Occlusive disease

   a. Embolectomy or bypass of the occluded vessel to prevent infarction
   b. If infarction has occurred, resection of that part of the bowel should be performed.
   c. Total parenteral nutrition may be needed and continued indefinitely if a large portion of the bowel is resected.

2. Nonocclusive disease: Correct or alleviate underlying problems.

   a. Hypovolemia
   b. Heart failure
   c. Digitalis toxicity

3. The goal is to restore intestinal perfusion, reverse ischemia, and prevent infarction.
4. Once circulating volume has been restored, vasodilator therapy can be initiated.
5. Begin antibiotic coverage before surgery if peritonitis is suspected (broad-spectrum for gram-negative bacteria and anaerobes).
6. Vasodilator drugs can also be administered via an intra-arterial catheter placed during arteriography.

   a. Papaverine (Paverine, Pavabid)
   b. Glucagon, 0.25–1 mg IV
   c. Vasodilator prostaglandins

7. Stent placement for stenosis or occlusions has been effective as an adjunct therapy to angioplasty or as a primary method of treatment for chronic mesenteric ischemia.

References

1. Balian, A., Veyradier, A., Naveau, S., Wolf, M., Montembault, S., Giraud, V., Borotto, E., Henry, C., Meyer, D., & Chaput, J.C. (1999). Prothrombin 2021-G/A mutation in two patients with mesenteric ischemia. *Digestive Diseases & Sciences, 44*, 1919–1923.
2. Chan, F.P., Li, K.C., Heiss, S.G., & Razavi, M.K. (1999). A comprehensive approach using MR imaging to diagnose acute segmental mesenteric ischemia in a porcine model. *American Journal of Roentgenology, 173*, 523–529.
3. Ferri, F.F. (1995). *Practical guide to the care of the medical patient* (3rd ed.). St. Louis: Mosby.
4. Grendell, J.H., McQuaid, K.R., & Friedman, S.L. (1996). *Current diagnosis and treatment in gastroenterology*. Stamford, CT: Appleton & Lange.
5. Hector Dunphy, L.M. (1999). *Management guidelines for adult nurse practitioners*. Philadelphia: F.A. Davis.
6. Hirsch, C.G., & Caswell, D. (1999). Gastrointestinal disorders. In A. Gawlinski & D. Hamwi (Eds.), *Acute care nurse practitioner: Clinical curriculum and certification review*. Philadelphia: W.B. Saunders.
7. Kohn, A., Cerro, P., Milite, G., De Angelis, E., & Prantera, C. (1999). Prospective evaluation of transabdominal bowel sonography in the diagnosis of intestinal obstruction in Crohn's disease. *Inflammatory Bowel Diseases, 5*, 153–157.
8. Rakel, R.E. (1996). *Saunders manual of medical practice*. Philadelphia: W.B. Saunders.
9. Seidel, S.A., Bradshaw, L.A., Ladipo, J.K., Wikswo, J.P., & Richards, W.O. (1999). Noninvasive detection of ischemic bowel. *Journal of Vascular Surgery, 30*, 367–369.
10. Sheeran S.R., Murphy, T.P., Khwaja, A., Sussman, S.K., & Hallisey, M.J. (1999). Stent placement for treatment of mesenteric artery stenoses or occlusions. *Journal of Vascular & Interventional Radiology, 10*, 861–867.
11. Tierney, L.M., McPhee, S.J., & Papadakis, M.A. (1999). *Current medical diagnosis & treatment* (38th ed.). Stamford, CT: Appleton & Lange.

GASTROINTESTINAL BLEEDING

Charlene M. Myers, MSN, RN, CS, ACNP, CCRN

I. ESOPHAGEAL VARICES[2–4, 6, 7, 10]

A. Definition

1. Dilated submucosal veins that may develop in patients with underlying portal hypertension and can result in severe gastrointestinal (GI) bleeding.
2. Varices can rupture at any moment and become a medical emergency.
3. Three out of ten patients will die from the initial hemorrhage.
4. Overall mortality reaches nearly 60% as rebleeding claims the lives of another three out of ten.

B. Etiology

1. Cirrhosis—Most common
2. A portal venous pressure of at least 12 mmHg is needed for varices to bleed (normal pressure is 2–6 mmHg).
3. Bleeding from esophageal varices usually occurs in the distal 5 cm of the esophagus and upper portion of the stomach.
4. Aspirin, used alone on in combination with other NSAIDs, has been associated with a first variceal bleeding episode in patients with cirrhosis.

C. Clinical manifestations

1. Hematemesis
2. Melena
3. Hematochezia (indicates massive bleed, >1000 mL)
4. Abdominal discomfort
5. Signs and symptoms of hypovolemia or shock

D. Diagnostics/Laboratory findings

1. CBC

   a. Hemoglobin/hematocrit—Normal, then decreased related to hemoconcentration/volume resuscitation
   b. WBCs—Elevated, related to the body's attempt to restore homeostasis
   c. Platelets—Increased, then decreased related to attempts to restore homeostasis, and finally reflects true blood loss

2. Electrolyte panel

   a. K^+—Decreases as a result of emesis, then increases

b. Na^{++}—Decreases, then increases as a result of hemo-concentration/fluid resuscitation

c. Ca^{++}—Normal or decreased

d. Hyperglycemia—Stress response

e. BUN/Creatinine ratio—Elevated related to poor perfusion to the liver and kidneys

f. Lactate levels—Elevated (lactic acidosis related to anaerobic metabolism)

g. AST/ALT ratio and bilirubin level are usually abnormal in patients with underlying chronic liver disease.

h. Albumin—Low

i. Prolonged prothrombin time (PT) and partial thromboplastin time (PTT).

j. Arterial blood gases—Respiratory alkalosis/metabolic acidosis

3. Endoscopy—After stabilization, to identify the source of the bleed

4. Barium studies—Can be performed to define the presence of peptic ulcers, bleeding sites, tumors, and inflammation

E. Management

1. Emergency resuscitation

a. Insert two large-bore (16-gauge) IVs and central venous pressure (CVP) line access.

b. Laboratory studies: Blood type and crossmatch, PT/PTT, CBC, electrolyte panel, renal and liver function tests

c. Infuse crystalloids (lactated Ringer's or normal saline) for treatment of hypotension until blood products can be administered. (Note: Overzealous hydration increases portal pressure and can exacerbate or cause rebleeding of varices).

i. Maintain

- Systolic blood pressure >110 mmHg
- CVP ≤10 mmHg
- Pulmonary capillary wedge pressure ≤8 mmHg (if pulmonary artery catheter is in place)

ii. Administer fresh frozen plasma for coagulopathies.

d. Administer oxygen at 5–10 L/min.

e. Insert a Foley catheter.

f. NPO—Insert nasogatric tube.

g. Consult a surgeon and a gastroenterologist.

2. Sixty to eighty percent of patients will stop bleeding spontaneously, but without therapy, over half will rebleed within a week.

3. Emergency endoscopy—Sclerotherapy using agents such as ethanolamine or tetradecyl sulfate, or band ligation

4. Vasopressin—Vasoconstrictor that decreases portal pressures by reducing the splanchnic flow (successful in only 50% of cases).

   a. Dose: 0.2–0.4 units/min to a maximum of 0.8 units/min
   b. Taper down over 24 h after the bleeding is controlled.

   - Use only in a peripheral line—not a central line, owing to severe coronary spasms that may result.

   c. Monitor for vasopressin-induced side effects
      i. Chest pain
      ii. Sweating
      iii. Paleness

5. Octreotide (Sandostatin), 25–100 μg/h, works as vasopressin but without the side effects.
6. Vitamin K—10 mg IM for cirrhotics with coagulopathies
7. Lactulose—30 mL b.i.d. for patients with severe liver disease to prevent encephalopathy (causes induction of 2–3 stools/day)
8. Balloon tamponade may be necessary to control bleeding.

   - Sengstaken-Blakemore (SB) tube (3 ports), or
   - Minnesota tube (4 ports)

   a. Normal inflation pressure is 20–45 mmHg.
   b. Inflation pressures must be continuously monitored.
   c. Balloons should be deflated every 8–12 h.

   - The esophageal balloon must be deflated before the gastric tube is removed to prevent tube displacement upward and occlusion of the airway.

   d. Keep scissors at the bedside.
   e. Possible complications
      i. Gastric balloon rupture—Occlusion of airway
      ii. Esophageal rupture—Characterized by severe back pain
      iii. Ulcerations of the esophageal or gastric mucosa

F. Prevention of rebleeding

1. Routine follow-up with endoscopy
2. Beta blockers

   a. Propranolol or labetalol, 20 mg b.i.d., increased gradually until heart rate falls by 25% or reaches 55 beats per min.
   b. Average dose: 60 mg b.i.d.
   c. Used frequently in combination with sclerotherapy

3. Transjugular intrahepatic portosystemic stent (TIPS)—For patients with recurrent bleeds despite the above therapies

4. Portosystemic shunts—Usually reserved for patients for whom beta blockers have failed or who are noncompliant. (TIPS is used more commonly than portosystemic shunt.)
5. Liver transplantation

II. UPPER GASTROINTESTINAL BLEEDING[1, 2, 4–7, 9, 10]

A. Definition

1. Acute upper gastrointestinal bleeding refers to loss of blood within the intraluminal gastrointestinal tract from any location between the upper esophagus and the duodenum at the ligament of Treitz.
2. Patient history is very important in determining the time of onset of bleeding, severity, and possible causes.

B. Etiology

1. Peptic ulcer disease (PUD)
2. Esophageal and gastric varices as a result of portal hypertension
3. Mallory-Weiss tear
4. Vascular abnormalities
5. Neoplasm
6. Gastric or duodenal erosion
7. Aortoenteric fistula
8. Dieulafoy's vascular malformation—A submucosal artery usually located in the proximal stomach abnormally close to the mucosa that causes erosion of the epithelium and may result in massive upper tract bleeding
9. Hematobilia—Blood in the bile or bile ducts
10. Ménétrier's disease

   a. Gastritis of unknown cause
   b. Marked by excessive proliferation of the stomach mucosal folds

C. Clinical manifestations

1. Hematemesis (bright red or "coffee grounds")
2. Melena, in the majority of cases as evidenced by 50–100 mL of blood in the upper gastrointestinal (UGI) tract; hematochezia in massive UGI bleeds (>1000 mL)
3. Signs and symptoms of hypovolemic shock, such as hypotension and tachycardia, are present in severe cases or acute loss (e.g., >40% blood volume).
4. Orthostatic changes are noted in patients with a loss of 20% or more of blood volume.
5. Skin pallor
6. Spider angiomata, palmar erythema, and icterus suggest chronic liver disease.

7. Nasogastric tube aspirate—Bright red blood indicates active bleeding and is associated with a higher mortality than is melena.

D. Diagnostics/Laboratory findings

1. Blood type and crossmatch for at least four units of packed red blood cells.
2. Hemoglobin and hematocrit—Poorly reflect the degree and severity of blood loss
3. PT/PTT, platelet count, electrolytes, BUN/creatine, liver enzymes
4. ECG in the elderly and in patients with coronary artery disease (CAD) may indicate ischemia related to severe anemia.
5. Barium studies are of little value.
6. Endoscopy is both diagnostic and therapeutic. Endoscopic evaluation of the UGI tract should be considered in asymptomatic patients who have a positive fecal occult blood test and a negative colonoscopy, especially if they are anemic.

E. Management

1. Rapid clinical evaluation and assessment of hemodynamic status (i.e., ABCs)
2. Endotracheal intubation may be indicated.
3. Consult a gastroenterologist and a surgeon.
4. Patients with significant blood loss

   a. Insert two large-bore IV lines (16-gauge) or a central line for fluid resuscitation.
   b. Blood transfusion for high-risk patients
      i. Keep hematocrit >30 mL/dL
      ii. Young/healthy patients: Maintain hematocrit >20 mL/dL
   c. Coagulopathies: Fresh frozen plasma and vitamin K
   d. Low platelet counts: Transfuse platelets.

5. Nasogastric tube placement—Tap water lavage

   a. If aspirate does not clear after 2–3 L, continued active bleeding is assumed.
   b. More urgent resuscitation and endoscopic interventions are indicated.

6. Endoscopy—Should be considered in all patients with UGI bleeding

   a. Should be performed as an emergency procedure in a patient with an active hemorrhage after stabilization
   b. Active, self-limiting bleeds: Perform within 24 h, unless
      i. Portal hypertension or aortoenteric fistula is suspected
      ii. Bleeding recurs after initial stabilization

  c. Patients with chronic blood loss may have elective endoscopy.

  d. Treatment options include

   i. Thermal coagulation (i.e., cauterization)

   ii. Injection therapy with epinephrine or sclerosant

   iii. Band ligation

7. Acute pharmacologic therapies

  a. IV H_2 blockers to keep gastric pH >4.0

   i. Cimetidine (Tagamet), 37.5–50 mg/h, or

   ii. Ranitidine (Zantac), 6.25 mg/h, or

   iii. Famotidine (Pepcid), 1 mg/h

   iv. Double dose if gastric pH remains low (<7)

  b. Proton pump inhibitors such as omeprazole (Prilosec) or lansoprazole (Prevacid) are not recommended.

  c. Octreotide, 50–250 μg/h, reduces splanchnic arterial flow and portal pressures.

   i. Has been shown to decrease the risk of rebleeding without significant side effects

   ii. Used for bleeding related to portal hypertension

  d. Vasopressin, 0.2 units/min

   i. May increase to 0.8 units/min if there are no signs of ischemia

   ii. Do not stop abruptly or use in patients with coronary artery disease (CAD).

   iii. Prolonged use, over 12 h, is not recommended.

  e. Nitroglycerin 2% ointment, 15–30 mg q4h, may be used concomitantly.

8. Balloon tamponade

9. Surgery is indicated

  a. For severe bleeding or rebleeding in which two endoscopic treatments have failed

  b. For massive exsanguinating hemorrhage in which resuscitative efforts have failed

  c. When more than 6–8 units of blood were needed in the first 24-h period

  d. For slow, continuous bleeding lasting more than 48 h

  e. For nonsurgical patients, consult an interventional radiologist for arteriography/embolization.

III. LOWER GASTROINTESTINAL BLEEDING[2, 4, 6–8, 10]

A. Definition

1. Bleeding that originates below the ligament of Treitz, such as in the small intestine or colon

2. Up to 10% of patients presenting with hematochezia have an UGI source of bleeding (e.g., PUD).

B. Etiology

1. Diverticulosis (40% of patients)
2. Vascular ectasias

   a. Painless bleeding ranging from acute hematochezia to chronic occult blood loss
   b. Most common in patients >70 years of age, or in patients with chronic renal failure

3. Neoplasms

   a. Benign or malignant
   b. Usually manifest by chronic, occult blood loss
   c. Sometimes evidenced by periodic hematochezia
   d. Occasionally manifest by massive lower-tract bleeding

4. Inflammatory bowel disease (i.e., ulcerative colitis)

   a. Abdominal pain
   b. Tenesmus
      i. Spasmodic contraction of the anal sphincter
      ii. Pain
      iii. Persistent desire to empty the bowel, with involuntary ineffectual straining efforts
   c. Urgency

5. Anorectal disease

   a. Small amounts of bright red blood on the toilet tissue, streaking in the stool, or dripping into the toilet
   b. Rarely results in significant blood loss
   c. Painless bleeding is indicative of internal hemorrhoids.
   d. Painful bleeding may indicate anal fissure.

6. Ischemic colitis

   a. Seen in the elderly who have a history of atherosclerosis
   b. Results in hematochezia or bloody diarrhea
   c. Usually with associated with pain and cramps

7. Others

   a. Radiation-induced colitis
   b. Infectious colitis
      i. *Shigella* spp.
      ii. *Campylobacter* spp.
      iii. *Escherichia coli*
   c. Other systemic conditions (rare)

C. Clinical manifestations

1. Most patients with lower gastrointestinal (LGI) bleeding present with hematochezia, although occasionally melena will be present in bleeding in the upper small intestine.

2. Chronic blood loss

   a. Pallor
   b. Tachycardia
   c. Postural hypotension

3. Acute blood loss

   a. Altered mental status
   b. Hypotension
   c. Shock
   d. Gross evidence of rectal blood loss

4. Rule out vaginal and urethral bleeding in females.

D. Diagnostics/Laboratory studies

1. Rule out upper GI source by placing a nasogastric tube.
2. CBC

   a. Anemia—When loss has been subacute or chronic
   b. CBC may be normal in acute and massive bleeds related to hemoconcentration.

3. Serum iron, total iron-binding capacity (TIBC), ferritin: Help confirm iron deficiency when patient is anemic and GI blood loss is suspected
4. Fecal occult blood test: In stable patients whose GI blood loss is questionable
5. Anoscopy and sigmoidoscopy
6. Colonoscopy—Should be performed in all patients with significant LGI bleeding within 6–24 h after admission to the hospital after the colon has been cleansed
7. Arteriography or technetium Tc 99m-labeled red blood cell scintigraphy

E. Management

1. Resuscitate hemodynamically compromised patients.

   a. Place two large-bore (16-gauge) IVs and/or pulmonary artery catheter.
   b. Administer lactated Ringer's solution or normal saline and/or blood products.
   c. Monitor heart rate, blood pressure, mean arterial pressure, pulmonary capillary wedge pressure/central venous pressure
   d. Titrate infusion rate to maintain perfusion.

2. Discontinue aspirin and all NSAIDs. Treat the cause of the bleeding.
3. Blood type and crossmatch for four units of packed red blood cells

4. Colonoscopic therapies—Electrocoagulation is useful in treating vascular ectasias of the colon.
5. Angiographic techniques

   a. Intra-arterial vasopressin
   b. Embolization

6. Surgery

   a. Depends on the nature and location of the bleeding
   b. Usually a segmental or subtotal colectomy is indicted.

References

1. Bini, E.J., Rajapaksa, R.C., Valdes, M.T., & Weinshel, E.H. (1999). Is upper gastrointestinal endoscopy indicated in asymptomatic patients with a positive fecal occult blood test and negative colonoscopy? *American Journal of Medicine, 106*, 613–618.
2. Ferri, F.F. (1995). *Practical guide to the care of the medical patient* (3rd ed.). St. Louis: Mosby.
3. Giacchino, S., & Houdek, D. (1998). Ruptured varices! Act fast. *RN, 61*, 33–36.
4. Grendell, J.H., McQuaid, K.R., & Friedman, S.L. (1996). *Current diagnosis and treatment in gastroenterology.* Stamford, CT: Appleton and Lange.
5. Hector Dunphy, L.M. (1999). *Management guidelines for adult nurse practitioners.* Philadelphia: F.A. Davis.
6. Hirsch, C.G., & Caswell, D. (1999). Gastrointestinal disorders. In A. Gawlinski & D. Hamwi (Eds.), *Acute care nurse practitioner: Clinical curriculum and certification review* (pp. 618–722). Philadelphia: W.B. Saunders.
7. Krumberger, J.M., & Hammer, B. (1997). Gastrointestinal alterations. In J.C. Hartshorn, M.L. Sole, & M.L. Lamborn (Eds.), *Introduction to critical care nursing* (pp. 425–472). Philadelphia: W.B. Saunders.
8. Martin, F.L. (1997). Ulcerative colitis: How to manage this chronic inflammatory disease and prevent systemic complications. *American Journal of Nursing, 97*, 38–39.
9. Rakel, R.E. (1996). *Saunders manual of medical practice.* Philadelphia: W.B. Saunders.
10. Tierney, L.M., McPhee, S.J., & Papadakis, M.A. (1999). *Current medical diagnosis & treatment* (38th ed.). Stamford, CT: Appleton & Lange.

Management of Patients with Genitourinary Disorders

URINARY TRACT INFECTIONS

Charlene M. Myers, MSN, RN, CS, ACNP, CCRN

I. URINARY TRACT INFECTIONS

A. Definition[1, 2]

The presence of microorganisms in the urine that have the potential to invade the tissues of the urinary tract and adjacent structures such as the bladder, urethra, prostate, renal parenchyma (kidneys), and collecting system

B. Etiology/Incidence[3, 4, 6, 9, 10]

1. Urinary tract infections (UTIs) account for 7 million office visits annually.
2. UTIs are more common in women than in men.
3. *Escherichia coli* is the most common causative organism (70–80% of all cases), followed by *Staphylococcus saprophyticus* (5–15% of cases).

   a. Nosocomial infections may include *Proteus* spp., *Klebsiella* spp., *Enterobacter* spp., *Pseudomonas*, staphylococci, and *E. faecalis.*
   b. In patients who are critically ill and chronically catheterized, *Candida* spp., have become a common cause.

4. Contributing factors in women

   a. Short urethra
   b. Sexual intercourse
   c. Use of a diaphragm
   d. Diabetes
   e. Permanent indwelling catheter

5. Contributing factors in men

   a. Prostatic enlargement resulting in urine residual
   b. Neuropathic bladder
   c. Calculi
   d. Prostatitis
   e. Permanent indwelling catheter

C. Clinical manifestations[1–6, 9, 10]

1. Lower urinary tract (cystitis/urethritis/prostatitis)

   a. Dysuria
   b. Frequency
   c. Urgency

d. Nocturia
e. Suprapubic pain
f. Hematuria with bacteriuria
g. Malodorous urine
h. Incontinence
i. Fever and chills are uncommon but may be present.
j. No flank or costovertebral pain

2. Upper urinary tract (pyelonephritis, renal abscess)

a. Flank pain
b. Fever
c. Hematuria
d. Nausea and vomiting
e. Mental status changes (in elderly patients)
f. Malaise
g. Shaking chills (rigors)
h. Tachypnea
i. Tachycardia
j. If symptoms last for more than 3 days, abscess formation should be considered.

D. Laboratory findings/Diagnostics[1, 3, 4, 8–10]

1. Clean-catch urinalysis with culture and sensitivity testing
2. Pyuria: Presence of >10 leukocytes/mL
3. Bacteriuria: More than 100,000 bacteria/mL indicates active infection.

a. Bacterial counts of 10,000–100,000/mL can also indicate infection, especially if accompanied by pyuria.
b. In urine specimens obtained by suprapubic aspiration or in-and-out (I & O) catheterization, bacterial colony counts of 100–10,000/mL indicate infection.

4. Leukocyte esterase dipstick test: Positive (purple in 60 s)— May be false-negative in uncomplicated UTI
5. Nitrate dipstick test: Positive for protein, blood, nitrates (pink in 30 s)—May be false-negative in uncomplicated UTI
6. CBC: Leukocytosis with a left shift in acute pyelonephritis
7. Occasional erythrocytes and white cell casts and mild proteinuria may be present in acute pyelonephritis.
8. Elevated erythrocyte sedimentation rate in pyelonephritis
9. Blood culture may be indicated for suspected pyelonephritis or sepsis.
10. To rule out obstruction, calculi, and papillary necrosis in men with UTIs and in women with recurrent UTIs, consider

a. Intravenous pyelogram
b. Cystoscopy
c. Ultrasound

E. Management[1–4, 6, 7, 9, 10]

1. Lower UTI (cystitis/urethritis/prostatitis)

   a. Single-dose regimen: Three-day course is preferred because of high relapse rates related to single-dose regimen.
      i. Trimethoprim-sulfamethoxazole (Bactrim DS), 160/800 mg, two tablets p.o.
   b. Uncomplicated lower UTI
      i. Three-day course: Trimethoprim-sulfamethoxazole (TMP-SMZ) (Bactrim DS), 160 mg/800 mg b.i.d.
      ii. Ciprofloxacin (Cipro), 500 mg p.o. b.i.d. for 3 days, or
      iii. Amoxicillin/clavulanate (Augmentin), 500 mg p.o. t.i.d. for 3 days
   c. Standard oral regimens
      i. Sulfisoxazole (Gantrisin), 2 g p.o., then 1–2 g p.o., q.i.d. for 10 days
      ii. Nitrofurantoin (Macrobid), 50 mg p.o. q.i.d. for 7–10 days
      iii. Cephalexin (Keflex), 500 mg p.o. q.i.d. for 7–10 days
      iv. TMP-SMZ, 160 mg/800 mg p.o. b.i.d. for 7–10 days
      v. Ciprofloxacin, 250 mg p.o. b.i.d. for 7–10 days
      vi. Nitrofurantoin, 100 mg p.o. b.i.d.
      vii. Doxycycline (Doxy), 100 mg p.o. b.i.d. on day one; then 100–200 mg/day
      viii. Ampicillin (Ampicin), 250–500 mg p.o. q.i.d. (30% of infections are resistant, so should not be used as sole therapy.)

2. Uncomplicated upper UTI

   a. TMP-SMZ for 14 days
   b. Ciprofloxin for 14 days
   c. Norfloxin (Noroxin) for 14 days
   d. Intravenous
      i. Ticarcillin-clavulanate (Timentin), 3.1 g q4–6h
      ii. Ampicillin-clavulanate, 1.5– 3 g q6h
      iii. Cefazolin (Ancef, Kefzol), 0.25– 1.5 g q6h
      iv. Cephalothin, 0.5 g q6h, or 2 g q4h
      v. Ceftazidime (Fortaz), 1–2 g q6–12h
      vi. Ceftriaxone (Rocephin), 1–2 g q12h
      vii. Gentamicin (Garamycin), 3–5 mg/kg/day given q8h

3. Patients with toxemia and/or elderly patients with acute bacterial pyelonephritis

   a. Should be hospitalized and aminoglycoside therapy should be initiated.
      i. Gentamicin, 3–5 mg/kg/day q8h
      ii. Adjust dosage according to renal function.

    b. A cephalosporin should be added depending on allergies, such as
       i. Cefazolin, 1 g q8h
       ii. Ceftriaxone, 1 g q24h
       iii. Ciprofloxacin, 400 mg q12h
    c. Ampicillin, 2 g q6h, should be added to cover *Enterococcus* if gram-positive cocci are present on cultures or Gram's stain.
    d. Imipenem/cilastatin
       i. Covers a very broad spectrum of bacteria, including
         (1) Gram-positive
         (2) Gram-negative
         (3) Anaerobic
       ii. Also active against enterococci and *Pseudomonas aeruginosa*
       iii. Has been associated with candidal superinfections
    e. Aztronam is active only against gram-negative bacteria, including *Pseudomonas aeruginosa*. A good agent to use in patients
       i. With nosocomial infections when aminoglycosides are contraindicated
       ii. Who are penicillin-sensitive

4. Quinolones cannot be used during pregnancy nor sulfonamides near time of delivery. Cephalexin is a reasonable choice.
5. Phenazopyridine hydrochloride (Pyridium), 200 mg p.o. t.i.d. for 2 days, may be added for discomfort associated with irritation.
6. Aseptic techniques are essential if indwelling catheters are required.

    a. Modification of the catheter material to confer antimicrobial activity may play an important part in the prevention of catheter-related infections.
    b. The new technology of the Erlanger silver catheter has been shown to effectively reduce the number of catheter-related infections, as silver has antimicrobial activity against both gram-positive and gram-negative bacteria.

7. Increase water intake and decrease carbonated drink intake.
8. Instruct females to void after sexual intercourse.
9. Discuss means of contraception other than the diaphragm.
10. Consider prophylaxis in patients with recurrent lower UTIs.
11. Repeat urinalysis with culture and sensitivity tests after therapy.
12. Emphasize compliance with medication and follow-up.

References

1. Crutchfield, N.S. (1998). Interstitial cystitis: A diagnostic and therapeutic dilemma. *Advance for Nurse Practitioners, 6,* 54–56.

2. DiPiro, J.T. (1998). Infectious diseases. In B.G. Wells, J.T. Dipiro, T.L. Schwinghammer, & C.W. Hamilton (Eds.), *Pharmacotherapy handbook* (pp. 592–606). Stamford, CT: Appleton & Lange.

3. Ferri, F.F. (1995). *Practical guide to the care of the medical patient* (3rd ed.). St. Louis: Mosby.

4. Hector Dunphy, L.M. (1999). *Management guidelines for adult nurse practitioners.* Philadelphia: F.A. Davis.

5. Malterud, K., & Baerheim, A. (1999). Peeing barbed wire: Symptom experiences in women with lower urinary tract infection. *Scandanavian Journal of Primary Health Care, 17,* 49–53.

6. Rakel, R.E. (1996). *Saunders manual of medical practice.* Philadelphia: W.B. Saunders.

7. Rosch, W., & Lugauer, S. (1999). Catheter-associated infections in urology: Possible use of silver-impregnated catheters and the Erlanger silver catheter. *Infection, 27* (Suppl 1), S74–S77.

8. Semeniuk, H., & Church, D. (1999). Evaluation of the leukocyte esterase and nitrate urine dipstick screening tests for detection of bacteriuria in women with suspected uncomplicated urinary tract infections. *Journal of Clinical Microbiology, 37,* 3051–3052.

9. Sherman, M.B. (1999). Renal disorders. In A. Gawlinski & D. Hamwi (Eds.), *Acute care nurse practitioner: Clinical curriculum and certification review.* Philadelphia: W.B. Saunders.

10. Tierney, L.M., McPhee, S.J., & Papadakis, M.A. (1999). *Current medical diagnosis & treatment* (38th ed.). Stamford, CT: Appleton & Lange.

RENAL INSUFFICIENCY/ FAILURE

Charlene M. Myers, MSN, RN, CS, ACNP, CCRN

I. ACUTE RENAL FAILURE

A. Definition[10]

A sudden decrease in renal function resulting in the retention of nitrogen waste products such as urea nitrogen and creatinine

B. Classification/Etiology[1-6, 9-11]

1. Prerenal

   a. Characterized by diminished renal perfusion resulting from a decrease in the blood supplying the kidneys. There is no nephron damage.
   b. Causes
      i. Intravascular volume depletion

         • Hemorrhage
         • Gastrointestinal losses (e.g., diarrhea, vomiting, large amount of nasogastric tube aspirate)
         • Urinary losses (e.g., diabetes insipidus, diuretics)
         • Skin losses (third spacing, large surface area burns, and/or wounds)

      ii. Vasodilatory states
         (1) Sepsis
         (2) Anaphylaxis
         (3) Drugs
            (a) ACE inhibitors, which may inhibit intrinsic renal autoregulation
            (b) NSAIDs, which may decrease renal blood flow
      iii. Decreased cardiac output
         (1) Congestive heart failure
         (2) Myocardial infarction
         (3) Cardiogenic shock
      iv. Vasoconstrictive states (catecholamines)
       v. Uncontrolled hypertension/atherosclerosis
      vi. Liver disease
   c. Results in increased tubular sodium and water reabsorption (in an attempt to re-expand circulating blood volume)
      i. Oliguria
      ii. Decreased urine sodium (<20 mEq/L)
      iii. High urine osmolality (>500 mOsm/L)

iv. Fractional excretion of sodium (FE_{Na^+}) $<1\%$:

$$Fe_{Na^+} = \frac{\text{Urine sodium/Plasma sodium}}{\text{Urine creatinine/Plasma creatinine}}$$

   v. Urine specific gravity: Increased (>1.020)
- d. The BUN:creatinine ratio (BUN/Cr) will exceed $20:1$.
- e. Urinary sediment: Hyaline casts

2. Intrarenal (intrinsic)

- a. Abrupt decrease in glomerular filtration rate (GFR) owing to tubular cell damage as a result of renal ischemia or nephrotoxic injury
- b. Acute tubular necrosis
  - i. Ischemic
    - Decreased cardiac output
    - Prolonged hypotension
    - Volume depletion
    - Catecholemines
    - Volume shift
    - Liver disease ("hepatorenal syndrome")
  - ii. Nephrotoxic
    - Endogenous (e.g., hemoglobin, myoglobin)
    - Exogenous (aminoglycosides, contrast media, ethylene glycol)
- c. Acute tubulointerstitial nephritis: Caused by
  - i. Bacterial pylonephritis
  - ii. Drug-induced hypersensitivity to
    - (1) Penicillins
    - (2) Cephalosporins
    - (3) Diuretics
    - (4) NSAIDs
- d. Urinalysis: Urinary sediment, with
  - i. Renal tubular epithelial cells
  - ii. Cellular debris
  - iii. Pigmented granular casts
  - iv. Renal tubular cell casts
  - v. "Muddy brown" coarse granular casts (See Table 42–1.)
- e. Urine volume
  - i. Anuria: <100 mL/24 h
  - ii. Oliguria: $100–400$ mL/24 h
  - iii. Nonoliguria: >400 mL/24 h
  - iv. Polyuria: >6 L/24 h
- f. Urine osmolality: Isotonic (≤350 mOsm)
- g. Urine specific gravity: Fixed ($1.0008–1.012$)
- h. Urine Na >40 mEq/L

TABLE 42–1. URINARY ABNORMALITIES IN RENAL FAILURE

	PRERENAL	POSTRENAL (ACUTE)	INTRINSIC RENAL (ACUTE)	INTRINSIC RENAL (CHRONIC)
Urinary volume	↓	Absent-to-wide fluctuation	Oliguric or nonoliguric	1000 mL + until end stage
Urinary creatinine	↑ (U/P Cr ± 40)	↓ (U/P Cr ± 20)	↓ (U/P Cr <20)	↓ (U/P Cr <20)
Osmolarity	↑ (±400 mOsm/kg)	(<350 mOsm/kg)	(<350 mOsm/kg)	(<350 mOsm/kg)
Degree of proteinuria	Minimum	Absent	Varies with cause of renal failure: Modest with ATN Nephrotic range common with acute glomerulopathies, usually <2 g/24 h with interstitial disease*	Varies with cause of renal disease (from 1–2 g/day to nephrotic range)

410

| Urinary sediment | Negative, or occasional hyaline cast | Negative or hematuria with stones or papillary necrosis Pyuria with infectious prostatic disease | ATN: Muddy brown Interstitial nephritis: lymphocytes, eosinophils (in stained preparations), and WBC casts RPGN: RBC casts Nephrosis: Oval fat bodies | Broad casts with variable renal "residual" acute findings |

↑, Increased; ↓, decreased; U/P, urine/plasma; clearance $= \dfrac{\text{Urinary concentration} \times \text{Urinary volume}}{\text{Plasma concentration}}$; Cr, creatinine; ATN, acute tubular necrosis; RPGN, rapidly progressing glomerulonephritis.

*Except NSAID-induced allergic interstitial nephritis with concomitant "nil disease."

(From Ferri, F.F. [1998]. *Practical guide to the care of the medical patient* [4th ed.] [p. 656]. St. Louis: Mosby, with permission.)

     i. FE_{Na+} >1%
     j. BUN/Cr: 10–15:1
     k. Low serum Na (<135 mEq)

3. Postrenal

    a. Associated with conditions causing obstruction of urinary flow and, consequently, decrease in GFR
    b. Mechanical
       i. Calculi
       ii. Tumors
       iii. Urethral strictures
       iv. Benign prostatic hyperplasia
       v. Blood clots
       vi. Occluded Foley catheter
    c. Functional
       i. Neurogenic bladder
       ii. Diabetic neuropathy
       iii. Spinal cord disease
    d. Urine volume may fluctuate between anuria and polyuria.
    e. Urine osmolality: Isotonic (<350 mOsm) (initially may be high)
    f. Urine specific gravity: Fixed (1.0008–1.012)
    g. Urine Na: >40 mEq/L (initially may be low)
    h. FE_{Na+}: >1%
    i. Urinary sediment
       i. Normal or red cells
       ii. White cells
       iii. Crystals
    j. BUN/Cr: 10–15:1
    k. In-and-out catheter may reveal an increased postvoid residual volume, and renal ultrasound may demonstrate hydronephrosis.
    l. A plain film x-ray (kidney, ureter, and bladder) of the abdomen will document the presence of two kidneys and also provide a check for kidney stones. See Table 42–2.
    m. CT scan or MRI may also identify obstruction.
    n. Retrograde urography may be utilized to provide information on the ureters and lower urinary tract.
    o. Renal biopsy with special immune stains and electron microscopy may assist in determining the cause of renal failure.

C. Management[1, 3, 5, 6, 8–10]

1. Adjust intake to output based on fluid status. Take the use of diuretics into consideration.
2. Appropriate fluid challenges in contracted patients

TABLE 42–2. SERUM AND RADIOGRAPHIC ABNORMALITIES IN RENAL FAILURE

	PRERENAL	POSTRENAL (ACUTE)	INTRINSIC RENAL (ACUTE)	INTRINSIC RENAL (CHRONIC)
BUN	↑ 10:1 > Cr	↑ 20–40/day	↑ 20–40/day	Stable, ↑ varies with protein intake
Serum creatinine	N/Moderate ↑	↑ 2–4/day	↑ 2–4 day	Stable ↑ (production equals excretion)
Serum potassium	N/Moderate ↑	↑ varies with urinary volume	↑ ↑ (particularly when patient is oliguric)	Normal until end stage, unless tubular dysfunction (type 4 RTA)
			↑ ↑ ↑ with rhabdomyolysis	
Serum phosphorus	N/Moderate ↑	Moderate ↑	↑	Becomes significantly elevated when serum creatinine surpasses 3 mg/dL
		↑ ↑ with rhabdomyolysis		
		N/ ↓ with PO$_4^{-3}$		
Serum calcium	N		Poor correlation with duration of renal disease ↓ (poor correlation with duration of renal failure)	Usually ↓
Renal size by ultrasound	N/ ↑	↑ and dilated calices	N/ ↑	↓ and with ↑ echogenicity
Fe$_{Na}$*	<1	<1 → >1	>1	>1

↑, Increase; ↓ decrease; N, normal; ↑ ↑, large increase; U, urine; P, plasma; Na, sodium; Cr, creatinine; RTA, renal tubular acidosis.
*FE$_{Na}$ = U$_{Na}$/P$_{Na}$ U$_{Cr}$/P$_{cr}$ × 100.
(From Ferri, F.F. [1998]. *Practical guide to the care of the medical patient* [4th ed.] [p. 653] St. Louis, Mosby, with permission.)

413

3. Maximize cardiac function and maintain optimal blood pressure for renal perfusion.
4. Discontinue offending drugs.
5. Monitor for complications.

    a. Electrolyte imbalances
        i. Hyperkalemia
        ii. Hypernatremia
        iii. Hyponatremia
        iv. Hypocalcemia
        v. Metabolic acidosis
        vi. Hypermagnesemia
        vii. Hyperphosphatemia
    b. Volume overload: Pulmonary edema
    c. Uremia: Pericarditis
    d. Infection
    e. Gastrointestinal bleeding

6. Anticipate the need for dialysis.

    a. Intravascular volume overload: Pulmonary edema
    b. Hyperkalemia (Sodium polystyrene sulfonate [Kayexalate] adds 1 mEq Na^+ for each 1 mEq K^+ removed via the gastrointestinal tract.)
    c. Acidosis/alkalosis
    d. Uremia (symptomatic syndrome resulting from increase in nitrogenous wastes [azotemia])
        i. Central nervous system disturbances
        ii. Gastrointestinal indications (nausea/vomiting/anorexia)
        iii. Level of azotemia (elevation of waste products): BUN 100–200 mg/dL
    e. Specific drug/Toxin

7. Adjust all medications: Assume GFR is <10 mL/min (normal: 80–120 mL/min).
8. Adjust diet: Low protein/Na/K.

II. CHRONIC RENAL FAILURE

A. Definition[10]

1. Progressive azotemia over weeks, months, or years
2. Isosthenuria is common.
3. Hypertension is common in the majority.
4. Ultrasound studies show evidence of bilateral small kidneys.
5. X-rays show evidence of renal osteodystrophy.

B. Etiology[1–4, 6, 9–11]

1. Glomerular disease
2. Polycystic kidney disease

3. Hypertensive nephropathy
4. Diabetic nephropathy
5. Tubulointerstitial nephritis
6. Obstructive nephropathies
7. Renal artery stenosis

C. Stages

1. The progression of chronic renal failure occurs in three stages.
2. Each stage reflects an increasing loss of nephrons.
3. Stage I—Diminished renal reserve

   a. Fifty percent functional nephron loss
   b. Patient is asymptomatic.
   c. Serum creatinine is within the high normal range (2 mg/dL).

4. Stage II—Renal insufficiency

   a. Nephron loss of 75–80%
   b. Patient exhibits mild azotemia (elevated BUN/Cr) and impaired ability to concentrate urine.
   c. Anemia
   d. Creatinine level around 4 mg/dL

5. Stage III—End-stage renal disease (ESRD)

   a. Ninety percent nephron loss
   b. Homeostasis can no longer be maintained, and all body systems are affected.
   c. Requires renal replacement therapy for the patient to survive
   d. Creatinine around 8 mg/dL
   e. Monitor GFR. The normal is 80–120 mL/min.
      i. Formula for calculation:

$$\text{GFR} = \frac{(140 - \text{age}) \times \text{wt (kg)}}{S_{Cr} \times 72}$$

      ii. Renal replacement is instituted when GFR falls to between 5 and 10 mL/min.
   f. Creatinine clearance is used by many practitioners as a more accurate method of estimating GFR.

$$\text{i. } C_{cr} = \frac{[\text{Urine}_{Cr}] \times (\text{volume of urine per 24 h})}{[\text{Serum}_{Cr}] \times 1440}$$

      ii. Normal

         • *Males:* 97–137 mL/min/1.73m^2
         • *Females:* 88–128 mL/min/1.73m^2

D. Clinical manifestations[1, 5–9, 11]

1. General

   a. Fatigue
   b. Weakness

2. Skin

   a. Pruritus
   b. Easy bruising
   c. Pallor, ecchymosis
   d. Excoriations
   e. Edema
   f. Xerosis
   g. Sallow complexion (ill, yellow appearing)

3. Ear, nose, and throat

   a. Metallic taste in the mouth
   b. Epistaxis
   c. Urinous breath

4. Pulmonary

   a. Shortness of breath
   b. Rales
   c. Pleural effusion

5. Cardiovascular

   a. Dyspnea on exertion
   b. Retrosternal pain on inspiration and pericardial friction rub caused by pericarditis related to uremia
   c. Hypertension caused by volume overload
   d. Cardiomegaly

6. Gastrointestinal

   a. Anorexia
   b. Nausea and vomiting

7. Genitourinary

   a. Impotence
   b. Iso-osmolar urine: The urine has an osmolarity similar to plasma osmolality despite variations in fluid intake, which indicates a marked impairment in renal concentrating ability.

8. Neurologic

   a. Irritability
   b. Inability to concentrate
   c. Decreased libido
   d. Stupor

e. Asterixis
f. Myoclonus
g. Peripheral neuropathy associated with diabetes if present

E. Management of common problems in chronic renal failure[1, 3, 5, 6, 8–10]

1. Fluid overload

   a. Monitor weight, standing blood pressure, urine Na^+ excretion, creatinine clearance (CrCl), and serum creatinine.
   b. Decrease Na^+ and fluid intake.
   c. Diuretics
      i. Hydrochlorothiazide (HydroDIURIL), 25–100 mg/day in 1–2 doses
         (1) As a diuretic, may be given q.o.d. or 3–5 days a week
         (2) Found to be ineffective in moderate to severe cases
      ii. Furosemide (Lasix), 20–80 mg/day initially
         (1) Up to 600 mg may be necessary.
         (2) Doses up to 1 g/day have been used in congestive heart failure and renal failure.
         (3) Remains effective when the GFR is less than 25 mL/min
      iii. Other agents that may be used
         (1) Metolazone (Zaroxolyn), 0.5–10 mg p.o. daily
         (2) Bumetanide (Bumex), 0.5–2 mg once/day (may repeat at 4–5 h intervals, if needed, to a maximum of 10 mg/day)
         (3) Torsemide (Demadex), 10–20 mg once a day, p.o./IV (may increase up to 200 mg/day as needed)

2. Hypertension

   a. Determine the patient's optimal Na^+ and H_2O intact. Excess Na^+/H_2O increases the level of hypertension.
   b. Antihypertensive agents that maintain renal blood flow and reduce glomerular pressure and proteinuria are preferred.
   c. If proteinuria is present, ACE inhibitors and calcium channel blockers may be superior to conventional treatment in decreasing proteinuria and glomerular hypertension.
   d. Antihypertensives
      i. ACE inhibitors
      ii. Calcium channel blockers
      iii. Direct vasodilators (hydralazine [Apresoline], minoxidil [Loniten])

      iv. Peripheral alpha blockers (doxazosin mesylate [Cardura], prazosin [Minipress])

      v. Beta blockers (propranolol [Inderal])

      vi. Central alpha blockers (clonidine hydrochloride [Catapres])

3. Protein catabolism

   a. Limit protein intake (1 g/kg/day).

   b. Provide adequate calories.

   c. Avoid stresses of trauma, infection, and immobilization if possible.

   d. Physical activity should be moderate.

   e. Thyroid hormone, steroids, and tetracycline increase catabolism and must be avoided.

   f. Anabolic agents may help some patients avoid a negative nitrogen balance (help stimulate erythropoiesis):

      i. Fluoxymesterone (Halotestin)

      ii. Nandrolone decanoate (Deca-Durabolin)

4. Acidosis: Alkalinizing agents are indicated when plasma HCO_3 is <20 mEq/L.

   a. $NaHCO_3$: 1 g = 13 mEq Na; generally used in emergencies because it may cause volume overload secondary to Na^+

   b. Sodium citrate (Shohl's solution, Bicitra): 1 mEq/mL of Na^+

   c. Sodium and potassium citrate and citric acid (Polycitra): Monitor K^+ levels, and avoid in patients with hyperkalemia.

5. Hyperkalemia

   a. Avoid foods and medications high in K^+.

   b. Avoid hypercatabolic states.

   c. Medical emergency if K^+ >7.0 mEq/L

      i. Administer hypertonic glucose, insulin, and HCO_3.

      ii. Calcium gluconate IV to modify myocardial irritability

      iii. Correct acidosis.

      iv. Administer K^+ ion exchange resins to remove excess potassium ions.

        • Kayexalate, 30–60 g/day (1 g resin = 1 mEq K^+ out = 1 mEq Na^+ in)

      v. Hemodialysis

      vi. Monitor ECG for flat P waves, peaked T waves, PR interval >.20 s, QRS complex >.10 s, and bradycardia.

6. Hyperphosphatemia (choose one or more from the following)

   a. Phosphate-binding agents (i.e., aluminum compounds such as Amphojel, given with meals)
   b. Calcium carbonate, 650 mg t.i.d.
      i. Phosphate binding agent
      ii. Prevents aluminum toxicity
   c. Calcium acetate, 667 mg (2–6 tabs) t.i.d., with meals
   d. Hemodialysis

7. Hypocalcemia

   a. Maintain phosphorus level <6 mg/dL.
   b. Calcium carbonate supplements
   c. 1,25-OH$_2$ vitamin D in extreme cases

8. Hypermagnesemia: Avoid Mg^{++}-containing laxatives/antacids.

9. Anemia

   a. Iron
   b. Vitamin supplements as needed
   c. Erythropoietin, 2–3 injections/week (30–150 units), SC/IV

10. Neurologic problems

    a. Anticonvulsants
       i. Dilantin
       ii. Phenobarbital
    b. Sedatives
       i. Chloral hydrate
       ii. Benadryl

11. Renal osteodystrophy

    a. Prevent acidosis, hypocalcemia, hyperphosphatemia; control hyperparathyroidism
    b. Correct low Ca (<6.5 mg/dL).
       i. Administer calcium supplement such as calcium carbonate and calcium gluconate, 1–2 g/day.
       ii. Titrate as necessary to control serum phosphate and calcium levels.
    c. Correct high phosphorus levels (>5mg/dL). Administer phosphate-binders (i.e., aluminum hydroxide gel), 2–4.8 g t.i.d. or q.i.d. with meals.
    d. Correct acidosis (HCO_3 < 15 mEq/dL). Administer $NaHCO_3$, 2–5 mEq/kg, as a 4–8 h infusion (for emergency situations), or 650 mg p.o. t.i.d., and titrate as needed.

  e. Administer vitamin D if Ca stays <6 mg/dL, bone pain
     is a problem, alkaline phosphatase levels increase, and
     x-rays reveal evidence of osteomalacia.

F. Management options

1. Hemodialysis
2. Peritoneal dialysis
3. Renal transplantation

III. MODIFICATION OF DRUG DOSAGES

A. Types of drugs

1. Type A: Eliminated entirely by the kidney
2. Type B: Eliminated entirely by extrarenal mechanism
3. Type C: Eliminated both by renal and extrarenal mechanisms

B. Decreased renal function results in

1. Abnormal excretion rates
2. Abnormal metabolism rates of certain drugs
3. Abnormal sensitivity to certain drugs

C. Before administration of any drug to a patient in renal failure, consider:

1. Does this drug depend on the kidney for excretion?
2. Does an excess blood level affect the kidney or cause nephrotoxicity?
3. Does the effect of the drug alter electrolyte imbalance?
4. Is the patient susceptible to the drug because of kidney
   disease?

D. Modification of drug doses:

1. Serum Cr is >10 mg/mL; renal function is 15% of normal:
   Major modification is needed.
2. Serum Cr is 3–10 mg/mL; renal function is 15–20% of normal: Modest changes are needed.

References

1. Hamilton, C.W. (1998). Renal disorders. In B.G. Wells, J.T. Dipiro, T.L.
   Schwinghammer, & C.W. Hamilton (Eds.), *Pharmacotherapy handbook*
   (pp. 908–918). Stamford, CT: Appleton & Lange.
2. Bracco, A., Garrido, S., & Valdecantos, J. (1999). Kidney revascularization and function recovery in patients in dialysis. *Medicina, 58,* 747–754.
3. Couchoud, C., Pozet, N., Labeeuw, M., & Pouteil, C. (1999). Screening
   early renal failure: Cut-off values for serum creatinine as an indicator
   of renal impairment. *Kidney International, 55,* 1878–1884.
4. Eckardt, K.U. (1999). Renal failure in liver disease. *Intensive Care Medicine, 25,* 5–14.
5. Ferri, F.F. (1995). *Practical guide to the care of the medical patient* (3rd ed.).
   St. Louis: Mosby.

6. Hektor Dunphy, L.M. (1999). *Management guidelines for adult nurse practitioners*. Philadelphia: F.A. Davis.
7. Rakel, R.E. (1996). *Saunders manual of medical practice*. Philadelphia: W.B. Saunders.
8. Sherman, M.B. (1999). Renal disorders. In A. Gawlinski & D. Hamwi (Eds.), *Acute care nurse practitioner: Clinical curriculum and certification review*. Philadelphia: W.B. Saunders.
9. Sosa-Guerrero, S., & Gomez, N.J. (1997). Dealing with end stage renal disease. *American Journal of Nursing, 97*, 44–50.
10. Tierney, L.M., McPhee, S.J., & Papadakis, M.A. (1999). *Current medical diagnosis & treatment* (38th ed.). Stamford, CT: Appleton & Lange.
11. Zanchetti, A., & Stella, A. (1999). Cardiovascular disease and the kidney: An epidemiologic overview. *Journal of Cardiovascular Pharmacology, 33* (Suppl 1), S1–S6.

BENIGN PROSTATIC HYPERTROPHY

Charlene M. Myers, MSN, RN, CS, ACNP, CCRN

I. BENIGN PROSTATIC HYPERTROPHY (BPH)

A. Definition[2, 4, 7]

1. Enlargement of the prostate gland, a condition commonly seen in men over age 50
2. A progressive condition that can cause obstruction of the urethra with interference in urine flow

B. Etiology/Incidence[2, 5, 7]

1. Incidence is age-related

   a. Twenty percent in men aged 41–50 years
   b. More than 80% in men older than 80 years

2. Exact cause is unknown.
3. The condition may be a response of the prostate gland to androgen hormones over time.
4. Dietary fat may play a role.

C. Clinical manifestations[2, 4, 5, 7–9]

1. Irritative symptoms—Consequence of bladder dysfunction

   a. Frequency
   b. Dysuria
   c. Urgency
   d. Nocturia
   e. Incontinence

2. Obstructive symptoms

   a. Hesitancy
   b. Straining
   c. Starting and stopping
   d. Dribbling
   e. Retention

3. Focal or uniform enlargement

   a. On digital rectal examination (DRE), the prostate may be enlarged.
   b. It should feel smooth and rubbery.
   c. Focal enlargement, nodularity, or extreme hardness may represent malignancy, and further investigation is indicated.

422

    i. Transrectal ultrasound
    ii. Biopsy

4. Palpable bladder consistent with urinary retention

D. Laboratory findings[2, 3, 6, 9]

1. Urinalysis

    a. Pyuria suggests infection.
    b. Hematuria may be a sign of malignancy.

2. Urine culture to rule out urinary tract infection if there are irritative symptoms
3. BUN/CR to assess for renal insufficiency
4. Prostate-specific antigen (PSA)—Values >10 ng/mL suggest prostate cancer.
5. Transrectal ultrasound if there is a palpable nodule or elevated PSA

E. Management[1, 2, 4, 5, 7–9]

1. Mild symptoms

    a. Patient may recover spontaneously over time.
    b. Avoid medication that can worsen symptoms.
        i. Decongestants and other sympathomimetics (These act on alpha receptors to increase prostate muscle tone, which increases dynamic obstruction.)
        ii. Anticholinergics (antihistamines), bowel antispasmodics, tricyclic antidepressants, and antipsychotics, which decrease bladder muscle contraction, increasing urine retention

2. Mild to moderate symptoms

    a. Alpha blockers will relax muscle fibers in the prostate gland and capsule and in the internal urethral sphincter, thereby facilitating emptying of the bladder.
        i. Terazosin (Hytrin), 1 mg at bedtime, increasing up to 10 mg at bedtime as necessary or tolerated
        ii. Prazosin (Minipress), 1–5 mg p.o. b.i.d., may also be used.
        iii. Hypotension and dizziness are the main side effects.
    b. Hormonal manipulation
        i. Finasteride (Proscar), 5 mg/day
        ii. Estrogens, antiandrogens, or gonadotropin-releasing hormone (GnRH) can be used, but only if Finasteride is not tolerated because of adverse effects.
    c. Combination of alpha blockers and hormonal manipulation
    d. Avoid medications that increase obstructive symptoms (as noted previously).

3. Severe symptoms

   a. Surgery may be necessary if significant urinary symptoms exist.

   b. Types of surgeries

     i. Transurethral resection of the prostate (TURP)

       (1) Low mortality (1%), but moderate morbidity (18%)

       (2) Should bring about improvement in the signs and symptoms of BPH

       (3) Repeat resection is needed in <10% of cases.

       (4) Retrograde ejaculation may occur following procedure.

       (5) Uncommon complications

         (a) Bladder neck contracture

         (b) Urethral stricture disease

         (c) Incontinence

     ii. Open prostatectomy

     iii. Transurethral incision of the prostate

       (1) No tissue is resected.

       (2) Antegrade ejaculation is usually maintained.

       (3) Can usually be performed as an outpatient procedure

       (4) May benefit BPH associated with smaller glands, especially in younger men

   c. Balloon dilation is being evaluated. There appears to be a high recurrence of symptoms with this procedure.

   d. Transurethral laser resection and thermotherapy are being evaluated for efficacy.

   e. Ethanol injection therapy of the prostate (ETP)

     i. A new technique that can be performed as an outpatient procedure

     ii. Appears to be safe and cost-effective

     iii. Dehydrated ethanol is injected transurethrally with lumbar or sacral and urethral anesthesia.

     iv. There is evidence of improvement of symptoms, peak urinary flow rate, residual volume, and quality of life scores 3 months after therapy.

   f. Urethral stents may be used for patients who are not candidates for standard surgery.

     i. Can be performed under local anesthesia

     ii. Preferred to chronic catheterization or suprapubic cystostomy

References

1. Goya, N., Ishikawa, N., Ito, F., Ryoji, O., Tokumoto, T., Toma, H., & Yamaguchi, Y. (1999). Ethanol injection therapy of the prostate for benign prostatic hyperplasia: Preliminary report on application of a new technique. *Journal of Urology, 162,* 383–386.

2. Hektor Dunphy, L.M. (1999). *Management guidelines for adult nurse practitioners*. Philadelphia: F.A. Davis.

3. Karakiewicz, P.I., & Aprikian, A.G. (1998). Clinical basics: Prostate cancer: 5. Diagnostic tools for early detection. *CMAJ-JAMC, 159*, 1139–1146.

4. Kennedy-Malone, L., Fletcher, K.R., & Plank, L.P. (2000). *Management guidelines for gerontological nurse practitioners*. Philadelphia: F.A. Davis.

5. Rakel, R.E. (1996). *Saunders manual of medical practice*. Philadelphia: W.B. Saunders.

6. Ropiquet, F., Giri, D., Lamb, D., & Ittmann, M. (1999). FGF7 and FGF2 are increased in benign prostatic hyperplasia and are associated with increased proliferation. *Journal of Urology, 162*, 595–599.

7. Sherman, M.B. (1999). Renal disorders. In A. Gawlinski & D. Hamwi (Eds.), *Acute care nurse practitioner: Clinical curriculum and certification review*. Philadelphia: W.B. Saunders.

8. Stoevelaar, H.J., Van De Beek, C., Casparie, A.F., McDonnell, J., & Nijs, H.G.T. (1999). Treatment choice for benign prostatic hyperplasia: A matter of urologist preference? *Journal of Urology, 161*, 133–138.

9. Tierney, L.M., McPhee, S.J., & Papadakis, M.A. (1999). *Current medical diagnosis & treatment* (38th ed.). Stamford, CT: Appleton & Lange.

RENAL ARTERY STENOSIS

Charlene M. Myers, MSN, RN, CS, ACNP, CCRN

I. RENAL ARTERY STENOSIS

A. Definition[3]

1. A progressive disease in which there is interruption of vascular supply to the kidney that may lead to gradual loss of renal function
2. Compensatory contralateral hypertrophy may temporarily maintain renal function.

B. Etiology[3, 5]

1. Occurs in about 5% of patients with hypertension and is one form of hypertension that can be corrected surgically
2. Atherosclerosis
3. Fibromuscular dysplasia

C. Clinical manifestations[3, 5]

1. Renal artery stenosis should be considered in the following circumstances:

   a. If the onset of hypertension (usually sudden) is below age 20 or after the age of 50
   b. Epigastric or renal artery bruits
   c. Atherosclerotic disease of the aorta or peripheral arteries
   d. Abrupt deterioration in renal function after administration of ACE inhibitors
   e. Metabolic acidosis

D. Diagnostics[1, 2, 3, 5]

1. Renal arteriography is the definitive diagnostic test.
2. ACE inhibitor test is probably the best noninvasive test.

   a. Radioisotope renography is performed before and after the administration of either captopril, 50 mg p.o., or enalaprilat, 2.5 mg IV.
   b. Study may show a smaller kidney with decreased function on the stenotic side.
   c. Uptake and clearance of the radiotracer are delayed.
   d. Exaggerated increase in plasma renin activity is present.
   e. Sensitivity and specificity is >95% in identifying hypertension related to renal stenosis compared with essential hypertension.

3. Doppler ultrasound, MRI, and intravenous pyelogram are preferred by some, except when stenosis is critical (>80–90%).
4. In the late 1990s, developments in renal magnetic resonance angiography (MRA) led to significant improvement in the technical success rate and diagnostic accuracy of cases of renal artery stenosis. Therefore, MRA will likely play an important role in the evaluation of patients with renovascular disease.

E. Management[3-5]

1. Treatment and control of blood pressure and renal perfusion
2. Percutaneous angioplasty for fibromuscular disease, followed by surgery if unsuccessful
3. Angioplasty or surgery for atherosclerotic disease, depending on the patient
4. ACE inhibitors have been successful in controlling hypertension related to renal artery stenosis.

   a. However, they have been associated with marked hypotension and deterioration of renal function in patients with bilateral renal artery stenosis.
   b. Monitor blood pressure and renal function closely during first few weeks of therapy.

References

1. Grist, T.M. (1999). Magnetic resonance angiography of renal arterial stenosis. *Coronary Artery Disease, 10,* 151–156.
2. Postma, C.T., Joosten, F.B., Rosenbusch, G., & Thien, T. (1997). Magnetic resonance angiography has a high reliability in the detection of renal artery stenosis. *American Journal of Hypertension, 10,* 957–963.
3. Sherman, M.B. (1999). Renal disorders. In A. Gawlinski & D. Hamwi (Eds.), *Acute care nurse practitioner: Clinical curriculum and certification review* (pp. 438–475). Philadelphia: W.B. Saunders.
4. Textor, S.C. (1997). Renal failure related to angiotensin-converting enzyme inhibitors. *Seminars in Nephrology, 17,* 67–76.
5. Tierney, L.M., McPhee, S.J., & Papadakis, M.A. (1999). *Current medical diagnosis & treatment* (38th ed.). Stamford, CT: Appleton & Lange.

NEPHROLITHIASIS

*Charlene M. Myers, MSN, RN, CS,
ACNP, CCRN*

I. RENAL CALCULI—NEPHROLITHIASIS

A. Definition[10]

1. Concretions of crystals in the urinary tract
2. Calculi may be composed of calcium oxalate, calcium phosphate, uric acid, struvite, or cystine.

B. Etiology[10]

1. Approximately 10% of the population will develop urinary calculi during their lifetime.

   a. More common in men
   b. Age of onset is usually the 30s.

2. Dehydration
3. Life stress
4. Supersaturation of urine with stone-forming salts

   a. Overexcretion of salt or reduced urine excretion
   b. May occur as a result of dietary overindulgence

5. Decreased stone inhibitors in urine

C. Types[1, 2, 6, 9]

1. Calcium stones constitute 80% of renal calculi; they can be caused by absorptive, reabsorptive, and renal disorders.

   a. Absorptive (Types I, II, and III)
      i. Secondary to inabsorption of calcium at the level of the small bowel (i.e., jejunum)
      ii. Treatment is focused on decreasing bowel absorption of calcium.
      iii. Type I: Cellulose phosphate, 10–15 g t.i.d. with meals, binds to calcium and impedes bowel absorption.
         (1) Use cautiously in postmenopausal women, as it can cause negative calcium balance and osteoporosis.
         (2) May also result in hypomagnesemia
         (3) Follow-up every 6–8 months
      iv. Thiazide therapy is an alternative to the preceding in treatment of type I absorptive hypercalciuria.
         (1) Decreases renal excretion of calcium
         (2) Increases bone density by 1%/year
         (3) Has limited long-term (<5 years) use

    v. Type II is diet-dependent. Decreasing dietary calcium by 50% (i.e., by 400 mg/day) decreases the hypercalciuria.

    vi. Type III is secondary to a renal phosphate leak that results in increased vitamin D synthesis and secondarily in increased small-bowel absorption of calcium.

       (1) Can be reversed by orthophosphates, 0.5 g t.i.d.

       (2) Inhibits vitamin D synthesis but not intestinal absorption

  b. Resorptive

    i. Secondary to hyperparathyroidism

    ii. Hypercalcemia, hypophosphatemia, and elevated levels of parathyroid hormones are present.

    iii. Surgical resection of the adenoma, which leads to hyperparathyroidism, cures the disease and stones.

  c. Renal hypercalciuria

    i. The renal tubules are unable to reabsorb filtered calcium efficiently, and hypercalciuria occurs.

    ii. Hydrochlorothiazides are effective as long-term therapy.

2. Uric acid calculi

  a. Frequently have urinary pH values <5.5 (average urinary pH is 5.85)

  b. Increasing the pH to >6.5 can dramatically increase solubility and dissolve large stones.

  c. Potassium citrate (liquid, crystals, or tablets—10 mEq), two tablets p.o. t.i.d. or q.i.d.

  d. Many patients have gout.

    i. If hyperuricemia is present, allopurinol (Zyloprim) should be initiated at 200–800 mg/day.

    ii. Doses >300 mg should be divided and given b.i.d.

3. Struvite calculi

  a. Magnesium-ammonium-phosphate stones

  b. Commonly seen in women with recurrent urinary tract infections

  c. Radiodense

  d. Urinary pH is high (>7.0–7.5) = alkalotic.

  e. Secondary to urease-producing organisms (e.g., *Proteus, Pseudomonas, Providencia, Klebsiella*, staphylococci, *Mycoplasma*)

  f. Stones are soft and amenable to percutaneous nephrolithotomy.

  g. They can recur rapidly.

  h. Acetohydroxamic acid is an effective urease inhibitor; however, it is poorly tolerated because of gastrointestinal side effects.

4. Cystine calculi

    a. Result of abnormal excretion of cystine, ornithine, lysine, and arginine

    b. Cystine is the only amino acid that becomes insoluble in urine.

    c. Difficult to manage

    d. Increase fluid intake.

    e. Alkalinize the urine to pH >7.5.

    f. Administer penicillamine and tiopronin.

D. Clinical manifestations[3, 7, 8, 10]

1. Acute flank pain (i.e., colic-like)
2. Nausea and vomiting
3. Pain not relieved by position
4. Costovertebral angle (CVA) tenderness
5. If the flank pain increases in intensity and radiates downward to the groin, this indicates that the stone has passed to the lower third of the ureter.
6. Frequency, urgency, and dysuria suggest that the stone is in the portion of the ureter within the bladder wall.
7. Oliguria and acute renal failure (ARF) may occur when both collecting systems are obstructed by stones.
8. Hematuria

E. Diagnostics/Laboratory findings[1, 5, 10]

1. X-ray studies

    a. Plain films of the abdomen will reveal opaque calculi.

    b. Nonopaque stones, such as a uric acid stone, can be visualized on ultrasound and/or intravenous pyelogram (IVP).

2. An excretory or retrograde pyelogram permits exact definition of stones and reveals the presence or absence of obstruction.
3. Noncontrast CT has proved to be an accurate, safe, rapid technique to assess acute flank pain and the evaluation of choice for patients who would otherwise require IVP for diagnosis.
4. Urinalysis reveals blood.
5. Increased WBC count
6. Hypercalcemia, hypercalciuria (24-h urine sample)
7. Urine culture: Positive for urease-producing organisms

F. Management[1, 4, 10]

1. Relieve pain, nausea, and vomiting.
2. Restore fluid if necessary.
3. Remove stone or allow for spontaneous passage (small stones <5–6 mm in size).
4. Larger stones require removal.

5. Extracorporeal, percutaneous ultrasonic, or endoscopic lithotripsy can be used to cause fragmentation of stone in the kidney by using high-intensity shock waves.
6. Larger fragments are removed by cystoscopy or open surgery.
7. After removal, the goal is stone prevention:

   a. Adequate fluid intake (Assure patient has >2 L fluids/24 h)
   b. Dietary adjustments
      i. Reduce animal protein (red meat).
      ii. Increase vegetable fiber.
      iii. Prohibit dairy products.
      iv. Limit intake of table salt.
   c. Adjust the pH to >7. A pH >8 will dissolve cystine crystals.
   d. Recurrence rate is approximately 20–50%.
   e. Regular medical prophylaxis may effectively prevent stone recurrence in patients with a history of recurrence, calcium oxalate dihydrate stones, hypercalciuria, and hyperuricuria.
      i. Dietary advice for all patients
      ii. Renal leak hypercalciuria: 50 mg hydrochlorothiazide (HCTZ), p.o. daily, and 5 g potassium citrate powder p.o. three times daily after meals
      iii. Absorptive stones
         (1) Calcium-restricted diet and potassium citrate
         (2) Patients with hypocitraturic calcium oxalate nephrolithiasis receive potassium citrate.
      iv. Uric acid and calcium oxalate calculi with hyperuricuria or gouty diathesis: 100 mg allopurinol, p.o. b.i.d., as well as potassium citrate
      v. Infected stones: Potassium citrate and appropriate antibiotics
      vi. Cost effectiveness, patient compliance, and gastrointestinal upset may limit patient acceptability and clinical use of medical prophylaxis.

References

1. Curhan, G.C., Willett, W.C., Speizer, F.E., & Stampfer, M.J. (1998). Beverage use and risk for kidney stones in women. *Annals of Internal Medicine, 128,* 534–540.
2. Ferri, F.F. (1995). *Practical guide to the care of the medical patient* (3rd ed.). St. Louis: Mosby.
3. Hektor Dunphy, L.M. (1999). *Management guidelines for adult nurse practitioners.* Philadelphia: F.A. Davis.
4. Lee, Y.H., Huang, W.C., Tsai, J.Y., & Huang, J.K. (1999). Prophylaxis for preventing upper urinary tract calculi: A midterm followup study. *Journal of Urology, 161,* 1453–1457.

5. Niall, O., Russell, J., MacGregor, R., Duncan, H., & Mullins, J. (1999). A comparison of noncontrast computerized tomography with excretory urography in the assessment of acute flank pain. *Journal of Urology, 161,* 534–537.

6. Pak, C. (1998). Kidney stones. *Lancet, 351,* 1797–1801.

7. Rakel, R.E. (1996). *Saunders manual of medical practice.* Philadelphia: W.B. Saunders.

8. Sherman, M.B. (1999). Renal disorders. In A. Gawlinski & D. Hamwi (Eds.), *Acute care nurse practitioner: Clinical curriculum and certification review* (pp. 44–50). Philadelphia: W.B. Saunders.

9. Tierney, L.M., McPhee, S.J., & Papadakis, M.A. (1999). *Current medical diagnosis & treatment* (38th ed.). Stamford, CT: Appleton & Lange.

10. Tiselius, H. (1999). Crystalluria in patients with calcium stone disease. *Journal of Urology, 161,* 1432.

Management of Patients with Endocrine Disorders

DIABETES MELLITUS
Thomas W. Barkley, Jr., DSN, RN, CS, ACNP

I. DIABETES MELLITUS: OVERVIEW OF PRINCIPLES[4, 9]

A. Definition[4, 10, 20]

1. A group of metabolic diseases resulting from a breakdown in the body's ability either to produce and/or to utilize insulin
2. Characterized by hyperglycemia and associated with numerous acute and chronic complications

   a. Acute complications
      i. Diabetic ketoacidosis
      ii. Hyperglycemic hyperosmolar nonketotic coma
   b. Chronic complications
      i. Neuropathy
      ii. Nephropathy
      iii. Retinopathy
      iv. Cardiovascular disease
      v. Peripheral vascular disease

B. Incidence/Predisposing factors[10, 17]

1. Approximately 14 million Americans have diabetes.
2. Affects approximately 5% of the United States population
3. Affects approximately one fifth (18%) of individuals aged 65–74
4. Approximately 50% of all individuals with diabetes mellitus are undiagnosed.
5. Ethnic minorities, with native Americans at highest risk
6. Others with a family history of diabetes mellitus

C. Classifications of diabetes mellitus and other forms of glucose intolerance[4, 5, 14, 20]

1. Type 1 (previously, insulin-dependent or juvenile-onset diabetes)—See section II.
2. Type 2 (previously, non–insulin-dependent or adult-onset diabetes mellitus)—See section III.
3. Secondary diabetes related to:

   a. Hormonal excess
      i. Cushing's syndrome
      ii. Acromegaly
      iii. Hyperthyroidism
      iv. Pheochromocytoma

    b. Medications
        i. Glucocorticoids
        ii. Diuretics
        iii. Phenytoin (Dilantin)
        iv. Oral contraceptives
    c. Pancreatic disease
        i. Pancreatitis
        ii. Pancreatectomy
    d. Other genetic factors
        i. Beta cell defects
        ii. Neoplasia
        iii. Other genetic syndromes
            (1) Down syndrome
            (2) Turner's syndrome

4. Gestational diabetes
5. Impaired glucose homeostasis

    a. Impaired fasting glucose
    b. Impaired glucose tolerance

D. Laboratory/Diagnostic testing[2, 3, 4, 10, 15]

1. According to the Expert Committee on the Diagnosis and Classification of Diabetes Mellitus, the diagnosis of diabetes mellitus and/or impaired glucose homeostasis may be made from positive findings from *any two* of the following tests *on different days:*

    a. Symptoms of diabetes mellitus
        i. Polyuria
        ii. Polydipsia
        iii. Unexplained weight loss
    PLUS
    b. Random or casual (any time of day without regard to time since the last meal) plasma glucose concentration ≥200 mg/dL (11 mmol/L)
    OR
    c. Fasting plasma glucose (FPG) = ≥ 126 mg/dL (7.0 mmol/L)
    OR
    Two-hour postprandial glucose (PPG) ≥ 200 mg/dL (11.1 mmol/L) after a 75-g glucose load

2. Impaired glucose homeostasis/Impaired fasting glucose[4, 10, 15]

    a. *Fasting plasma glucose (FPG):* 111–125 mg/dL (6.1–7.0 mmol/L)
    b. *Two-hour postprandial glucose (PPG):* 140 to <200 mg/dL (7.75 to <11.1 mmol/L)
    c. If FPG is <126 mg/dL, yet diabetes is suspected, an oral glucose tolerance test may be conducted.

d. However, because of the possibility of numerous inaccuracies, clinicians employ repeated fasting plasma glucose levels as a more definitive means of diagnosing diabetes, rather than utilizing the oral glucose tolerance test.

e. Although seldom used and not recommended for routine clinical use, the oral glucose tolerance test procedure includes

   i. After an overnight fast, a 75-g load of glucose solution is given to a patient who has been receiving at least 150–200 g of carbohydrates each day for 3 days prior to the test.

   ii. According to the Expert Committee on the Diagnosis and Classification of Diabetes, diagnosis is made using the following criteria when evaluating the standard oral glucose tolerance test:

   - *Fasting plasma glucose:*
   - Normal ≤110 mg/dL
   - Impaired fasting glucose (IFG) = 111–125 mg/dL
   - Diabetes mellitus ≥126 mg/dL
   - *Two hours after the glucose load:*
   - Normal <140 mg/dL
   - Impaired glucose tolerance ≥140 mg/dL but <200 mg/dL
   - Diabetes mellitus ≥200 mg/dL

3. Urinalysis: Although less used today because of the wide availability of glucose meters, monitor for:

   a. Glycosuria—Easily detected by Diastix or Clinistix paper strip testing

   b. Ketonuria—Quantitatively evident in Type 1 patients via nitroprusside tests such as Acetest or Ketostix.

4. BUN and urinary creatinine
   a. Baseline
   b. To rule out dehydration (i.e., elevated)

5. Glycosylated hemoglobin (HbA$_{1c}$)

   a. Elevated in approximately 85% of patients with diabetes before diagnosis

   b. Indicative of a patient's glycemic control over the past 2–3 months

   c. Not used for the initial diagnosis of diabetes mellitus because of the low sensitivity of the test

   d. Although the test has low sensitivity, the test is quite specific; therefore, measurements are conducted in known diabetic patients at 3–4 month intervals to adjust therapy, as needed.

e. Goal values are approximately 5.5–7.0%, with higher levels indicating higher blood glucose levels and thus poorer glucose control.

E. Recommendations for diabetes screening for asymptomatic patients[2, 4, 10, 15]

1. Test at age 45 and every 3 years thereafter.
2. Test before age 45 and more frequently than every 3 years if the patient has one or more of the following risk factors:

   a. Obesity: ≥120% of desired body weight OR BMI ≥ 27 kg/m²
   b. First-degree relative with diabetes mellitus
   c. Member of a high-risk ethnic group
      i. African American
      ii. Hispanic
      iii. Native American
      iv. Asian
   d. History of gestational diabetes mellitus or delivering a baby weighing more than 4032 g (9 lb)
   e. Hypertension (blood pressure ≥140/90 mmHg, with some guidelines citing ≥135/85 mmHg)
   f. High-density lipoprotein cholesterol ≤35 mg/dL (0.90 mmol/L) and/or triglyceride level ≥250 mg/dL (2.83 mmol/L)
   g. History of impaired glucose tolerance (IGT) or impaired fasting glucose (IFG) on prior tests.

F. Management: Diet, exercise, and foot care for diabetic patients[1, 4, 7, 8, 18, 20]

Note: Treatment plans for all diabetic patients must be highly individualized. The following points provide general guidelines that may be tailored to the needs of each patient.

1. Teach patients about the benefits of diet therapy, including:

   a. American Diabetic Association (ADA) diets found at www.eatright.org OR www.ada.org
   b. Refer patient to a dietician, as appropriate.
   c. Total carbohydrate intake should be 55–60% of total caloric intake.
   d. Fiber should = 25 g/1000 calories.
   e. Fats should = 20–30% of total calories (individualized according to serum lipid levels).
   f. Protein should = 10–20% of total calories.
   g. Meal schedules for diabetic patients
      i. Type 1 patients should be encouraged to have three meals each day and three snacks on a consistent schedule consistent with insulin regimens.

    ii. Type 2 patients should be taught to have meals 5 h apart, with few or no snacks.

    iii. Teach patients who are on insulin how to use the Diabetic Exchange List.

  h. Artificial sweeteners may be encouraged instead of sugar.

  i. Alcohol intake should be limited to modest use (e.g., ≤2 drinks per day).

  j. Optimal glycemic control and weight reduction, as needed, are both important goals of therapy.

2. Encourage exercise—an essential component of care for all diabetic patients.

  a. Encourage at least 30 min of exercise every other day; allow for a period of warm-up (5–10 min) and cool-down (5–10 min).

  b. Teach the patient to use silica gel or air midsoles and polyester or cotton-blend socks to keep feet as dry as possible. Wearing proper footwear and monitoring for blisters is of paramount importance.

  c. Monitor for dehydration; encourage extra fluids.

  d. Teach the patient to inject insulin at a body site far from that being exercised, if possible (e.g., abdomen instead of legs or arms).

  e. Additional carbohydrates should be ingested prior to exercise.

  f. Teach that exercise diminishes the need for insulin.

3. Foot care: Patients should be taught the importance of foot care in preventing infection, gangrene, and/or the need for amputation.

  a. The most important prevention strategy for foot complications is to examine the feet for injuries each day with a mirror, including the bottoms of the feet and between the toes.

  b. Report any new problems such as broken skin, ulcers, or blisters immediately—that is, tell the patient not to wait until his/her next appointment.

  c. Keep nails trimmed regularly by an experienced health care provider.

  d. Wash feet daily with lukewarm water and a mild soap. Pat feet dry with a soft cloth. Apply lotion after washing.

  e. Wear only shoes prescribed by a health care professional.

  f. Always wear protective shoes and socks. Do not wear socks only.

  g. Cease smoking.

G. Complications[4, 11, 23–25]

1. Diabetic retinopathy

   a. Occurs in approximately 15% of diabetic patients after 15 years—increasing 1% each year after diagnosis
   b. The most common cause of all blindness
   c. Annual ophthalmology examinations are indicated.

2. Cardiovascular disease

   a. Diabetes adds an independent risk factor to atherosclerotic development.
   b. The prevalence of hypertension is 2 times greater in Type 2 diabetics than in the general population.

3. Cataracts—Increased incidence among diabetic patients
4. Glaucoma—Occurs in approximately 6% of diabetic patients
5. Neuropathy (peripheral and autonomic)

   a. Most common complication
   b. Poorly understood
   c. May involve loss of sensation as well as pain along autonomic and peripheral tracks

6. Nephropathy—End-stage renal disease has a 40% incidence in Type 1 diabetes patients, a <20% incidence in Type 2 patients.
7. Infections

   a. Chronically common in diabetic patients
   b. Watch for necrobiosis lipoidica diabeticorum lesions over the anterior legs and dorsal surfaces of the ankles, which may predispose patients to infection.
   c. Yeast infections are also common.

8. Gangrene of the feet—Incidence is 20 times higher among diabetic patients.
9. Diabetic ketoacidosis (Type 1 patients)—See Chapter 47.
10. Hyperosmolar hyperglycemic nonketosis (HHNK)—See Chapter 47.

II. TYPE 1 DIABETES MELLITUS

A. Predisposing factors/General comments: Type 1 Diabetes[3, 4, 10, 16, 21]

1. Fifteen per 100,000 individuals with diabetes are diagnosed with this type each year.
2. Most commonly seen in whites
3. African Americans have the lowest incidence of this type in the United States.

4. Males and females are affected equally.
5. Genetic predisposition
6. Approximately 70% acquire Type 1 before age 20.
7. Virtual absence of circulating insulin
8. Islet cell antibodies may be found in approximately 90% of patients within the first year of diagnosis.
9. Development of this type of diabetes is strongly associated with the presence of human leukocyte antigens, HLA-DR3 or HLA-DR4.
10. Absence of C-peptide
11. Ketone development usually occurs.
12. Usually develops acutely over a period of days to weeks

B. Subjective/Physical examination findings: Type 1 Diabetes[4, 14]

1. Polyuria
2. Polydipsia
3. Polyphagia
4. Weight loss
5. Skin and genital infections
6. Nocturnal enuresis
7. Weakness/fatigue
8. Blurred vision
9. Changes in levels of consciousness (irritability to coma)
10. Loss of subcutaneous fat and muscle wasting

C. Laboratory/Diagnostic testing: Type 1 Diabetes[4, 9, 10, 12, 14, 15]
Refer to section I.D. Laboratory/Diagnostic testing. Essential criteria:

1. Polyuria, polydipsia, weight loss, and random serum glucose ≥200 mg/dL
2. Plasma glucose ≥126 mg/dL after an overnight fast for at least 8 h—performed on more than one occasion
3. Ketonemia, ketonuria, or both

D. Management: Type 1 Diabetes[1–6, 14, 16, 18–20, 22]
Note: Treatment plans for all diabetic patients must be highly individualized. The following points provide general guidelines that may be tailored to the needs of each patient.

1. Physician/endocrinologist referral—especially indicated for newly diagnosed patients and those with comorbidities
2. For Type 1 diabetic patients, particularly those diagnosed by the findings of ketones and/or young age of onset, *conventional use* of insulin may be used initially, especially during the early phases of their diagnosis.

   a. Conventional split dose mixtures
      i. The morning dose of insulin is ⅔ NPH and ⅓ Regular.

  ii. The evening dose is ½ NPH and ½ Regular.
  iii. Therefore, a 70-kg patient would receive 35 U of insulin each day: 10 U Regular insulin and 15 U NPH every morning and 5 U Regular and 5 U NPH every evening.

3. Intensive therapy (used for patients who cannot maintain normal levels with conventional therapy without becoming hypoglycemic at night)

 a. Reducing/omitting the evening insulin dose and adding a portion at bedtime:
  i. 10 U Regular insulin with 15 U NPH every morning—*THEN*
  ii. 5 U of Regular insulin before the evening meal—*AND*
  iii. 5 U NPH insulin at bedtime
 b. Intensive therapy may be necessary several years following the diagnosis of Type 1 diabetes, and may be the preferred method prescribed by some clinicians.

4. Home testing

 a. Blood glucose levels should be monitored q.i.d. (i.e., before breakfast, lunch, dinner, and bedtime).

5. Calculating insulin dosages[16, 18]

 a. As a general rule, the initiation of insulin commonly begins by prescribing 0.5 U/kg/day—giving ⅔ of the dose in the morning and the remaining ⅓ in the evening. Note that dosages may be slightly lower for thinner patients and slightly higher for those who are obese.
 b. If serum glucose values remain >140 mg/dL before the evening meal, dosages are changed by adding 2–5 U approximately every 3 days until the patient is well regulated.
 c. Once afternoon postprandial glucose values are controlled (<140 mg/dL), fasting plasma levels are checked. If fasting levels are elevated, ⅔ of the insulin dose will be administered before breakfast with the remaining ⅓ given before dinner until the fasting glucose level reaches 120–140 mg/dL.
 d. Following achievement of afternoon and before-breakfast glucose regulation, late-morning glucose levels are assessed and Regular insulin may be added to the morning injection to keep glucose levels <140 mg/dL. Note: Regular insulin usually does *not* exceed 50% of the amount of insulin given at one time.

6. Examples of insulin administration schedules
Again, treatment plans must be highly individualized based on the needs of the patient. However, the following examples may be useful as a guide in practice.

   a. Two (2) injection regimen: Regular and NPH or Lente insulin in conventional split doses before breakfast and dinner; usually ⅔ of total daily dose administered in the morning
   b. Three (3) injection regimen: Regular and NPH or Lente insulin mixed in the morning before breakfast, Regular insulin before dinner, and NPH or Lente insulin at bedtime; used to prevent the dawn phenomenon and the Somogyi effect
   c. Four (4) injection regimen: Lispro (Humalog) before meals (sometimes Regular insulin instead) and NPH or Lente insulin at bedtime
   d. Insulin pump regimen: Using either Humalog or Regular insulin, administering 50% of total daily needs at a basal hourly rate, then boluses before meals and before bedtime snack

7. Types of insulin with most common examples (Table 46–1)
Note: In addition to Type 1 diabetic patients, insulin (usually beginning with NPH single-dose therapy) is indicated for Type 2 patients whose glucose levels fail to be adequately controlled by diet, exercise, and oral antidiabetic agents.

8. Sliding scales

   a. Used when round-the-clock therapy fails to maintain adequate glucose control
   b. Considering individual weight, height, and activity calculations, a recommended initial example ordering regular insulin to be used on a sliding-scale basis might include:

Blood Glucose Level	Regular Insulin Dose
150–199 mg/dL	2 units
200–250 mg/dL	5 units
251–300 mg/dL	7 units
301–350 mg/dL	10 units
351–400 mg/dL	12 units

9. Monitoring control of glucose

   a. Patient testing
      i. Patients should be taught to document home glucose readings and bring their documentation to appointments with their clinician.
      ii. The acute care nurse practitioner should target optimal parameters for nonpregnant diabetic patients (Table 46–2).

TABLE 46–1. TYPES OF INSULIN WITH MOST COMMON EXAMPLES

ULTRA-SHORT-ACTING (CLEAR PREPARATIONS)

Insulin	Type	Onset	Peak	Duration
Lispro (Humalog)	human analog	15–30 min	1 h	2–4 h

SHORT-ACTING (CLEAR PREPARATIONS)

Insulin	Type	Onset	Peak	Duration
Regular	human	30–60 min	2–3 h	5–7 h
Regular Humulin	human	30–60 min	2–3 h	5–7 h

INTERMEDIATE-ACTING

Insulin	Type	Onset	Peak	Duration
NPH Humulin	human	30–90 min	4–12 h	18–24 h
NPH Novolin	human	30–90 min	4–12 h	18–24 h
Lente Humulin	human	1–2.5 h	8–12 h	18–24 h
Lente (30% semilente & 70% ultralente)	human	1–2.5 h	8–12 h	18–24 h

LONG-ACTING WITH SLOW ONSET OF ACTION

Insulin	Type	Onset	Peak	Duration
Ultralente Humulin	human	4–8 h	16–18 h	>36 h

PREMIXED

Insulin	Type	Onset	Peak	Duration
Novolin 70/30 (70% NPH & 30% Regular)	human	30 min	2–12 h	24 h
Humulin 70/30 (70% NPH & 30% Regular)	human	30 min	2–12 h	24 h
Humulin 50/50 (50% NPH & 50% Regular)	human	30 min	2–12 h	24 h

    b. Hemoglobin A_{1c}
       i. Measurements are indicated every 3–4 months to assess glucose control.

10. Management of poorly controlled early morning glucose
    Note: Diagnosed by monitoring 3 AM blood glucose levels

    a. Somogyi effect
       i. Nocturnal hypoglycemia develops, stimulating a surge of counter-regulatory hormones (Somogyi ef-

TABLE 46–2. THERAPEUTIC TARGETS FOR NONPREGNANT DIABETIC PATIENTS

PARAMETERS	NORMAL	GOAL	SIGNALS POSSIBLE INTERVENTION*
Premeal glucose (mg/dL)	<110	80–120	<80 or >140
Bedtime glucose (mg/dL)	<120	100–140	<100 or >160
HbA$_{1c}$† (%)	<6	<7	>8
LDL cholesterol (mg/dL)	<130	<100‡	>130‡
HDL cholesterol (mg/dL)	>35	>35	<35
Fasting triglycerides (mg/dL)	<150	<150	>250–300
Blood pressure (mmHg)	<140/90	<130/85	>130/85

LDL = low-density lipoprotein; HDL = high-density lipoprotein.
* Targets may vary depending on assessment of risk-benefit ratio.
† Targets need to be adjusted for local laboratory differences in assay method and non-diabetic reference ranges.
‡ Less than 100 for patients with coexisting cardiovascular disease.
(From Goldman, L., & Bennett, J. C. [Eds.] [1999]. *Cecil textbook of medicine* [21st ed.]. Philadelphia: W.B. Saunders, with permission.)

fect) that raise blood sugar, resulting in elevated early morning glucose levels.
   ii. The patient is *hypoglycemic* at 3 AM and rebounds with an elevated blood sugar at 7 AM.
   iii. Treatment: Reduce or omit the bedtime dose of insulin.
   b. Dawn phenomenon
      i. Decreased sensitivity to insulin occurs nocturnally owing to the presence of growth hormone, which spikes at night.
      ii. Blood sugar becomes progressively elevated throughout the night, resulting in elevated glucose levels at 7 AM.
      iii. Treatment: Add or increase the bedtime dose of insulin.
   c. Waning of insulin levels—Insufficient dosing of intermediate-acting insulin may also cause elevated early morning glucose levels.
      i. Treatment: Increase the amount of intermediate-acting insulin at bedtime.

11. Major complications

    a. Diabetic ketoacidosis—See Chapter 47.

    b. Hypoglycemia

III. TYPE 2 DIABETES MELLITUS

A. Predisposing factors/General comments: Type 2 Diabetes[3, 4, 10, 14, 18, 21]

1. Affects 3.5% of the general population
2. More than 90% of all diabetic patients have Type 2 diabetes mellitus.
3. Usually seen in adults, especially after age 45
4. Circulating insulin exists enough to prevent ketoacidosis, but is inadequate to meet the patient's insulin needs.
5. Caused either by tissue insensitivity to insulin or by an insulin secretory defect that results in resistance and/or impaired production of insulin
6. Obesity is associated with approximately 75–80% of Type 2 diabetes patients in the United States.
7. Ketone production does not usually occur with Type 2 patients.
8. Associated with "Syndrome X" phenomenon characterized by findings such as

    a. Obesity—especially truncal

    b. Hypertension

    c. Abnormal lipid profile—especially high-density lipoproteins ≤ 35 mg/dL and triglycerides ≥ 250 mg/dL

    d. Hyperinsulinism and/or insulin resistance

9. Usually develops insidiously and, other than being hyperglycemic, the patient may be asymptomatic

B. Subjective/Physical examination findings: Type 2 diabetes[3, 4, 21, 14]

1. Polyuria
2. Polydipsia
3. Frequent infections, including vulvovaginitis and pruritis
4. Acute weight loss, yet the patient is often overweight
5. Fatigue
6. Blurred vision (recurrent)
7. Peripheral neuropathy

C. Laboratory/Diagnostic testing: Type 2 diabetes[3, 4, 10, 14, 15, 21]

1. Note the essential critieria listed in section II.B.

TABLE 46–3. ORAL ANTIDIABETIC MEDICATIONS

ORAL AGENT	DURATION	STARTING DOSE	DAILY DOSAGE	COMMENT(S)
Sulfonylureas: First Generation				
Tolbutamide (Orinase)	6–10 h	500 mg/day	500 mg q.i.d. (before meals and at h.s.)	Very safe choice for patients with normal liver function
Tolazamide (Tolinase)	20 h	100 mg/day	100–250 mg per day single dose or in 2 divided doses; max dose = 1 g per day	Especially useful when tolbutamide (Orinase) does not control morning hyperglycemia
Acetohexamide (Dymelor)	12–24 h	250 mg	250–1500 mg per day or b.i.d.	Increases risk of hypoglycemia if taken with certain foods (e.g., garlic, celery, juniper berries, ginseng); taken either before the AM meal or before both the AM and PM meals
Chlorpropamide (Diabinese)	24–72 h	100 mg	100–500 mg per day	Contraindicated in patients with renal insufficiency; may cause hyponatremia and alcohol-induced flushing; less commonly prescribed today than second-generation sulfonylureas

Table continued on following page

TABLE 46–3. ORAL ANTIDIABETIC MEDICATIONS *Continued*

ORAL AGENT	DURATION	STARTING DOSE	DAILY DOSAGE	COMMENT(S)
Sulfonylureas: Second Generation				
Glipizide (Glucotrol)	10–24 h	5 mg	40 mg per day single dose or in 2 divided doses	Should be taken on an empty stomach 30 min prior to meals
Glyburide (DiaBeta, Micronase)	24 h	2.5 mg	20 mg per day	Contraindicated in the elderly, those with hepatic or renal impairment, and those at serious risk for hypoglycemia (may cause prolonged hypoglycemia)
Glimepiride (Amaryl)	24 h	1 mg	8 mg per day	Prescribed once each day as either monotherapy or in combination with insulin
Biguanides				
Metformin HCl (Glucophage)	12–24 h	500 mg	500–2250 mg in b.i.d. or q.i.d. dosing	"Insulin sparing" agent that does not cause weight gain in diabetics; therefore, extremely popular with obese patients and in combination with a sulfonylurea
Alpha-Glucosidase Inhibitors				
Acarbose (Precose)	6–12 h	25 mg once or twice daily	100 mg t.i.d.	May cause flatulence; dosage should be increased slowly to reduce GI side effects

Miglitol (Glyset)	2–4 h	25 mg t.i.d. at the first bite of each meal; if severe GI side effects occur, may start at 25 mg each day	50 mg t.i.d. at the first bite of each meal; maximum dose = 100 mg t.i.d.	Increases risk of hypoglycemia if taken with certain foods (e.g., garlic, celery, juniper berries, ginseng); contraindicated in Type 1 diabetes; use cautiously in patients with renal insufficiency
Nonsulfonylurea Insulin Stimulator/Meglitinide				
Repaglinide (Prandin)	<1 h	0.5 mg 30 min or less before meals if HbA_{1c} <8%; 1–2 mg of HbA_{1c} >8%	0.5–4.0 mg before meals; maximum dose = 16 mg per day	Use cautiously in patients with hepatic or renal impairment; contraindicated in Type 1 diabetic patients
Thiazolinediones				
Rosiglitazone maleate (Avandia)	No data	2 or 4 mg b.i.d.	2 or 4 mg b.i.d.	May be taken with or without food; after 12 weeks of therapy, may increase the dosage to 8 mg; may be used in combination with metformin and/or insulin
Pioglitazone hydrochloride (Actos)	No data	15 or 30 mg every day	15 or 30 mg every day	May be used as monotherapy or in combination with metformin and/or insulin; minor GI upset may occur; monitor liver enzymes

D. Management: Type 2 Diabetes[1–8, 14, 18–20, 23–25]

Note: Treatment plans for all diabetic patients must be highly individualized. The following points provide general guidelines that may be tailored to the needs of each patient.

1. Physician/endocrinologist referral—especially indicated for newly diagnosed diabetic patients and those with comorbidities
2. Diet and exercise—Refer to section I.F.
3. Oral pharmacologic agents should be initiated upon failure of diet and exercise to control glucose levels.

   i. Insulin therapy is reserved until Type II patients fail oral therapy.
   ii. Note: The use of insulin therapy is common after 12–15 years of oral therapy.

4. Oral antidiabetic choices (five classes) (Table 46–3):[2, 11, 13, 14, 19, 22]

   a. Sulfonylureas
      i. Most widely prescribed agents; they stimulate pancreas to release more insulin.
      ii. First generation preparations are less commonly prescribed today because second generation preparations are more effective and have less-serious side effects
      iii. Note: Alcohol, chloramphenicol, methyldopa, miconazole, MAO inhibitors, salicylates, sulfonamides, warfarin, and phenylbutazone may potentiate hypoglycemic effects of sulfonylureas.
   b. Biguanides
   c. Alpha-glucosidase inhibitors
   d. Nonsulfonylurea insulin stimulator
   e. Thiazolinediones

5. Major complication

   a. Hyperosmolar hyperglycemic nonketosis (HHNK)—See Chapter 47.

References

1. American Diabetes Association (2000). Diabetes mellitus and exercise. American Diabetes Association: Clinical Practice Recommendations 2000, July 31, volume 23, supplement 1, http://www.journal.diabetes.org/FullText/Supplements/DiabetesCare/Supplement100/s50.htm.
2. American Diabetes Association (2000). Standards of medical care for patients with diabetes mellitus. Clinical Practice Recommendations 2000, July 31, volume 23, supplement 1, http://www.journal.diabetes.org/FullText/Supplements/DiabetesCare/Supplement100/s32.htm.
3. American Diabetes Association (2000). Diabetes Info: Standards of CARE. http://www.diabetes.org/ada/c30a.asp.
4. American Diabetes Association (2000). Report of the expert committee on the diagnosis and classification of diabetes mellitus. July 26, 2000,

Clinical Practice Recommendations 2000, July 26, Volume 23, Supplement 1, http://www.journal.diabetes.org/FullText/Supplements/DiabetesCare/Supplement100/s4.htm.

5. Baker, K.L., Hardwick, D.F., & Agana-Defensor, R. (1999). Endocrine anatomy and physiology. In L. Bucher & S. Melander (Eds.), *Critical care nursing* (pp. 603–611). Philadelphia: W.B. Saunders.

6. Berger, M., & Muhlhauser, I. (1999). Diabetes and patient-oriented outcomes. *Journal of the American Medical Association, 281,* 1676–1678.

7. Diabetes Foot Clinic Staff (July, 2000). General Foot Care. http://www.celos.psu.edu/dfc/patients—module1.html.

8. American Diabetes Association (2000). Nutrition recommendations and principles for people with diabetes mellitus. Clinical Practice Recommendations 2000, July 31, Volume 23, Supplement 1, http://www.journal.diabetes.org/FullText/Supplements/DiabetesCare/Supplements100/s43.htm.

9. Davies, M. (1999). New diagnostic criteria for diabetes—Are they doing what they should? *The Lancet, 354,* 610–611.

10. Expert Committee (1997). Report of the expert committee on the diagnosis and classification of diabetes mellitus. *Diabetes Care, 20,* 1183–1197.

11. Ferri, F.F. (Ed.). (1999). *Ferri's clinical advisor.* St. Louis: Mosby.

12. Garber, A.J. (1998). Diabetes Mellitus. In J.H. Stein (Ed.), *Internal medicine* (5th ed.) (pp. 1850–1874). St. Louis: Mosby.

13. Karch, A.M. (Ed.). (2000). *Lippincott's nursing drug guide 2000.* Philadelphia: J.B. Lippincott.

14. Karam, J.H. (2000). Diabetes mellitus and hypoglycemia. In L.M. Tierney, S.J. McPhee, & M.A. Papadakis (Eds.), *Current medical diagnosis & treatment* (39th ed.) (pp. 1152–1197). New York: Lange Medical Books/McGraw-Hill.

15. Mayfield, J. (1998). Diagnosis and classification of diabetes mellitus: New criteria. *American Family Physician, 58,* 1355–1362, 1368–1370.

16. Miller, S.K. (2000). Management of patients with endocrine disorders. *Acute care nurse practitioner certification review.* Potomac, MD: Health Leadership Associates.

17. Noble, J. (Ed.). (1999). *Primary care medicine.* St. Louis: Mosby.

18. Salerno, S.M. (1999). Endocrine disorders. In V.L. Millonig & S.K. Miller (Eds.), *Adult nurse practitioner certification review guide* (pp. 329–372). Potomac, MD: Health Leadership Associates.

19. Sengwald, J.M. (1999). Update on diabetes medications. *Journal of Emergency Medicine, 25,* 28–30.

20. Sherwin, R.S. (2000). Diabetes mellitus. In J. Bennett & F. Plum (Eds.), *Cecil textbook of medicine* (20th ed.) (pp. 1263–11285). Philadelphia: W.B. Saunders.

21. Schultz, R.M. (1999). Diabetes mellitus. In M.R. Dambro (Ed.), *Griffith's 5 minute clinical consult* (pp. 310–311). Philadelphia: Lippincott, Williams & Wilkins.

22. Turkoski, B.B., Lance, B.R., & Bonfiglio, M.F. (1999). *Drug information handbook for nursing 1999–2000* (2nd ed.). Hudson, OH: Lexi-Comp Inc.

23. Turner, R.C., Cull, C.A., Frughi, V., & Holman, R.R. (1999). Glycemic control with diet, sulfonylurea, metformin, or insulin in patients with Type 2 diabetes mellitus: Progressive requirement for multiple therapies (UKPDS 49). *Journal of the American Medical Association, 28,* 2005–2012.

24. UK Prospective Diabetes Study (UKPDS) Group (1998a). Intensive blood-glucose control with sulphonylureas or insulin compared with conventional treatment and risk of complications in patients with type 2 diabetes (UKPDS 33). *The Lancet, 352,* 837–853.

25. UK Prospective Diabetes Study (UKPDS) Group (1998b). Effect of intensive blood-glucose control with metformin on complications in overweight patients with type 2 diabetes (UKPDS 34). *The Lancet, 352,* 854–865.

DIABETIC EMERGENCIES

Thomas W. Barkley, Jr., DSN, RN, CS,
ACNP

I. DIABETIC KETOACIDOSIS (DKA)

A. Definition[3, 7]

1. A state of intracellular dehydration as a result of elevated blood glucose levels
2. Hyperglycemia increases serum osmolality, causing a shift of intracellular water into the intravascular space.
3. In addition to hyperglycemia, DKA is characterized by hyperketonemia and an acidotic pH.

B. Incidence/Predisposing factors[1, 9, 12, 13, 15, 17]

1. Accounts for approximately 14% of all hospital admissions among diabetic patients; while usually occurring in Type 1 diabetes patients, it may occur in Type 2 patients as well.
2. Occurs in approximately 46/10,000 diabetic patients
3. Increasing incidence among patients with insulin pumps
4. Mortality rate is approximately 5%.
5. Poor patient compliance—Common causes include

   a. Lack or omission of insulin; classically, the patient stops taking or fails to appropriate insulin.
   b. Too much food or insufficient exercise without an appropriate amount of insulin
   c. Failure to consume extra fluids and insulin during illness or acute stress

6. Pancreatitis
7. Sepsis/infection
8. Surgery or trauma in the patient with diabetes mellitus

C. Subjective/Physical examination findings[1, 8, 9, 12, 14, 17]

1. Polyuria (including nocturia)
2. Polydipsia
3. Nausea
4. Vomiting
5. Weight loss
6. Sunken eyes and poor turgor
7. Diminished vision
8. Headache
9. Abdominal pain related to bloating from gastric atony, leading to constipation

10. Weakness/fatigue
11. Altered level of consciousness ranging from drowsiness to coma
12. Flushed, dry skin
13. Fast, labored, deep breathing (i.e., Kussmaul's respirations)
14. Tachycardia with weak, rapid pulse
15. Acetone (fruity) breath odor
16. Hypotension—especially orthostatic
17. Usually hypothermia is present if without infection; DKA patients with infections are usually normothermic or hyperthermic.

D. Laboratory/Diagnostic testing[1, 9, 11, 13, 19]

1. Serum glucose levels >250 mg/dL and frequently >300 mg/dL
2. Arterial pH usually <7.3 and P_{CO_2} <40 mmHg, indicating metabolic acidosis; HCO_3 < 15 mEq/L
3. Ketones present in serum and urine
4. Hyperkalemia related to hydrogen ions shifting intracellularly in an attempt to buffer the acidosis; subsequently, hydrogen ions are exchanged for potassium ions
5. Increased BUN level related to dehydration
6. Glycosuria
7. Increased hematocrit level related to dehydration
8. Leukocytosis—WBC count may be 25,000/μL.
9. Serum hyperosmolality (>280 mOsm/L) is common. Note: Osmolality >320–330 mOsm/L usually results in coma. To effectively measure serum osmolality:

$$mOsm/L = 2[Na(mEq/L) + K (mEq/L) + Glucose/18]$$

Note: Serum osmolality is approximately 2 × the Na value.
10. Expect an *increased* anion gap = Na − (HCO_3 + Cl)

   a. Normal anion gap is 7–17 mEq/L
   b. Note that the higher the anion gap, the higher the patient's acuity.

11. Hypercholesterolemia may be present.
12. Hypertriglyceridemia may be present.
13. Hyperamylasemia may be present.

E. Management[1, 3, 8–10, 14]

1. Critical care monitoring is indicated. Consider invasive monitoring (e.g., central venous pressure/pulmonary arterial catheter) based on the patient's history of cardiovascular and/or pulmonary disease (e.g., congestive heart failure, pulmonary edema).
2. Parenteral fluid replacement should be initiated with 0.9% normal saline (NS) at 1000 mL/h for 1 h, followed by an ad-

ministration of 300–500 mL/h for 4 h to correct a usual fluid deficit of 4–8 L.

   a. Once dehydration improves, 250 mL/h is recommend.
   b. Expect to order approximately 4–8 L fluid to be administered during the first 24 h of treatment.

3. Potassium values should be closely monitored during fluid resuscitation.
4. Isotonic fluids are generally used until the patient is hemodynamically stable.
5. Once the patient is hemodynamically stable, hypotonic solutions (e.g., ½ NS) are used to promote intracellular hydration.
6. As the patient's glucose levels fall to approximately 250 mg/dL, IV fluids are changed to dextrose-containing agents such as D_5½NS to prevent hypoglycemia and cerebral edema caused by lowering glucose too rapidly.
7. Watch for potassium imbalance (i.e., hypokalemia post treatment) and dysrhythmias. Potassium chloride, 20–30 mEq/L IV, should be added to IV fluids within the first 2–3 h of therapy unless potassium levels are >5.0 mEq/L.
8. Administer a loading dose of 0.1 U/kg units of *regular* insulin IV followed by a continuous insulin drip (1 : 1) at 0.1 U/kg/h.

   a. If plasma levels of glucose do not fall 10% within the first hour of therapy, a second loading dose is indicated.
   b. Once the metabolic acidosis has been corrected, SC insulin therapy may be initiated.

9. Sodium bicarbonate is rarely needed but may be administered via 1–2 ampules per liter of hypotonic saline if pH ≤7.0 or serum bicarbonate levels are <9 mEq/L. Once pH reaches 7.1 and there are no signs of cardiac irritability, bicarbonate should be discontinued to avoid over compensation.
10. Monitor for other electrolyte disturbances following treatment (e.g., hypophosphatemia if diuresis and acidosis totally deplete phosphorus levels).

II. HYPEROSMOLAR HYPERGLYCEMIC NONKETOSIS (HHNK)

A. Definition/General comments[7]

1. A state of greatly elevated serum glucose, hyperosmolality, and severe dehydration without ketone production
2. Usually occurs in patients who are able to produce enough insulin (Type 2 diabetics) to prevent ketoacidosis but who cannot produce enough insulin to prevent severe hyperglycemia, osmotic diuresis, and extracellular fluid depletion

3. Since lipolysis from adipose tissue is inhibited, ketone production does not occur.

    a. Osmotic diuresis related to hyperglycemia leads to the severe dehydration.

    b. Intracellular dehydration occurs, causing cerebral dehydration and neurologic signs and symptoms.

4. Mortality rate may approach 30–50%

B. Incidence/Predisposing factors[4, 7, 11, 15]

1. Recent onset of mild diabetes
2. Patient receiving TPN or high-calorie feedings
3. Patient receiving thiazide, steroid, or hypertonic solution administration
4. Illness, trauma, or stress
5. Diet-controlled diabetes
6. Pancreatitis
7. Increased incidence in diabetic patients of advanced age

C. Subjective/Physical examination findings[7, 11, 14]

1. Weakness
2. Neurologic changes that may be the most obvious presenting signs

    a. Disorientation
    b. Lethargy
    c. Seizures
    d. Stupor
    e. Coma

3. Flushed/dry skin, dry mucous membranes, poor turgor (dehydration)
4. Polyuria
5. Hypotension
6. Tachycardia
7. Shallow breathing

D. Laboratory/Diagnostic testing[4, 5, 7, 9, 13, 16]

1. Blood glucose levels $\geq$600 mg/dL (commonly >1000 mg/dL)
2. Elevated serum osmolarity (>310 mOsm/L [normal = 275–295 mOsm/L]) resulting in osmotic diuresis and severe dehydration. Refer to calculations in section I.D. of this chapter.
3. Elevated BUN and creatinine
4. Elevated serum sodium (to retain water, the kidneys try to conserve sodium)
5. Relatively normal pH, >7.30; relatively normal sodium bicarbonate level, >15 mEq/L (ketosis does not occur).
6. Anion gap is normal—Refer to section I.D. of this chapter.

E. Management[2, 4, 5, 9, 14]

1. Critical care monitoring is indicated. Consider invasive monitoring (e.g., central venous pressure/pulmonary arterial catheter) based on the patient's history of cardiovascular and/or pulmonary disease (e.g., congestive heart failure, pulmonary edema).
2. Massive fluid replacement. Isotonic fluids are used until the patient becomes hemodynamically stable.
3. If the patient is not hypotensive or once serum sodium level reaches 145 mEq/L, hypotonic solutions are used to hydrate the intracellular compartment (e.g., ½NS).
   a. Expect to order approximately 4–6 L in the first 8–10 h of therapy.
   b. Overall fluid volume deficit may be 6–10 L.
4. Monitor for complications of too much fluid replacement.
   a. Cardiac failure
   b. Cerebral edema
   c. Seizures
5. Less insulin is required to control HHNK than to control DKA.
   a. An initial bolus of 15 U of regular insulin IV and 15 U SC may suffice.
   b. Subsequent doses range from approximately 10–20 U SC q4h.
   c. Some clinicians advocate regular insulin at 1–2 U/h IV by continuous infusion (1 : 1) until glucose reaches approximately 300 mg/dL.
6. Fluid resuscitation and initial insulin as described above should make a continuous infusion of insulin unnecessary.
7. Continuous monitoring of electrolytes (Na, K, HCO_3, Cl, phosphorus) is necessary with replacement, as needed.
8. Cardiac monitoring for dysrhythmias—especially monitor potassium levels.
9. Frequent blood glucose monitoring and clear documentation of glucose levels (e.g., bedside flow sheet)

III. HYPOGLYCEMIA

A. Definition
A state of decreased serum glucose from a variety of causes

B. Incidence/Predisposing factors[1, 11, 18]

1. Frequently occurs in Type 1 diabetes mellitus (i.e., in patients on insulin therapy)
2. Too much insulin

3. Lack of food intake
4. Excessive exercise, especially without adequate food intake
5. Diarrhea and vomiting
6. Alcohol consumption

C. Subjective/Physical examination findings[1, 11, 18]

1. Dizziness
2. Weakness
3. Neurologic changes including confusion, seizures, coma
4. Tremor, nervousness, anxiety
5. Sweating, pallor, cold skin
6. Tachycardia, palpitations
7. Visual disturbances, including diplopia
8. Paresthesias

D. Diagnostic/Laboratory testing

1. Blood glucose ≤45–50 mg/dL. Note: In diabetic patients, symptoms of hypoglycemia may occur at higher glucose levels and correlate with the rapidity of falling glucose values.
2. Urine negative for sugar and acetone

E. Management[1, 6, 8, 11]

1. In the acute care facility, a blood glucose level should first be drawn.
2. Give approximately 10–20 g of carbohydrate such as *one* of the following:

   a. 4 oz sweetened carbonated beverage or unsweetened fruit juice
   b. 1 tbs honey
   c. 5 pieces of hard candy with sugar
   d. 4 oz. regular soft drink

3. If the patient is unable to swallow:

   a. $D_{50}W$ per IV in the acute care facility followed by an IV continuous infusion of D_5W, as needed, to maintain glucose levels >100 mg/dL
   b. Glucagon, 1 mg, IM in the deltoid if away from the acute care facility and IV access is not possible

4. Give crackers and milk or other protein and complex carbohydrate snack following the event.
5. Continue to monitor glucose levels as necessary; patients taking oral antiglycemic agents should be closely followed for 24–48 h.

References

1. Abercrombie, S.A. (1999). Diabetic ketoacidosis. In M.R. Dambro (Ed.), *Griffith's 5 minute clinical consult* (pp. 314–315). Philadelphia: Lippincott, Williams & Wilkins.

2. Ferri, F.F. (Ed.). (1999). *Ferri's clinical advisor*. St. Louis: Mosby.

3. Freeland, B.S. (1998). Emergency: Diabetic ketoacidosis. *American Journal of Nursing, 98*, 52.

4. Genuth, S.M. (1997). Diabetic ketoacidosis and hyperglyemic hyperosmolar coma. *Current Therapy in Endocrinology & Metabolism, 6*, 438–447.

5. Guthrie, D.W. (1996). Patients with disorders of glucose metabolism. In J.M. Clochesy, C. Breu, S. Cardin, A.A. Whittaker, & E.B. Rudy (Eds.), *Critical care nursing* (2nd ed.) (pp. 1107–1121). Philadelphia: W.B. Saunders.

6. Hart, S.P., & Frier, B.M. (1998). Causes, management and morbidity of acute hypoglycemia in adults requiring hospital admission. *QJM: Monthly Journal of the Association of Physicians, 91*, 505–510.

7. Hinnen, D., & Childs, B. (1999). Diabetic ketoacidosis and hyperglycemic hyperosmolar nonketotic coma. In L. Bucher & S. Melander (Eds.), *Critical care nursing* (pp. 628–642). Philadelphia: W.B. Saunders.

8. Horn, M.M. (1997). Diabetic ketoacidosis. In J.H. Keen & P.L Swearingen (Eds.), *Mosby's Critical Care Nursing Consultant*. St. Louis: Mosby.

9. Karam, J.H. (2000). Diabetes mellitus and hypoglycemia. In L.M. Tierney, S.J. McPhee, & M.A. Papadakis, (Eds.), *Current medical diagnosis & treatment* (38th ed.) (pp. 1152–1197). Stamford, CT: Appleton & Lange.

10. Kitabchi, A.E., & Wall, B.M. (1999). Management of diabetic ketoacidosis. *American Family Physician, 60*, 455–464.

11. Krumberger, J.M., & Waite, L.G. (1997). Endocrine alterations. In J.C. Hartshorn, M.L. Sole, & M.L. Lamborn (Eds.), *Introduction to critical care nursing* (2nd ed.) (pp. 473–521). Philadelphia: W.B. Saunders.

12. Mcdermot, P.A. (1998). Diabetic emergencies and sick day rules. *Home Care Provider, 3*, 298, 301.

13. Miller, S.K. (2000). Management of patients with endocrine disorders. *Acute care nurse practitioner certification review*. Potomac, MD: Health Leadership Associates.

14. Murphy, D. (1998). Acute complication of diabetes mellitus. *Nurse Practitioner Forum, 9*, 69–73.

15. Padmore, E. (1998). Predisposing factors in diabetic emergencies. *Accident & Emergency Nursing, 6*, 160–163.

16. Shin, S.J., Lee. Y.J., Hsaio, P.J., & Tsai, J.H. (1999). Increased urinary atrial natriuretic peptide-like immunoreactivity excretion but decreased plasma atrial natriuretic peptide concentration in patients with hyperosmolar-hyperglycemic nonketotic syndrome. *Diabetes Care, 22*, 1181–1185.

17. Thelan, L.A., Urden, L.D., Lough, M.E., & Stacy, K.M. (1998). *Critical care nursing: Diagnosis and management* (3rd ed.). St. Louis: Mosby.

18. Waickus, C.M., de Bustros, A., & Shakil, A. (1999). Recognizing factitious hypoglycemia in the family practice setting. *Journal of the American Board of Family Practice, 12*, 133–136.

19. Woolliscroft, J.O. (1996). *Handbook of current diagnosis & treatment*. Philadelphia: Mosby.

THYROID DISEASE

Thomas W. Barkley, Jr., DSN, RN, CS, ACNP

I. HYPERTHYROIDISM (THYROTOXICOSIS)

A. Definition[10–12]

A condition of excess secretion of thyroxine (T_4) and thiodothyronine (T_3) resulting from a variety of clinical disorders

B. Etiology/Predisposing factors/Incidence[4, 6, 12]

1. Graves' disease—the most common cause; associated with goiter and ocular changes
2. Subacute thyroiditis
3. Thyroid-stimulating hormone (TSH) pituitary tumor
4. Toxic nodular goiter or thyroid carcinoma
5. Other autoimmune causes

   a. Pernicious anemia
   b. Diabetes mellitus
   c. Myasthenia gravis

6. Most commonly seen between 20 and 40 years of age
7. Higher incidence among women, with an 8 : 1 female to male ratio
8. May also occur in patients on high-dose amiodarone (Cordarone) therapy. Note: High-dose amiodarone therapy may also cause signs of hypothyroidism as well.

C. Subjective/Physical examination findings (thyrotoxic manifestations)[1, 2, 5, 6, 9]

1. Hypermetabolism
2. Heat intolerance
3. Fatigue
4. Anxiety
5. Nervousness
6. Manic behavior
7. Confusion/restlessness
8. Emotional lability
9. Fine tremors
10. Diaphoresis
11. Hyperreflexia of deep tendon reflexes
12. Resting tachycardia/palpitations/atrial fibrillation
13. Exertional dyspnea
14. Low-grade fever
15. Increased appetite

16. Weight loss
17. Frequent bowel movements
18. Smooth, warm, moist, velvety skin with occasional pruritus
19. Fine/thin hair
20. Exophthalmos
21. Eyelid lag
22. Infrequent blinking
23. Graves' ophthalmopathy—Noted in 20–40% of cases

D. Laboratory/Diagnostic findings[2, 5, 7, 10, 12]

1. TSH assay—Most sensitive test, and levels are *low* in most cases of hyperthyroidism
2. Serum T_3, T_4, thyroid resin uptake, and free thyroxine index (FTI) values are elevated. Note: T_4 may be normal, but T_3 will be elevated.
3. Elevated erythrocyte sedimentation rate
4. Serum antinuclear antibodies (ANA) level usually elevated without evidence of systemic lupus erythematosus or other autoimmune disease
5. May see hypercalcemia and anemia on complete blood cell count with decreased granulocytes
6. For investigating the most common causes of hyperthyroidism, results of thyroid radioactive uptake tests may be used:

   a. High iodine uptake is usually indicative of Graves' disease.
   b. Low iodine uptake is usually indicative of subacute thyroiditis.

7. MRI of the orbits is used to assess Graves' ophthalmopathy, as indicated.

E. Management[3, 5, 10, 11]

1. Physician/endocrinologist consultation for newly diagnosed patients and those with comorbidities
2. Symptomatic relief: Propranolol (Inderal), 10 mg p.o., (may increase dosage to 80 mg) q.i.d.
3. Antithyroid medications are used for mild cases of hyperthyroidism and in patients with small goiters who are afraid of using isotopes. However, there is a high rate of recurrence of the disease after 1 year.

   a. Methimazole (Tapazole), 30–60 mg every day in three divided doses
   b. Propylthiouracil, 300–600 mg every day in four divided doses

4. Radioactive iodine (^{131}I)

   a. Used to destroy goiters

b. Usually takes 3–4 months for the patient to become euthyroid

5. Thyroid surgery to remove the gland
   a. Not a common modality
   b. Used for
      i. Pregnant patients
      ii. Patients suspected of having cancer
   c. Lugol's solution, 2–3 drops p.o. every day for 10 days, to reduce the vascularity of the thyroid preoperatively by blocking the release of hormones from the thyroid gland.
   d. The patient must be euthyroid before the gland is removed.

6. Subacute thyroiditis—Best treated with propranolol (symptomatically)

II. THYROID STORM (THYROTOXIC CRISIS)

A. Definition[3, 13]

1. A deadly, hypermetabolic state caused by inadequately controlled hyperthyroidism
2. This crisis manifests with exacerbated thyrotoxic symptoms.

B. Predisposing factors/Incidence/General comments for patients with existing diagnosed or undiagnosed hyperthyroidism[3, 5, 13]

1. Trauma
2. Major stress
3. Infection
4. Subtotal thyroidectomy or other thyroid surgery
5. Uncontrolled diabetes
6. Antithyroid drug overdose
7. Pregnancy
8. Thyrotoxic crisis is a rare disorder.

C. Subjective/Physical examination findings[2, 8, 12, 14]

1. Fever (100°–105.8°F)
2. Dilated vessels/flushing
3. Profuse diaphoresis (fluid loss may equal 4 L/24 h)
4. Marked tachycardia (supraventricular tachycardia possible)/palpitations
5. Mental status changes
   a. Extreme agitation
   b. Delirium
   c. Psychosis
   d. Stupor/coma
6. Gastrointestinal disturbances: Hyperdefecation may be an early sign of thyroid storm.

7. Hyperglycemia
8. Others—Refer to section I.C. Subjective/Physical exmination findings (Thyrotoxic manifestations).

D. Laboratory/Diagnostic findings[2, 5, 7, 12]

1. Refer to section I.D. Laboratory/Diagnostic findings.

E. Management[2, 5, 13]

1. Basic measures

   a. Supportive care including decreasing environmental stimuli
   b. Hypothermic measures, antipyretics (e.g., acetaminophen)
   c. Avoid acetylsalicylic acid (aspirin) therapy because it interferes with the binding of T_4 and thryoid-binding globulin, potentially resulting in exacerbated hypermetabolism.

2. Pharmacologic therapy (3 classes)

   a. Agents that inhibit synthesis of thyroid hormone (antithyroid drugs)
      i. Propylthiouracil, 150–250 mg q6h OR
      ii. Methimazole (Tapazole), 15–25 mg q6h WITH the following 1 h later:
   b. Agents that inhibit the release of thyroid hormone (iodine preparations)
      i. Lugol's solution, 10 drops p.o. t.i.d., OR
      ii. Sodium iodine, 1 g slowly IV WITH
   c. Agents that block the effects of thyroid hormone (i.e., beta adrenergic blockers)
      i. Propranolol (Inderal), 0.5–2.0 mg IV q4h, or 20–120 mg p.o. q6h WITH
      ii. Hydrocortisone, 50 mg q6h, followed by rapid tapering of the dosage as the patient improves

3. Surgery and treatment with radioactive iodine is delayed until the patient becomes euthyroid.

III. HYPOTHYROIDISM (MYXEDEMA COMA)

A. Definition[10]
A condition of decreased metabolism resulting from a deficient amount of circulating thyroid hormone

B. Incidence/Predisposing factors/Etiology[7, 11, 12]

1. Most common thyroid disease
2. Affects all ages
3. Women have a higher incidence, especially those with a history of thyroiditis or other autoimmune disorder (e.g., systemic lupus erythematosus, rheumatoid arthritis).

4. Causes

    a. Worldwide, hypothyroidism is most commonly related to iodine deficiency.

    b. In the United States, autoimmune thyroiditis processes (e.g., Hashimoto's) are the primary causal factor.

5. Deficiency of pituitary TSH

    a. Pituitary tumor

    b. Hypophysectomy damage

6. Hypothalamic deficiency of thyroid-releasing hormone (TRH)
7. Thyroidectomy
8. Failure to take thyroid medication
9. High-dose amiodarone (Cordarone) therapy. Note: High-dose amiodarone therapy may also cause signs of hyperthyroidism as well.

C. Subjective/Physical examination findings[5, 8, 11]

1. Extreme fatigue
2. Changes in level of consciousness (i.e., confusion → depression → coma)
3. Puffiness of face/eye
4. Hypoventilation
5. Bradycardia
6. Hypothermia
7. Hypoglycemia
8. Anorexia
9. Decreased bowel sounds
10. Weight gain
11. Constipation
12. Dry, cracked skin
13. Coarse, brittle hair
14. Brittle nails
15. Cold intolerance
16. Myxedema in extremities and periorbital edema
17. Decreased deep tendon reflexes
18. Paresthesias
19. Decreased sweating
20. Enlarged tongue
21. Ataxia
22. Hair loss
23. Hoarseness

D. Diagnostic/Laboratory findings[2, 5, 7, 8, 12]

1. Elevated TSH level
2. Low or low normal T_4 level
3. Decreased resin T_3 uptake. T_3 is not a reliable test for hypothyroidism.

4. Hypoglycemia
5. Hyponatremia
6. Anemia (normochromic, normocytic)
7. Elevated transaminases
8. Hypercholesterolemia and elevated triglyceride levels

E. Management[2, 5, 8]

1. Hypothyroidism

   a. Levothyroxine (Synthroid)
      i. For patients < *60 years old and without coronary artery disease:* 50–100 µg every day, increasing dosage by 25 µg every 1–2 weeks until symptoms stabilize and the patient becomes euthyroid
      ii. For patients > *60 years old with coronary artery disease:* 25–50 µg every day, increasing dosage by 25 µg every 1–2 weeks until symptoms stabilize and the patient becomes euthyroid

2. Myxedema coma

   a. Oxygen supplementation and mechanical ventilation for hypercapnia is almost always needed.
   b. Fluid replacement (i.e., isotonic/hypertonic for severe hyponatremia, adding glucose to relieve hypoglycemia) as needed
   c. Consider fluid restriction and 3% normal saline for severe hyponatremia.
   d. Consider $D_{50}W$ for severe hypoglycemia.
   e. IV thyroid replacement:
      i. Levothyroxine, one dose of 400 µg IV, then 100 µg every day
      ii. If adrenal insufficiency is suspected, hydrocortisone (Solu-Cortef), 100 mg IV bolus, then 25–50 mg q8h to avoid excessive hyperadrenalism-like affects associated with rapid thyroid replacement
   f. Slow rewarming with blankets. Note: Hyperthermia blankets are contraindicated because rapid vasodilation may further hypotension and lead to circulatory collapse.
   g. Patient teaching including the need for levothyroxine replacement (usually 100–200 µg/day) for life
   h. Follow-up patient teaching to prevent future episodes

References

1. Baird, M.S. (1997). Hypothyroidism. In J.H. Keen & P.L Swearingen (Eds.), *Mosby's critical care nursing consultant* (pp. 232–233). St. Louis: Mosby.
2. Brown, D. (1999). Thyroid crisis and myxedema coma. In L. Bucher & S. Melander (Eds.), *Critical care nursing* (pp. 603–611). Philadelphia: W.B. Saunders.

3. Dambro, M.R. (Ed.). (1999). *Griffith's 5 minute clinical consult*. Philadelphia: Lippincott, Williams & Wilkins.

4. Ferri, F.F. (Ed.). (1999). *Ferri's clinical advisor*. St. Louis: Mosby

5. Fitzgerald, P.A. (2000) Endocrinology. In L.M. Tierney, S.J. McPhee, & M.A. Papadakis, (Eds.), *Current medical diagnosis & treatment* (39th ed.) (pp. 1079–1151). Stamford, CT: Appleton & Lange.

6. Haddad, G. (1998). Is it hyperthyroidism? You can't always tell from the clinical picture. *Postgraduate Medicine, 104*, 42–59.

7. Helfand, M., & Redfern, C.C. (1998). Screening for thyroid disease: An update. *Annals of Internal Medicine, 129*, 144–158.

8. Krumberger, J.M., & Waite, L.G. (1997). Endocrine alterations. In J.C. Hartshorn, M.L. Sole, & M.L. Lamborn (Eds.), *Introduction to critical care nursing* (pp. 473–521). Philadelphia: W.B. Saunders.

9. Levey, G.S., & Klein, I. (1998). Disorders of the thyroid. In J.H. Stein (Ed.), *Internal medicine* (pp. 1797–1817). Philadelphia: Mosby.

10. Miller, S.K. (2000). Management of patients with endocrine disorders. *Acute care nurse practitioner certification review*. Potomac, MD: Health Leadership Associates.

11. Noble, J. (Ed.) (1999). *Primary care medicine*. St. Louis: Mosby.

12. Salerno, S.M. (1999). Endocrine disorders. In V.L. Millonig & S.K. Miller (Eds.), *Adult nurse practitioner certification review guide* (pp. 329–372). Potomac, MD: Health Leadership Associates.

13. Thelan, L.A., Urden, L.D., Lough, M.E., & Stacy, K.M. (1998). *Critical care nursing: Diagnosis and management* (3rd ed.). St. Louis: Mosby.

14. Woolliscroft, J.O. (1996). *Handbook of current diagnosis & treatment*. Philadelphia: Mosby.

CUSHING'S SYNDROME

*Thomas W. Barkley, Jr., DSN, RN, CS,
ACNP*

I. CUSHING'S SYNDROME[6]

A. Definition/General comments[6, 9]

1. A group of symptoms resulting from hypercortisolism due to numerous causes
2. Excess adrenocorticotropic hormone (ACTH) secretion by the pituitary comprises 90% of Cushing's syndrome and is therefore referred to as Cushing's disease.

B. Incidence/Predisposing factors[3, 7, 9, 10]

1. Excess ACTH production from the pituitary; approximately 70% of cases of Cushing's syndrome are caused by benign pituitary adenomas.
2. Adrenal neoplasms account for approximately 10–15% of cases; women are affected more often than men at a 5:1 ratio.
3. Non-pituitary neoplasms such as small-cell lung cancer account for approximately 15% of cases.
4. Excessive glucocorticoid administration including prolonged use

C. Subjective/Physical examination findings[3, 4, 5, 8]

1. Obesity—Central with muscle wasting
2. Moon face
3. Emotional lability

   a. Depression
   b. Anxiety
   c. Irritability

4. Buffalo hump
5. Acne
6. Purple striae
7. Protuberant abdomen
8. Hirsutism
9. Fragile ecchymotic skin on thin extremities
10. Hypertension
11. Weakness
12. Backache
13. Headache
14. Amenorrhea/impotence

15. Polyuria
16. Hyperglycemia
17. Osteoporosis

D. Diagnostic/Laboratory findings[1, 2, 3, 8]

1. Hyperglycemia as evidenced by impaired glucose tolerance testing
2. Glycosuria
3. Hypokalemia
4. Hypernatremia
5. Leukocytosis
6. Elevated serum and free urinary cortisol
7. Screening test utilizing dexamethasone

   a. Administer dexamethasone, 1 mg, at 11 PM and check serum cortisol at 8 AM the next day.
   b. Cortisol levels < 5 μg/dL exclude the diagnosis of Cushing's syndrome with 98% accuracy.

8. Although less commonly used today, testing of 24-h urine for cortisol and creatinine may be useful.

   a. An extremely elevated 24-h urine cortisol level is indicative of Cushing's syndrome, *OR*
   b. A cortisol to creatinine ratio of > 95 μg cortisol/1 g creatinine also helps confirm the diagnosis.

9. Dexamethasone suppression test

   a. Dexamethasone, 0.5 mg, is ordered p.o. q6h for 48 h.
   b. On day 2, urine is collected.
   c. A free urinary cortisol level > 20 μg/day or urine 17-hydroxycorticosteroid > 4.5 mg/day is diagnostic.

10. Midnight cortisol level > 7.5 μg/dL is diagnostic but requires

    a. The patient to have been in the same time zone for 3 days
    b. The patient being without food for the previous 3 h
    c. Indwelling arterial line preferred for serum collection

11. Elevated serum ACTH (normal = 20–100 pg/mL)

F. Management[3, 8]

1. Depends on the cause; therefore, treat the underlying cause.

   a. Transsphenoidal resection for pituitary adenomas
   b. Laparoscopic or more extensive surgery for adrenal neoplasms
   c. Resection of ACTH-secreting tumors
   d. Discontinuation or at least reduction of drugs that may cause the disease (i.e., glucocorticoids)

2. Manage fluid and electrolyte imbalances.
3. Manage other complications, such as osteoporosis, as indicated.

References

1. Clutter, W.E. (1998). Endocrine diseases. In C.F. Carey, H.H. Lee, & K.F. Woeltje (Eds.), *The Washington manual of medical therapeutics* (pp. 418–432). Philadelphia: Lippincott, Williams & Wilkins.
2. Finding, J.W., & Raff, H. (1999). Newer diagnostic techniques and problems in Cushing's disease. *Endocrinology and Metabolism Clinics of North America, 28*, 191–210.
3. Fitzgerald, P.A. (2000) Endocrinology. In L.M. Tierney, S.J. McPhee, & M.A. Papadakis, (Eds.), *Current medical diagnosis & treatment* (39th ed.) (pp. 1079–1151). Stamford, CT: Appleton & Lange.
4. Gill, G.N. (1996). Endocrine and reproductive diseases. In J.C. Bennett & F. Plum (Eds.), *Cecil textbook of medicine* (20th ed.) (pp. 1176–1350). Philadelphia: W.B. Saunders.
5. Katz, J. & Bouloux, P.M. (1999). Cushing's: How to make the diagnosis. *Practitioner, 243*, 118–122.
6. Miller, S.K. (2000). Management of patients with endocrine disorders. *Acute care nurse practitioner certification review.* Potomac, MD: Health Leadership Associates.
7. Molchan, S. (1999). The importance of early Cushing disease diagnosis. *Archives of Dermatology, 135*, 474.
8. Newell-Price, J., & Grossman, A. (1999). Diagnosis and management of Cushing's syndrome. *The Lancet, 353*, 2087–2088.
9. Noble, J. (Ed.). (1998). *Primary care medicine.* St. Louis: Mosby.
10. Young, W.F. (1999). Cushing's disease and syndrome. In M.R. Dambro (Ed.), *Griffith's 5 minute clinical consult* (pp. 276–277). Philadelphia: Lippincott, Williams & Wilkins.

PRIMARY ADRENOCORTICAL INSUFFICIENCY (ADDISON'S DISEASE) AND ADRENAL CRISIS

Thomas W. Barkley, Jr., DSN, RN, CS, ACNP

I. ADRENAL CRISIS (ACUTE ADRENAL INSUFFICIENCY)[12]

A. Definition[10]

A condition characterized by a deficiency of cortisol, androgens, and aldosterone as the result of destruction of the adrenal cortices

B. Incidence/Predisposing factors[2–4, 6, 9, 11, 16]

1. Incidence is 40–60/1,000,000 individuals.
2. Female to male ratio is 2:1.
3. Sudden withdrawal of glucocorticoids (deficiency)
4. Extreme stress
5. Trauma
6. Adrenal hemorrhage, post adrenalectomy
7. Sepsis
8. Tuberculosis

C. Etiology[12]

1. Autoimmune destruction of the adrenal gland
2. Bilateral adrenal hemorrhage (e.g., as a result of anticoagulant therapy)
3. Metastatic cancer
4. Pituitary failure resulting in decreased levels of adrenocorticotropic hormone (ACTH)

D. Chronic subjective/Physical examination findings[1, 3, 5, 7, 12, 16]

1. Weakness/fatigue
2. Headache
3. Nausea
4. Vomiting
5. Abdominal pain with accompanying diarrhea
6. Hyperpigmentation in the buccal mucosa and skin creases related to excess ACTH

   a. Apparent in knuckles, knees, posterior neck, elbows, and palmar creases
   b. Signifies a deficiency in cortisol, not in ACTH

7. Sparse axillary hair
8. Hypotension
9. Arthralgias
10. Weight loss

E. Acute subjective/Physical examination findings[12]

1. Marked and rapid worsening of the preceding chronic findings
2. Fever
3. Hypovolemia/hypotension
4. Changes in mental status/level of consciousness

F. Diagnostic/Laboratory findings[1, 7, 12, 13, 15]

1. Hyponatremia
2. Hyperkalemia
3. Hypoglycemia
4. Elevated erythrocyte sedimentation rate
5. Neutropenia (approximately $5000/\mu L$)
6. Eosinophil count $>300/\mu L$
7. Lymphocytosis in approximately 50% of patients
8. Plasma cortisol <5 mg/dL at 8 AM
9. Hypercalcemia may be present.
10. Elevated BUN—Related to extracellular fluid volume decreasing from aldosterone deficiency
11. Metabolic acidosis

    a. Related to hypotension, decreased renal function and decreased hydrogen ion excretion caused by a lack of aldosterone

12. Positive cultures of blood, urine, and/or sputum if the patient is predisposed to bacteria.
13. Simplified cosyntropin (synthetic ACTH) test

    a. Cosyntropin, 0.25 mg IV, is administered. Note: For patients undergoing glucocorticoid treatment, hydrocortisone must be discontinued at least 8 h prior to the test.
    b. Plasma cortisol levels are checked 30–60 min following administration.
    c. Normally, cortisol levels rise to at least 20 $\mu g/dL$.
    d. If the patient has primary adrenal disease, serum ACTH levels will not rise.

14. Chest and abdominal x-rays
15. Abdominal computed tomographic scan, as indicated.

G. Management[1, 5, 7, 8, 12–14]

1. Outpatient management

    a. Consult endocrinologist/specialist.

b. Glucocorticoid and mineralocorticoid replacement therapy, as needed
    i. Hydrocortisone, 15–25 mg p.o. q.d. in two divided doses (⅔ given in the morning and the remaining ⅓ administered in late afternoon)
    ii. If additional therapy is needed, fludrocortisone acetate (Florinef Acetate) may be initiated at 0.05–0.3 mg p.o. q.d. or every other day.
        (1) Note: Dosage should be increased if orthostatic hypotension, weight loss, or hyperkalemia occurs.
        (2) Dosage should be decreased if hypertension, edema, or hypokalemia develops.
c. Teach the patient signs and symptoms of adrenal crisis. Encourage wearing of a medical alert bracelet.

2. Acute management

a. Consult endocrinologist/specialist.
b. Once the diagnosis of adrenal crisis is suspected, a cortisol level should be immediately drawn and hydrocortisone (Solu-Cortef), 100–300 mg, should be administered IV with normal saline for pharmacologic and fluid replacement therapy.
c. Following the initial administration, hydrocortisone phosphate (hydrocortisone sodium phosphate) or hydrocortisone sodium succinate, 100 mg IV, should be ordered.
    i. Continuous IV infusions of hydrocortisone at 50–100 mg should be given q6h during the first day of therapy.
    ii. On the second day of therapy, hydrocortisone, 50–100 mg, should be given q8h and the dosage adjusted and tapered congruent with the patient's clinical picture.
d. Volume may also be replaced by using D_5NS at 500 mL/h for 4 h and then tapered, as indicated.
e. Initiate potassium replacement therapy. Even though the level may be high initially, there is usually a total body deficit.
f. Consider broad-spectrum antibiotics while cultures are pending, since bacterial infections are frequently a causative factor in adrenal crises.
g. Once the patient has stabilized, hydrocortisone, 10–20 mg p.o., may be ordered q6h and reduced to a satisfactory maintenance level.
    i. Most patients require a b.i.d. regimen of 10–20 mg p.o. in the morning and 5–10 mg p.o. in the evening.
h. Treat underlying cause.

References

1. Baker, K.L., Hardwick, D.F., & Agana-Defensor, R. (1999). Endocrine anatomy and physiology. In L. Bucher & S. Melander (Eds.), *Critical care nursing* (pp. 603–611).

2. Betterle, C. Volpato, M., Rees Smith, B., Furmaniak, J., Chen, S., Zanchetta, R., Greggio, N.A., Pedini, B., Boscaro, M., & Prescotto, F. (1997). Adrenal cortex and steroid 21-hydroxylase autoantibodies in children with organ-specific autoimmune disease: Markers of high progression to clinical Addison's disease. *Journal of Clinical Endocrinology and Metabolism, 82*, 939–942.

3. Denner, A.G. (1996). Adrenal crisis. In S.D. Melander (Ed.), *Review of critical care nursing: Case studies and applications* (pp. 279–282). Philadelphia, W.B. Saunders.

4. Derex, L., Giraud, P., Hanss, M., Riche, H., Nighoghossian, N., & Trouillas, P. (1998). Spontaneous intracerebral hemorrhage revealing Addison's disease. *Cerebrovascular Disease, 8*, 240–243.

5. DiGregorio, G.J., & Barbieri, E.J. (1998). *Handbook of commonly prescribed drugs* (13th ed.). West Chester, PA: Medial Surveillance, Inc.

6. Ferri, F.F. (Ed.). (1999). *Ferri's clinical advisor*. St. Louis, Mosby.

7. Fitzgerald, P.A. (2000). Endocrinology. In L.M. Tarn, S.J. McPhee, & M.A. Papadakis (Eds.), *Current medical diagnosis & treatment* (39th ed.) (pp. 1079–1151). Stamford, CT: Appleton & Lange.

8. Gill, G.N. (1996). Endocrine and reproductive diseases. In J.C. Bennett & F. Plum (Eds.), *Cecil textbook of medicine* (pp. 1176–1350). Philadelphia, W.B. Saunders.

9. Kellerman, R., & Gerstberger, M. (1999). Addison's disease. In M.R. Dambro (Ed.), *Griffith's 5 minute clinical consultant* (pp. 12–13). Philadelphia, Lippincott, Williams & Wilkins.

10. Kendall, J., & Loriaux, D.L. (1998). Disorders of the adrenal cortex. In J.H. Stein (Ed.), *Internal medicine* (pp. 1817–1826). St. Louis, Mosby.

11. Kenderseki, A., Micic, D., Sumarac, M., Zoric, S., Macut, D., Colic, M., Skaro-Millic, A., & Bogdanovich, Z. (1999). White Addison's disease: What is the possible cause? *Journal of Endocrinology Investigation, 22*, 395–400.

12. Miller, S.K. (2000). Management of patient with endocrine disorders. *Acute care nurse practitioner certification review*. Potomac, MD: Health Leadership Associates.

13. Noble, J. (Ed.). (1998). *Primary care medicine*. St. Louis: Mosby.

14. Phornphutkul, C., Boney, C., Gruppuso, P.A. (1998). A novel presentation of Addison's disease: Hypoglycemia unawareness in an adolescent with insulin-dependent diabetes mellitus. *The Journal of Pediatrics, 132*, 882–884.

15. Thelan, L.A., Urden, L.D., Lough, M.E., & Stacy, K.M. (1998). *Critical care nursing: Diagnosis and management* (3rd ed.). St. Louis, Mosby.

16. Woolliscroft, J.O. (1996). *Handbook of current diagnosis & treatment*. Philadelphia, Mosby.

PHEOCHROMOCYTOMA

Thomas W. Barkley, Jr., DSN, RN, CS, ACNP

I. PHEOCHROMOCYTOMA

A. Definition/General comments[5, 9, 11, 12]

1. A rare but serious condition

   a. Results from excessive catecholamine release (norepinephrine and epinephrine), usually from an adrenal medullary tumor
   b. Characterized by paroxysmal or sustained hypertension

2. Tumors may also arise along the sympathetic nervous system chain as well as in the thorax, the bladder, and the brain.

B. Etiology/Incidence/Predisposing factors[1, 7]

1. Almost always caused by an adrenal medullary tumor, of which approximately 10% are malignant
2. Pheochromocytomas are found in less than 0.1% of hypertensive patients.
3. Familial causes account for approximately 10% of cases.

C. Subjective/Physical examination findings[6, 8, 10–12]

1. Hypertension, which may be labile
2. Hyperglycemia
3. Diaphoresis
4. Severe headache
5. Palpitations—Related to supraventricular tachycardia
6. Anxiety
7. Tachycardia
8. Tremor
9. Weight loss
10. Increased appetite
11. Nausea
12. Weakness
13. Dyspnea
14. Heat intolerance
15. Postural hypotension
16. Mild temperature elevation

D. Diagnostic/Laboratory findings[2, 3, 5, 6, 10–12]

1. Glycosuria may be present.
2. Hyperglycemia may be present.

3. Thyroid-stimulating hormone, T_4, free T_4, and T_3 levels are normal.
4. Assay of urinary catecholamines (total and fractionated), metanephrines, vanillylmandelic acid (VMA), and creatinine
   a. A 24-h urine collection is preferred, but an overnight collection may be sufficient.
   b. Results indicating pheochromocytoma have

   • Greater than 2.2 μg of metanephrine per mg of creatinine *AND*
   • More than 5.5 μg of VMA per mg of creatinine

   c. Be aware of numerous pharmacolgic agents, foods, disorders, and chemicals that may affect the tests for the disorder, including

   • Alcohol
   • Sympathomimetics
   • Vasodilators
   • Levodopa
   • Methylxanthines such as aminophylline
   • Various disease states, such as Guillain-Barré syndrome, hypoglycemia, quadriplegia, intracranial lesions, and acute psychosis, among others
   • Isoproterenol
   • Methyldopa
   • Lithium

5. Direct assay of epinephrine and norepinephrine in blood and urine

   a. Most sensitive test for patients manifesting paroxysmal hypertension
   b. High epinephrine levels are associated with tumors localized in the adrenal gland.

6. CT and/or MRI scan for localization of the pheochromocytoma

E. Management[4–8, 10, 11]

1. Surgery to remove tumor; usually, laparoscopy is used

   a. For acute treatment preoperatively, phentolamine (Regitine), 1–2 mg IV q5min until the patient becomes stabilized; then 1–5 mg IV q12–24h.
   b. For p.o. therapy, alpha-adrenergic blocking agents are indicated such as phenoxybenzamine (Dibenzyline), 10 mg p.o. q12h.
      i. Increase the dose for approximately 3 days until the hypertension is controlled.
      ii. Maintenance doses range from 40 to 120 mg every day.

c. Consider autotransfusion of 1–2 units of packed red blood cells 12 h preoperatively to reduce the risk of postoperative hypotension.

2. Postoperatively, monitor for

a. Hypotension from depleted catecholamines
b. Adrenal insufficiency if a large part of the gland is removed
c. Hemorrhage, because the adrenal gland is highly vascular
d. Check urinary catecholamine levels at 1–2 weeks postoperatively in case metastatic tumors exist.

References

1. Arshinoff, S. (1997). The many faces of pheochromocytoma. *Canadian Medical Association Journal, 157,* 1516.
2. Clarke, M.R., Weyant, R.J., Watson, C.G., & Carty, S.E. (1999). Prognostic markers in pheochromocytoma. *Human Pathology, 29,* 486–487.
3. Eisenhofer, G., Lenders, J.W., Linehan, W.M., Walther, M.M., Goldstein, D.S., & Keiser, H.R. (1999). Plasma normetanephrine and metanephrine for detecting pheochromocytoma in von Hippel-Lindau disease and multiple neoplasia type 2. *New England Journal of Medicine, 340,* 1872–1879.
4. Finkstedt, G., Gasser, R.W., Hofle, G., Lhotta, K., Kolle, D., Gschwendtner, A., & Janetschek, G. (1999). Pheochromocytoma and sub-clinical Cushing's syndrome during pregnancy: Diagnosis, medical pre-treatment and cure by laparoscopic unilateral adrenalectomy. *Journal of Endocroniological Investigation, 22,* 551–557.
5. Fitzgerald, P.A. (2000). Endocrinology. In L.M. Tierney, S.J. McPhee, & M.A. Papadakis, (Eds.), *Current medical diagnosis & treatment* (39th ed.) (pp. 1079–1151). Stamford, CT: Appleton & Lange.
6. Gill, G.N. (1996). Endocrine and reproductive diseases. In J.C. Bennett & F. Plum (Eds.), *Cecil textbook of medicine* (20th ed.) (pp. 1176–1350). Philadelphia, W.B. Saunders.
7. Inoue, K., Ohmori, K., & Nishimura, K. (1999). A case of pheochromocytoma detected by hypertensive crisis immediately after drip infusion urography. *Hinyokika Kiyo, 45,* 331–333.
8. Matthews, M.R., Al-kasspooles, M.F., Caruso, D.M., Phillips, B.J., Malone, J.M., & Canulla, M.V. (1999). Management of a trauma patient with incidental pheochromocytoma. *The Journal of Trauma, 46,* 738–740.
9. Miller, S.K. (2000). Management of patients with endocrine disorders. *Acute care nurse practitioner certification review.* Potomac, MD: Health Leadership Associates.
10. O'Conner, D.T. (1996). Adrenal medulla. In J.C. Bennett, & F. Plum, (Eds.), *Cecil textbook of medicine* (20th ed.) (pp. 1253–1257). Philadelphia, W.B. Saunders.
11. Walther, M.M., Keiser, H.R., & Lineham, W.M. (1999). Pheochromocytoma: Evaluation, diagnosis and treatment. *World Journal of Urology, 17,* 35–39.
12. Woolliscroft, J.O. (1996). *Handbook of current diagnosis & treatment.* Philadelphia, Mosby.

SYNDROME OF INAPPROPRIATE ANTIDIURETIC HORMONE

Thomas W. Barkley, Jr., DSN, RN, CS, ACNP

I. SYNDROME OF INAPPROPRIATE ANTIDIURETIC HORMONE (SIADH)

A. Definition/Etiology[2, 3, 11, 13]

1. A grouping of symptoms that occur from the secretion of antidiuretic hormone (ADH) independent of volume-dependent stimulation or osmolality
2. ADH is released either from the posterior pituitary gland or from malignant tumors and results in severe water retention despite a low serum osmolality.

B. Incidence/Predisposing factors/Etiology[5, 7, 10, 12, 15, 16]

1. Effects 1–2% of patients with cancer
2. Central nervous system disorders such as brain tumors, hemorrhages, head trauma including skull fractures, meningitis, Guillain-Barré syndrome, systemic lupus erythematosus
3. Chronic lung disease including chronic obstructive pulmonary disease and tuberculosis, bacterial pneumonia, aspergillosis, bronchiectasis
4. Malignancies such as bronchogenic, pancreatic, prostatic, and renal carcinoma, leukemia, malignant lymphoma
5. Pharmacologic agents that either increase ADH production or potentiate ADH action, such as antidepressants, NSAIDs, carbamazepine (Tegretol)
6. Other conditions, including AIDS, physiologic stress, and pain

C. Subjective/Physical examination findings[4–6, 8–10, 15, 16]

1. Neurologic changes from hyponatremia (mild headache to seizures)
2. Hypothermia may be present.
3. Concentrated urine (ADH stimulates kidneys to reabsorb water)
4. Decreased urinary output
5. Decreased deep tendon reflexes
6. Weight gain and edema
7. Vomiting and abdominal cramping
8. Thyroid, cardiac, renal, adrenal, and liver function are without disease.

D. Diagnostic/Laboratory findings[1, 3, 8, 9, 10, 14, 15]

1. Hyponatremia—yet the patient is euvolemic.
2. Decreased serum osomolality (<280 mOsm/kg)
3. Increased urine osmolality (>150 mOsm/kg)
4. Decreased BUN (<10 mg/dL)
5. Increased urine Na (>20 mEq/L)

E. Management[3, 8, 9, 14, 15]

1. Treat the underlying cause.
2. Symptomatic patients (usually when Na <120 mEq/L)

   a. Restrict water intake to approximately 500 mL/day.
   b. Increase serum Na only by 1–2 mEq/L/h within the first day of therapy to avoid potential demyelination of nerves, cerebral edema, and seizures.
   c. Rate of Na administration should be reduced to 0.5–1 mEq/L/h once neurologic deficits improve.
   d. Goal of therapy should be to reach a Na value of 125–130 mEq to avoid over correction.
   e. Hypertonic 3% saline with furosemide (Lasix), 0.5–1 mg/kg IV, is indicated in symptomatic patients.
      i. If furosemide is not administered with hypertonic saline to the euvolemic patient, Na levels will temporarily increase, yet excess sodium will be excreted.
   f. To determine the amount of 3% saline to administer:

      • Check a random urinary Na after furosemide diuresis has begun.
      • The excreted Na is replaced with 3% saline at 1–2 mL/kg/h, and then the infusion rate is adjusted based on urinary output and urinary sodium.

   g. Seizure precautions should be employed for any patient with a markedly low serum Na level.

3. Asymptomatic patients

   a. Restrict water intake to 800–1000 mL/day.
   b. Increase the serum Na approximately 0.5 mEq/L/h using normal saline (0.9%) IV with furosemide, 0.5–1 mg/kg, in patients with Na values <120 mEq/L.
   c. Replace urinary sodium as described in section E.2.f.
   d. Seizure precautions, as indicated
   e. Demeclocycline (Declomycin), 300–600 mg p.o. b.i.d.
      i. May be used in patients who cannot follow fluid restriction and/or in those who require additional treatment
      ii. Inhibits the effect of ADH in the kidneys
      iii. Note: May take 1–2 weeks for best effect
      iv. May increase the risk of renal failure

References

1. Bouman, W.P., Pinner, G., & Johnson, H. (1998). Incidence of selective serotonin reuptake inhibitor (SSRI)-induced hyponatraemia due to the syndrome of inappropriate antidiuretic hormone (SIADH) secretion in the elderly. *Internation Journal of Geriatric Psychiatry, 13,* 12–15.
2. Caruthers, B. (1997). Diabetes insipidus: An overview. *Surgical Technologist, 29,* 41–43.
3. Demura, R. (1999). The role of antidiuretic hormone in hyponatremia in adrenal insufficiency—Is the guideline for the diagnosis of syndrome of inappropriate secretion of the antidiuretic hormone appropriate? *Internal Medicine, 38,* 426–432.
4. Farmer, B. (1996). Syndrome of inappropriate antidiuretic hormone. In S.D. Melander (Ed.), *Review of critical care nursing: Case studies and applications* (pp. 295–304). Philadelphia, W.B. Saunders.
5. Ferri, F.F. (Ed.). (1999). *Ferri's clinical advisor.* St. Louis, Mosby
6. Fitzgerald, P.A. (2000). Endocrinology. In L.M. Tierney, S.J. McPhee, & M.A. Papadakis (Eds.), *Current medical diagnosis & treatment* (39th ed.) (pp. 1079–1151). Stamford, CT: Appleton & Lange.
7. Girault, C., Richard, J.C., Chevron, C., Goulle, J.P., Droy, J.M., Bonmarchand, G., & Leroy, J. (1997). Syndrome of inappropriate secretion of antidiuretic hormone in two elderly women with elevated serum fluoxetine. *Journal of Toxicology-Clinical Toxicology, 35,* 93–95.
8. Heater, D.W. (1999a). If ADH goes out of balance: Diabetes insipidus. *RN, 62,* 44–46.
9. Heater, D.W., (1999b). If ADH goes out of balance: SIADH. *RN, 62,* 47–50.
10. Kamoe, L., Kurokawa, K.H., Kasai, H., Mazusawa, A., Ebe, T., Sasaki, H., Matuzuki, Y., Seino, Y., Takahashi, M., Togashi, K., Miyamura, H., Sato, Y., & Kaneko, H. (1998). Aymptomatic hyponatemia due to inappropriate secretion of antidiuretic hormone as the first sign of a small cell lung cancer in an elderly man. *Internal Medicine, 37,* 907–908.
11. Kokko, J.P. (1996). Disorders of fluid volume, electrolyte, and acid-base balance. In J.C. Bennett & F. Plum (Eds.), *Cecil textbook of medicine* (20th ed.) (pp. 533–538). Philadelphia: W.B. Saunders.
12. Lieh-Lai, M.W., Stanitski, D.F., Sarnaik, A.P., Uy, H., Rossio, N.F. Simpson, P.M., & Stanitski, C.L. (1999). Syndrome of inappropraite antidiuretic hormone secretion in children following spinal fusion. *Critical Care Medicine, 27,* 622–627.
13. Miller, S.K. (2000). Management of patients with endocrine disorders. *Acute care nurse practitioner certification review.* Potomac, MD: Health Leadership Associates.
14. Noble, J. (Ed.). (1998). *Primary care medicine.* St. Louis: Mosby.
15. Okuda, T., Kurokawa, K., & Papadakis, M.A. (1999). Fluid and electrolyte disorders. In L.M. Tierney, S.J. McPhee, & M.A. Papadakis (Eds.), *Current medical diagonsis & treatment* (38th ed.) (pp. 840–843). Stamford, CT: Appleton & Lange.
16. Sterns, R.H. (1999). The syndrome of inappropriate antidiuretic hormone secretion of unknown origin. *American Journal of Kidney Diseases, 33,* 161–163.

DIABETES INSIPIDUS

Thomas W. Barkley, Jr., DSN, RN, CS, ACNP

I. DIABETES INSIPIDUS (DI)[1, 4, 8, 9]

A. Definition

1. A syndrome occurring from a deficiency of or insensitivity to antidiuretic hormone (ADH), resulting in volume depletion secondary to the inability to concentrate urine
2. Three types

    a. Central (neurogenic)—Deficiency of ADH production or release
    b. Nephrogenic—Renal insensitivity to ADH
    c. Psychogenic

B. Incidence/Predisposing factors[2, 3, 9]

1. Central—Due to damage to the hypothalamus or the pituitary that results in a deficiency of ADH production or release

    a. Idiopathic
    b. Trauma
    c. More commonly seen with neurosurgical patients
        i. Brain tumors
        ii. Intracranial hemorrhage
        iii. Aneurysms
        iv. Pituitary tumors
    d. Infections
        i. Meningitis
        ii. Tuberculosis
        iii. Syphillis
    e. Anoxic encephalopathy
    f. Vasopressinase-induced
        i. Seen in the puerperium and last trimester of pregnancy
        ii. Associated with preeclampsia or liver dysfunction

2. Nephrogenic—Due to a defect in the renal tubules that results in renal insensitivity to ADH, thereby interfering with water reabsorption; unresponsive to vasopressin

    a. Familial X-linked trait
    b. Renal disease (e.g., acquired via pyelonephritis or a defect in the renal tubules)

c. Chronic hypokalemia or hypocalcemia
d. Certain medications may induce nephrogenic DI, e.g.,
  i. Lithium
  ii. Methicillin

3. Psychogenic—Refer to specialist.

C. Subjective/Physical examination findings[4-6, 10]

1. May be physically asymptomatic (with central DI) OR
2. Changes in level of consciousness
3. Thirst (extreme) with cravings for ice water; the patient may report 5–20 L/day of fluid intake.
4. Hypotension
5. Tachycardia
6. Increased urinary output (2–20 L/24 h)
7. Nocturia may be present
8. Low urine specific gravity (<1.006)
9. Poor turgor
10. Elevated temperature/fever
11. Other findings indicative of the underlying cause

D. Diagnostic/Laboratory findings[3-5, 10]

1. Although less commonly used today, 24-h urine collection:

  a. Polyuria (output >300 mL/h)
  b. Urine hyposomolality (dilute and odorless)
  c. Check glucose and creatinine as well.

2. Serum levels of glucose, BUN, potassium, sodium, and calcium should be monitored frequently.
3. Hypernatremia
4. Severe dehydration
5. If central DI is suspected, a vasopressin (desmopressin) challenge test should be ordered.

  a. Desmopressin acetate, 0.05–0.1 mL (5–10 μg) intranasally, or 1 μg SC or IV, is administered.
  b. Urine volume is measured 12 h before and after the administration.
  c. Sodium levels are checked for hyponatremia.
  d. If the response is questionable or marginal, the dose is doubled.
  e. Patients with central DI have a *positive* test result (i.e., thirst markedly decreases as well as polyuria; sodium usually remains normal).
  f. The test result is *negative* in patients with nephrogenic DI (i.e., there is no improvement in the patient's clinical condition).

6. If the cause remains unclear, MRI may be used to assess for a mass/lesion.

E. Management[3-5, 7]

1. Fluid replacement
2. For central DI, desmopressin (DDAVP, exogenous ADH) should be used—It increases water reabsorption by the kidneys and also has vasoconstrictive properties.

   a. Desmopressin (100 μg/mL solution), 0.05–0.10 mL q12–24h intranasally; the dose may then be individualized, OR
   b. Desmopressin (4 μg/mL), 1–4 μg IV, IM, or SC q12–24h, OR
   c. Desmopressin (0.1- or 0.2-mg tablets), 0.1 mg every day, increased to a maximum dose of 0.2 mg q8h

3. Reduce aggravating factors such as corticosteroids (increase water clearance) to improve polyuria.
4. Hydrocholorothiazide, 50–100 mg/day with a potassium supplement, may be ordered for both central and nephrogenic DI.
5. Chlorpropamide (Diabinese) may be used to decrease thirst sensation in patients with continued hypernatremia. Note: Chlorpropamide may cause hypoglycemia.
6. Nephrogenic DI may be managed with a combination of indomethacin-hydrochloride, indomethacin-desmopressin, or indomethacin-amiloride. Acutely, 50 mg of indomethacin q8h is usually effective.

References

1. Calvo, B., Bilbao, J.R., Rodriguez, A., & Castano, L. (1999). Molecular analysis in familial neurohypophyseal diabetes insipidus: Early diagnosis of an asymptomatic carrier. *Journal of Clinical Endocrinology and Metabolism, 84*, 3351–3354.
2. Coufal, F., Linarello, L., James, H.E., & Krous, H. (1998). Suprasellar germinoma associated with Cushing's disease and diabetes insipidus in a child. *Pediatric Neurosurgery, 29*, 19–22.
3. Ferri, F.F. (Ed.). (1999). *Ferri's clinical advisor*. St. Louis: Mosby.
4. Fitzgerald, P.A. (2000). Endocrinology. In L.M. Tierney, S.J. McPhee, & M.A. Papadakis (Eds.), *Current medical diagnosis & treatment* (39th ed.) (pp. 1079–1151). Stamford, CT: Appleton & Lange.
5. Heater, D.W. (1999). If ADH goes out of balance: Diabetes insipidus. *RN, 62*, 42–46.
6. Krumberger, J.M., & Waite, L.G. (1997). Endocrine alterations. In J.C. Hartshorn, M.L. Sole, & M.L. Lamborn (Eds.), *Introduction to critical care nursing* (2nd ed.) (pp. 473–521). Philadelphia: W.B. Saunders.
7. Noble, J. (Ed.). (1998). *Primary care medicine*. St. Louis: Mosby.
8. Phatouros, C.C., Higashida, R.T., Malek, A.M., Smith, W.S., Dowd, C.F., & Halbach, V.V. (1999). Embolization of the meningohypophyseal trunk as a cause of diabetes insipidus. *American Journal of Neuroradiology, 20*, 1115–1118.
9. Thelan, L.A., Urden, L.D., Lough, M.E., & Stacy, K.M. (1998). *Critical care nursing: Diagnosis and management* (3rd ed.). St. Louis: Mosby.
10. Woolliscroft, J.O. (1996). *Handbook of current diagnosis & treatment*. Philadelphia: Mosby.

Management of Patients with Musculoskeletal Disorders

ARTHRITIS

Colleen R. Walsh, MSN, RN, ONC,
CS, ACNP

I. OSTEOARTHRITIS

A. Definition[2–4, 6, 8, 12]

1. Osteoarthritis (OA) is a progressive joint disorder characterized by slow destruction of the normal collagen architecture followed by attempts of chondrocytes to produce replacement articular cartilage of joint surfaces.
2. OA is classified as noninflammatory, although inflammatory changes occur due to synovial response to reactive new bone formation.
3. OA is classified as either primary or secondary.

B. Etiology/Incidence/Predisposing factors[1–4, 6–11]

1. Thought to be "wear and tear" syndrome; 16 million affected in the United States
2. People >60 years of age have a 60% chance of developing OA.
3. Both sexes are affected equally between the ages of 45 and 55.

   a. After age 55, women are more likely to be affected.
   b. Black women have twice the incidence of white women.

4. Men have more OA in hips; women have OA more in hands and fingers.
5. Some evidence suggests OA may be genetically inherited as an autosomal recessive trait.
6. Increased age
7. Metabolic abnormalities, such as Paget's disease
8. Height and weight, such as abnormal height or increased weight-to-height ratio (i.e., obesity)
9. Mechanical stressors, such as repetitive microtrauma associated with sports injuries, ballet dancing, repetitive physical tasks
10. Prior trauma, especially sprains, dislocations, and fractures
11. Genetic/congenital, such as congenital hip dysplasia; increased incidence of Heberden's nodules in OA in distal interphalangeal (DIP) joint caused by a single gene that has not yet been identified
12. Chemicals, such as organic or heavy metals that stimulate cartilage injuring enzyme activity

13. Neurologic disorders, such as diabetic neuropathy, Charcot's, neuropathic joints
14. Hematologic/endocrine disorders, such as hemochromatosis and acromegaly

C. Subjective findings[2–4, 6, 8, 9, 12, 13]

1. Pain in one or more joints, usually weight bearing, such as hips and knees, but also central and peripheral joints such as fingers, hands, wrists
2. Stiffness of affected joints after prolonged sitting that quickly dissipates upon arising; ''grating'' sensation during any range of motion (ROM); usually worsens as day progresses
3. Feeling of instability, locking or buckling of the knees, especially when climbing or descending stairs

D. Physical findings[2–4, 6, 9, 12, 14, 15]

1. Bony induration or enlargement of affected joints; some may have effusions with warmth and redness
2. Heberden's nodules—enlargements on DIP joints
3. Bouchard's nodules—enlargements on proximal interphalangeal (PIP) joints
4. Angular deformities of affected joints (valgus and varus), especially the knees
5. Limited ROM with palpable/audible crepitus
6. Pain on palpation of the joint line

E. Laboratory/Diagnostic findings[3, 4, 6, 9, 13, 16, 18]

1. Plain x-rays show narrowing of joint space with cyst formations.
2. Anteroposterior and lateral knee films should be taken bilaterally and standing to detect and measure degrees of varus/valgus deformity if they exist.
3. Synovial fluid analysis demonstrates clear, yellow fluid with normal white blood cell (WBC) count ($<1000/mm^3$) and glucose levels that approximate patient's serum glucose.
4. No laboratory test is specific for OA; complete blood count and biochemical panel should be drawn to detect any hematologic and/or renal impairment when considering therapy with nonsteroidal anti-inflammatory drugs (NSAIDs).
5. Bone scan, magnetic resonance imaging, and computed tomography should be considered if there is question of infection or spur formations, or if compression of soft tissue structure is suspected.

F. Management[1–4, 6, 7, 12, 13]

1. Goals
   a. Relieve symptoms.
   b. Maintain or improve function.

   c. Limit disability as much as possible.
   d. Avoid drug toxicity.

2. Multidisciplinary team approach is best
3. Weight reduction if applicable
4. Rest and joint protection: May require occupational therapy consultation
5. Heat and cold therapy; physical therapy evaluation
6. Aspirin (ASA), 650 mg p.o. q.i.d. as initial therapy
7. Acetaminophen, 650 mg p.o. t.i.d. if ASA-allergic
8. Intra-articular joint injection: Hyaluronic acid, a disaccharide that is the major component of the proteoglycan aggregates needed for functioning of cartilage, is injected weekly for 3 weeks into affected joint and can provide pain relief with increased ROM

   a. Sodium hyaluronate (Hyalgan)
   b. Hylan G-F (Synvisc)

9. NSAIDs

   a. Act by inhibiting the enzyme cyclooxygenase (COX), which is required for the synthesis of prostaglandins and thromboxanes.
      i. Two isoforms have been identified: COX-1 and COX-2.
      ii. COX-1 is thought to be found tissue-wide and is thought to protect gastric mucosa.
      iii. COX-2 is mainly induced at the inflammation site.
   b. Older NSAIDs act by blocking both COX isoforms, leading to possible gastric ulceration. COX-2 drugs are selective, thus providing more gastric protection.
      i. Rofecoxib (Vioxx), 12.5–25 mg p.o. q.d.
      ii. Celecoxib (Celebrex), 100–200 mg p.o. q.d.

       • Concurrent use of zafirlukast, fluconazole, and fluvastatin may increase serum concentration of celecoxib.

   c. See Tables 54–1 and 54–2 for comparison list of NSAIDs.

10. Glucosamine: Over-the-counter preparation sold as a nutritional supplement in the United States. At this time, no long-term studies have been conducted to demonstrate that it helps with OA, and since it increases insulin resistance, it should not be used in persons with Type 2 diabetes
11. Surgical options: Refer to orthopedist for definitive surgical treatment.

   a. Total joint replacement
   b. Arthrotomy/arthroscopy for joint debridement
   c. Osteotomy

Text continued on page 500

TABLE 54-1. PHARMACOLOGIC MANAGEMENT OF RHEUMATOID ARTHRITIS

DRUG	DOSE	SIDE EFFECTS	NURSING CONSIDERATIONS
Salicylates Aspirin: plain, buffered enteric-coated	1000–6000 mg/d in 2–4 divided doses Increase dosage by 1–2 tablets/d until tinnitus develops; then decrease by 1–2 tablets/d until tinnitus stops	Salicylism (tinnitus, nausea, vomiting, drowsiness) GI irritation and bleeding	Give with milk, food, or antacid Consider use of enteric-coated tablets for high-risk persons Enteric-coated tablets should not be crushed or taken with milk Teach patients to report black tarry stools Keep salicylate levels between 15 and 25 mg/dL Instruct patients to report tinnitus so dose can be adjusted Hearing disorders from high-dose aspirin are usually reversible within 24 h by decreasing dose Use aspirin carefully in hearing-impaired older adults. They may fail to notice changes in hearing (fullness, tinnitus, muffled sounds)

Nonacetylated Salicylates

Drug	Dose	Adverse Effects	Considerations
Magnesium salicylate (Magan)	1500–4000 mg/d in 2–4 divided doses	Salicylism	Sodium-free Monitor serum magesium levels if high doses are used in patients with renal failure
Diflunisal (Dolobid)	500–1500 mg/d in 2 divided doses	CNS effects, tinnitus, GI disturbances (nausea, vomiting) Hypersensitivity syndrome	Full anti-inflammatory effects may not occur for several weeks in some persons Not hydrolyzed to salicylate in body, so serum salicylate levels cannot be used to guide therapy Instruct patient to report eye problems immediately to physician. Severe eye complications have been reported
Meclofenamate sodium (Meclomen)	200–400 mg/d in 4 divided doses	Severe diarrhea (dose related), GI distress, edema, CNS effects	Instruct patient to report weight gains greater than 3–4 lb/wk Monitor patients with renal impairment closely because drug is excreted primarily by kidneys Not generally used as initial drug because of GI side effects

Table continued on following page

TABLE 54–1. PHARMACOLOGIC MANAGEMENT OF RHEUMATOID ARTHRITIS *Continued*

DRUG	DOSE	SIDE EFFECTS	NURSING CONSIDERATIONS
Nonsteroidal Anti-inflammatory Agents (NSAIDs)		GI irritation, fluid retention/edema, diarrhea, interstitial nephritis, CNS changes (dizziness, blurred vision, headaches), hematologic changes, bone marrow depression, prolonged bleeding time, skin reactions/rashes	NSAIDs are generally better tolerated that acetylsalicylic acid Therapeutic response may not be seen for up to 2 wk Instruct patients to drive with caution until response to drug is known Give with milk, food, or a full glass of water Teach patients to report GI distress (heartburn, dyspepsia, nausea, vomiting, abdominal pain) Monitor baseline hematologic, renal, liver, auditory, and ophthalmic functions. Repeat periodically if patient is on high doses of NSAIDs Instruct patient to report increased bleeding, severe pruritus, weight gain over 5 lb/wk, persistent headaches, blurred vision Instruct patient to avoid alcohol because of increased risk of GI toxicity

Indoles Indomethacin (Indocin)	50–200 mg/d in 2–4 doses	High incidence of adverse reactions in elderly patients	Effective for short-term treatment of active synovitis Single evening dose may be used for severe morning stiffness
Sulindac (Clinoril)	300–400 mg/d in 2 divided doses	Retinal damage with long-term use	Tablet can be safely crushed for those with impaired swallowing Teach patient to report any changes in vision Patients should have ophthalmoscopic examination before beginning therapy
Tolmetin (Tolectin)	800–1600 mg/d in 4–6 doses	See NSAIDs; also, higher incidence of mild edema, hypertension	Tablets can be crushed (or capsules may be opened) and mixed with food Monitor blood pressure, weight, presence of edema
Proprionic Acid Derivatives Ibuprofen (Motrin)	1200–3200 mg/d in 3–6 doses	See NSAIDs; also, amblyopia, blurred vision, reduced visual fields	Food slows absorption; best given on an empty stomach Patients with visual disturbances should have complete ophthalmoscopic examinations

Table continued on following page

TABLE 54–1. PHARMACOLOGIC MANAGEMENT OF RHEUMATOID ARTHRITIS *Continued*

DRUG	DOSE	SIDE EFFECTS	NURSING CONSIDERATIONS
Naproxen (Naprosyn)	250–1500 mg/d in 2 doses	See NSAIDs	Visual disturbances usually disappear when drug is discontinued Best absorption occurs when taken on an empty stomach 30 min before meals or 2 h after meals Give with milk or food if patient has GI distress
Fenoprofen (Nalfon)	1200–3200 mg/d in 3–4 divided doses	See NSAIDs	Peak effect of drug is not often seen for 2 wk
Ketoprofen (Orudis)	100–400 mg/d in 3–4 doses	See NSAIDs	Dosage should be decreased by one-half in elderly patients or those with renal failure
Oxicams Piroxican (Feldene)	20 mg/d (1 dose)	Higher incidence of GI bleeding	Long half-life permits daily dose Adverse side effects may be delayed 7–10 d after starting therapy Instruct patient to take missed dose if discovered 8 h before next dose is due. Otherwise, patient should omit dose

Drug	Dose	Side/Adverse Effects	Nursing Considerations
Pyrazoles			
Phenylbutazone (Butazolidin)	200–800 mg/d in 1–4 doses	Bone marrow depression and blood dyscrasias, skin rash, dizziness, fluid retention	Drug is usually discontinued if effectiveness is not noted within 1 wk Significant hematologic changes can occur during or after therapy Instruct patient in importance of follow-up laboratory work
Oxyphenbutazone (Tandearil)	400–600 mg/d in divided doses	GI distress (reactivation of peptic ulcer), bone marrow depression, anemia, agranulocytosis	Monitor CBC before beginning therapy Monitor weight and peripheral edema
Antimalarials			
Hydroxychloroquine (Plaquenil)	200–400 mg/d (maintenance dose)	Retinal or visual field changes, CNS (vertigo, headaches, confusion), blood dyscrasias, skin rash, pruritus, skeletal muscle weakness, GI distress	Give with food or milk to decrease GI distress Schedule patient for baseline and every-3-mo ophthalmoscopic examinations and blood counts Instruct patient to report any visual changes, unexplained bruising or bleeding, skin eruptions or weakness Inform patient that full effectiveness of drug may not be seen for 6 mo

Table continued on following page

TABLE 54–1. PHARMACOLOGIC MANAGEMENT OF RHEUMATOID ARTHRITIS *Continued*

DRUG	DOSE	SIDE EFFECTS	NURSING CONSIDERATIONS
Chloroquine (Aralen)	20 mg/d (1 dose)	See Hydroxychloroquine	Instruct patient to avoid driving until response to drug is known Inform patient that drug can cause urine to be rusty yellow or brown
Gold Compounds Gold sodium thiomalate (Myochrysine) Aurothioglucose (Solganal)	*Initial intramuscular dose:* 10 mg/wk *Second dose:* 25 mg/wk *Subsequent doses:* 25–50 mg/wk until total dose administered is 0.5–1 g With improvement, maintenance doses are 25–50 mg q2wk for up to 20 wk, then 25–50 mg q3–4wk	*Major:* blood dyscrasias, renal impairment, proteinuria, dermatitis Also, CNS effects (sweating, flushing, dizziness), GI effects (metallic taste, stomatitis, nausea, vomiting, diarrhea, hepatitis)	Gold sodium thiomalate is water based; aurothioglucose is oil based Gold is usually given with NSAIDs until improvement is seen Baseline blood counts and urinalyses are essential, followed by periodic monitoring Analyze urine for hematuria/proteinuria before each injection Teach patient to report early signs of toxicity: rash, pruritus, stomatitis, metallic taste. Drug is usually discontinued if these appear

			Monitor for allergic reactions, which can occur at any time during therapy
			Give deep into gluteus muscle
			Instruct patient to remain flat for 30 min postinjection to avoid dizziness, sweating, flushing
Auranofin (Ridaura)	6–9 mg/d in 2–3 divided doses	See intramuscular gold; also, diarrhea (dose related), cough, dyspnea	Administer with food/fluids
			Instruct patients with diarrhea to increase fiber. An antidiarrheal agent may be useful
			Inform patient that benefits are not often seen for 3–4 mo
			Assess for jaundice, unexplained bleeding, mouth ulcers, metallic taste, unexplained cough, dyspnea
			Instruct patients to avoid the sun because pruritus and dermatitis appear to be related to sun exposure
Third-Level Agents (Disease-Modifying Drugs)			
Penicillamine (Cuprimine, Depen)	250–750 mg/d	Thrombocytopenia, leukopenia, nephrotic syndrome, skin reactions, GI upset, altered taste	Monitor CBC, liver function, urine, and platelets weekly for 8–10 wk, then monthly

Table continued on following page

TABLE 54–1. PHARMACOLOGIC MANAGEMENT OF RHEUMATOID ARTHRITIS *Continued*

DRUG	DOSE	SIDE EFFECTS	NURSING CONSIDERATIONS
			Give on empty stomach (30 min before meals or 2 h after meals)
			Instruct patient to report fever, sore throat, chills, bruising, bleeding
Methotrexate	7.5–40 mg/wk (either single dose or 3 separate doses 8–12 h apart)	Bone marrow suppression, ulcerative stomatitis, GI upset (diarrhea, nausea, vomiting), alopecia, cirrhosis/hepatotoxicity	Instruct patient to refrain from alcohol because it increases drug-associated hepatotoxicity
			Monitor hepatic and renal function every week
			Teach patient to report mouth sores and inflamed gums
Azathioprine (Imuran)	Minimum: 1 mg/kg/d Maximum: 2.5 mg/kg/d	Bone marrow depression, blood dyscrasias, bladder toxicity, GI disturbance, dermatitis, alopecia, altered immunity (susceptibility to infection)	Monitor blood work and urinalyses weekly
			Give drug in divided doses to decrease nausea and GI upset
			Inform women of childbearing age of need to use contraceptives. Drug is highly toxic to fetus
			Instruct patient to avoid persons with colds. Report signs of infection (chills, fever, sore throat), which

		could indicate agranulocytosis Therapeutic effects are not usually seen for 6–8 wk
Corticosteroids Hydrocortisone (Cortef) Prednisolone (Delta-Cortef) Prednisone (Deltasone)	Highly individualized, but as low a dose as possible. Doses generally range between 2.5 and 7.5 mg/d or every other day (low-dose therapy)	Osteoporosis, fractures, avascular necrosis, gastric ulcers, susceptibility to infection, hyperglycemia, hypertension, cataracts, glaucoma, thinning of skin, hirsutism, acne, moon face, edema, menstrual disorders, emotional lability	Give entire daily dose between 6:00 AM and 8:00 AM when natural steroid levels are lowest Doses should be tapered as soon as patient's condition permits Instruct patients not to stop drug abruptly Monitor elderly patients carefully because they are at much higher risk for side effects (fluid retention, elevated blood pressure, peripheral edema) Teach patients to avoid sources of infection Avoid use of tape on skin Handle patient gently to prevent bruises, skin tears

GI, Gastrointestinal; CNS, central nervous system; CBC, complete blood count. (From Holmes, S.B. [1998]. Autoimmune and inflammatory disorders. In A.B. Maher, S.W. Salmond, & T.A. Pellino [Eds.], *Orthopaedic nursing* [2nd ed.] [pp. 368–371]. Philadelphia: W.B. Saunders, with permission.)

TABLE 54-2. EXPERIMENTAL DRUG THERAPY IN RHEUMATOID ARTHRITIS

DRUG	DESCRIPTION	COMMENTS
Alkylating agents	Highly potent suppressors of immune function. Alkylating agents were derived from sulfur mustard gases used in World War I and II. Their primary mode of action is the alkylation of nucleic acids, which results in inactivation of DNA. The formation of electrophilic bonds leads to crosslinking and abnormal base pairing, thus preventing DNA replication	Beneficial in patients with severe refractory disease

Cyclophosphamide (Cytoxan)	Has antineoplastic, alkylating, and immunosuppressive actions. Suppresses cell-mediated and humoral immunity	Usual oral dose: 50–150 mg/d
		Usual IV dose: 0.5–2 mg/kg/d
		Dosage decreased in renal failure
		IV boluses every 3–4 wk appear to be the least toxic
		Clinical response may not be seen for 3–6 mo
		Many toxicities and adverse effects:
		  GI—nausea, vomiting, diarrhea, hepatotoxicity
		  GU—hemorrhagic cystitis, nephrotoxicity
		  Metabolic—hyperkalemia, weight gain
		  Hematologic—thrombocytopenia, leukopenia, neutropenia, interference with wound healing
		  Other—dizziness, facial flushing, secondary neoplasms, pulmonary emboli, alopecia, nail changes

Agent	Description
Mechlorethamine (nitrogen mustard, Mustargen)	Usually given in daily IV doses of 1–3 mg Drug is powerful vesicant: Use great care to avoid extravasation or direct contact with skin Major dose-limited toxicities are bone marrow suppression, nausea, and vomiting Other adverse effects include alopecia, diarrhea, stomatitis, and sterility
Chlorambucil (Leukeran)	Considered the least toxic and slowest acting of the alkylating agents Not widely used in the United States Usual dose is 4–12 mg/d Higher risk for development of leukemia Has milder incidence of nausea and vomiting
Sulfasalazine (SASP)	A sulfonamide thought to be converted by the intestines to sulfapyridine (an antibacterial agent) and 5-aminosalicylic acid (an anti-inflammatory agent) Developed in late 1940s to treat RA. Early trials comparing SASP to gold and salicylates showed that drug was not effective Current research reports drug has efficacy as a second-line agent May be more effective than gold Most common side effect is GI intolerance Slow acting; clinical effectiveness is not seen for up to 6 mo Dose varies from 500 mg/d to 2–3 g/d
Fish oil derivatives (omega-3 fatty acids) Cyclosporine	Inhibit the formation of prostaglandins and leukotrienes Directly inhibits T cell function Study indicates fish oil is moderately effective in treating RA Usual dose: 5–10 mg/kg/d Highly toxic to kidneys
Combination agents	Several second-line and third-line therapy combinations have been tried Combination studies under investigation include oral plus IM gold, hydroxychloroquine and methotrexate, oral gold and methotrexate azathioprine and methotrexate

See alkylating agents

IV, Intravenous; GI, gastrointestinal; GU, genitourinary; RA, rheumatoid arthritis; IM, intramuscular. (From Holmes, S.B. [1998]. Autoimmune and inflammatory disorders. In A.B. Maher, S.W. Solmond, & T.A. Pellino [Eds.], *Orthopaedic nursing* [2nd ed.] [p. 372]. Philadelphia, W.B. Saunders, with permission.)

   d. Autogenous cartilage implantation and osteochondral
      grafting

II. RHEUMATOID ARTHRITIS

A. Definition[5–8, 10, 11, 14]

1. Rheumatoid arthritis (RA) is a chronic, systemic autoimmune
   disease of unknown etiology that causes inflammation of connective tissue.
2. Synovium of joints is primarily affected first, then spreads to
   articular cartilage, tendons, ligaments, and other soft tissues
   including renal, cardiovascular, hematopoietic, and pulmonary structures.

B. Etiology/Incidence/Predisposing factors[5, 6, 8, 10, 11, 17]

1. Approximately 6 million people in the United States are affected; 75% are women; female to male ratio is 3 : 1. Two
   thirds of those affected have moderate to severe disease.
2. Cause is unknown; probably multifactorial, with genetic, environmental, hormonal, and reproductive components
3. Exposure to Epstein-Barr virus, bacteria, and mycoplasma
4. Autoimmune response in genetically predisposed individuals
   with defects in HLA-DR4, HLA-DQ, and HLA-DP areas of
   histocompatability complex
5. Decreased reproductive hormones after birth exacerbate
   disease.
6. The proinflammatory cytokine tumor necrosis factor-alpha
   (TNF-alpha) is thought to play a dominant role in the pathogenesis of RA.

C. Subjective findings[4–6, 8–11]

1. Symmetrical joint and muscle pain, which is usually worse in
   the morning and improves as the day progresses
2. Weakness, fatigue
3. Anorexia
4. Weight loss
5. Generalized malaise

D. Physical examination findings[5, 6, 9–11, 15]

1. Articular

   a. Swelling of joints with typical "boggy" feel on palpation.
      Most frequently seen in metacarpophalangeal (MCP)
      joints, wrists, and PIP joints
   b. Warmth and redness of skin over affected joints
   c. Multiple, symmetrical joint involvement
   d. Joint deformity, especially PIP, DIP, MCP of hands
   e. Multiple nodules on volar aspect of forearms

2. Extra-articular
   a. Pleural effusions
   b. Scleritis and episcleritis: Inflammation of the scleras and surrounding ophthalmologic structures
   c. Arteritis
   d. Pericarditis, conduction defects, myocarditis
   e. Splenomegaly (Felty's syndrome)
   f. Pulmonary nodules and fibrosis

E. Laboratory/Diagnostic studies[5, 6, 8, 9, 11, 18]

1. Granulocytopenia (Felty's syndrome): Neutrophil count $<500/\mu L$
2. Anemia (hypochromic, microcytic)

   a. Low hemoglobin count (normal: 14–18 g/dL in males and 12–16 g/dL in females)
   b. Low serum ferritin and low or normal total iron-binding capacity

3. May have positive rheumatoid factor, although nonspecific
4. Antinuclear antibody may be elevated.
5. Erythrocyte sedimentation rate is usually elevated
6. Radiographs demonstrate joint swelling, then progressive cortical thinning, osteopenia, joint space narrowing.

   • Radiographs of cervical spine are needed to detect cervical spine instability due to atlantoaxial (C1–C2) subluxation.

7. Synovial fluid: Yellow turbid fluid with friable mucin clot; elevated WBC up to $100,000/mm^3$; normal glucose
8. RA is a clinical diagnosis, not a laboratory or radiologic diagnosis.

F. Management[5, 6, 8–12, 17]

1. Multidisciplinary team approach is best.
2. "Traditional" stepwise pyramid for treatment of RA now has been rejected. Early diagnosis, referral, and treatment with disease modifying antirheumatic drugs (DMARDs) have been advocated.
3. Early referral to rheumatoligist is recommended.
4. DMARDs used in treatment of RA:

   a. Methotrexate, 5.0–7.5 mg on "pulse" schedule; i.e., Thursday, Friday, Saturday
      i. Implications: Monitor liver function studies with baseline tests and monitoring of AST, ALT, and albumin every 4–6 weeks.
   b. Cyclosporine (unlabeled use therapy)
      i. An immunomodulatory agent that blocks the production and release of several cytokines including interleukin-2.

    ii. Used for RA unresponsive to methotrexate and gold preparations.

    iii. Dose is usually 2.5 mg/kg/day and increased to 5 mg/kg/day.

    iv. Implications: May cause nephrotoxicity, which is dose dependent.

    v. Obtain baseline renal function measurements and monitor monthly.

c. Gold preparations: Auranofin, aurothioglucose, and aurothiomalate are parenteral preparations used for moderate to severe RA.

    i. Implications: Can cause serious side effects including thrombocytopenia, proteinuria, and hematuria

    ii. Drugs should be ordered and monitored by a rheumatologist.

d. Hydroxychloroquine: An antimalarial drug whose mechanism of action is unknown

    i. Implications: Low side effect profile, but one major possible side effect is retinal damage.

    ii. Patients should have baseline eye examination with follow-up exams every 6 months.

    iii. Drug should be ordered and monitored by a rheumatologist.

e. Sulfasalazine: Used for moderate RA, but mechanism of action is unknown; is used in combination with methotrexate and cyclosporine

    i. Implications: Major toxicities include leukopenia, thrombocytopenia, hemolysis agranulocytosis, aplastic anemia, and eosinophilic pneumonia.

    ii. Drug should be ordered and monitored by a rheumatologist.

f. Leflunomide: Mechanism of action is to disrupt T-cell proliferation and is indicated for moderate to severe RA. Loading dose of 100 mg p.o. for 3 days with recommended maintenance dose of 20 mg daily

    i. Implications: Can cause elevated liver enzymes; therefore, baseline followed by monthly, liver function tests should be done until levels are stable

    ii. Drug should be ordered and monitored by a rheumatologist.

g. Etanercept: Acts by inhibiting the binding of both TNF-alpha and TNF-beta to the cell-surface TNF receptor. Can be used in conjunction with methotrexate and other DMARDs. Dose is 25 mg SC twice weekly

    i. Implications: Low toxicity profile with upper respiratory tract symptoms, such as cough, rhinitis, sinusitis, and pharyngitis.

    ii. Drug must be given subcutaneously.

h. See Table 54–1 for NSAIDs.

5. Physical/occupational therapy for assistive devices and durable medical equipment
6. Surgery: Refer to orthopedist
   a. Arthrotomy/arthroscopy for joint debridement
   b. Osteotomy
   c. Total joint replacement; hand joint replacements

References

1. Anonymous. (1999). Rofecoxib for osteoarthritis and pain. *Medical Letter on Drugs and Therapeutics, 41*, 59–61.
2. Adams, M.E. (1999). Hype about glucosamine. *The Lancet, 354*, 353–354.
3. Altizer, L.L. (1998). Degenerative disorders. In A.B. Maher, S.W. Salmond, & T.A. Pellino (Eds.), *Orthopaedic nursing* (2nd ed.) (pp. 480–544). Philadelphia: W.B. Saunders.
4. Apgar, B. (1999). Celecoxib for patients with arthritis and osteoarthritis. *American Family Physician, 60*, 296.
5. Arriola, E.R., & Le, N.P. (1999). Treatment advances in rheumatoid arthritis. *Western Journal of Medicine, 170*, 278–281.
6. Brashers, V.L. (1998). *Clinical application of pathophysiology: Assessment, diagnostic reasoning and management.* St. Louis: Mosby.
7. Bryant, G.G. (1998). Modalities for immobilization. In A.B. Maher, S.W. Salmond, & T.A. Pellino (Eds.), *Orthopaedic nursing* (2nd ed.) (pp. 296–322). Philadelphia: W.B. Saunders.
8. Holmes, S.B. (1998). Autoimmune and inflammatory disorders. In A.B. Maher, S.W. Salmond, & T.A. Pellino (Eds.), *Orthopaedic nursing* (2nd ed.). (pp. 480–544). Philadelphia: W.B. Saunders.
9. Irvine, S., Munro, R., & Porter, D. (1999). Early referral diagnosis, and treatment of rheumatoid arthritis: Evidence for changing medical practice. *Annals of the Rheumatic Diseases, 58*, 510–514.
10. Jarvis, C. (1996). *Physical examination and health assessment* (2nd ed.). Philadelphia: W.B. Saunders.
11. Kaplan, D. (1999). The latest approaches to rheumatoid arthritis treatment. *Patient Care, 33*, 69–73.
12. Klippel, J.H. (1997). *Primer on the rheumatic diseases* (11th ed.). Atlanta: The Arthritis Foundation.
13. LaPrade, R.F., & Swiontkowski, M.F. (1999). New horizons in the treatment of osteoarthritis of the knee. *Journal of the American Medical Association, 281*, 876–878.
14. Leslie, M. (1999). Hyaluronic acid treatment for osteoarthritis of the knee. *Nurse Practitioner, 24*, 38–42.
15. Mourad, L.A. (1998). Alteration of musculoskeletal function. In K.L. McCance, & S.E. Huether (Eds.), *Pathophysiology: The biological basis for disease in adults and children* (3rd ed.) (pp. 1435–1485). St. Louis: Mosby.
16. Moye, C.E. (1998). Diagnostic modalities for orthopaedic disorders. In A.B. Maher, S.W. Salmond, & T.A. Pellino (Eds.), *Orthopaedic nursing* (2nd ed.). Philadelphia: W.B. Saunders.
17. Schhadlich, H., Erman, J., Biskop, M., Falk, W., et al. (1999). Anti-inflammatory effects of systemic anti-tumor necrosis factor alpha treatment in human/murine SCID arthritis. *Annals of the Rheumatic Diseases, 58*, 428–438.
18. Skinner, H.B. (1995). *Current diagnosis and treatment in orthopedics.* Stanford, CT: Appleton & Lange.

SUBLUXATIONS AND DISLOCATIONS

Colleen R. Walsh, MSN, RN, ONC, CS, ACNP

I. SUBLUXATIONS

A. Definition[2, 4, 5, 8, 9]

1. Partial loss of the articulation of the bone ends within the joint capsule caused by partial displacement or separation of the bone end from its position in the joint
2. Also defined as a partial dislocation, caused by disruption of the joint ligaments

B. Etiology/Incidence/Predisposing factors[2, 8, 9]

1. Trauma, usually blunt force
2. Congenital
3. Pathologic
4. Neuromuscular diseases, such as muscular dystrophy, cerebrovascular accidents (CVAs)
5. Inflammatory joint diseases, such as rheumatoid arthritis
6. Ligamentous laxity: Condition in which ligamentous structures are loose, stretched, or injured and can lead to injury or dislocation
7. Commonly seen in persons <20 years of age
8. Often associated with fractures
9. Common sites

   a. Acromioclavicular joint
   b. Shoulder
   c. Elbow
   d. Wrist
   e. Hip
   f. Knee
   g. Ankle

C. Subjective findings[2, 5, 8, 9]

1. Patient gives detailed description of mechanism of injury.
2. Pain over affected area
3. The patient may give history of repeated subluxations with decreasing trauma associated with each subluxation.

D. Physical examination findings[2–5, 8]

1. Swelling around peripheral joints
2. May have obvious joint deformity
3. Loss of range of motion (ROM)

E. Laboratory/Diagnostic findings[2, 4, 6–8]

1. X-rays reveal area and extent of subluxation.
2. Complete blood count may show elevated white blood cells (WBC) (>10,000 mm/L) as result of stress response to trauma.

F. Management[1, 2, 4, 5, 8]

1. Early reduction of subluxation; many reduce spontaneously
2. Immobilization: Cast, splint, sling, brace
3. Physical therapy for muscle strengthening exercises
4. Nonsteroidal anti-inflammatory drugs (NSAIDs) for pain and swelling
5. Rarely need narcotics except in cases of multiple trauma

II. DISLOCATIONS

A. Definition[2, 4, 5, 8, 9]

1. Complete loss of the articulation of the bone ends within the joint capsule
2. Caused by complete displacement or separation of the bone end from its position in the joint

B. Etiology/Incidence/Predisposing factors[2, 8, 9]

1. High-energy blunt force trauma
2. Congenital
3. Pathologic
4. Neuromuscular diseases, such as muscular dystrophy
5. Inflammatory joint diseases, such as rheumatoid arthritis
6. Ligamentous laxity: Condition in which ligamentous structures are loose, stretched, or injured and can lead to injury or dislocation
7. Seen in all age groups, but more frequent in persons <35 years old
8. Very commonly associated with fractures
9. Common sites

   a. Shoulder
      i. Anterior: Associated with humeral fracture
      ii. Posterior: Spontaneously due to ligament laxity
      iii. Superior: Fall on outstretched arm
      iv. Inferior: Neuromuscular disorder, e.g., CVA, brachial plexus injury
   b. Elbow
   c. Wrist
   d. Hip
   e. Knee
   f. Ankle

C. Subjective findings[2–5]

1. Pain over affected area, usually severe
2. History of mechanism of injury

D. Physical examination findings[2–5, 8]

1. Obvious joint deformity
2. Shortening and abnormal posture of affected limb
3. Swelling
4. May see contusion or laceration over affected joint due to blunt force trauma
5. Decreased or absent peripheral pulses distal to joint
6. Decreased or absent ROM of joint or distal to joint
7. Decreased or absent sensation distal to joint due to peripheral nerve damage/compression

E. Laboratory/Diagnostic findings[2–4, 6–9]

1. WBC is elevated due to stress response to trauma ($>10,000$ mm^3/L).
2. X-rays demonstrate dislocation.

    a. Should order anteroposterior and lateral films for all dislocations
    b. May consider oblique films for dislocations associated with fractures
    c. Inlet/outlet views for all pelvic trauma

3. Computed tomography scan is indicated for pelvic trauma to rule out hip or sacral dislocation.
4. Always order arteriogram for posterior knee dislocation due to high incidence of popliteal artery injury.
5. Consider compartment pressure measurements in knee dislocations with vascular compromise that are >8 h since injury.

F. Management[1, 2, 4, 8, 9]

1. Early anatomic reduction is essential.

    a. Closed, manual reduction is primarily used in dislocations without fractures.
    b. Surgical reduction may be necessary if fractures are associated with dislocation.

2. Postreduction immobilization is essential

    a. Splints
    b. Casts
    c. Immobilizers
    d. External fixation devices for knee dislocations associated with vascular injury and repair
    e. Slings

   f. Elevation of extremity with application of cold compresses to reduce swelling

3. Surgical repair of ligamentous structures
4. Physical therapy for muscle strengthening exercises
5. Occupational therapy for assistive devices if neurovascular injury occurs
6. Narcotics for short-term use

   a. Oxycodone/acetaminophen (Tylox), 5–7.5 mg (1–2 tablets) p.o. q4–6h p.r.n.
   b. Meperidine (Demerol), 50–100 mg p.o. q4–6h p.r.n.
   c. Codeine/acetaminophen (Tylenol #3 or #4), 1–2 tablets p.o. q4–6h p.r.n.

7. NSAIDs: See Tables 54–1 and 54–2 for comprehensive list
8. May need antispasmodic for severe muscle spasms

   a. Diazepam (Valium), 2–10 mg p.o. q6–8h p.r.n.
   b. Cyclobenzaprine (Flexeril), 10 mg p.o. t.i.d. p.r.n.

9. Skeletal traction therapy in select cases

References

1. Bryant, G.G. (1998). Modalities for immobilization. In A.B. Maher, S.W. Salmond, & T.A. Pellino (Eds.), *Orthopaedic nursing* (2nd ed.) (pp. 296–322). Philadelphia: W.B. Saunders.
2. Inverson, L.D., & Swiontkowski, M.F. (1995). *Manual of acute orthopaedic therapeutics* (2nd ed.). Boston: Little, Brown.
3. Jarvis, C. (1996). *Physical examination and health assessment* (2nd ed.). Philadelphia: W.B. Saunders.
4. Lewis, S.M., Collier, I.C., & Heitkemper, M.L. (1996). *Medical-surgical nursing* (4th ed.). St. Louis: Mosby.
5. Mourad, L.A. (1998). Alteration of musculoskeletal function. In K.L. McCance, & S.E. Huether (Eds.), *Pathophysiology: The biological basis for disease in adults and children* (3rd ed.) (pp. 1435–1485). St. Louis: Mosby.
6. Moye, C.E. (1998). Diagnostic modalities for orthopaedic disorders. In A.B. Maher, S.W. Salmond, & T.A. Pellino (Eds.), *Orthopaedic nursing* (2nd ed.). Philadelphia: W.B. Saunders.
7. Pellino, T.A., Polacek, L.A., Preston, M.A.S., Bell, N.L., & Evans, R.L. (1998). Complications of orthopaedic disorders and orthopaedic surgery. In A.B. Maher, S.W. Salmond, & T.A. Pellino (Eds.), *Orthopaedic nursing* (2nd ed.) (pp. 212–260). Philadelphia: W.B. Saunders.
8. Skinner, H.B. (1995). *Current diagnosis and treatment in orthopedics*. Stanford, CT: Appleton & Lange.
9. Snyder, P.E. (1998). Fractures. In A.B. Maher, S.W. Salmond, & T.A. Pellino (Eds.), *Orthopaedic nursing* (2nd ed.) (pp. 663–719). Philadelphia: W.B. Saunders.

SOFT TISSUE INJURY

*Colleen R. Walsh, MSN, RN, ONC,
CS, ACNP*

I. SOFT TISSUE INJURY

A. Definition[2–6, 8, 9]

1. Any injury that occurs in nonosseous structures of the musculoskeletal system
2. These soft tissues are

   a. Muscles
   b. Ligaments
   c. Tendons
   d. Bursa
   e. Cartilage

B. Classifications

1. Contusions
2. Hematomas
3. Lacerations/tears
4. Strains—Muscles
5. Sprains—Ligaments

   a. First degree—Mild
   b. Second degree—Moderate
   c. Third degree—Severe; these often are complex, unstable injuries and need to be referred to the physician for definitive care/surgery.

6. Ruptures

   a. Both muscles and ligaments
   b. Need immediate referral to the physician for definitive care/surgery
   c. Characterized by
      i. Instability
      ii. Inability to move injured extremity
      iii. Swelling.

C. Etiology/Incidence/Predisposing factors[2, 3, 5, 8, 9]

1. Trauma

   a. Blunt
   b. Rotational
   c. Shear forces

2. Exercise
3. Overuse syndromes
4. Sports
5. Autoimmune diseases such as systemic lupus erythematosus (SLE), scleroderma, and rheumatoid arthritis (RA)
6. Soft tissue injury is commonly seen in all age groups; more frequent in persons <35 years old
7. Obesity

D. Subjective findings[2, 3, 5, 8, 9]

1. Pain
2. Swelling
3. History of precipitating event
4. Feeling of instability of joint

E. Physical examination findings[2–5, 8, 9]

1. Muscle tears/ruptures

   a. Decreased or absent range of motion (ROM) of joint/joints affected by the muscle
   b. Swelling with hematoma formation
   c. Ecchymosis of skin over muscle
   d. Palpable discontinuity of muscle belly with obvious defect on careful palpation
   e. Abnormal contour of muscle

2. Ligaments

   a. Strains
      i. Pain on palpation and ROM
      ii. Mild swelling
      iii. Rarely, hematoma formation
   b. Sprains
      i. Pain on palpation and ROM
      ii. Moderate swelling with decreased ROM
      iii. Possible hematoma formation
      iv. *Lachman's test:* Possible joint laxity of the anterior/posterior cruciate ligaments during special maneuvers; sensation of the joint acting hypermobile during stressing maneuvers
         (1) The examiner grasps the tibia with one hand while stabilizing the femur with the other hand.
         (2) The patient relaxes the leg while the examiner holds the knee flexed at 30 degrees and pulls forward/pushes backward on the tibia.
         (3) Excessive motion determines a positive sign.
      v. *McMurray's test:* Indicates an injured/torn meniscus by production of a pronounced audible or palpable "click" during manipulation of the tibia with the knee flexed and then abruptly straightened

    c. Ruptures

       i. Complete instability of joint

      ii. Large amount of swelling almost immediately after injury

     iii. Ecchymosis

     iv. Inability to perform adequate examination owing to pain and guarding by patient

      v. Minimal or no ROM

     vi. Need immediate referral to a physician for definitive treatment

    vii. Area should be immobilized with a splint to prevent further injury.

   viii. Neurovascular integrity should be monitored closely owing to potential vascular disruption.

3. Tendons

    a. Swelling

    b. Possible hematoma formation

    c. Decreased or absent ROM of affected joint

    d. Limited examination owing to pain and patient guarding

4. Cartilage

    a. Moderate swelling of joint, usually several hours after injury occurs

    b. Palpable and/or audible "click" during special maneuvers such as McMurray's test

    c. Pain on palpation over joint lines

    d. Limited examination owing to pain and guarding by patient

5. Bursa

    a. Swelling of bursa with "boggy" feeling on palpation

    b. Erythema over bursa

    c. May see abrasion over bursa

    d. Possible decreased ROM due to swelling

F. Laboratory/Diagnostic findings[2, 3, 5, 6–9]

1. Possible white blood cell elevation ($>10,000/mm^3$), especially with bursitis.
2. Joint aspiration demonstrates bloody fluid.
3. Complete blood count may show decreased hemoglobin and hematocrit if large blood loss is associated with massive soft tissue injuries.
4. Plain x-rays may demonstrate soft tissue swelling.
5. Magnetic resonance imaging of joint, especially knee, demonstrates location and degree of injury.

G. Management[1-3, 5, 8, 9]

1. RICE (Rest, Ice, Compression, Elevation) of injured part
2. Immobilization may be necessary, depending on location, severity, and type of injury.

   a. Casts
   b. Splints
   c. Immobilizers
   d. Slings

3. Surgery may be necessary if

   a. Rupture of tendons, muscles, or ligaments
   b. Grade III ligament sprains with joint instability
   c. Septic bursa: Incision and drainage performed

4. Physical therapy for muscle strengthening and ROM
5. Pharmacologic interventions

   a. Nonsteroidal anti-inflammatory drugs: See Tables 54–1 and 54–2
   b. May need antispasmodic for severe muscle spasms
      i. Diazepam (Valium), 2–10 mg p.o. q6–8h as needed
      ii. Cyclobenzaprine (Flexeril), 10 mg p.o. t.i.d. as needed
   c. Narcotics for short-term use
      i. Oxycodone/acetaminophen (Tylox), 5–7.5 mg (1–2 tablets) p.o. q4–6h as needed
      ii. Meperidine (Demerol), 50–100 mg p.o. q4–6h as needed
      iii. Codeine/acetaminophen (Tylenol #3 or #4), 1–2 tablets p.o. q4–6h as needed
   d. Broad-spectrum antibiotics for septic bursitis that will cover most common gram-positive organisms
      i. Cephalexin (Keflex), 250–500 mg p.o. q.i.d. for 7–10 days
      ii. Cefazolin (Ancef), 1 g IV q8h for 48–72 h after incision and drainage, then continue with cephalexin (Keflex), for a total of 10 days of treatment
   e. Aminoglycosides for suspected anaerobic, gram-negative bacilli; immunocompromised patients at greatest risk
      i. Gentamycin (Garamycin), 3–5 mg/kg/day IV
      ii. Newest recommendations are that total dose should be given once a day to prevent renal impairment, although q8h dosing is still common.
      iii. Duration of therapy is variable depending on patient response

References

1. Bryant, G.G. (1998). Modalities for immobilization. In A.B. Maher, S.W. Salmond, & T.A. Pellino (Eds.), *Orthopaedic nursing* (2nd ed.) (pp. 296–322). Philadelphia: W.B. Saunders.

2. Holmes, S.B. (1998). Autoimmune and inflammatory disorders. In A.B. Maher, S.W. Salmond, & T.A. Pellino (Eds.), *Orthopaedic nursing* (2nd ed.) (pp. 480–544). Philadelphia: W.B. Saunders.

3. Iverson, L.D., & Swiontkowski, M.F. (1995). *Manual of acute orthopaedic therapeutics* (2nd ed.). Boston: Little, Brown.

4. Jarvis, C. (1996). *Physical examination and health assessment* (2nd ed.). Philadelphia: W.B. Saunders.

5. Lewis, S.M., Collier, I.C., & Heitkemper, M.L. (1996). *Medical-surgical nursing* (4th ed.). St. Louis: Mosby.

6. Mourad, L.A. (1998). Alteration of musculoskeletal function. In K.L. McCance & S.E. Huether (Eds.), *Pathophysiology: The biological basis for disease in adults and children* (3rd ed.) (pp. 1435–1485). St. Louis: Mosby.

7. Moye, C.E. (1998). Diagnostic modalities for orthopaedic disorders. In A.B. Maher, S.W. Salmond, & T.A. Pellino (Eds.), *Orthopaedic nursing* (2nd ed.). Philadelphia: W.B. Saunders.

8. Skinner, H.B. (1995). *Current diagnosis and treatment in orthopedics*. Stamford, CT: Appleton & Lange.

9. Snyder, P.E. (1998). Fractures. In A.B. Maher, S.W. Salmond, & T.A. Pellino (Eds.), *Orthopaedic nursing* (2nd ed.) (pp. 663–719). Philadelphia: W.B. Saunders.

FRACTURES

Colleen R. Walsh, MSN, RN, ONC, CS, ACNP

I. FRACTURES

A. Definition[4, 7, 8, 11, 12]

Break or disruption in the continuity of a bone

B. Classification[4, 6, 7, 10, 11]

1. Closed: No break in skin over fracture
2. Open: Varying amounts of skin or soft tissue injury over fracture

   a. Type I: Wound <1 cm, minimal contamination
   b. Type II: Wound >1 cm, moderate contamination, moderate soft tissue damage
   c. Type III: High degree of contamination, severe fracture with instability, extensive soft tissue damage
      i. Type IIIA: Soft tissue coverage is adequate; fracture is severely comminuted.
      ii. Type IIIB: Extensive injury to or loss of soft tissue; moderate amount of periosteal stripping with exposed bone
      iii. Type IIIC: Any open fracture associated with vascular injury and is not dependent on amount of skin or tissue loss

3. Incomplete or complete
4. Simple or comminuted
5. Traumatic or pathologic
6. Intra-articular or extra-articular
7. Type of fracture line

   a. Transverse
   b. Spiral
   c. Oblique
   d. Compression

C. Etiology/Incidence/Predisposing factors[2–4, 6, 9–11]

1. High energy trauma, such as crush, blunt, or deceleration forces
2. Rotational forces
3. Osteoporosis/osteopenia
4. Tumors of bone
5. Metabolic disorders, such as rickets and renal osteodystrophy

6. Drugs, such as corticosteroids (prednisone) and phenytoin (Dilantin)
7. Nutritional deficiencies, such as vitamin D, malabsorption syndromes, inflammatory bowel diseases
8. Infectious disorders, such as tuberculosis and osteomyelitis
9. Congenital disorders
10. Neuromuscular disorders, such as spinal cord injuries and muscular dystrophy

D. Subjective findings[4, 6, 9–11]

1. Pain is usually moderate to severe.
2. Patient gives history of trauma event.

E. Physical examination findings[4–7, 10, 11]

1. Pain on palpation over fracture site
2. May have deformity of limb; not always immediately visible
3. Palpable and audible crepitus
4. May see diminished or absent distal pulses
5. Swelling
6. Ecchymosis or frank bleeding
7. Decreased or absent range of motion distal to fracture
8. Neurologic injury distal to fracture
9. Specific fracture findings: Always determine the mechanism of injury!

   a. Cervical spine: Always treat as if fracture exists until proved otherwise
   b. Shoulder: Inability to abduct or adduct arm
   c. Humerus (proximal): Ecchymosis, deformity, inability to abduct arm
   d. Humerus (midshaft): Neurovascular compromise, radial nerve palsy, abnormal positioning
   e. Humerus (distal): Neurovascular compromise, inability to flex or extend the elbow
   f. Forearm (proximal): Swelling, inability to flex or extend the elbow
   g. Forearm (midshaft): May have some swelling or tenderness on pronation/supination
   h. Forearm (distal): Deformity around wrist, inability to flex or extend wrist
   i. Wrist: "Dinner fork" deformity; inability to flex or extend wrist
   j. Hand/finger: Pain; may have obvious deformity
   k. Hip, proximal femur: Shortening with external rotation of leg
   l. Femur (midshaft, distal): Possible shortening with internal or external rotation of leg
   m. Tibia (proximal): Plateau fractures with swelling, or may be occult

n. Tibia (midshaft): Swelling; may see exposed bone or lacerations
o. Tibia (distal): External/internal rotation of foot
p. Ankle: Malposition of foot, ecchymosis, swelling
q. Foot/toe: Ecchymosis, swelling
r. Thoracic/lumbar spine: Always treat as if a fracture exists until it is ruled out
s. Pelvis: Leg shortening; positive pelvic rock test (grasp anterior and posterior iliac crests simultaneously and try to rock the pelvis back and forth)

- Caution with this maneuver: If anteroposterior pelvis x-ray is positive for sacral fracture or dislocation, serious, even fatal bleeding can occur if a clot becomes dislodged!

F. Laboratory/Diagnostic findings[1, 5, 8, 9, 11, 12]

1. X-ray evidence of fracture

a. Always order anteroposterior (AP) and lateral x-ray films
b. Oblique films for complex fractures of humerus, femur, or ankle
c. Mortise view of ankle fractures to check talus
d. Three-dimensional computed tomography scan if pelvic or spinal fractures are found on plain films
e. Magnetic resonance imaging if spinal cord injury is suspected

2. Leukocytosis without left shift
3. Serial CBCs to monitor blood loss from fracture site
4. Urinalysis in crush injuries looking for myoglobinuria
5. Electrolytes, especially elevated K^+, due to necrosis of muscle tissue
6. Arteriogram if diminished or absent distal pulses

G. Management[1, 2, 5, 7, 8, 11, 12]

1. Acute interventions

a. Follow tenets of trauma care: ABCs (airway, breathing, circulation) are first priority.
b. Musculoskeletal examination is part of secondary survey.
c. Fluid resuscitation with normal saline or Ringer's lactate
d. Cover open wounds with saline dressings until the patient is taken to the operating room for debridement.
e. Early, anatomic reduction of fracture is mandatory, with adequate immobilization of fracture after reduction.
f. Formal surgical irrigation and debridement of open fracture is mandatory for adequate healing and prevention of infection.

g. Pharmacologic therapy
  i. Any open fracture requires antibiotics.
  ii. Cefazolin (Kefzol), 1 g IV q8h. If both penicillin and cephalosporin allergy exist, give vancomycin (Vancocin), 1 g IV q12h.
  iii. Depending on the environment in which the injury occurred, may need to add gentamycin (Garamycin), 3–5 mg/kg/day, either in 3 divided doses or 1 single dose
  iv. Clindamycin (Cleocin), 600 mg IV q8h if clostridia is suspected
  v. Narcotics for pain: May use patient-controlled analgesia pump with morphine sulfate or meperidine (Demerol)
  vi. Oxycodone/acetaminophen (Tylox), 1–2 tablets p.o. q4–6h p.r.n. as needed
  vii. Acetaminophen/codeine (Tylenol #3/4), 1–2 tablets p.o. q4–6h p.r.n. as needed
  viii. Tetanus toxoid

2. Reduction of fractures

  a. Referral to orthopedist in all fractures except for minor, nondisplaced fractures
  b. Toe fractures can be "buddy-taped" to toes on either side of fracture to immobilize; this is mainly a comfort measure.
  c. Radius/ulna fractures: Can be placed in splint with Ace bandage wrap if simple hairline or greenstick fracture
  d. Always order postreduction/splinting AP and lateral radiographs to check for displacement during splinting.

References

1. Bassam, D., Cephas, G.A., Ferguson, K.A., Beard, L.N., & Young, J.S. (1998). Protocol for the initial management of unstable pelvic fractures. *American Surgeon, 64,* 862–867.
2. Bryant, G.G. (1998). Modalities for immobilization. In A.B. Maher, S.W. Salmond, & T.A. Pellino (Eds.), *Orthopaedic nursing* (2nd ed.) (pp. 296–322). Philadelphia: W.B. Saunders.
3. Holmes, S.B. (1998). Autoimmune and inflammatory disorders. In A.B. Maher, S.W. Salmond, & T.A. Pellino (Eds.), *Orthopaedic nursing* (2nd ed.) (pp. 480–544). Philadelphia: W.B. Saunders.
4. Hunt, A.H. (1998). Metabolic conditions. In A.B. Maher, S.W. Salmond, & T.A. Pellino (Eds.), *Orthopaedic nursing* (2nd ed.) (pp. 431–479). Philadelphia: W.B. Saunders.
5. Iverson, L.D., & Swiontkowski, M.F. (1995). *Manual of acute orthopaedic therapeutics* (2nd ed.). Boston: Little, Brown.
6. Jarvis, C. (1996). *Physical examination and health assessment* (2nd ed.). Philadelphia: W.B. Saunders.

7. Lewis, S.M., Collier, I.C., & Heitkemper, M.L. (1996). *Medical-surgical nursing* (4th ed.). St. Louis: Mosby.

8. Mourad, L.A. (1998). Alteration of musculoskeletal function. In K.L. McCance, & S.E. Huether (Eds.), *Pathophysiology: The biological basis for disease in adults and children* (3rd ed.) (pp. 1435–1485). St. Louis: Mosby.

9. Moye, C.E. (1998). Diagnostic modalities for orthopaedic disorders. In A.B. Maher, S.W. Salmond, & T.A. Pellino (Eds.), *Orthopaedic nursing* (2nd ed.). Philadelphia: W.B. Saunders.

10. Pellino, T.A., Polacek, L.A., Preston, M.A.S., Bell, N.L., & Evans, R.L. (1998). Complications of orthopaedic disorders and orthopaedic surgery. In A.B. Maher, S.W. Salmond, & T.A. Pellino (Eds.), *Orthopaedic nursing* (2nd ed.) (pp. 212–260). Philadelphia: W.B. Saunders.

11. Skinner, H.B. (1995). *Current diagnosis and treatment in orthopedics*. Stanford, CT: Appleton & Lange.

12. Snyder, P.E. (1998). Fractures. In A.B. Maher, S.W. Salmond, & T.A. Pellino (Eds.), *Orthopaedic nursing* (2nd ed.) (pp. 663–719). Philadelphia: W.B. Saunders.

COMPARTMENT SYNDROME

Colleen R. Walsh, MSN, RN, ONC, CS, ACNP

I. COMPARTMENT SYNDROME

A. Definition[3–5, 7–10, 12–14]

1. Condition where increased tissue pressure within a limited space compromises the circulation and function of the contents within that space
2. A compartment consists of bone, blood vessels, nerves, muscles, and soft tissue lying within a fascial envelope. Fascia is a nonexpanding tissue that contributes to the syndrome.
3. Of the body's 46 compartments, 38 are in the arms and legs.

B. Etiology/Incidence/Predisposing factors[3, 4, 7–10, 12–14]

1. Space limiting envelope

   a. Circumferential dressings
   b. Casts
   c. Splints
   d. Eschar and/or scars

2. Increased intracompartmental contents owing to

   a. Bleeding/hemorrhage
   b. Coagulation disorders
   c. Iatrogenic: Infiltrated intravenous sites, improper positioning
   d. Venous pooling/obstruction
   e. Increased capillary filtration
      i. Trauma/surgery
      ii. Crush syndrome
      iii. Tissue ischemia
      iv. Thermal/electrical burns
      v. Snake/spider bites

C. Subjective findings[4, 6–10, 12–14]

1. Pain out of proportion to injury
2. History of trauma event

D. Physical examination findings[4–8, 10, 12–14]

The six Ps

1. Pain on passive stretch of affected compartment
2. Paresthesias along dermatomal patterns

3. Paralysis of affected limb
4. Pulses

   a. Early: Bounding distal pulses
   b. Late: Pulselessness

5. Pallor of affected limb late in course—Rubor early in course of syndrome
6. Polar: Limb becomes ice cold.

   • Swelling may not be evident by palpation or inspection, but affected limb may feel tense to palpation.

E. Laboratory/Diagnostic findings[1, 3, 4–8, 10, 11–14]

1. White blood cell count may be elevated ($>14,000/mm^3$).
2. Electrolytes may demonstrate elevated K^+ levels.
3. Electrocardiogram may demonstrate classic hyperkalemic changes with peaked T waves.
4. Urinalysis may show positive myoglobin.
5. Elevated compartment pressure readings >40 mmHg are clinically diagnostic.
6. Creative phosphokinase (CPK) and lactate dehydrogenase (LDH) levels elevated: CPK >130 units/L; LDH >150 units/L
7. Elevated levels of serum inflammatory mediators
8. Acute compartment syndrome is a clinical diagnosis based on a high index of suspicion, signs, and symptoms.

F. Management[2, 4, 5, 7, 8, 12–14]

1. Nonsurgical

   a. Position limb at level of heart; do not elevate limb.
   b. May consider diuretics, but rarely used; furosemide, 20–40 mg IV or p.o.
   c. Continuous neurovascular function checks
   d. Mannitol is occasionally used as osmotic diuretic.

2. Surgical

   a. Fasciotomy of affected compartment
   b. Delayed closure of fasciotomy wounds (5–7 days)
   c. Skin grafting procedures
   d. Amputation may be necessary owing to sepsis

3. Restorative

   a. Functional splinting
   b. Active/passive range of motion exercises

References

1. Breit, G.A., Gross, J.H., Watenpaugh, D.E., et al. (1997). Near-infrared spectrometry for monitoring of tissue oxygenation of exercising skeletal

muscle in a chronic compartment syndrome model. *Journal of Bone and Joint Surgery, 79A*, 838–843.

2. Bryant, G.G. (1998). Modalities for immobilization. In A.B. Maher, S.W. Salmond, & T.A. Pellino (Eds.), *Orthopaedic nursing* (2nd ed.) (pp. 296–322). Philadelphia: W.B. Saunders.

3. Dabney, D., Greif, F., Yaniv, M, et al. (1998). Thrombaxame A_2 in post ischemic acute compartment syndrome. *Archives of Surgery, 133*, 953–956.

4. Iverson, L.D., & Swiontkowski, M.F. (1995). *Manual of acute orthopaedic therapeutics* (2nd ed.). Boston: Little, Brown.

5. James, M.D., & Bregis, R.M. (1998). Mannitol treatment for acute compartment syndrome. *Nephron, 79*, 492.

6. Jarvis, C. (1996). *Physical examination and health assessment* (2nd ed.). Philadelphia: W.B. Saunders.

7. Kalb, R.L. (1999). Preventing the sequelae of compartment syndrome. *Hospital Practice, 34*, 105–107.

8. Lewis, S.M., Collier, I.C., & Heitkemper, M.L. (1996). *Medical-surgical nursing* (4th ed.). St. Louis: Mosby.

9. Mittal, R., & Gupta, V. (1998). Compartment syndrome of the thigh and the role of skin scars: Case report and review of the literature. *Journal of Trauma, 45*, 395–396.

10. Mourad, L.A. (1998). Alteration of musculoskeletal function. In K.L. McCance & S.E. Huether (Eds.), *Pathophysiology: The biological basis for disease in adults and children* (3rd ed.) (pp. 1435–1485). St. Louis: Mosby.

11. Moye, C.E. (1998). Diagnostic modalities for orthopaedic disorders. In A.B. Maher, S.W. Salmond, & T.A. Pellino (Eds.), *Orthopaedic nursing* (2nd ed.). Philadelphia: W.B. Saunders.

12. Pellino, T.A., Polacek, L.A., Preston, M.A.S., Bell, N.L., & Evans, R.L. (1998). Complications of orthopaedic disorders and orthopaedic surgery. In A.B. Maher, S.W. Salmond, & T.A. Pellino (Eds.), *Orthopaedic nursing* (2nd ed.) (pp. 212–260). Philadelphia: W.B. Saunders.

13. Skinner, H.B. (1995). *Current diagnosis and treatment in orthopedics*. Stanford, CT: Appleton & Lange.

14. Snyder, P.E. (1998). Fractures. In A.B. Maher, S.W. Salmond, & T.A. Pellino (Eds.), *Orthopaedic nursing* (2nd ed.) (pp. 663–719). Philadelphia: W.B. Saunders.

BACK PAIN SYNDROMES

59

*Colleen R. Walsh, MSN, RN, ONC,
CS, ACNP*

I. LOW BACK PAIN

A. Definition[2, 3, 7, 9–12, 16, 17]

1. Low-back pain (LBP) is any pain perceived by the patient as originating from the lumbosacral region of the spinal column.
2. Pain usually in the lower back that causes discomfort, limited range of motion, varying degrees of neurologic symptoms, and inability to participate in or perform activities of daily living
3. May be localized or radiate to lower extremities
4. LBP is the leading cause of lost workdays in the United States.
5. It is important to distinguish the causes of back pain, as each back syndrome presents with varying symptoms, and treatment options differ for each of the four major syndromes:

   a. Back strain
   b. Disk herniation—See section II. Herniated Disk.
   c. Osteoarthritis/disk degeneration: Osteophyte (bone spur) formation of the vertebral bodies
   d. Spinal stenosis: Narrowing of the spinal foramen leading to encroachment on the spinal nerve roots

B. Etiology/Incidence/Predisposing factors[1–4, 8, 9, 12, 16, 17]

1. Most Americans experience LBP at least once in their lives.
2. Common causes

   a. Mechanical strain
   b. Obesity
   c. Poor body mechanics
   d. Trauma
   e. Repetitive twisting, bending, or lifting
   f. Herniated lumbar disks
   g. Spondylolysis: Defect in neural arch of vertebral body
   h. Spondylolisthesis: Forward subluxation of vertebral body due to defect in the neural arch of the vertebral body
   i. Spinal stenosis: Narrowing of the spinal canal or the foramen in which spinal nerves exit the spinal cord
   j. Degenerative disk disease
   k. Osteoarthritis of the spine
   l. Rarely, tumors

C. Subjective findings[2, 3, 9, 10, 16, 17]

1. Pain in lower back region; may have radicular (radiating) component in affected nerve dermatome
2. Numbness along specific dermatome
3. Bowel, bladder, or sexual dysfunction

   • If present, bowel/bladder dysfunction requires immediate referral for possible emergency surgical intervention

4. Cauda equina syndrome: Gradual to sudden weakness and/or inability to lift or move legs; bowel and/or bladder incontinence or retention; and loss of or diminished sensation in legs

   • May be first symptom of spinal cord compression from metastatic lesion to spine
   • Cauda equina syndrome is a surgical emergency and requires emergency referral.

D. Physical examination findings[2, 3, 7, 9–12, 14, 16, 17]

1. Back strain: Paraspinal muscle spasms, listing to one side, decreased range of motion (ROM), positive bilateral straight leg raise test

   a. Straight leg raise: With the patient in supine position, lift one leg at a time, forcefully dorsiflex the foot, and ask the patient if there is pain down the leg (radiculopathy).
   b. Crossover straight leg raise: If the patient has a herniated disk, the crossover straight leg raise test will cause radicular pain down the affected leg even if the other leg is raised.
   c. Simultaneous bilateral straight leg raise: This test reproduces the back pain but does not cause radicular pain.

2. Herniated disk—See section II. Herniated Disk.
3. Osteoarthritis: Decreased ROM, muscle spasm, possible positive bilateral straight leg raise, but rarely with radicular component
4. Spinal stenosis: Often called "neurogenic claudication" owing to back, buttock, and leg pain during ambulation

   a. Pain is relieved with rest and sitting: thought to be relieved by sitting when the spine is flexed and the spinal nerve roots have less compression
   b. Positive straight leg raises with radicular component: Often multilevel in lower lumbar spine

5. Weak rectal tone

E. Laboratory/Diagnostic findings[2, 6, 7, 9, 10, 13, 16, 17]

1. Serum blood work usually within normal limits

2. Plain x-rays (anteroposterior [AP] and lateral) to rule out bony defects; scoliosis, bone spurs
3. Magnetic resonance imaging best for soft tissue structures; demonstrates disk bulge
4. Computed tomography (CT) scan for detailed bony imaging
5. Myelography of spine with/without CT scan to show filling defects along spinal nerve roots

F. Management[2–4, 6–9, 14, 16, 17]

1. Nonsurgical
   a. Rest for 1–2 days only
   b. Alternate ice/heat therapy
   c. Nonsteroidal anti-inflammatory drugs (NSAIDs) for mild to moderately severe injuries
      i. Act by inhibiting the enzyme cyclooxygenase (COX), which is required for the synthesis of prostaglandins and thromboxanes.
         (1) Two isoforms have been identified: COX-1 and COX-2.
         (2) COX-1 is thought to be found tissue-wide and is thought to protect gastric mucosa.
         (3) COX-2 is mainly induced at the inflammation site.
      ii. Older NSAIDs act by blocking both COX isoforms, leading to possible gastric ulceration. COX-2 drugs are selective, thus providing more gastric protection.
      iii. Rofecoxib (Vioxx), 12.5–25 mg p.o. daily
      iv. Celecoxib (Celebrex), 100–200 mg p.o. b.i.d.
      v. Concurrent use of zafirlukast, fluconazole, and fluvastatin may increase serum concentration of celecoxib.
      vi. See Tables 54–1 and 54–2 for management with NSAIDs.
   d. May need antispasmodic for severe muscle spasms
      i. Diazepam (Valium), 2–10 mg q6–8h as needed
      ii. Cyclobenzaprine (Flexeril), 10 mg p.o. t.i.d. as needed
   e. Narcotics may be needed for short-term acute back strain to promote mobility.
   f. Physical therapy for toning, strengthening muscles
   g. Weight loss program
   h. Epidural steroid injections: Done by anesthesia directly into the affected nerved sheath; refer the patient to pain management center for treatment.

2. Surgical
   a. Foramenotomy for nerve root decompression in spinal stenosis
   b. Depending on number and level of disks, may require spinal fusion with bone grafts
   c. See section II. Herniated Disk

II. HERNIATED DISK

A. Definition[2–5, 7, 9, 10, 12, 14, 16, 17]

1. Bulging or protrusion of the nucleus pulposus through a defect in the annulus of cervical, thoracic, or lumbar intervertebral disks
2. May encroach on peripheral nerves exiting the spinal cord

B. Etiology/Incidence/Predisposing factors[1–3, 5, 7–10, 12, 14–17]

1. Degeneration of the nucleus pulposus, which is the portion of the disk that contains gelatinous material enclosed in a fibrous band
2. Dehydration of the disk
3. Trauma
4. Forceful coughing or sneezing (e.g., Valsalva maneuver)
5. Sedentary lifestyle
6. Obesity
7. Peak incidence at 35–45 years of age
8. Ninety percent located at L4–L5 and L5–S1

C. Subjective findings[2, 3, 5, 7, 9–11, 15–17]

1. Radicular pain along specific dermatomal pattern
2. Numbness or sense of weakness along affected dermatome
3. Bowel, bladder, or sexual dysfunction

   • Requires immediate referral for possible surgical interventions

D. Physical examination findings[2, 5, 7, 9–12, 15–17]

1. All physical findings dependent on the spinal nerve root affected
2. Decreased or absent reflexes innervated by specific nerve
3. Atrophy of muscles innervated by affected nerve in chronic compression
4. Antalgic gait; limp
5. Proprioception (position sense) decreased
6. Possible positive straight leg raise test: Radicular or sciatic pain
7. Limited ROM of spine
8. Positive pelvic rock test: Test for sacroiliac joint dysfunction.

   a. Place one hand over each anterior-superior iliac spine and attempt to "open and close" the pelvis.
   b. Positive test if patient feels pain in either or both sacroiliac joints

E. Laboratory/Diagnostic findings[2, 6, 7, 9, 10, 13, 16, 17]

1. Radiographic studies most commonly used

   a. AP and lateral plain x-rays of the spine

b. CT scan with and without contrast dye; good for detecting bony defects in the spinal canal or foramen

c. MRI scan with and without contrast dye; good for detecting soft tissue defects, such as herniated disks

d. Myelogram: Consists of injection of contrast dye into the spinal canal to detect filling defects in myelin sheaths

2. Electromyelography (EMG): Consists of stimulating various nerves with low-voltage electrical impulses to test for nerve innervation to muscles

3. Nerve conduction studies: Also uses electrical impulses to test amplitude and waveform of different spinal nerves

4. Serum blood work is usually within normal limits.

F. Specific lumbar nerve root findings

1. L4 root: Indicative of pathology in disk between L4 and L5

   a. Motor: Quadriceps muscles weak and/or atrophic; difficulty extending the quadriceps of the knee
   b. Sensory: Pain radiating into medial malleolus; numbness along the same path, especially the medial aspect of the knee
   c. Reflex: Diminished or absent knee jerk
   d. Screening examination: Have patient squat and rise

2. L5 root: Indicative of pathology in disk between L5 and S1

   a. Motor: Weakness of the dorsiflexion mechanism of great toe and foot (extensor hallicis longus)
   b. Sensory: Pain radiating into lateral calf; numbness of dorsum of foot and lateral calf
   c. Reflex: None at this level
   d. Screening examination: Have patient walk on heels of feet

3. S1 root: Indicative of pathology in disk between S1 and S2

   a. Motor: Weakness of plantar flexion of great toe and foot
   b. Sensory: Pain along buttocks, lateral leg, and lateral malleolus; numbness on lateral aspect of foot and in posterior calf (gastrocnemius muscles)
   c. Reflex: Diminished or absent Achilles reflex
   d. Screening examination: Have patient walk on toes

G. Management[2–4, 6–9, 14, 16, 17]

1. Nonsurgical

   a. Functional bracing with an orthotic device
   b. Rest for 1–2 days only in mild disk bulges/herniations
   c. Physical therapy for muscle strengthening
   d. Alternate heat/ice therapy
   e. Weight loss program

    f. Education in proper body mechanics
    g. Transcutaneous electric nerve stimulator
    h. NSAIDs for mild to moderately severe injuries
       i. Act by inhibiting the enzyme cyclooxygenase (COX), which is required for the synthesis of prostaglandins and thromboxanes.
         (1) Two isoforms have been identified: COX-1 and COX-2.
         (2) COX-1 is thought to be found tissue-wide and is thought to protect gastric mucosa.
         (3) COX-2 is mainly induced at the inflammation site.
      ii. Older NSAIDs act by blocking both COX isoforms, leading to possible gastric ulceration. COX-2 drugs are selective, thus providing more gastric protection.
      iii. Rofecoxib (Vioxx), 12.5–25 mg p.o. daily
      iv. Celecoxib (Celebrex), 100–200 mg p.o. q.d.
      v. Concurrent use of zafirlukast, fluconazole, and fluvastatin may increase serum concentration of celecoxib.
      vi. See Tables 54–1 and 54–2 for management with NSAIDs
    i. May need antispasmodic for severe muscle spasms
      i. Diazepam (Valium), 2–10 mg q6–8h as needed
      ii. Cyclobenzaprine (Flexeril), 10 mg p.o. t.i.d. as needed
    j. Narcotics for short-term use
      i. Oxycodone/acetaminophen (Tylox), 5–7.5 mg (1–2 tables) p.o. q4–6h as needed
      ii. Meperidine (Demerol), 50–100 mg p.o. q4–6h as needed
      iii. Codeine/acetaminophen (Tylenol #3 or #4), 1–2 tablets p.o. q4–6h as needed
    k. Eqidural steroid injections: Done by anesthesia directly into the affected nerve sheath; refer the patient to pain management center for treatment

2. Surgical

    a. Laparoscopic diskectomy
    b. May require hemilaminectomy
    c. Depending on number and level of disks, may require spinal fusion with bone grafts

References

1. Adams, M.A., & Dolan, P. (1997). Could sudden increase in physical activity cause degeneration of intervertebral discs? *The Lancet, 350,* 734–735.
2. Altizer, L.L. (1998). Degenerative disorders. In A.B. Maher, S.W. Salmond, & T.A. Pellino (Eds.), *Orthopaedic nursing* (2nd ed.) (pp. 480–544). Philadelphia: W.B. Saunders.

3. Anonymous. (1999). Information from your family doctor: When you have a herniated disc. *American Family Physician, 59,* 586–587.

4. Bryant, G.G. (1998). Modalities for immobilization. In A.B. Maher, S.W. Salmond, & T.A. Pellino (Eds.), *Orthopaedic nursing* (2nd ed.) (pp. 296–322). Philadelphia: W.B. Saunders.

5. Fautrel, B., Rozenberg, S., Koeger, A.C., Willer, J.C., & Bourgwois, P. (1998). L5-S1 disc origin for a pyramidal syndrome? *The Lancet, 352,* 1679–1680.

6. Hermantin, F.U., Peters, T., Quartararo, L., & Kambin, P. (1999). A prospective, randomized study comparing the results of open discotomy with those of video-assisted arthroscopic microdiscectomy. *American, Journal of Bone and Joint Surgery, 81,* 958–968.

7. Humphreys, C.S., & Eck, J.C. (1999). Clinical evaluation and treatment options for herniated lumbar discs. *American Family Physician, 59,* 575–582.

8. Hunt, A.H. (1998). Metabolic conditions. In A.B. Maher, S.W. Salmond, & T.A. Pellino (Eds.), *Orthopaedic nursing* (2nd ed.) (pp. 431–479). Philadelphia: W.B. Saunders.

9. Iverson, L.D., & Swiontkowski, M.F. (1995). *Manual of acute orthopaedic therapeutics* (2nd ed.). Boston: Little, Brown.

10. Jarvis, C. (1996). *Physical examination and health assessment* (2nd ed.). Philadelphia: W.B. Saunders.

11. Lewis, S.M., Collier, I.C., & Heitkemper, M.L. (1996). *Medical-surgical nursing* (4th ed.). St. Louis: Mosby.

12. Mourad, L.A. (1998). Alteration of musculoskeletal function. In K.L. McCance, & S.E. Huether (Eds.), *Pathophysiology: The biological basis for disease in adults and children* (3rd ed.) (pp. 1435–1485). St. Louis: Mosby.

13. Moye, C.E. (1998). Diagnostic modalities for orthopaedic disorders. In A.B. Maher, S.W. Salmond, & T.A. Pellino (Eds.), *Orthopaedic nursing* (2nd ed.). Philadelphia: W.B. Saunders.

14. Postacchini, F. (1999). Management of herniation of the lumbar disc. *American, Journal of Bone and Joint Surgery, 81,* 567–577.

15. Prochet, F., Vader, J.P., & Larequi-Lauber, M. (1999). The assessment of appropriate indications for laminectomy. *American, Journal of Bone and Joint Surgery, 81,* 234–240.

16. Rodts, M.F. (1998). Disorders of the spine. In A.B. Maher, S.W. Salmond, & T.A. Pellino (Eds.), *Orthopaedic nursing* (2nd ed.) (pp. 545–584). Philadelphia: W.B. Saunders.

17. Skinner, H.B. (1995). *Current diagnosis and treatment in orthopedics.* Stamford, CT: Appleton & Lange.

Management of Patients with Hematologic Disorders

ANEMIAS

Sylvia R. Love, MED, MSN, RN, CS, ACNP, ANP

I. INITIAL ANEMIA WORKUP

A. Definition of anemia[6, 11, 14]

1. Reduction below normal blood levels of erythrocytes, hemoglobin (Hgb), or volume of red blood cells (RBCs), caused by blood loss, bone marrow failure/impaired production, or hemolysis/destruction of RBCs
2. The inability of the blood to supply adequate oxygen for proper functioning of the human body

B. Incidence/Predisposing factors[1, 6, 11, 14]

1. In the healthy person, about 1% of the fully mature circulating RBCs are lost daily.
2. Common among the elderly
   a. Occurs in >33% of outpatients
   b. Hgb and hematocrit (Hct) decrease slightly with age but remain in the normal adult range.
3. Anemia is a sign, not a diagnosis.
4. Adults residing at higher altitudes have normal values higher than those of adults residing at lower altitudes.
5. Plasma volume expansion in fluid-retaining states can mimic the appearance of anemia, and conversely, states of dehydration can mimic the appearance of a normal Hct when the patient may actually be anemic.

C. Subjective findings[3, 6, 11, 14]

1. Complaints are related to tissue hypoxia, such as
   a. Dyspnea on exertion that previously had not caused any problems
   b. Headaches
   c. Tinnitus
   d. Syncope
   e. Dizziness
   f. Fatigue, weakness
   g. Sleep disturbance
   h. Mood disturbance
   i. Impaired concentration
   j. Jaundice and hepatosplenomegaly
   k. Neurologic manifestations
   l. May have increased frequency of angina pectoris

2. Dementia or intermittent claudication may be exacerbated.
3. Anorexia and weight loss
4. If the anemia has developed very slowly, the patient may be asymptomatic.

D. Physical examination findings[3, 11, 16]

1. Skin and mucous membrane pallor
2. Tachycardia and increased pulse pressure (may be minimal if anemia is slow, progressive)
3. Systolic ejection murmurs
4. Venous hums
5. Peripheral edema
6. Retinal hemorrhages (flame-like) in severe anemia associated with thrombocytopenia

E. Laboratory/Diagnostic findings[1, 11, 14, 16]

1. Initially, consider ordering

   a. Complete blood count (CBC) with differential or Hct with mean corpuscular volume (MCV)
   b. Reticulocyte count (absolute)
   c. Platelet count (or estimate of platelets on smear)
   d. Wright-stained blood smear
   e. Serum ferritin, serum iron, and total iron binding capacity (TIBC)

F. Evaluation/Management[6, 11, 14]

1. A diagnosis of the specific cause of anemia should be made before transfusion, if possible.
2. Evaluate Hgb and Hct against normal ranges of patient population.
3. Evaluate reticulocyte count:

   a. Absolute reticulocyte count not elevated = anemia of marrow failure. This is the most common cause of anemia.
   b. Elevated absolute reticulocyte count indicates erythropoietic response to anemia = probable blood loss or hemolysis.

4. Evaluate peripheral blood smear for characteristics.
5. Classify RBC indices according to the size or MCV of the erythrocytes.

   a. Microcytosis = decreased MCV (MCV < 80 fL)
   b. Normocytosis = normal MCV (MCV 80–100 fL)
   c. Macrocytosis = increased MCV (MCV > 100 fL)

6. Classify RBCs by variation in size from the normal red cell size using the red cell indices in concert with the red cell distribution width (RDW) rating.

   a. Normal RDW = 11.5–14.5%
   b. Increased RDW may indicate anisocytosis resulting from a heterogeneous mix of cells or poikilocytosis from a variation in cell mix. The type of cell is then specified.

7. Consider bone marrow smear and biopsy. Interpretation requires a differential count of

   a. Myeloid, lymphoid, erythroid series, and maturational characteristics
   b. Iron stain

8. Specific studies are indicated to rule out specific disease processes such as

   a. Hgb electrophoresis (hemoglobinopathies, thalassemia syndromes)
   b. Antiglobulin testing (hemolytic anemias)
   c. Osmotic fragility test (hereditary spherocytosis)
   d. Sucrose hemolysis test or acidified serum test (known as Ham's test) (paroxysmal nocturnal hemoglobinuria)
   e. Tests for RBC enzymes (hemolytic anemias, G-6-PD deficiency, PK deficiency)
   f. Serum iron and iron-binding capacity (iron-deficiency anemia)
   g. Folate and vitamin B_{12} measurements (megaloblastic anemias)

II. PERNICIOUS ANEMIA

A. Definition[1, 4, 12, 19]

1. A megaloblastic anemia
2. Caused by a lack of intrinsic factor produced by the parietal cells of the gastric mucosa, which prevents vitamin B_{12} absorption, resulting in vitamin B_{12} deficiency
3. Autoimmune in origin

B. Incidence/Predisposing factors[1, 4, 12, 16, 19]

1. May be inherited as an autosomal recessive disorder.

   a. More common in people of northern European ancestry
   b. Rare in African Americans and Asians

2. May be caused by atrophic gastritis, antibodies to gastric parietal cells, autoimmune histamine-fast achlorhydria
3. Occurs in about 1% of people, usually older adults > age 60
4. Antibodies to intrinsic factor (IF) are found in about 50% of patients with disease.
5. The patient may have or develop other, associated autoimmune diseases including

   a. IgA deficiency
   b. Rheumatoid arthritis
   c. Graves' disease
   d. Myxedema
   e. Thyroiditis
   f. Idiopathic adrenocortical insufficiency

    g. Hypoparathyroidism
    h. Agammaglobulinemia
    i. Vitiligo
    j. Tropical sprue
    k. Celiac disease
    l. Crohn's disease
    m. Ileum and small intestine infiltrate disorders

6. It takes approximately 3 years to deplete the liver stores of vitamin B_{12} after absorption ceases.
7. Predisposition to gastric polyps and stomach cancer

C. Subjective findings[1, 4, 12, 14, 19]

1. Weakness and tiredness
2. Bleeding gums
3. Nausea, appetite loss, and weight loss
4. Sore tongue in about 50% of patients
5. Tingling of hands and feet
6. Difficulty maintaining balance
7. Yellowish tinge to eyes and skin
8. Shortness of breath
9. Poor memory
10. Headache
11. Depression

D. Physical examination findings[1, 4, 12, 14, 19]

1. Patient is usually pale and may be mildly icteric.
2. Abnormal reflexes
3. Babinski's sign is positive.
4. Romberg's sign is positive.
5. Vibratory sensation and proprioception are lost or decreased in lower extremities.
6. Paresthesia and numbness of extremities
7. Ataxia
8. Sense of smell is lost or diminished.
9. Patient may exhibit loss of glossal papillae with tenderness (smooth tongue).
10. Depression or dementia may be present.
11. Splenomegaly
12. Tinnitus
13. Hepatomegaly
14. Tachycardia
15. Congestive heart failure

E. Laboratory/Diagnostic findings[1, 4, 12, 14, 19]

1. Vitamin B_{12} deficiency is a megaloblastic anemia.

    a. Macrocyte with MCV is usually 110–140 fL, but can be in normal range if concurrent with iron deficiency or thalassemia.
    b. RDW is increased.

2. Hct may be 10–15 mL/dL low.
3. Peripheral blood smears usually exhibit macro-ovalocytes, anisocytosis, and poikilocytosis with hypersegmented neutrophils present (more than four lobes, sometimes six lobes).
4. Reticulocyte count is usually reduced.
5. In severe cases, pancytopenia is present with WBC and platelet count reduced.
6. Serum folate is usually increased in vitamin B_{12} deficiency.
7. Decreased serum vitamin B_{12} (less than 100 pg/mL)
8. Red cell folate is usually decreased in vitamin B_{12} deficiency.
9. Serum ferritin is increased.
10. Lactate dehydrogenase (LDH) may be elevated. (Often it is mistakenly assumed that the anemia is hemolytic.)
11. Consider ordering:

    a. Anti-IF and anti-parietal cell antibodies (presence affirms deficiency)
    b. Schilling's test (only when it is unclear why the patient is vitamin B_{12}-deficient because of the expense of the test)
    c. Gastric analysis for achlorhydria

12. Megaloblastosis of the bone marrow characteristically is present.

F. Management[1, 4, 14]

1. Parenteral vitamin B_{12}, 100–1000 μg subcutaneously daily for 7 days, then once a week for 1 month, then monthly for the remainder of life
2. Folic acid should not be given without vitamin B_{12} owing to the potential for fulminant neurologic deficit.
3. Hypokalemia may coincide with the first week of vitamin B_{12} replacement.
4. Central nervous system signs and symptoms are reversible if of short duration (<6 months), and if replacement therapy is initiated aggressively and promptly.
5. Endoscopy every 5 years even if asymptomatic (opinion varies in the literature)

III. VITAMIN B_{12} DEFICIENCY

A. Definition[1, 4, 12, 19]

1. A megaloblastic anemia caused by a deficiency of vitamin B_{12}
2. Usually a result of a deficiency of hydrochloric acid or pancreatic enzymes that causes an inability to metabolize vitamin B_{12}

B. Incidence/Predisposing factors[1, 4, 12, 16, 19]

1. Vegans and strict vegetarians are at risk.
2. Major cause is malabsorption as a result of diseases of the ileum or enteritis.

3. Blind loop syndrome
4. Drugs such as alcohol, anesthetics, metformin, nitrous oxide, and the antituberculosis drug para-aminosalicylic acid (PASA)
5. Hemodialysis
6. Fish tapeworm (*Diphyllobothrium latum*)
7. Since storage of vitamin B_{12} is normally high and body utilization is low, deficiency takes about 2–7 years to develop in the case of malabsorption.
8. Nutritional vitamin B_{12} deficiency is rare in the United States.

C. Subjective findings[1, 4, 12, 14, 19]

Same as in pernicious anemia (see preceding)

D. Physical examination findings[1, 4, 12, 14, 19]

Same as in pernicious anemia (see preceding)

E. Laboratory/Diagnostic findings[1, 4, 12, 14, 19]

1. Same as with pernicious anemia (see preceding) except as follows:
2. Anti-IF and anti-parietal cell antibodies (specific for pernicious anemia)
3. Schilling's test (only when it is unclear why the patient is vitamin B_{12}-deficient, not to prove the existence of the anemia, because of the expense of the test)

F. Management[1, 4, 19]

1. As in pernicious anemia (see preceding) if severe deficiency
2. Treatment of the underlying cause will normalize vitamin B_{12} levels:

   a. In blind loop syndrome, tetracycline, 250–500 mg q6h or 500 mg–1 g q12h, for 10 days normalizes vitamin B_{12} levels.
   b. In fish tapeworm, common in Scandinavian countries, give vitamin B_{12} alone or intrinsic factor and vitamin B_{12}.

IV. IRON DEFICIENCY

A. Definition[2, 9, 12]

1. State in which iron stores in the body are inadequate to preserve homeostasis
2. Microcytic anemia is characterized by small, pale RBCs and depleted iron stores.

B. Incidence/Predisposing factors[5, 8, 10, 12]

1. The most common anemia worldwide

   a. Accounts for 60% of anemias in patients over age 65
   b. Usually mild, but may become moderate or even severe

2. Common cause is blood loss from gastrointestinal and genito-urinary systems (particularly with menses).
3. Gastric or small-bowel surgery without adequate iron supplements
4. Blood donations
5. Iron requirements increase during pregnancy, upsetting iron balance.
6. Chronic aspirin use may precipitate iron loss without documented lesion.
7. Menorrhagia or other uterine bleeding
8. Chronic hemoglobinuria; traumatic hemolysis secondary to abnormally functioning cardiac valve
9. Repeated pregnancies with breast feeding

C. Subjective findings[5, 9, 10, 12]

1. Initially may be asymptomatic
2. Fatigue
3. Exertional dyspnea
4. Dizziness
5. Headache
6. Exercise intolerance
7. May develop pica (usually craving for substances such as ice, but may be for other items such as starch, paint, or clay)

D. Physical examination findings[5, 9, 10, 12]

1. Pallor (skin and conjunctiva)
2. Red and smooth tongue
3. May have spoon-shaped, brittle nails (koilonychia)
4. May have cheilosis (cracking corners of the mouth)
5. Tachycardia
6. Palpitation
7. Peripheral paresthesias
8. May have apical systolic "hemic" heart murmur

E. Laboratory/Diagnostic findings[3, 5, 9, 10]

1. Peripheral smear

   a. Staging of deficiency
      i. Stage 1—Depletion of body stores but laboratory test results may be normal
      ii. Stage 2—May have normal hemoglobin but depleted iron stores per laboratory test values
      iii. Stage 3—Iron depletion, slight anemia, normal MCV
      iv. Stage 4—Severe iron deficiency, hypochromic RBCs, and low MCV with marked anemia
   b. Microcytosis, poikilocytosis, and hypochromia appear as deficiency worsens.

2. An elevated RDW in the absence of any other RBC abnormalities is a major diagnostic indicator.
3. Reticulocyte count is disproportionately decreased in relation to the degree of anemia.
4. Ferritin level <10–12 μg/dL; TIBC >300 μg/dL
5. Serum iron (usually low, below 50 mg/dL) test ordered for transferrin saturation ratio (serum iron to TIBC); if ratio <15%, then iron deficiency is present.
6. Platelet count may be elevated (as high as 1.5 million/mm³).
7. Bone marrow biopsy is indicated when preceding are inconclusive.

   a. Gold standard is bone marrow iron stain.
   b. Decreased or absent marrow iron stores indicate deficiency.
   c. Deficiency is reported as Prussian blue–negative on bone marrow stain.

8. Consider ordering:

   a. Stool
      i. For guaiac testing
      ii. For ova and parasites (O & P)
   b. Gastrointestinal endoscopy
   c. Clotting studies

F. Management[3, 5, 10, 12, 17]

1. Determine the cause and amount of blood loss and treat the underlying disorder.
2. Oral ferrous sulfate, 300–325 mg t.i.d., 1 h before meals for 6 months

   • Enteric-coated or sustained-release iron preparations are not well absorbed and should be avoided.

3. For uncomplicated iron deficiency anemia, a polysaccharide iron complex (Hytinic, Niferex, Niferex-150, Nu-Iron, Nu-Iron-150) may be considered.

   a. They are associated with fewer adverse reactions.
   b. Dosage for adults: 50–100 mg of elemental iron t.i.d.

4. Follow-up in 2–4 weeks with CBC count

   a. Hgb should be normalized at 2 months.
   b. Six months of treatment is recommended to build iron stores.

5. Transfusion of packed RBCs may be necessary if anemia is symptomatic (1 mL of transfused RBCs delivers 1 mg iron).

6. Parenteral iron intravenously or deep intramuscularly is reserved for intolerance of or noncompliance with oral supplements.

   a. Anaphylaxis may occur.
      i. A test dose of 0.5 mL should be given before initiation of therapy.
      ii. Diphenhydramine (Benadryl) and epinephrine should be readily available.
   b. Painful injections need to be given in large muscles of the buttocks.
      i. Injections may stain the skin.
      ii. No more than 1 mL in each buttock per day should be given.
   c. Intravenous administration may cause phlebitis.
   d. Administration can be according to the following formula:

   $$\text{milligrams of iron} = (\text{normal Hgb} - \text{patient's Hgb}) \times \text{weight (kg)} \times 2.21 + 1000$$

   e. Iron dextran (Imferon), 50 mg/mL, can be administered IM or IV; IV administration should not exceed 1 mL/min and 2 mL/day.

7. Within 7–10 days a reticulocyte response and increase in hematocrit should occur.
8. Failure to respond to therapy within 5–8 weeks warrants evaluation for compliance, impaired absorption, gastric or bowel pathology, blood loss, or incorrect diagnosis.

V. FOLIC ACID DEFICIENCY

A. Definition[12, 16]

1. A megaloblastic anemia
2. Decreased red blood cells and hemoglobin content due to impaired production related to decreased serum folate

B. Incidence/Predisposing factors[1, 12, 16, 19]

1. Usually result of

   a. Inadequate dietary intake
   b. Lack of absorption
   c. Inadequate conversion of folate to tetrahydrofolate

2. Nutritional folate deficiency usually related to alcoholism, anorexia, old age with inadequate dietary intake, or special diets
3. Malabsorption of folic acid found with celiac disease, tropical sprue, and gluten-sensitive enteropathy
4. Increased utilization of folic acid during pregnancy, malignancy, or hemolysis

5. May be drug-induced by

    a. Methotrexate
    b. Pyrimethamine
    c. Phenytoin
    d. Alcohol
    e. Isoniazid
    f. Oral contraceptives

6. Normal body store of folate is 5000 to 20,000 μg.
7. Clinical signs of folate deficiency can occur in about 4 months.

C. Subjective findings[1, 4, 12]

1. Fatigue
2. Pallor
3. Mouth/tongue pain
4. Symptoms may not be present until anemia is severe.

D. Physical examination findings[1, 4, 12]

1. Patient may show signs of malnutrition.
2. Patient may or may not show the following:

    a. Glossitis
    b. Stomatitis
    c. Gastrointestinal symptoms
    d. Hyperpigmentation
    e. Infertility
    f. Orthostatic hypotension
    g. Weight loss
    h. Neurologic symptoms are less common but do occur.

E. Laboratory/Diagnostic findings[1, 2, 16]

1. Serum folate <4 μg/L (rises and falls rapidly with dietary intake)
2. RBC folate is a better indicator of tissue levels (<100 ng/mL).
3. MCV usually >115 fL^3 or may gradually increase over several months to years and remain in normal range

F. Management[12, 16, 19]

1. Care should be given to ensure a correct diagnosis. Administration of folate can exacerbate the neurologic symptoms of vitamin B_{12} deficiency.
2. Oral folate, 1–5 mg/day for 3–4 months
3. Folate should be given along with vitamin B_{12} when both are deficient.

4. After the initiation of folate:

   a. Peak of reticulocytosis is in 6–8 days, followed by a slow increase in Hgb.

   b. Total correction should be seen within 2 months.

VI. ANEMIA OF CHRONIC DISEASE (ACD)

A. Definition[3, 8, 11, 12, 16, 17]

1. An anemia that is

   a. Gradual in onset

   b. Usually normochromic and normocytic

   c. Accompanies

      i. Chronic infections or chronic inflammation

      ii. Connective tissue diseases such as rheumatoid arthritis

      iii. Underlying malignancies

   d. The anemia resolves when the underlying disorder clears.

2. Inability of the reticuloendothelial cells to recirculate iron from phagocytosed, fully mature RBCs, with tissue iron stores normal or increased rather than absent

3. Anemia is occasionally hypochromic, microcytic.

B. Incidence/Predisposing factors[8, 12, 16, 17]

1. Second most common anemia after iron deficiency

   a. Accompanies any chronic infection

   b. Seen with inflammation, particularly connective tissue (immune) disorders

   c. Common in

      i. Acute inflammatory disorders

      ii. Protein-energy malnutrition

      iii. Burns

      iv. Myocardial infarction

2. Seen with

   a. Chronic renal disease

   b. Liver disease with or without alcoholism

   c. Endocrine disorders

      i. Hypothyroidism

      ii. Hypopituitarism

      iii. Hypogonadism

      iv. Hyperparathyroidism

3. Anemia develops within 1–2 months of the onset of illness.

4. Degree of anemia usually coincides with the severity of the underlying disease.

5. Usually manifested in individual in whom primary disease is obvious

6. Any infection due to a bacterium or a fungus that lasts more than 2 weeks can cause anemia.
7. Commonly confused with iron deficiency anemia

C. Subjective findings[8, 11, 12, 17]

1. Frequently occurs without symptoms
2. If anemia is severe, the patient may complain of the following:

   a. Fatigue
   b. Shortness of breath
   c. Weight loss
   d. Lightheadedness
   e. Loss of appetite

3. The patient may complain only of symptoms related to the underlying chronic disease.

D. Physical examination findings[8, 11, 12, 17]

Primarily those of the underlying disease

E. Laboratory/Diagnostic findings[8, 9, 11, 12, 16, 17]

1. Mild to moderate anemia with Hgb concentration <10 g/dL is extremely unusual.
2. RBCs are usually normocytic and normochromic, but occasionally are hypochromic, microcytic.
3. Reticulocyte count is less than 1% or a low absolute number.
4. Normal or increased iron stores differentiate anemia of chronic disease (ACD) from iron deficiency anemia.

   a. Serum ferritin is usually high in ACD (>100 ng/mL).
   b. TIBC is usually depressed in ACD (<250 μg/mL).

5. RBC morphology varies very little from normal: RDW is usually normal in ACD.
6. Sideroblasts are absent in bone marrow, but iron stores are normal or increased.
7. Leukocytosis and thrombocytosis are often seen in the peripheral smear if infection or malignancy is present.
8. Consider ordering erythrocyte sedimentation rate (ESR) to assess the severity of inflammation associated with the underlying chronic illness.

F. Management[8, 12, 16, 17]

1. In premenopausal women, a therapeutic trial of oral iron may be given with re-evaluation of CBC in 2–3 weeks to rule out iron deficiency anemia.

   a. A 1.5 g/dL or greater rise in Hgb concentration should have occurred.

b. Failure warrants further investigation.
c. Not appropriate for postmenopausal women or men of any age

2. No specific therapy exists. Oral iron is of no benefit in this anemia.
3. Identification and treatment of underlying disease are required. If the disorder is reversible, the anemia should resolve.
4. Recombinant human erythropoietin is used for individuals with chronic diseases such as renal disease/failure and rheumatoid arthritis to increase hematopoiesis.

a. Dosage for adults is individualized: Starting dose is 50–100 units/kg IV three times a week.
b. Nondialysis or continuous peritoneal dialysis patients may receive doses SC or IV.
c. Dose is adjusted in 2–8 weeks, based on response to therapy.
d. Target Hct range 30–33 mL/dL (max 36 mL/dL)
e. Hct should not increase more than 4 points in any 2-week period to reduce risk of hypertension or seizures.

VII. THALASSEMIA

A. Definition[7, 12, 13]

1. A group of inherited disorders that are a result of a defective production of the globin portion of the hemoglobin, characterized by hypochromic, microcytic anemia.
2. Cooley's anemia is the name commonly used for severe thalassemia (thalassemia major).

B. Incidence/Predisposing factors[7, 12, 15]

1. The word *thalassemia* is derived from the Greek word for *sea*.

a. The disorder was first recognized in Mediterranean coastal regions among individuals of Italian or Greek ancestry.
b. Worldwide distribution of thalassemia is associated with that of malignant malaria.
c. Thalassemia affords a protective effect against *Plasmodium falciparum* malaria in indigenous areas.

2. Many genetic mutations make up the β-thalassemia syndromes. General classifications include:

a. Thalassemia minor
b. Thalassemia intermedia
c. Thalassemia major (Cooley's anemia), or homozygous β-thalassemia

3. α-thalassemia classified into four types:

  a. Silent carrier state: α-thalassemia-2 trait (asymptomatic)
  b. Mild, microcytic, hypochromic anemia: α-thalassemia-1 trait
  c. Moderately severe hemolytic anemia usually not requiring chronic transfusions: Three genes affected
  d. Nonfunctional: All four genes affected; results in hydrops fetalis and Bart's hemoglobin

4. The most common form is thalassemia trait.

  a. Represented in the heterozygous form of either α- or β-thalassemia
  b. In areas where the thalassemia trait is common, the homozygous form is more prevalent.

5. In the U.S., β-thalassemia is most prevalent among ethnic groups originating from the Mediterranean area and parts of Africa and Asia.
6. In the U.S., α-thalassemia is the most prevalent among patients of Asian ancestry.
7. About 1000 patients with severe forms of thalassemia are known in the U.S.
8. Gallstones occur in 15% of patients over age 15.

C. Subjective findings[12, 15, 18]

1. Heterozygous β-thalassemia silent carriers
2. Pallor
3. Fatigue
4. Dark urine
5. Poor growth

D. Physical examination findings[3, 12, 13, 16]

1. Hepatosplenomegaly
2. Cardiac failure/dilation
3. Jaundice
4. Cooley's anemia facies (marked osteoporosis and cortical thinning)

  a. Erythroid overgrowth of the marrow may distort the bones of the head, face, rib cage, and pelvis.
  b. Predisposed to pathologic fractures of long bones and vertebrae

5. Growth retardation with delayed or absent adolescent growth spurt and delayed menarche, oligomenorrhea, or amenorrhea

  a. Delayed secondary sexual characteristics
  b. Hypogonadism

E. Laboratory/Diagnostic findings[3, 7, 12, 16, 18]

1. Hallmark is microcytic, hypochromic anemia.
2. Usually manifests as a decrease in Hgb, Hct, MCV, and mean corpuscular hemoglobin (MCH) in conjunction with normal to increased RBC, normal to mildly decreased mean corpuscular hemoglobin concentration (MCHC), and normal RDW
3. Wright's stain

   a. Homozygous β-thalassemia and double heterozygous non–α-thalassemia exhibit extreme anisocytosis and poikilocytosis with bizarre shapes, target cells, ovalocytes, and large numbers of nucleated RBCs.
   b. Heterozygous β-thalassemia
      i. Exhibits hypochromic and microcytic cells with mild to moderate anisocytosis and poikilocytosis
      ii. Target cells are frequent, with basophilic stippling.

4. Indirect bilirubin level

   a. Increased in both thalassemia major and thalassemia intermedia
   b. Ranges from 1–6 mg/dL
   c. Indirect bilirubin levels in thalassemia intermedia exceed those in thalassemia major.

5. Osmotic fragility of red cells—May be used as inexpensive screening for thalassemia carrier state
6. Hgb electrophoresis is used to confirm the diagnosis— Cellulose acetate electrophoresis is preferred to starch gel electrophoresis or citrate agar gel electrophoresis.

   a. HbA_2: If elevated, is consistent with heterozygous β-thalassemia
   b. HbF: If HbF and HbA_2 levels are normal, microcytosis with minimal or no anemia suggests α-thalassemia.

7. Restriction endonuclease mapping of the α-globin genes is the only definitive test for α-gene deletion.

   a. Expensive and time-consuming
   b. Usually reserved for special circumstances involving prenatal diagnosis

8. Consider ordering:

   a. Evaluation of iron status to rule out iron deficiency anemia and assess for iron load
      i. Serum iron level
      ii. TIBC
      iii. Serum ferritin level
   b. Free erythrocyte protoporphyrin (FEP) if lead poisoning suspected

9. Skull x-ray may show "hair on end" appearance in a homozygous β-thalassemia patient.

F. Management[13, 16, 18]

1. Severe β-thalassemia

    a. Blood transfusion support

        i. Each unit of packed RBCs contains about 200 mg iron.

        ii. Multiple transfusions predispose a patient to manifestations of hemochromatosis at an early age.

        iii. Thalassemia intermedia patients, who may not receive transfusions, are also at risk, but at a later age.

    b. Iron chelation therapy with severe beta-thalassemia

        i. Deferoxamine (Desferal) given parenterally, 2–6 g, 5–6 nights a week, with a 30–40 mg excretion of iron daily in older patients.

          (1) Usually given IM

          (2) Abdominal SC pump infusion slowly over a period of 8–12 h nightly is most effective.

        ii. Chelation therapy via a Hickman catheter at 3–4 g/day over 18–20 h may be self-administered by well-motivated patients.

    c. Goal for Hgb levels—9–10 g/dL with chelation therapy

    d. Concurrent administration of vitamin C (150–250 mg/day) orally may enhance iron excretion.

        i. Use cautiously with older patients.

        ii. May enhance iron toxicity

2. Observation for leukopenia and thrombocytopenia as indicators for splenic enlargement and potential need for splenectomy

3. Allogeneic bone marrow transplantation

References

1. Allen, R.H. (1996). Megaloblastic anemias. In J.C. Bennett & F. Plum (Eds.), *Cecil textbook of medicine* (pp. 843–851). Philadelphia: W.B. Saunders.

2. Abrams, W.B., Beers, M.H., & Berkow, R. (Eds.). (1995). *The Merck manual of geriatrics* (2nd ed.) (pp. 860–861). Whitehouse Station, N.J.: Merck Research Laboratories.

3. Andreoli, T.E., Bennett, J.C., Carpenter, C.C., & Plum, F. (1997). *Cecil essentials of medicine* (4th ed.) (pp. 381–397). Philadelphia: W.B. Saunders.

4. Bottner, W.A. (1996). Megaloblastic anemia. In R.E. Rakel (Ed.), *Saunders manual of medical practice* (pp. 577–578). Philadelphia: W.B. Saunders.

5. Duffy, T.P. (1996). Microcytic and hypochromic anemias. In J.C. Bennett & F. Plum (Eds.), *Cecil textbook of medicine* (pp. 839–843). Philadelphia: W.B. Saunders.

6. Glassman, A.B. (1997). Anemia: Diagnosis and clinical considerations. In D.M. Harmening (Ed.), *Clinical hematology and fundamentals of hemostasis* (3rd ed.) (pp. 71–79). Philadelphia: F.A. Davis.

7. Harrison, C.R. (1997). Thalassemia. In D.M. Harmening (Ed.), *Clinical hematology and fundamentals of hemostasis* (3rd ed.) (pp. 193–210). Philadelphia: F.A. Davis.

8. Julius, C.J. & Gwaltney-Krause, S. (1997). Anemia associated with systemic, nonhematologic disorders. In D.M. Harmening (Ed.), *Clinical hematology and fundamentals of hemostasis* (3rd ed.) (pp. 244–261). Philadelphia: F.A. Davis.

9. Leclair, S.J. (1997). Iron metabolism and hypochromic anemias. In D.M. Harmening (Ed.), *Clinical hematology and fundamentals of hemostasis* (3rd ed.) (pp. 97–115). Philadelphia: F.A. Davis.

10. Lee, T.C. (1996). Iron deficiency anemia. In R.E. Rakel (Ed.), *Saunders manual of medical practice* (pp. 575–576). Philadelphia: W.B. Saunders.

11. Lindenbaum, J. (1996). An approach to the anemias. In J.C. Bennett & F. Plum (Eds.), *Cecil textbook of medicine* (pp. 823–831). Philadelphia: W.B. Saunders.

12. Linker, C.A. (1997). Blood. In L.M. Tierney, Jr., S.J. McPhee, & J.A. Papadakis (Eds.), *Current medical diagnosis & treatment* (36th ed.) (pp. 463–518). Stamford, CT: Appleton & Lange.

13. Mankad, V.N. (1996). Thalassemia syndromes. In R.E. Rakel (Ed.), *Saunders manual of medical practice* (pp. 585–586). Philadelphia: W.B. Saunders.

14. Memoli, D. (1996). Anemia workup. In R.E. Rakel (Ed.), *Saunders manual of medical practice* (pp. 572–574). Philadelphia: W.B. Saunders.

15. Nienhuis, A.W. & Benz, E.J., Jr. (1996). The thalassemias. In J.C. Bennett & F. Plum (Eds.), *Cecil textbook of medicine*. (pp. 877–882). Philadelphia: W.B. Saunders.

16. Pechet, L. (1996). Anemias and other red cell disorders. In J. Noble (Ed.), *Textbook of primary care medicine* (2nd ed.) (pp. 722–734). St. Louis: Mosby.

17. Richer, S. (1997). A practical guide for differentiating between iron deficiency anemia and anemia of chronic disease in children and adults. *The nurse practitioner, 22,* 82–101.

18. Steinberg, M.H. (1994). Hemoglobinopathies and thalassemia. In Stein, J.H. (Ed.), *Internal medicine* (4th ed) (pp. 852–863). St. Louis: Mosby-Year Book.

19. Taghizadeh, M. (1997). Megaloblastic anemias. In D.M. Harmening, (Ed.), *Clinical hematology and fundamentals of hemostasis* (3rd ed) (pp. 116–134). Philadelphia: F.A. Davis.

SICKLE CELL DISEASE/CRISIS

Sylvia R. Love, MED, MSN, RN, CS, ACNP, ANP

I. SICKLE CELL DISEASE/CRISIS

A. Definition[3, 5, 8]

1. Sickle cell anemia (SS) is an uncompensated hemolytic anemia, with shortened red blood cell (RBC) survival; increased RBC production (erythropoiesis) is insufficient to balance the increased rate of destruction.
2. An inherited disorder caused by abnormal properties conveyed to sickle cell erythrocytes by mutant sickle cell hemoglobin

B. Incidence/Predisposing factors[1, 2, 5, 8]

1. In the United States, African Americans are primarily affected. Persons of African, Mediterranean, Southeast Asian, Caribbean, South and Central American, and East Indian origin may also be affected.
2. The sickle cell trait confers a protective effect against *Plasmodium falciparum* malaria.
3. Presence of the trait is associated with sudden death in military recruits.
4. Sickle cell trait is accompanied by increased risk for development of pneumonia or acute chest syndrome.
5. Mean age of death

   a. Hemoglobin SS (HbSS) sickle cell disease
      i. Women = 46
      ii. Men = 43
   b. Sickle cell hemoglobin C (HbSC) disease
      i. Women = 63
      ii. Men = 60

6. Prevalence

   a. HbSS sickle cell disease, the most severe form, is seen in about 1 in 375 patients.
   b. Hemoglobin SC is seen in about 1 in 835 patients.
   c. Hemoglobin S–β-thalassemia is seen in about 1 in 1667 patients.

7. Sickle cell trait, HbAS, is found in about 1 in 12 African Americans.

   a. Not part of the sickle cell disease syndrome
   b. Life expectancy is the same as in the general population.

8. Pain

   a. One third of patients with SS rarely have pain.
   b. One third are hospitalized for pain two to six times a year.
   c. One third have six or more pain-related hospitalizations per year.

9. Common neurologic complications in 25% of SS patients include

   a. Transient ischemic attacks (TIAs)
   b. Cerebral infarction
   c. Cerebral hemorrhage
   d. Seizures
   e. Unexplained coma

C. Subjective findings[2, 6, 8]

1. Symptoms usually relate to increased cell viscosity and subsequent vaso-occlusion that result in the following:

   a. Generalized pain in long bones, joints
   b. Fever, fatigue, malaise
   c. Abdominal pain, nausea, vomiting, decreased appetite
   d. Swelling in hands, feet, joints
   e. Priapism

2. Depression (particularly in adolescents—due to low self-esteem and maturation delays)

D. Physical examination findings[1, 5, 6, 8]

1. Chronic hemolytic anemia
2. Tachycardia
3. Fever
4. Tachypnea
5. Splenomegaly

   a. Frequently seen with HbSC
   b. Usually nonpalpable with HbSS

6. Hepatomegaly
7. Jaundice (sclera) with darkened urine
8. Cardiomegaly
9. Retinopathy
10. Adolescents may exhibit physical immaturity.

    a. Delay in sex organ development and maturation; menarche delayed until age 15–17
    b. Delayed adolescent growth in both height and weight
    c. Decreased physical endurance compared with peers

11. Leg ulcers near the medial or lateral malleolus may occur spontaneously or as a result of trauma.

E. Laboratory/Diagnostic findings[1, 2, 8]

1. Hemoglobin electrophoresis will confirm:

   a. Hemoglobin genotype (cellulose acetate and citrate agar gel) for sickle cell disease
   b. Hemoglobin F (fetal) and A_2 for presence of thalassemia

2. HbSS patients are anemic; hematocrit is usually 20–30 mL/dL.
3. Reticulocyte count markedly elevated (10–25%); if not, then anemia source other than sickle cell disease should be sought.
4. WBC count is usually elevated (12,000–15,000 μg/L).
5. Sickled cells (5–50%) are found on the peripheral blood smear.
6. Elevated levels of

   a. Serum unconjugated (indirect) bilirubin
   b. Serum transaminase
   c. Alkaline phosphatase

7. Serum creatinine level is lower than normal (unless in renal failure) because of increased glomerular filtration rate of the kidneys, which cannot concentrate urine.
8. The urine may contain protein.
9. Decreased levels of

   a. Plasma protein C
   b. Plasma protein S

10. Elevated levels of

    a. Factor VIII activity
    b. Von Willebrand's factor antigen
    c. Thrombin

11. Platelet counts are moderately elevated.
12. Consider:

    a. Ordering x-ray studies of painful bones
    b. To rule out aseptic necrosis, may need
       i. Computed tomography (CT)
       ii. Magnetic resonance imaging (MRI)

F. Management[1, 2, 4–8]

1. Keep the patient well hydrated.

   a. Maintain oral fluid intake at 3–4 L/day.
   b. Administer IV fluids for dehydration, acute illness.
   c. Avoid iatrogenic fluid overload.

2. Administer oxygen to hypoxic patients with $Pao_2 < 60$–70 mmHg. Use humidified O_2, 40%.

3. Give non-narcotic analgesics such as nonsteroidal anti-inflammatory drugs or acetaminophen.

   a. May be given for mild to moderate pain, or
   b. Give with narcotic analgesic to enhance analgesia

4. For moderate/severe pain, give narcotic analgesics.

   a. Morphine (drug of choice), 0.15 mg/kg q3–4h IV, SC, IM, or PCA
   b. Use of meperidine is controversial; it may be vigorously avoided in some centers.

5. For mild pain, use narcotic analgesics such as codeine, oxycodone, or propoxyphene (drug of choice), 65 mg q4h p.o., or 100 mg as napsylate.

6. Alternative drugs, usually used in combination with analgesics, include

   a. Antihistamines
   b. Tricyclic antidepressants

7. Use phenothiazines for nausea and vomiting.

8. Hospitalization is indicated for

   a. Persistent pain unrelieved by analgesics for longer than 8 h
   b. Sepsis and persistent fever
   c. Central nervous system disorders
      i. Increased lethargy
      ii. Headaches
   d. Acute chest syndrome
   e. Surgical emergency
   f. Pregnancy-related complications
   g. Priapism (may require exchange transfusion or surgical shunting by urologist)

9. If chest complications occur, consider

   a. Oxygen supplementation
   b. Antibiotics
   c. Complete-exchange transfusion (if the patient is arterial hypoxic)

10. Preventive measures for the adult should include

   a. Folic acid, 1 mg p.o., daily supplementation
   b. Pneumococcal vaccine
   c. Hepatitis vaccine (if result of hepatitis B antibody screen is negative)
   d. Foot care and protective shoes may prevent chronic leg ulcers.
   e. Annual and repeated health care visits as needed, with two to three visits a year for those over age 30 (dictated by patient status)

    f. Annual retinal evaluation begun at school age; if no sickle cell-related findings, repeat visits as adult every 2–3 years.

    g. History of priapism should be sought at each visit, with early treatment.

11. Genetic counseling should be offered.

    a. Birth control options should be presented to adolescents with sickle cell disease.

    b. Oral contraceptives are not contraindicated.

12. Patients should avoid temperature extremes and physical overexertion that leads to dehydration.

13. In HbSS, aliphatic butyrate salts and hydroxyurea increase the level of fetal hemoglobin.

    a. Hydroxyurea, 500–750 mg/d, is used to reduce occurrence of painful crises.

    b. Erythropoietin is mentioned in the literature on sickle cell disease, but the effective dosage schedules are unclear.

14. Successful cure of SS has been accomplished with allogeneic bone marrow transplantation, but this is not considered conventional therapy at present in the United States.

References

1. Andreoli, T.E., Bennett, J.C., Carpenter, C.C., & Plum, F. (1997). Disorders of red cells. *Cecil essentials of medicine* (4th ed.) (pp. 381–397). Philadelphia: W.B. Saunders.
2. Bobo-Mosley, L. (1996). Sickle cell disease. In R.E. Rakel (Ed.), *Saunders manual of medical practice* (pp. 581–584). Philadelphia: W.B. Saunders.
3. Bookchin, R.M., & Lew, V.L. (1996). Pathophysiology of sickle cell anemia. *Hematology/Oncology Clinics of North America, 10,* 1241–1253.
4. Charache, S. (1996). Experimental therapy. *Hematology/Oncology Clinics of North America, 10,* 1373–1382.
5. Embury, S.H. (1996). Sickle cell anemia and associated hemoglobinopathies. In J.C. Bennett & F. Plum (Eds.), *Cecil textbook of medicine* (pp. 882–893). Philadelphia: W.B. Saunders.
6. Kinney, T.R., & Ware, R.E. (1996). The adolescent with sickle cell anemia. *Hematology/Oncology Clinics of North America, 10,* 1255–1264.
7. Koshy, M., & Dorn, L. (1996). Continuing care for adult patients with sickle cell disease. *Hematology/Oncology Clinics of North America, 10,* 1265–1272.
8. Linker, C.A. (1999). Blood. In L.M. Tierney, Jr., S.J. McPhee, & M.A. Papadakis (Eds.), *Current medical diagnosis & treatment* (38th ed.) (pp. 485–537). Stamford, CT: Appleton & Lange.

COAGULOPATHIES

Sylvia R. Love, MED, MSN, RN, CS, ACNP, ANP

I. IDIOPATHIC THROMBOCYTOPENIA PURPURA (ITP)

A. Definition[3, 11]

1. Disorder in which antibody-sensitive platelets are destroyed by the spleen
2. An autoimmune disorder in which IgG autoantibody binds to platelets, facilitating their destruction by the spleen

B. Incidence/Predisposing factors[3, 11, 12]

1. In children

    a. Usually precipitated by a viral illness
    b. Self-limiting
    c. Results in bruising and mucosal bleeding

2. In adults

    a. Usually chronic
    b. Requires periodic treatment

3. Disease of young persons; women aged 20–40 outnumber men 2:1.
4. Spontaneous recovery occurs in only 5% of adult cases.
5. Thrombocytopenia may be induced by

    a. Heparin
    b. Sulfonamides
    c. Thiazides
    d. Quinine
    e. Cimetidine
    f. Gold

6. Thrombocytopenia purpura is a common secondary manifestation of

    a. Systemic lupus erythematosus (SLE) in 14–26% of patients
    b. Chronic lymphocytic leukemia (CLL)

7. About two thirds of patients require no further treatment after splenectomy. Response is achieved within 10 days.
8. Thirteen thousand new cases of adult ITP are believed to occur each year in the United States.

C. Subjective findings[11, 12]

1. Presenting complaint is usually mucosal or epidermal bleeding.
   a. Epistaxis
   b. Oral bleeding
   c. Menorrhagia
   d. Purpura
   e. Petechiae

2. Patient is usually systemically well.

D. Physical examination findings[11]

1. Patient is afebrile and usually appears well, with no abnormal findings on examination except those related to bleeding.
2. Spleen is nonpalpable.

E. Laboratory/Diagnostic findings[11, 14]

1. Thrombocytopenia is the hallmark of the disease; may be <10,000 platelets/μL.
2. No definitive test for ITP exists; diagnosis is by exclusion.
3. Other hematopoietic cell lines are normal, although platelets are enlarged (megathrombocytes).
4. Ten percent of patients have coexistent autoimmune hemolytic anemia (Evans' syndrome).
   a. Anemia, reticulocytosis, and spherocytes are seen on peripheral smear.
   b. No fragmented cells (schistocytes) should be seen.
5. An antinuclear antibody (ANA) test may help point to an autoimmune process.
6. Consider ordering
   a. Monoclonal antibody immobilization of platelet antigens (MAIPA)
      i. Considered the most sensitive and specific antibody test
      ii. Immunoglobin G (IgG) platelet antibodies are present in 90% of patients.
   b. Bone marrow biopsy (normal or increased megakaryocytes) to exclude myelodysplasia
   c. All patients with decreased platelet counts should have the peripheral blood smear reviewed to confirm the automated count and to rule out EDTA artifact from the test.
      i. Platelet clumping may be seen in purple-top tube with EDTA.
      ii. Platelet count should be repeated using blue-top tube with sodium citrate or green-top tube with heparin.
   d. Determine blood type, specifically Rh status, if WinRho treatment (described subsequently, under F. Management) is considered as a treatment option.

F. Management[3, 4, 9, 11, 12, 14]

1. Treatment may not be needed until the platelet count is less than 20,000/μL, unless the patient is symptomatic.

   a. Initial treatment is with prednisone, 1–2 mg/kg/day.
   b. Bleeding often diminishes within 1 day of treatment.
   c. Elevation of platelets is usually seen within 2–3 days.

2. High-dose IV gamma globulin (400 mg/kg for 3–5 days) is highly effective.

   a. Very expensive treatment (approximately $5000)
   b. Usually produces response in 1–5 days
   c. Usually reserved for emergency situations
   d. In HIV-related ITP, gamma globulin (2 mg/kg/day in divided doses) is preferred to steroids.

3. Splenectomy is highly effective.

   a. Indicated when prednisone therapy fails
   b. Pneumococcal vaccine should be considered several weeks prior to splenectomy to minimize complications from sepsis.

4. Chemotherapy is used for those who fail to respond to splenectomy and prednisone therapy.

   a. Danazol, 600 mg/day in two to four divided doses, for 2 months
   b. Or immunosuppressive agents
      i. Vincristine, 1–2 mg for adults for 5–7 days, three courses
      ii. Vinblastine, 0.1 mg/kg, maximum dose 10 mg, for 5–7 days, three courses
      iii. Azathioprine, 50–250 mg, with the average 150 mg, for 3–26 months (average 10 months)
      iv. Cyclophosphamide, 50–200 mg/day for 1–9 months; used in refractory cases

5. Platelet transfusion is used in life-threatening bleeding only.
6. Most serious complication of ITP: Spontaneous intracranial hemorrhage

   a. Less than 1% of patients are afflicted with this disorder.
   b. Patients are at risk when platelet count is less than 5000/μL.

7. New treatment for Rh-positive patients

   a. Intravenous anti-D (Rh$_0$[D]) immune globulin (WinRho SDF), at about 50 μg/kg, given in a single dose, has been found to be effective with about half the expense of IV gamma globulin.

    b. Dosage-regimen studies are still ongoing.

    c. Follow-up platelet counts should be obtained in about 1 week.

    d. Retreatment is given when the platelet count is less than $30,000/\mu L$.

    e. This treatment is not the first-line therapy, nor is it indicated for refractory ITP.

II. DISSEMINATED INTRAVASCULAR COAGULATION (DIC)

A. Definition[1, 2, 6, 10, 15]

1. An acquired coagulation disorder that occurs as a secondary process concomitant with a pathophysiologic disease or a clinical state

2. A hemorrhagic syndrome

    a. Caused by the consumption of many coagulation factors and platelets

    b. An abnormal stimulus results in the formation of excess thrombin, which in turn causes

       i. Fibrinogen consumption

      ii. Irreversible platelet aggregation

     iii. Activation of the fibrinolytic system

3. Other names

    a. Consumptive coagulopathy

    b. Diffuse intravascular coagulation

B. Incidence/Predisposing factors[2]

1. Infection is the most common cause; 10–20% of cases are caused by gram-negative sepsis.

2. Often associated with

    a. Obstetric complications

    b. Malignant neoplasms

    c. Liver disease

    d. Trauma

    e. Burns

3. Transfusion of ABO-incompatible red blood cells

C. Subjective findings[2, 11, 15]

1. Bleeding complications are most common.

    a. The patient may exhibit mild symptoms, such as oozing from venipuncture sites or wounds.

    b. Typically, bleeding is from multiple sites.

2. The patient may complain of bleeding that is

    a. Oral

    b. Gingival

c. Gastrointestinal
d. Genitourinary

D. Physical examination findings[11, 15]

1. Acute DIC

   a. Tachycardia
   b. Hypotension
   c. Edema

2. Other possible findings

   a. Spontaneous bruising
   b. Gastrointestinal bleeding
   c. Respiratory tract bleeding
   d. Hematuria
   e. Persistent bleeding at venipuncture sites or wounds
   f. Skin necrosis
   g. Venous thromboembolism

3. Thrombosis

   a. May be superficial or deep venous (Trousseau's syndrome)
   b. Digital ischemia and gangrene may be the most common forms.
   c. Thrombosis is most common in cancer patients.

E. Laboratory/Diagnostic findings[1, 10, 11]

1. No single laboratory test is diagnostic. Clinical states are not static.
2. Acute uncompensated DIC (active hemorrhage evident)

   a. Thrombocytopenia—Platelet count $<150,000/\mu L$ universal finding
   b. Prothrombin time (PT) and activated partial thromboplastin time (APTT) are prolonged by 70% and 50%, respectively.
   c. Fibrinogen, factor V, and factor VII levels are low.
   d. Fragmented red blood cells (schistocytes) are found on peripheral blood smear.

3. Subacute DIC

   a. PT and APTT are usually normal.
   b. Fibrinogen levels are usually normal.
   c. Thrombocytopenia and an elevated D-dimer may be the only abnormal laboratory values.

4. Chronic or compensated DIC

   a. Elevated fibrin degradation product levels (FDPs $>45 \mu g/mL$ or are present in a $>1:100$ dilution)
   b. D-Dimer is most sensitive (positive at $>1:8$ dilution) for differentiating DIC from primary fibrinolysis.

5. Consider ordering

   a. Blood cultures to rule out sepsis
   b. Repeat fibrinogen levels and partial thromboplastin time (PTT).
      i. Initially fibrinogen levels may be normal in DIC, since fibrinogen half-life is approximately 4 days.
      ii. Diagnosis is confirmed by rapidly falling fibrinogen levels.
   c. Factor VIII (usually in the normal range in coagulopathy associated with liver disease alone)

F. Management[1, 4, 7, 10, 11, 15]

1. Hematology referral for suspected cases
2. Diagnose and correct the underlying cause.

   a. Correct hypotension.
   b. Control sepsis.
   c. Deliver placenta or dead fetus.

3. When risks of hemorrhagic complication are significant, maintenance of blood volume and hemostatic function is indicated:

   a. Packed red blood cells
   b. Replacement therapy by platelet transfusion (goal: platelet count of 30,000–50,000/μL)
   c. Cryoprecipitate
      i. Goal: Plasma fibrinogen level of 150 mg/dL
      ii. One unit cryoprecipitate increases fibrinogen level approximately 6–8 mg/dL.
      iii. Fifteen units raise the level from 50 to 150 mg/dL.
   d. Fresh frozen plasma every 30 min in severe DIC

2. Supportive treatment includes prevention of hypoxemia and hemodynamic compromise.
3. Heparin therapy is controversial.

References

1. Andreoli, T.E., Bennett, J.C., Carpenter, C.C., & Plum, F. (1997). *Cecil essentials of medicine* (4th ed.) (pp. 411–421). Philadelphia: W.B. Saunders.
2. Ansell, J.E., Thane, M., & Parker, F. (1996). Hemorrhagic and thrombotic disorders. In J. Noble (Ed.), *Textbook of primary care medicine* (2nd ed.) (pp. 747–760). St. Louis: Mosby.
3. Blanchette, V., Freedman, J., & Garvey, B. (1998). Management of chronic immune thrombocytopenia purpura in children and adults. *Seminars in Hematology, 35* (Suppl 1), 36–51.
4. Bussel, J.B. (1998). Recent advances in the treatment of idiopathic thrombocytopenia purpura: The Anti-D clinical experience. *Seminars in Hematology, 35* (Suppl 1), 1–4.

5. Caruana, C.C., & Schwartz, S.L. (1997). Disorders of plasma clotting factors. In D.M. Harmening (Ed.), *Clinical hematology and fundamentals of hemostasis* (3rd ed.) (pp. 531–553). Philadelphia: F.A. Davis.

6. Daaleman, T.P. (1996). Disseminated intravascular coagulation. In R.E. Rakel (Ed.), *Saunders manual of medical practice*. (pp. 617–618). Philadelphia: W.B. Saunders.

7. Freilberg, A., & Mauger, D. (1998). Efficacy, safety, and dose response of intravenous anti-D immune globulin (WinRho SDF) for the treatment of idiopathic thrombocytopenia purpura in children. *Seminars in Hematology, 35* (Suppl 1), 23–27.

8. George, J.N., & Raskob, G.E. (1998). Idiopathic thrombocytopenia purpura: A concise summary of the pathophysiology and diagnosis in children and adults. *Seminars in Hematology, 35* (Suppl 1), 5–8.

9. Hong, F., Rolando, R., Price, H., Griffiths, A., Malinoski, F., & Woloski, M. (1998). Safety profile of WinRho Anti-D. *Seminars in Hematology, 35* (Suppl 1), 9–13.

10. Lazarchick, J., & Kizer, J. (1997). Interaction of the fibrinolytic, coagulation, and kinin systems and related pathology. In D.M. Harmening (Ed.), *Clinical hematology and fundamentals of hemostasis* (3rd ed.) (pp. 554–565). Philadelphia: F.A. Davis.

11. Linker, C.A. (1999). Blood. In L.M. Tierney, Jr., S.J. McPhee, & M.A. Papadakis (Eds.), *Current medical diagnosis & treatment* (38th ed.) (pp. 485–537). Stamford, CT: Appleton & Lange.

12. Scaradavou, A., & Bussel, J.B. (1998). Clinical experience with Anti-D in the treatment of idiopathic thrombocytopenia purpura. *Seminars in Hematology, 35* (Suppl 1), 52–57.

13. Schafer, A.I. (1994). Thrombocytopenia and disorders of platelet function. In J.H. Stein (Ed.), *Internal Medicine* (4th ed.) (pp. 796–804). St. Louis: Mosby.

14. Tarantino, M.D., & Goldsmith, G. (1998). Treatment of acute immune thrombocytopenia purpura. *Seminars in Hematology, 35* (Suppl 1), 28–35.

15. White, G.C., II (1994). Disorders of blood coagulation. In J.H. Stein (Ed.), *Internal Medicine* (4th ed.). (pp. 804–822). St. Louis: Mosby.

Management of Patients with Oncologic Disorders

LEUKEMIAS

*Sylvia R. Love, MED, MSN, RN, CS,
ACNP, ANP*

I. ACUTE LYMPHOCYTIC LEUKEMIA (ALL)

A. Definition[2, 9, 13]

1. Malignancy that causes hematopoietic progenitor cells to lose their ability to mature normally and differentiate
2. Cells proliferate in uncontrolled fashion and ultimately replace normal bone marrow, leading to decreased production of normal red blood cells (RBCs), white blood cells (WBCs), and platelets.

B. Incidence/Predisposing factors[1, 2, 9, 12, 14]

1. No clear cause
2. Constitutes 80% of all childhood leukemias, with peak onset ages 3–7 years, and 20% of adult leukemias
3. Acute lymphocytic leukemia (ALL) is the most common cancer and the leading cause of death in children under age 15.
4. Survivors of ALL are at risk for late sequelae of secondary brain tumors.
5. Childhood ALL survivors are at greater risk for reduced growth (secondary to cranial irradiation and resultant decreased bone mass), learning disabilities, and osteoporotic fractures in later life.

C. Subjective findings[2, 9]

1. Usually sudden onset of acute illness for days or weeks
2. Fever
3. Anorexia
4. Fatigue
5. Bone and joint pain
6. Dyspnea
7. Gum hypertrophy
8. Angina

D. Physical examination findings[2, 9]

1. Pale, with purpura and petechiae
2. Generalized lymphadenopathy
3. Gingival hypertrophy
4. Stomatitis
5. Hepatosplenomegaly
6. Bone tenderness, particularly in the sternum and tibia

E. Laboratory/Diagnostic findings[2, 4, 9, 13]

1. Pancytopenia with circulating blasts is the hallmark of the disease.
2. Blasts may be absent from the peripheral smear in 10% of cases.
3. Bone marrow is usually hypercellular; diagnosis requires that >30% of cells are blasts.
4. Anemia in most patients; decreases in RBC, hemoglobin (Hgb), and hematocrit (Hct) levels range from mild to severe.
5. Platelets are usually decreased but may be in the normal range.
6. Bone marrow biopsy is often essential to establish the diagnosis, owing to the variability of the preceding factors.
7. Hyperuricemia and azotemia are present
8. Terminal deoxynucleotidyl transferase (TdT) is present in 95% of cases.
9. Consider ordering:

   a. Human leukocyte antigen (HLA) typing at time of diagnosis (may be indicated in preparation for possible bone marrow transplantation)
   b. Bone marrow stains
      i. Periodic acid–Schiff (PAS)—positive
      ii. Sudan black—negative
      iii. Myeloperoxidase—negative
      iv. Terminal deoxynucleotidal transferase (TdT)—positive
   c. Chromosome analysis
   d. Multiparametric flow cytometry (confirms light microscopy diagnosis; may be useful for relapse prediction)
   e. Electron microscopy (rarely used except in poorly differentiated leukemia)
   f. Molecular genetic studies

F. Management[2, 13]

1. Hematology/Oncology referral for suspected cases
2. Treatment is usually supportive or to eradicate leukemic cell mass.

   a. Cures are infrequent except in children.
   b. In adults expect at least a 25% disease-free 5-year survival, and with aggressive regimens a 35–40% 5-year survival.

3. Supportive care may include the following when indicated:

   a. Transfusions of RBCs or platelets
   b. Hydration
   c. Aggressive antibiotic therapy for infection

    d. Allopurinol, 100–200 mg p.o. t.i.d., to prevent hyperuricemia and renal damage

    e. Acetazolamide, 500 mg/day, to promote alkalization of urine

4. If patients remain uremic, consider dialysis before initiation of chemotherapy.

5. Chemotherapy

    • Chemotherapy is given according to protocols.

    • Chemotherapy is divided into three phases:

1. Remission induction

2. Postremission therapy

3. CNS prophylaxis

    a. Remission induction

        i. Initial treatment is combination chemotherapy.

        ii. A number of combinations are used.

           (1) Usual drugs include vincristine and prednisone.

           (2) L-Asparaginase and/or daunorubicin is/are frequently added.

           (3) Intrathecal methotrexate and L-asparaginase is another standard combination.

        iii. Maintenance therapy usually includes 6-mercaptopurine and methotrexate.

    b. Postremission therapy

        i. Short courses of further chemotherapy are given.

        ii. Usually use chemotherapy agents not used to initiate therapy, such as

           (1) High-dose methotrexate

           (2) Cyclophosphamide

           (3) Cytarabine

        iii. Common maintenance therapies

           (1) Daily low dose of 6-mercaptopurine, or

           (2) Weekly or biweekly doses of methotrexate

    c. CNS prophylaxis: Intrathecal methotrexate alone or in combination with radiation therapy.

6. Bone marrow transplantation should be considered at the time of the first relapse or the second remission.

II. ACUTE MYELOGENOUS LEUKEMIA (AML)

A. Definition[9]

1. Malignancy of hematopoietic progenitor cell

2. An acute leukemia very similar to ALL, distinguished by morphologic examination and cytochemistry, differentiating myeloblasts from lymphoblasts

B. Incidence/Predisposing factors[1, 2, 9, 13]

1. No clear cause
2. Chromosomal abnormalities are found in a majority of patients with acute leukemias.
3. Predominant type of acute leukemia in adults: 80% of acute leukemias in individuals over age 20
4. Incidence increases with age: Median age is 50 years.
5. Increased incidence of associated disseminated intravascular coagulation (DIC), especially with acute promyelocytic leukemia (M3)

C. Subjective findings[2, 9]

1. Bleeding
2. Fever
3. Anorexia
4. Fatigue
5. Headache
6. Bone and joint pain
7. Bone tenderness—particularly in the sternum and tibia

D. Physical examination findings[2, 9, 13]

1. Occasional lymphadenopathy
2. Hepatosplenomegaly
3. Stomatitis and gingival hypertrophy
4. Purpura, petechiae, overt bleeding
5. Signs of infection

E. Laboratory/Diagnostic findings[2, 9]

1. Pancytopenia with circulating blasts
2. Anemia in most patients; RBCs, Hgb and Hct levels, and platelets usually decreased
3. Most patients have at least mild thrombocytopenia; about 25% have severe thrombocytopenia (<20,000 platelets per microliter).
4. Granules visible in blast cells
5. Presence of Auer's rods
6. Many myeloblasts
7. Disseminated intravascular coagulation: Elevation in prothrombin time (PT), partial thromboplastin time (PTT), decrease in fibrinogen level
8. Consider ordering:

   a. Human leukocyte antigen (HLA) typing at time of diagnosis in preparation for possible bone marrow transplantation
   b. Bone marrow stain: Result in AML is Sudan black—positive and myeloperoxidase—positive.
   c. Uric acid

    d. Metabolic profile
    e. PT, PTT, fibrinogen, and fibrin split products (FSP)

F. Management[2, 13]

1. Hematology/Oncology referral for suspected cases.
2. Supportive care includes

    a. Transfusions of RBCs or platelets
    b. Hydration
    c. Aggressive antibiotic therapy for infection
    d. Acetazolamide, 500 mg/day, to produce alkalinization of urine
    e. Allopurinol, 100–200 mg p.o. t.i.d., to prevent hyperuricemia and renal damage

3. If patient remains uremic, consider dialysis before initiating chemotherapy.
4. Chemotherapy is divided into remission induction therapy and consolidative and maintenance therapy.

    • Chemotherapy is given according to protocols.

    a. Remission induction therapy options include one of the following equivalent combination chemotherapy regimens:
        i. Dose-intensive cytarabine-based induction therapy
        ii. Cytarabine + daunorubicin
        iii. Cytarabine + idarubicin
        iv. Cytarabine + daunorubicin + thioguanine
        v. Mitoxantrone + etoposide
        vi. Treatment of central nervous system leukemia, if present: Intrathecal cytarabine or methotrexate
    b. Consolidative and maintenance therapy
        i. High-dose ara-C, $1–3 \text{ g/m}^2$ of body surface area twice daily, is preferred.
        ii. Therapy of M3 subtype is initiated with retinoic acid, then consolidative and maintenance therapy with traditional agents. (Making M3 diagnosis is crucial.)

5. Bone marrow transplantation should be considered at the time of the first relapse or the second remission (reserved for "salvage" therapy).

III. CHRONIC LYMPHOCYTIC LEUKEMIA (CLL)

A. Definition[8–10]

1. B-lymphocyte malignancy with progressive accumulation of immunoincompetent lymphocytes, leading to immunosuppression and bone marrow failure
2. Clonal malignancy of B lymphocytes

B. Incidence/Predisposing factors[3, 5, 6, 8–10, 15]

1. Most common type of leukemia in older adults
2. Primarily a disease of the elderly

    a. Ninety percent of patients over age 50
    b. Median age is 65.
    c. Poorer prognosis with increased age

3. Usually slow progression of disease, occasionally progressive
4. Etiology unknown; first-degree relatives of CLL patients have three times the normal risk of developing the disease.
5. Farmers have increased incidence of CLL.
6. Men are more often affected than women; 2:1 incidence.
7. Associated with warm-antibody autoimmune hemolytic anemias (AIHA)
8. Median survival is about 6 years.
9. Clinical stage is strongest predictor for survival.

C. Subjective findings[5, 6, 8, 9]

1. Frequently asymptomatic
2. As disease progresses patient may have

    a. Fatigue, malaise, lethargy
    b. Anorexia
    c. Early satiety
    d. Weight loss
    e. Occasionally, patients who exhibit infection have notable lymph node enlargement.

3. Fever is rare.
4. CLL patients have a stronger reaction to insect bites, but this phenomenon has not been explained.

D. Physical examination findings[6, 9, 10]

1. Lymphadenopathy is present in 80% of patients.

    a. Cervical, supraclavicular, and axillary nodes are most often involved.
    b. Nodes are usually mobile, nontender, and have a rubbery feel.

2. Hepatosplenomegaly is present in 50% of patients.
3. Progressive weight loss
4. Patients may exhibit nodular or diffuse skin infiltrations.

E. Laboratory/Diagnostic findings[6, 9]

1. Lymphocytosis is a hallmark of the disease.

    a. Minimum level is more than $5000/\mu L$.
    b. Usual range is $40,000–150,000/\mu L$.

2. Lymphocytes constitute 75–98% of circulating cells.
3. Smudge cells are usually seen on peripheral smear.
4. Hypogammaglobulinemia is present in 50% of cases, more commonly in advanced disease.
5. IgG, IgA, or IgM levels are low in 25% of patients at diagnosis; with disease progression, levels are low in 50–70% of patients.
6. Consider ordering when diagnosis is uncertain:

   a. Flow cytometry analysis to determine immunologic profile, identifying cellular antigens
   b. Bone marrow biopsy
      i. More than 30% lymphocytes seen in disease.
      ii. Either focal or diffuse infiltration can be seen on core biopsies.
      iii. Extent of marrow infiltration correlates directly with prognosis.

F. Management[5, 6, 8, 9]

1. Hematology/Oncology referral for suspected cases
2. History, physical examination, peripheral blood counts, and lymphocyte morphology are usually all that are required to diagnose CLL in the clinical setting.
3. No specific therapy for patients in early disease

   a. Treatment is usually not initiated until symptoms occur.
   b. Fatigue and malaise occasionally necessitate treatment.

4. Monitor for lymphadenopathy, anemia, thrombocytopenia. These require therapy whether or not symptoms occur.
5. Chemotherapy is given according to protocol. What constitutes the best initial treatment of CLL has become controversial.

   a. Clinical guidelines indicate that fludarabine is preferred by many as initial therapy as opposed to its prior place as second line therapy.
      i. Although studies have not shown significant differences in overall survival rates, a higher response rate that is more complete and lasting has been achieved with fludarabine.
      ii. Fludarabine (Fludara), 25–30 mg/m^2/day for 5 days, every 4 weeks for 4–6 months
   b. Standard therapy has been chlorambucil (Leukeran), 0.6–1 mg p.o. every 3–6 weeks (regimens vary widely).
      i. Dosage is adjusted based on development of thrombocytopenia or neutropenia, with maintenance continued for 6–12 months.

  ii. May be given on a pulse schedule (0.5–2 mg/kg) over 1–4 days every 4 weeks, or every 2 weeks at half the dosage

  iii. This treatment has been well tolerated, effective, and convenient.

6. COP regimen (used less often)

 a. Cyclophosphamide (Cytoxan), 100–300 mg/m^2 p.o. on days 1–5

 b. Vincristine (Oncovin), 2 mg IV on day 1

 c. Prednisone, 100 mg p.o. on days 1–5

7. Other commonly used agents include

 a. Cladribine ([2-chloro-2'-deoxyadenosine] Leustatin)

 b. Pentostatin ([2'-deoxycoformycin] Nipent)

8. Stage 0 or I disease median survival is 10 years.

9. Stage III or IV disease median survival is 2 years.

10. Splenectomy in very select cases

11. Radiation is usually limited to localized nodal masses, refractory to chemotherapy.

IV. CHRONIC MYELOGENOUS LEUKEMIA (CML)

A. Definition[6–9, 11]

1. Disorder characterized by myeloid cell overproduction; abnormal cells overcome and replace normal hematopoiesis.

2. Distinguished by presence of Philadelphia chromosome in the leukemic cells

3. Clonal stem cell disorder

4. Also known as chronic granulocytic leukemia (CGL) or chronic myeloid leukemia

B. Incidence/Predisposing factors[6–9]

1. Accounts for 7–15% of adult leukemias

2. Primarily a disorder of middle age

 a. Median age is 42 years.

 b. May occur in patients as young as 15 years or as old as 80

3. Ionizing radiation exposure increases risk of CML.

 • Atomic bomb survivors have a dose-related increased incidence of CML, peaking 5–12 years after exposure.

4. Etiology is unknown. Chromosomal abnormality is invariably associated with disease.

5. Children of CML parents have no greater incidence than does the general population.

6. Median survival is 3–4 years.

C. Subjective findings[6–9]

1. Insidious onset
2. Fatigue
3. Easy satiety
4. Weight loss
5. Diminished exercise tolerance
6. Common after disease progression:

   a. Low-grade fever
   b. Dizziness
   c. Irritability
   d. Increased sweating/night sweats
   e. Abdominal fullness (left upper quadrant)
   f. Bone pain
   g. Blurred vision
   h. Respiratory distress

D. Physical examination findings[6–9]

1. Splenomegaly in 60% of cases
2. Bone pain/sternal tenderness
3. Hepatomegaly (less common)
4. Bleeding and infection may be present in blast crisis.

E. Laboratory/Diagnostic findings[6, 8, 9]

1. WBC count grossly elevated (15,000–500,000/μL; frequently 150,000/μL at initial diagnosis)
2. Hgb and Hct levels initially are normal; they may decrease with disease progression.
3. Platelets may be increased initially; they will decrease with disease progression.
4. Vitamin B_{12} serum levels are usually elevated (sometimes >10 times normal).
5. Lactate dehydrogenase (LDH) and uric acid levels may be elevated.
6. Philadelphia chromosome is present in either peripheral blood or bone marrow.
7. Diagnosis established with:

   a. Characteristic finding is low to absent leukocyte alkaline phosphatase (LAP), also called neutrophilic alkaline phosphatase (NAP) (normal: males, 22–124 units/L; females, 33–149 units/L).
   b. Cytogenic bone marrow analysis (presence of Philadelphia chromosome)

F. Management[6, 7, 9, 11]

1. Hematology/Oncology referral for suspected cases
2. Immediate therapy is not indicated unless

   a. WBC count is less than 200,000/μL or
   b. There is evidence of
      i. Priapism
      ii. Confusion

    iii. Venous thrombosis
    iv. Visual blurring
    v. Dyspnea

3. Supportive therapy includes

    a. Hydration
    b. Allopurinol, 100 mg t.i.d., for hyperuricemia

4. Chemotherapy is given according to protocol.

    a. Initial therapy was formerly hydroxyurea (Hydrea), 2–4 g at first, with 0.5–2 g/day to follow to maintain WBC count at 5,000–10,000/μL.
    b. Recombinant alpha interferon, 5×10^6 units/m^2/day, as the treatment of choice in the chronic phase is becoming favored over hydroxyurea.
        i. Therapy is continued for 5 years or longer.
        ii. Premedicate with acetaminophen.
        iii. Insomnia, depression, fatigue symptoms are treated with antidepressants.

5. Allogeneic bone marrow transplantation (usually sibling-matched) is the only curative therapy. Treatment is

    a. More effective in younger patients
        i. In the early chronic phase
        ii. With matching, related donor
    b. Usually available for those <60 years old with a matching sibling donor

6. Median survival without bone marrow transplantation is 3–4 years.

7. Long-term survival rate for adults with transplantation is 60%, but 1-year mortality rate is increased owing to transplant side effects.

References

1. Andreoli, T.E., Bennett, J.C., Carpenter, C.C., & Plum, F. (1997). *Cecil essentials of medicine* (4th ed.) (pp. 358–366). Philadelphia: W.B. Saunders.
2. Appelbaum, F. (1996). The acute leukemias. In J.C. Bennett & F. Plum (Eds.), *Cecil textbook of medicine* (20th ed.) (pp. 936–940). Philadelphia: W.B. Saunders.
3. Byrd, J.C., Rai, K.R., Sausville, E.A., & Grever, M.R. (1998). Old and new therapies in chronic lymphocytic leukemia: Now is the time for a reassessment of therapeutic goals. *Seminars in Oncology, 25*, 65–74.
4. Ciudad, J.F., San Miguel, M.C., Vidriales, B., Valverde, B., Ocqueteau, M., Mateos, G., Caballero, M.D., Hernandez, J., Moro, M.J., Mateos, M.V., & Orfao, A. (1998). Prognostic value of immunophenotypic detection of minimal residual disease in acute lymphoblastic leukemia. *Journal of Clinical Oncology, 16*, 3374–3781.

5. Hays, K. & McCartney, S. (1998). Nursing care of the patient with chronic lymphocytic leukemia. *Seminars in Oncology, 25*, 75–79.
6. Holmer, L.D. (1997). Chronic leukemias. In D.M. Harmening (Ed.), *Clinical hematology and fundamentals of hemostasis* (3rd ed.) (pp. 346–373). Philadelphia: F.A. Davis.
7. Kantarjian, H.M., Giles, F.J., O'Brien, S.M., & Talpaz, M. (1998). Clinical course and therapy of chronic myelogenous leukemia with interferon-alpha and chemotherapy. *Hematology/Oncology Clinics of North America, 12*, 31–80.
8. Keating, M.J. (1996). The chronic leukemias. In J.C. Bennett & F. Plum (Eds.), *Cecil textbook of medicine* (20th ed.) (pp. 925–935). Philadelphia: W.B. Saunders.
9. Linker, C.A. (1999). Blood. In L.M. Tierney, Jr., S.J. McPhee, & J.A. Papadakis (Eds.), *Current medical diagnosis & treatment* (38th ed.) (pp. 485–537). Stamford, CT: Appleton & Lange.
10. Lowry, P.A. (1996). Hematologic malignancies. In J. Noble (Ed.), *Textbook of primary care medicine* (2nd ed.) (pp. 739–747). St. Louis: Mosby.
11. Miller, J.S. (1998). Innovative therapy for chronic myelogenous leukemia. *Hematology/Oncology Clinics of North America, 12*, 173–206.
12. Nysom, K., Holm, K., Michaelsen, K.F., Hertz, H., Muller, J., & Molgaard, C. (1998). Bone mass after treatment for acute lymphoblastic leukemia in childhood. *Journal of Clinical Oncology, 16*, 3752–3760.
13. Perkins, M.L., Odell, J.M., & Braziel, R.M. (1997). Introduction to leukemia and the acute leukemias. In D.M. Harmening (Ed.), *Clinical hematology and fundamentals of hemostasis* (3rd ed.) (pp. 294–323). Philadelphia: F.A. Davis.
14. Walter, A.W., Hancock, M.L., Pui, C.H., Hudson, M.M., Ochs, J.S., Rivera, G.K., Pratt, C.B., Boyett, J.M., & Kun, L.E. (1998). Secondary brain tumors in children treated for acute lymphoblastic leukemia at St. Jude Children's Research Hospital. *Journal of Clinical Oncology, 16*, 3761–3767.
15. Zwiebel, J.A., & Cheson, B.D. (1998). Chronic lymphocytic leukemia: Staging and prognostic factors. *Seminars in Oncology, 25*, 42–59.

LYMPHOMA

Sylvia R. Love, MED, MSN, RN, CS,
ACNP, ANP

I. STAGING

A. Ann Arbor Staging Classification parallels non-Hodgkin's and Hodgkin's disease[1, 13]

1. Stage I: Single lymph node or single extralymphatic origin
2. Stage II: Two or more lymph node regions or extralymphatic sites on the same side of the diaphragm
3. Stage III: Involvement of lymph node regions or extralymphatic sites on both sides of the diaphragm
4. Stage IV: Diffuse or disseminated involvement of more than one extralymphatic organ with or without associated lymph node involvement

   • Bone marrow involvement confers Stage IV designation.

B. Working Formulation (WF) funded by the National Cancer Institute[1, 2]

1. Low-grade lymphoma

   a. Small lymphocytic, plasmacytoid
   b. Follicular, predominantly small cleaved cell
   c. Follicular, mixed small cleaved and large cell

2. Intermediate-grade lymphoma

   a. Follicular, large cell
   b. Diffuse, small cleaved cell
   c. Diffuse, mixed small and large cell
   d. Diffuse, large cell

3. High-grade lymphoma

   a. Large cell immunoblastic
   b. Lymphoblastic
   c. Small, noncleaved cell Burkitt's, non-Burkitt's

C. The Revised European-American Lymphoma Classification (REAL)[1, 2, 9]

1. B-cell neoplasms

   a. Precursor B-cell neoplasms; precursor B-lymphoblastic leukemia/lymphoma
   b. Peripheral B-cell neoplasms
      i. B-cell chronic lymphocytic leukemia/prolymphocytic leukemia/small lymphocytic lymphoma

    ii. Lymphoplasmacytoid lymphoma/immunocytoma
   iii. Mantle cell lymphoma
   iv. Follicle center lymphoma, follicular lymphoma
     (1) Provisional cytologic grades
       (a) Grade I: Small cell
       (b) Grade II: Mixed small and large cell
       (c) Grade III: Large cell
     (2) Provisional subtype: Diffuse, predominantly small cell type
    v. Marginal zone B-cell lymphoma
     (1) Extranodal (mucosa-associated lymphoid tissue-type ± monocytoid B-cells)
     (2) Provisional subtype: Nodal (± monocytoid B-cells)
   vi. Provisional entity: Splenic marginal zone lymphoma (± villous lymphocytes)
   vii. Hairy cell leukemia
  viii. Plasmacytoma/plasma cell myeloma
   ix. Diffuse large B-cell lymphoma. Subtype: Primary mediastinal (thymic) B-cell lymphoma
    x. Burkitt's lymphoma
   xi. Provisional entity: High-grade B-cell lymphoma, Burkitt's-like

2. T-cell and putative NK-cell neoplasms

  a. Precursor T-cell neoplasms; precursor T-lymphoblastic lymphoma/leukemia
  b. Peripheral T-cell and NK-cell neoplasms
    i. T-cell chronic lymphocytic leukemia/prolymphocytic leukemia
    ii. Large granular lymphocytic leukemia (LGL)
     (1) T-cell type
     (2) NK-cell type
   iii. Mycosis fungoides/Sézary's syndrome
   iv. Peripheral T-cell lymphomas, unspecified
     (1) Provisional cytologic categories
       (a) Medium-sized cell
       (b) Mixed medium and large cell
       (c) Large cell
       (d) Lymphoepithelioid cell
     (2) Provisional subtype: Hepatosplenic $\gamma\delta$ T-cell lymphoma
    v. Angioimmunoblastic T-cell lymphoma, formerly known as angioimmunoblastic T-cell lymphoma with dysproteinemia (AILD)
   vi. Angiocentric lymphoma
   vii. Intestinal T-cell lymphoma (± enteropathy associated)

      viii. Adult T-cell lymphoma/leukemia (ATL/L)
       ix. Anaplastic large cell lymphoma (ALCL)
         (1) CD30+ type
         (2) T-cell type
         (3) Null-cell type
       x. Provisional entity: Anaplastic large-cell lymphoma, Hodgkin's-like

3. Hodgkin's disease

   a. Lymphocyte predominance
   b. Nodular sclerosis
   c. Mixed cellularity
   d. Lymphocyte depletion
   e. Provisional entity: Lymphocyte-rich classic Hodgkin's disease

II. NON-HODGKIN'S LYMPHOMA (NHL)

A. Definition[2, 12, 13]

Heterogeneous group of lymphocytic cancers predominantly of B-cell origin and lacking Reed-Sternberg cells that produce a diverse group of malignancies

B. Incidence/Predisposing factors[2, 7, 8, 13]

1. In most patients with NHL, the cause is unclear.
2. Average age of patients is early 40s.
3. Incidence is increased with HIV infection.
4. Incidence increased with viruses

   a. Epstein-Barr (EBV)
   b. HTLV-1

5. Associated with warm-antibody autoimmune hemolytic anemias (AIHA)
6. Sixth most common cause of cancer-related death in the U.S.
7. Because lymphomas are often diffuse at diagnosis, superior vena cava syndrome and cardiac tamponade should be anticipated, diagnosed, and treated.

C. Subjective findings[10, 12, 13]

1. Lymphadenopathy, painless, widespread, or isolated
2. Most patients are asymptomatic.
3. Fever
4. Night sweats
5. Weight loss
6. Abdominal fullness (common in Burkitt's lymphoma)
7. Skin ulcers

D. Physical examination findings[10, 12, 13]

1. Lymphadenopathy, isolated or widespread, painless
2. Extranodal sites of disease (skin ulcers).

   • Eighty percent of indolent lymphomas manifest as Stage IV disease (usually with bone marrow involvement).

3. Splenomegaly
4. Hepatomegaly

E. Laboratory/Diagnostic findings[10, 12–14]

1. Tissue biopsy of the largest node or involved organ that is accessible is definitive.

   a. Biopsy should be reviewed by an experienced pathologist.
   b. Needle-aspiration biopsy is not acceptable for initial diagnosis.

2. Peripheral blood is usually normal on light microscopy.
3. High-grade lymphomas may have malignant cells in spinal fluid.
4. Classification into three categories

   a. Indolent lymphomas: Small, well-differentiated cells
   b. Aggressive lymphomas: Larger, more immature cells
   c. Highly aggressive lymphomas: Larger, immature cells with diffuse pattern of growth

5. The recent REAL classification system lends itself to immunophenotypic studies and cytogenetic/molecular genetic studies.
6. Consider ordering:

   a. Complete blood count with differential and erythrocyte sedimentation rate (ESR; may help to follow clinical course)
   b. Lactate dehydrogenase (LDH) determination; useful marker for tumor bulk
   c. CT scan of chest and abdomen to aid in staging
   d. Bone marrow biopsy
   e. Gallium scan

F. Management[7, 10, 12, 13, 15, 16]

1. Hematology/Oncology referral for suspected cases.
2. Treatment is determined by the histologic type of the lymphoma and the age and underlying condition of the patient.
3. Timing of treatment, drugs to be used, and therapeutic goals vary with the individual patient.
4. Treatment is usually deferred until the patient is symptomatic in low-grade but not in high-grade lymphoma.

5. Irradiation or chemotherapy
    a. Leads to remission but not cure in low-grade lymphoma
    b. Accompanied by palliative therapy
6. Low-grade lymphoma is usually treated with cyclophosphamide (Cytoxan) or chlorambucil (Leukeran) with prednisone.
    a. Vincristine (Oncovin) may also be used.
    b. Prognosis is poorer if the patient is unable to receive full treatment doses because of age or underlying conditions.
7. Median survival is 6–10 years; overall prognosis is not favorable.
8. Intermediate-grade and high-grade lymphomas are more aggressive biologically, with potential for cure with aggressive chemotherapy.
9. Standard treatment
    a. CHOP: Cyclophosphamide, hydroxydaunomycin/doxorubicin (Adriamycin), vincristine (Oncovin), and prednisone given for six cycles
    b. Dosage is based on patient condition and body mass index.
10. Complete remission may occur in as many as 60–65% of patients.
11. Autologous (previously harvested from patient) and allogeneic (usually sibling) bone marrow transplantation in select patients in relapse
12. Rituximab (Rituxan), an unconjugated monoclonal antibody, has been approved for treatment of relapsed or refractory low-grade or follicular CD20+ B-cell NHL.
13. Salvage regimens include
    a. MINE: Mesna, ifosfamide, Novantrone (mitoxantrone), and etoposide
    b. ESHAP: Etoposide, cytarabine, cisplatin, prednisone
    c. ESHAP or cyclophosphamide, etoposide, procarboxide, and prednisone (±bleomycin)
    d. Dosage is based on condition and body mass index of patient.
14. Observe for sepsis.
    a. Usually caused by gram-negative bacteria, such as *Escherichia coli*, *Klebsiella* spp., and *Pseudomonas* spp.
    b. Endogenous flora usually cause infections in these patients, particularly if they are asplenic.

III. HODGKIN'S DISEASE
A. Definition[6, 8, 12, 13]

A group of cancers characterized by the presence of Reed-Sternberg giant cells in a background of benign inflammatory cells and/or fibrosis

B. Incidence/Predisposing factors[3, 5–8, 12, 13]

1. Cause is unclear; infection, genomic alterations, deregulation of growth factor gene, and immune defects are postulated.
2. Peaks at age 20–29 and again at age 60 or older; advanced age is associated with poor prognosis.
3. Male predominance under age 10, but equal male and female at the two age peaks
4. In the U.S., whites account for 90% of cases.
5. Disease is associated with

   a. Small family size
   b. High standard of living
   c. High level of maternal education

6. About 85% of adolescent patients treated can expect cure of their malignancy.
7. The primary Hodgkin's disease is the most common cause of mortality in these patients, with secondary malignancy neoplasms the second most common cause of death.
8. Associated with warm antibody autoimmune hemolytic anemias (AIHA)
9. Because lymphomas are often diffuse at diagnosis, superior vena cava syndrome and cardiac tamponade should be anticipated, diagnosed, and treated.

C. Subjective findings[6, 12, 13]

1. Manifests as a painless mass, usually in the neck
2. Patients may exhibit no symptoms (Group "A").
3. Group "B" symptoms include

   a. Unexplained fever of 101°F (38.5°C) or higher
   b. Drenching night sweats
   c. Weight loss of 10% or more in the previous 6 months

4. Milder versions of the preceding symptoms may be seen.
5. Generalized pruritus, weakness, malaise (unusual)
6. Pain in involved sites with alcohol ingestion (rare)

D. Physical examination findings[6, 12, 13]

1. About 90% of cases manifest as painless, nontender, cervical lymphadenopathy.
2. Can manifest in the adolescent or young adult as a large mediastinal mass on chest x-ray
3. The patient may have generalized pruritus.

E. Laboratory/Diagnostic findings[6, 8–10, 13]

1. Hallmark is presence of Reed-Sternberg cells on lymph node biopsy. Needle aspiration or needle biopsies are not adequate for diagnosis.

2. Staging is based on regions involved and presence or absence of symptoms.

   a. Stage I: One lymph node involved
   b. Stage II: Two lymph nodes involved on one side of diaphragm.
   c. Stage III: Lymph nodes involved on both sides of diaphragm
   d. Stage IV: Disseminated disease with bone marrow or liver involvement
   e. Stage A = No constitutional symptoms
   f. Stage B = Constitutional symptoms (see preceding Subjective findings)

3. Histopathologic (Rye) classification of Hodgkin's disease

   a. Lymphocyte predominance: LP
   b. Nodular sclerosis: NS
   c. Mixed cellularity: MC
   d. Lymphocyte depletion: LD

4. Anergic to typical skin antigen tests such as those of mumps and *Candida*

   • If the patient previously had a positive response to a tuberculin test, the response is now negative.

5. To facilitate staging, consider ordering

   a. Chest x-ray (About half of patients exhibit mediastinal adenopathy, often detected on routine chest x-ray.)
   b. CT of thorax, abdomen, and pelvis
   c. CBC count, ESR, Coombs' test, liver function tests, and albumin and LDH, calcium, and uric acid levels
   d. Lymphangiography, gallium scan
   e. Bilateral bone marrow biopsy (for patients with inadequate or equivocal lymphangiogram)
   f. Bone scan
   g. Consider the need for staging laparotomy if therapy will be changed by documentation of subdiaphragmatic disease.

F. Management[4, 6–8, 11–13]

1. Hematology/Oncology referral for suspected cases. Delays in receiving appropriate therapy have high medicolegal liability.
2. Radiation is the treatment of choice for pathologic Stage I and Stage II disease.
3. Consider ovarian transposition by laparoscopy to prevent iatrogenic ovarian failure and increase the possibility of pregnancy in the future.

4. Patients with advanced Hodgkin's disease (late Stage II, Stage III, or Stage IV) should receive

   a. Mechlorethamine, Oncovin (vincristine), procarbazine, prednisone (MOPP), or
   b. Adriamycin (doxorubicin), bleomycin, vinblastine, dacarbazine (ABVD), or
   c. MOPP alternating with ABVD
   d. Dosing is based on body mass index and condition of patient.

5. MOPP can result in infertility.

   a. Consider a sperm bank for males.
   b. Fertility concerns mandate ABVD.

6. Increased risk of pulmonary fibrosis with ABVD
7. Radiation/chemotherapy may be avoided out of concern for increases in late secondary leukemias or solid malignancies except in cases with massive mediastinal involvement.
8. Tumor bulk and stage appear to be the most important prognostic factors.

   a. The presence of Group "B" symptoms is a poor prognostic factor.
   b. Low Hct and high LDH levels are associated with higher rates of relapse.

9. Preoperative pneumococcal vaccine for splenectomy patients with daily prophylactic oral antibiotics and patient education in precautions for febrile illnesses
10. Relapsed patients who have received allogeneic (usually sibling-match) bone marrow transplants have shown a lower relapse rate compared with autologous (previously harvested from patient) stem cell recipients.
11. Observe for sepsis.

    a. Usually caused by gram-negative bacteria, such as *E. coli*, *Klebsiella* spp., and *Pseudomonas* spp.
    b. Endogenous flora usually cause infections in these patients, particularly if they are asplenic.

References

1. Andreoli, T.E., Bennett, J.C., Carpenter, C.C., & Plum, F. (1997). *Cecil essentials of medicine* (4th ed) (pp. 367–376). Philadelphia: W.B. Saunders.
2. Bilodeau, B.A., & Fessele, K.L. (1998). Non-Hodgkin's lymphoma. *Seminars in Oncology Nursing, 14,* 273–283.
3. Callaghan, M. (1998). Hodgkin's disease. *Seminars in Oncology Nursing, 14,* 262–272.
4. Classe, J.M., Mahe, M., Moreau, P., Rapp, M., Maisonneuve, H., Lemevel, A., Bourdin, S., Harousseau, J.L., & Cuilliere, J.C. (1998). Ovarian transposition by laparoscopy before radiotherapy in the treatment of Hodgkin's disease. *Cancer, 83,* 1420–1424.

5. Fernsler, J., & Fanuele, J.S. (1998). Lymphomas: Long-term sequelae and survivorship issues. *Seminars in Oncology Nursing, 14,* 321–328.

6. Fleisher, A.S. (1996). Hodgkin's disease. In R.E. Rakel (Ed.), *Saunders manual of medical practice* (pp. 607–609). Philadelphia: W.B. Saunders.

7. Hogan, D.K., & Rosenthal, L.D. (1998). Oncologic emergencies in the patient with lymphoma. *Seminars in Oncology Nursing, 14,* 312–320.

8. Hudson, M.M., Poquette, C.A., Lee, J., Greenwald, C.A., Shah, A., Luo, X., Thompson, E.I., Wilimas, J.A., Kun, L.E., & Crist, W.M. (1998). Increased mortality after successful treatment for Hodgkin's disease. *Journal of Clinical Oncology, 16,* 3592–3600.

9. Koeppen, H., & Vardiman, J.W. (1998). New entities, issues, and controversies in the classification of malignant lymphoma. *Seminars in Oncology, 25,* 421–434.

10. Krol, A.D., Hermans, J., Dawson, L., Snijder, S., Wijermans, P., Kluin-Nelemans, H.C., Kluin, P., van Krieken, J.H., & Noordijk, E.M. (1998). Treatment, patterns of failure, and survival of patients with stage I nodal and extranodal non-Hodgkin's lymphomas, according to data in the population-based registry of the Comprehensive Cancer Centre West. *Cancer, 83,* 1612–1619.

11. Laport, G.F., & Williams, S.F. (1998). The role of high-dose chemotherapy in patients with Hodgkin's disease and non-Hodgkin's lymphoma. *Seminars in Oncology, 25,* 503–517.

12. Linker, C.A. (1997). Blood. In L.M. Tierney, Jr., S.J. McPhee, & J.A. Papadakis, (Eds.), *Current medical diagnosis & treatment* (36th ed) (pp. 463–518). Stamford, CT: Appleton & Lange.

13. Lowry, P.A. (1996). Hematologic malignancies. In J. Noble (Ed.), *Textbook of primary care medicine* (pp. 739–747). St. Louis: Mosby.

14. Meisenber, B.R. (1996). Lymphoma. In R.E. Rakel (Ed.), *Saunders manual of medical practice* (pp. 605–606). Philadelphia: W.B. Saunders.

15. Skarin, A.T., & Dorfman, D.M. (1997). Non-Hodgkin's lymphomas: Current classification and management. *Journal of the American Cancer Society, 47,* 351–372.

16. Vose, J.M. (1998). Current approaches to the management of Non-Hodgkin's lymphoma. *Seminars in Oncology 25,* 483–491.

OTHER COMMON CANCERS

Sylvia R. Love, MED, MSN, RN, CS, ACNP, ANP

I. LUNG CANCER[1, 7, 13]

A. General comments/Incidence/Predisposing factors

1. Leading cause of cancer deaths among men and women in the U.S.
2. Accounts for 13.4% of all new cancers
3. More people die from lung cancer than from colon cancer, breast cancer, and prostate cancer combined.
4. Increased incidence with:

   a. Tobacco smoking
      i. Women who smoke have a greater risk of developing small cell rather than squamous cell lung cancer.
      ii. Men who smoke have a similar risk for both small and non–small types.
   b. Secondhand smoke
   c. Ionizing radiation
   d. Occupational exposure (may be additive or synergistic to tobacco)
      i. Asbestos
      ii. Chromium
      iii. Nickel
      iv. Hydrocarbons
      v. Chloromethyl ether

5. Less well established risks include:
   a. Air pollution
   b. Vitamin A and E deficiencies
   c. Cigar and pipe use

6. The average age of people found to have lung cancer is 60—unusual under the age of 40.
7. If found and treated early, before lymph node or other organ involvement, the 5-year survival rate is 42%.

B. Subjective findings

1. Ten to twenty-five percent of patients are asymptomatic at time of diagnosis.
2. Symptomatic lung cancer is generally advanced disease.
3. May have nonspecific complaints such as

   a. Weight loss
   b. Chest pain

    c. Dyspnea
    d. Loss of appetite

4. Symptoms confined to the lungs

    a. Cough
    b. Hemoptysis
    c. Hoarseness
    d. Wheezing
    e. Dyspnea
    f. Sputum production with or without fever
    g. Chest pain
    h. Recurring infections such as bronchitis and pneumonia

C. Physical examination findings

1. Central tumors may obstruct the following areas of the lungs:

    a. Segmental (left has eight segments, right has ten segments)
    b. Lobar (left has two lobes, right has three lobes)
    c. Main stem bronchi (and cause atelectasis and postobstructive pneumonitis)

2. Peripheral tumors may cause no abnormalities on physical examination.
3. Tumor invasion of pleural surface may cause pleural effusion.
4. Disease confined to the chest may include the following physical findings:

    a. Stridor hoarseness
    b. Changes on physical examination related to atelectasis
    c. Consolidation
    d. Diaphragm paralysis or effusion
    e. Superior vena caval obstruction
        i. Cyanosis
        ii. Engorgement of neck veins
        iii. Lack of pulsations
        iv. Enlarged neck circumference
        v. Pericardial disease
        vi. Tamponade

5. Lymphadenopathy, hepatomegaly, and clubbing are present in about 20% of patients.
6. Horner's syndrome may be present.

    a. Horner's syndrome is the result of neurologic damage to cervical nerve.
    b. It presents as unilateral miotic pupil, ptosis, and facial anhidrosis (inadequate perspiration).

7. Pancoast's syndrome may be present.

    a. Associated with tumor in apex of lung

    b. Symptoms include neuritic pain in the arm, atrophy of the muscles of the arm and hand caused by brachial plexus and sympathetic ganglia tumor.

8. Malignant pleural effusions associated with bronchogenic carcinoma.

D. Laboratory/Diagnostic findings

1. The only definitive test is biopsy.
2. Chest x-ray presentation varies with cell type.
3. Comparison of old films is very valuable.

    a. Central lesions tend to be

        i. Squamous cell carcinoma

        ii. Small cell carcinoma

    b. Peripheral lesions tend to be

        i. Adenocarcinoma

        ii. Large cell carcinoma

        iii. Bronchoalveolar cell carcinoma

    c. Cavitation tends to be

        i. Squamous cell carcinoma

        ii. Large cell carcinoma

    d. Early mediastinal-hilar involvement is usually indicative of small cell carcinoma.

4. Sputum cytology 80% + in centrally located lesions, <20% in peripheral nodules
5. Bronchoscopy may be used to obtain tissue for histologic confirmation.
6. Percutaneous needle aspiration
7. Pleural fluid, about 40–50% + in malignant pleural effusion
8. Mediastinal exploration (rare)
9. Open biopsy is used only occasionally to confirm diagnosis when less invasive diagnostics are negative.

E. Major treatments

1. Refer to oncology specialist.
2. Therapy dependent on

    a. Cell type

    b. Premorbid condition

    c. Underlying lung function

3. Small cell carcinoma (SCC)

    a. Almost always treated with chemotherapy

    b. Accounts for about 20% of all lung cancers

    c. Other names for small cell lung cancer are oat cell cancer and small cell undifferentiated.

4. SCC staged most often as

  a. Limited stage—One lung and in lymph nodes on the same side of the chest

    i. Most treated with chemotherapy such as cisplatin or carboplatin combined with etoposide.

    ii. Clinical trials using paclitaxel are in progress.

    iii. SCC commonly spreads to the brain.

    iv. Patients treated with chemotherapy with or without radiation usually experience remission, although only temporarily.

    v. One-year survival for limited stage SCC treated with chemotherapy and radiation is 60%, 30% at 2 years, and 10–15% by 5 years.

  b. Extensive stage—Both lungs, with spread to lymph nodes on the other side, or to distant organs

    i. Very poor prognosis when left untreated

    ii. Carboplatin or cisplatin along with etoposide are the usual chemotherapy drugs used.

    iii. Radiation therapy is sometimes used.

    iv. One-year survival is 20–30%, 5% by two years, 1–2% by 5 years.

5. Non–small cell carcinoma (NSCC) is the most common type of lung cancer, occurring in about 80% of lung cancers, and includes

  a. Squamous cell adenocarcinoma

  b. Bronchoalveolar cell

  c. Large cell

  d. Adenosquamous cell

6. NSCC staged with TNM system

  a. TNM = tumor, nodes, metastases

  b. Described in roman numerals 0–IV (0–4). The lower the number, the less the cancer has spread.

  c. Stage 0—Limited to lining of air passages

    i. Usually treated surgically with segmentectomy or wedge resection

    ii. Usually does not receive chemotherapy

    iii. Usually does not receive radiation

  d. Stage I—Invaded lung tissue

    i. Usually has lobectomy

    ii. May receive radiation therapy

    iii. Five-year survival with surgery about 60%

  e. Stage II—Invasion of lung tissue expanded

    i. Treatment usually same as in Stage I.

    ii. Five-year survival rates about 35% for patients with surgery.

f. Stage IIIA—Treatment depends on location of cancer in the lung and whether it has spread to lymph nodes.
    i. Surgery may be used alone.
    ii. May have chemotherapy or radiation
    iii. May have brachytherapy (selective placement of radio-active source in contact with or implanted into tumor tissues)
    iv. Five-year survival range 10–20%, better if without lymph node metastases.
g. Stage IIIB—Cancer has spread too widely to be completely removed surgically.
    i. May have chemotherapy or radiation
    ii. Five-year survival rate 10–20%
h. Stage IV—Cancer has spread to distant organs.
    i. Cure is not possible.
    ii. Therapy is palliative.
    iii. Chemotherapy may prolong life.
    iv. One-year survival is about 20–25%.

7. Localized disease commonly treated with
    a. Cisplatin
    b. Vinblastine

8. Advanced disease commonly treated with

    a. Cisplatin
    b. Vinorelbine

9. Surgical resection may involve solitary nodule in localized disease Stage I to IIIA.
10. Radiation therapy considered for nonsurgical candidates
11. Stage IIIB or IV usually receives

    a. Palliative radiation
    b. Experimental chemotherapy protocols

12. Therapeutic thoracentesis (if symptomatic) used with malignant pleural effusions.
13. Decision algorithms for lung cancer are anticipated to be available in 2001 on the American Cancer Society web site, www.cancer.org, and at the National Comprehensive Cancer Network web site, www.nccn.org.

II. COLORECTAL CANCER[6, 16]

A. General comments/Predisposing factors

1. Third most common cause of cancer (excluding skin cancer) in males and females in the U.S.
2. Ninety-five percent of colorectal cancers are adenocarcinomas.

3. Increased incidence in those
    a. Over the age of 50
    b. With a personal history of:
        i. Colorectal cancer
        ii. Colorectal adenomas
        iii. Inflammatory bowel disease
        iv. Peutz-Jeghers syndrome
        v. Breast cancer
        vi. Ovarian cancer
        vii. Endometrial cancer
        viii. Prostate cancer
        ix. Hereditary nonpolyposis colon cancer (HNPCC)
        x. High-fat and/or low fiber diet.
    c. With a family history of:
        i. Colorectal cancer
        ii. Cancer family syndrome
        iii. Gardner's syndrome

B. Subjective findings

1. Often asymptomatic until disease is advanced.
2. Bowel-specific symptoms include
    a. Change in bowel habits
    b. Bloody rectal discharge
    c. Abdominal discomfort
    d. Straining during a bowel movement.
3. Systemic symptoms are frequently insidious and may include
    a. Fatigue
    b. Weight loss
    c. Anemia
    d. Nausea
    e. Loss of appetite

C. Physical examination findings

1. Often external examination of the abdomen is unrevealing.
2. Abdominal examination may reveal
    a. Abdominal tenderness
    b. Discrete mass may be palpated dependent on tumor location and size.
3. Digital rectal examination, combined with stool guaiac testing, is the most important part of physical examination.

D. Laboratory/Diagnostic findings

1. Screening tests, recommended to begin at age 50 by both the American Cancer Society and the National Comprehensive Cancer Network, include
    a. Fecal occult blood testing (FOBT)
    b. Digital rectal examination (DRE)

   c. Flexible sigmoidoscopy
   d. Colonoscopy
   e. Double contrast barium enema

2. If there is reason to suspect colon or rectal cancer on history
and physical examination regardless of age, the following
should be considered:

   a. Digital rectal examination
   b. FOBT
   c. Colonoscopy
   d. Biopsy
   e. Complete blood count

3. May consider a serum carcinoembryonic antigen (CEA)

   a. Not recommended for screening
   b. Useful in monitoring therapy after surgery
   c. Elevation suggests recurrence.

4. Computed tomograpy (CT) may be ordered.
5. Chest x-ray may also be ordered.

E. Evaluation for metastasis may include

1. CT-guided needle biopsy
2. Magnetic resonance imaging (MRI)
3. Positron emission tomography (PET)
4. Angiography
5. Consultation with an enterostomal therapist

F. Major treatments in general include

1. Surgery (treatment of choice)

   a. Prior to surgery include
      i. Liver function tests
      ii. CEA level
      iii. Colonoscopy
      iv. Chest film

2. Chemotherapy

   a. Palliative
   b. Not proved curative
   c. 5-Fluorouracil (5-FU) is drug of choice for metastatic colorectal cancer. Frequently leucovorin is used in conjuction
with 5-FU to increase its effectiveness.
   d. Levamisole HCl (Ergamisol) is used to reduce the rate of
tumor recurrence.

3. Radiation therapy

   a. Not primary treatment
   b. May be used in conjunction with surgical excision of stage
B2 and C rectal tumors

    c. Owing to extensive lymphatic drainage in the rectum, rectal tumors tend to metastasize to regional lymph nodes early.

    d. Radiation therapy inhibits the metastases.

4. See algorithms for therapy for different stages of colorectal cancers at the American Cancer Society web site, www.cancer.org, or the National Comprehensive Cancer Network web site at www.ncc.org.

III. BREAST CANCER[3, 4, 9, 11]

A. General comments/Predisposing factors

1. Most common nonskin malignancy in females in the U.S.
2. Second only to lung cancer as cause of death in women
3. Increased incidence in

    a. Age over 50 with the mean and median age 60 and 61

    b. Personal history of

        i. Breast cancer

        ii. Colon cancer

        iii. Endometrial cancer

        iv. Ovarian cancer

        v. Nulliparity, low parity, or late first pregnancy

        vi. Greater than age 30 at first live birth

        vii. Early menarche, under age 12

        viii. Menopause after age 50

        ix. Cellular atypia or lobular carcinoma in situ on breast biopsy

    c. Family history of

        i. Breast cancer

        ii. Cancer family syndrome

4. Genetic mutations associated with breast cancer include

    a. *BRCA1*

    b. *BRCA2*

B. Subjective findings

1. Palpable, usually painless breast lump is detected by patient in most palpable breast cancers.
2. Nipple discharge (particularly if bloody and unilateral)
3. Focal breast pain with inflammation of the skin over the breast area may be associated with the cancer but may also be associated with other, benign breast conditions.
4. Less frequent symptoms are

    a. Breast pain

    b. Nipple discharge

    c. Erosion

    d. Retraction

e. Enlargement
f. Itching of the nipple
g. Redness
h. Generalized hardness
i. Enlargement of the breast
j. Shrinking of the breast

C. Physical examination findings

1. Early findings

   a. Single mass
   b. Nontender
   c. Firm to hard mass with ill-defined margins
   d. Mammographic abnormalities
   e. No palpable mass

2. Dominant breast masses should be considered highly suspicious for breast cancer.
3. Suspicion increased when

   a. Mass is hard or fixed to the overlying skin
   b. Overlying skin is dimpled or retracted.
   c. Unilateral bloody nipple discharge from the breast with the mass
   d. New onset of inverted nipple with or without evidence of mass
   e. Axillary adenopathy present (inconclusive finding)
   f. Breast enlargement, redness, edema, pain

D. Laboratory/Diagnostic findings

1. Confirmation of breast cancer requires cytology or histology finding

   a. Fine-needle aspiration (a negative finding is not conclusive to rule out cancer)
   b. Core-needle biopsy
   c. Open excisional biopsy is used in conjunction with planned surgical intervention.
   d. Stereotactically guided core-needle biopsy may also be used with occult nonpalpable breast lesions detected by mammography.

2. A consistently elevated erythrocyte sedimentation rate may be the result of disseminated cancer.
3. Liver and bone metastases may be associated with serum alkaline phosphatase elevation.
4. Hypercalcemia may be present in advanced disease—indication for bone scan.
5. Tumor markers used to follow disease process include

   a. Serum carcinoembryonic antigen (CEA)
   b. Serum CA15-3

6. Breast ultrasonography is used to distinguish fluid-filled cysts from solid tumor.
7. Breast tissue biopsy may be evaluated with

   a. Tumor hormone receptor (ER/PR) testing
      i. Estrogen receptors (ER)
      ii. Progesterone receptors (PR)
      iii. Primary tumors that are receptor-positive have more favorable response to therapy.
   b. HER-2/neu testing
   c. Cancer cell division
      i. SPF
      ii. Ki-67

8. Types of breast cancer include

   a. Carcinoma in situ (confined to ducts or lobules and has not invaded surrounding tissues or organs)
      i. Lobular carcinoma in situ (LCIS) usually does not become an invasive cancer.
      ii. Ductal carcinoma in situ (DCIS) is the most common type of noninvasive breast cancer.
   b. Infiltrating (or invasive) ductal carcinoma (IDC) is the most common of all breast cancers.
   c. Infiltrating (or invasive) lobular carcinoma (ILC)
   d. Medullary carcinoma
   e. Colloid carcinoma
   f. Tubular carcinoma
   g. Inflammatory breast carcinoma
   h. Adenoid cystic carcinoma

E. Major treatment

1. Immediate referral of suspected cases for biopsy.
2. Treatment can be curative or palliative.
3. Management of breast cancer is multifaceted, based on patient preference, medical expertise, and characteristics of the breast cancer.
4. Lumpectomy

   a. Breast-conserving surgery (BCS)
   b. Used in select women to remove the mass and limited surrounding tissue

5. Modified radical mastectomy

   a. Removal of the breast
   b. Axillary dissection
   c. Preservation of the pectoral muscles

6. Adjuvant therapy initially affects quality of life but is considered transient and minor overall.

   a. Indicated for positive axillary nodes such as
      i. Combination chemotherapy for women younger than 50 years of age
      ii. Tamoxifen for women older than 50 years of age

7. Melphalan and fluorouracil are commonly used.

   a. Postmenopausal women with estrogen receptor–positive tumors
   b. Adjuvant therapy indicated for negative axillary nodes
   c. May not require adjuvant therapy if tumor is less than 1 cm

8. Other common chemotherapy regimens

   a. CMF
      i. Cyclophosphamide
      ii. Methotrexate
      iii. Fluorouracil
   b. Adriamycin (doxorubicin) plus cyclophosphamide

9. Positive clinical trials include recombinant humanized monoclonal antibody—Herceptin
10. Decision algorithms for the different stages of breast cancer are available on the American Cancer Society web site, www.cancer.org, and at the National Comprehensive Cancer Network web site, www.nccn.org.

IV. CERVICAL CANCER[5, 14, 17]

A. General comments/Predisposing factors

1. Cervical cancer was once one of the most common causes of cancer death for American women, but it is much less common today.
2. When combined with cancers of the corpus uteri, cervical cancer is the fourth most common nonskin malignancy in females in the U.S.
3. Infection with human papillomavirus types 16, 18, 31, 33, 35, 45, 51, 52, and 56 has been strongly linked with cervical cancer.
4. Increased incidence with

   a. Early age at first intercourse
   b. Multiple sexual partners
   c. A promiscuous male partner
   d. History of genital warts
   e. Folate deficiency
   f. Immunosuppression
   g. Low socioeconomic status
   h. >5 years since last Pap smear
   i. Smoking

B. Subjective findings

1. Usually asymptomatic
2. Postcoital spotting
3. Abnormal uterine bleeding and vaginal discharge
4. Bloody or purulent, odorous, nonpruritic discharge may appear after invasion.
5. Late symptoms include

    a. Bladder dysfunction
    b. Rectal dysfunction
    c. Fistulas and pain

C. Physical examination findings

1. Direct visualization of the cervix

    a. Should begin when woman first engages in sexual intercourse
    b. Should be performed every 1–3 years based on risk factors

2. Cervical lesions may be visible on inspection as a tumor or ulceration.

D. Laboratory/Diagnostic findings

1. The Papanicolaou smear (Pap smear) interpretation most often used is the Bethesda Classification System. The Pap smear report is divided into three sections:

    a. The first section of the report is a statement of sample adequacy and is reported as
        i. Satisfactory for evaluation
        ii. Satisfactory for evaluation, but limited by (a reason is supplied in the report)
        iii. Unsatisfactory for evaluation
    b. The second section of the Bethesda system report contains either
        i. Within normal limits
        ii. Benign cellular changes
        iii. Epithelial cell abnormalities
    c. The third section is the description of diagnoses further explaining benign cellular changes or epithelial cell abnormalities.
        i. Benign cellular changes are further explained as reactive changes related to inflammation or infection.
        ii. Epithelial changes are further divided into
            (1) Squamous cell abnormalities such as:
                (a) I. Atypical squamous cells of undetermined significance (ASCUS)
                (b) II. Low-grade squamous intraepithelial lesions (LSIL)

(c) III. High-grade squamous intraepithelial lesions (ASIL) (this also includes squamous
carcinoma in situ).

(d) IV. Squamous cell carcinoma

(2) Glandular cell abnormalities:

(a) I. Benign endometrial cells

(b) II. Atypical glandular cells of undetermined
significance (AGUS)

(c) III. Adenocarcinoma in situ (AIS) and adenocarcinoma.

d. With vaginal smears only—A fourth section on the Pap
smear includes an evaluation of hormonal patterns related
to patient's age and history.

2. An abnormal Pap smear requires a consultation with a physician to determine procedure for follow-up.

3. A repeated Pap smear and a colposcopy are common methods of follow-up.

4. Follow-up is variable depending on cytopathology report
findings.

5. Acetic acid wash of the cervix is used as an adjunct to the
Pap smear, with whitened areas recommended to undergo
colposcopy.

6. Colposcopy is utilized to

a. Identify abnormal areas, extent of lesions
b. Obtain biopsy

E. Major treatments

1. Dysplasia on Pap smear warrants colposcopic examination of
the cervix.

2. Management is dependent on the specific findings of

a. Lesion grade
b. Size and involvement of the endocervical canal

3. The following therapies may be included

a. Cryotherapy—Freeze burn of abnormal cells
b. Laser ablation—Laser used to burn abnormal cells or to remove a small piece of tissue for study
c. Low-voltage loop electroexcision (LEEP, LEETZ)—Thin
electrically heated wire used as "knife" to remove tissue.
d. Cone biopsy—A cone-shaped piece of tissue is removed
from the cervix. May be by surgery or laser knife.
e. Simple hysterectomy—The surgical removal of the uterus,
leaving tissue near uterus such as parametria and uterosacral ligaments. Vagina and pelvic lymph nodes are also not
removed.

 f. Radical hysterectomy—Removes uterus, parametria, and uterosacral ligaments.

 g. Pelvic exenteration—Removes all of the organs and tissues as radical hysterectomy, but also may include bladder, vagina, rectum, and part of the colon.

 h. Radiation therapy

  i. External beam radiation—Radiation from outside the body

  ii. Brachytherapy—Radioactive source placed in contact with surface of tumor or inserted into tumor

 i. Chemotherapy

4. Follow-up

 a. Every 4–6 months for 1–2 years
 b. Repeat colposcopy is done for recurrent abnormalities.

5. Atypia on the Pap smear may warrant colposcopy.

 a. May be treated for an infection
 b. Re-examined with Pap smear in 3–4 months
 c. Persistent atypia warrants colposcopy.

6. Common therapies include:

 a. Carcinoma in situ (Stage 0)—In women who have completed childbearing, total hysterectomy is the treatment of choice.
 b. Invasive carcinoma
  i. Stage IA
   (1) Simple extrafascial hysterectomy
  ii. Stage IB and Stage IIA
   (1) Radical hysterectomy
   (2) Radiation therapy
  iii. Stage IIB and Stage III and Stage IV cancers are treated with radiation therapy.
  iv. Radical surgery without radiation is the preferred mode of therapy in younger women.

7. Decision algorithms for cervical cancer are anticipated to be available in 2001 on the American Cancer Society web site, www.cancer.org, and at the National Comprehensive Cancer Network web site, www.nccn.org.

V. OVARIAN CANCER[4, 14, 18]

A. General comments/Incidence/Predisposing factors

1. Leading cause of death from gynecologic cancer and the fifth most common cause of cancer deaths among women

2. Sixth most common nonskin malignancy in females in the U.S.
3. Half of all ovarian cancers found in women older than 65
4. Increased incidence of ovarian cancer in those with

   a. Personal history of
      i. Breast cancer
      ii. Endometrial cancer
      iii. Colon cancer
      iv. Infertility or use of fertility drugs
      v. Nulliparity
      vi. Perineal talc exposure
   b. Family history of
      i. Ovarian cancer
      ii. Breast cancer
      iii. Endometrial cancer
      iv. Colon cancer

5. Oral contraceptive use may reduce risk, including in those with a family history of ovarian cancer
6. Epithelial ovarian carcinomas (EOC) make up approximately 85–90% of ovarian cancers. EOCs are divided into the following types:

   a. Serous
   b. Mucinous
   c. Endometroid
   d. Clear cell

7. Germ cell tumors can be cancerous, although most are non-cancerous. The most common germ cell tumors are as follows:

   a. Teratoma—Can be subdivided into:
      i. Mature teratoma, which is also referred to as dermoid cyst (which may contain a variety of benign tissues such as bone and teeth) and usually occurs in the teens to the forties
      ii. Immature teratoma—A cancerous form that occurs in girls and young women, usually younger than 18
   b. Dysgerminoma—Most common ovarian cancer germ cell, but represents only about 2% of all ovarian cancers
   c. Endodermal sinus tumor (yolk sac tumor) and choriocarcinoma—Very rare tumors that usually grow and spread rapidly but respond to chemotherapy. They usually occur in girls and young women.
   d. Stromal tumors—Account for about 5% of ovarian cancers. They can occur in young women, but about half occur in women over age 50.

B. Subjective findings

1. Frequently asymptomatic
2. When symptoms appear, they usually indicate more advanced disease and may include

   a. Abdominal bloating
   b. Early satiety or anorexia
   c. Dyspepsia
   d. Pelvic pressure or pain
   e. Frequent urination
   f. Constipation
   g. Leg pain
   h. Unusual vaginal bleeding is a rare sign.

C. Physical examination findings

1. Pelvic mass
2. Abdominal distention
3. Pleural effusion
4. Ascites
5. Adenopathy
6. Cachexia

D. Laboratory/Diagnostic findings

1. Pelvic examination
2. Pelvic transvaginal ultrasonography
3. Color-flow Doppler of ovarian vessels
4. Serum tumor markers for epithelial tumors

   a. CA125 (also known as OC-125)
   b. CA72
   c. CA15-3
   d. Alpha-L-fucosidase levels
   e. Serum inhibin levels (elevated with mucinous-type tumors)

5. Germ cell tumors

   a. Serum beta-HCG or
   b. Alpha-fetoprotein levels elevated with various germ cell tumors

6. Preoperative staging tests may include

   a. Chest x-ray
   b. Complete blood count and serum chemistries
   c. Intravenous pyelogram
   d. Cystoscopy
   e. Proctoscopy
   f. MRI
   g. CT
   h. Barium enema (BE)

7. Surgery: Definitive diagnosis is made by histology on a surgical specimen.

E. Major treatments

1. Surgery (laparotomy) may be used to

   a. Stage the lesion
   b. Debulk the tumor
   c. Relieve bowel obstruction

2. Early-stage disease

   a. Includes Stage I (well differentiated)
   b. Includes Stage II (moderately differentiated)
   c. Usually involves no further treatment

3. Stage I, grade III; Stage II; and Stage IIIA often managed with

   a. Systemic chemotherapy (melphalan [Alkeran])
   b. Intraperitoneal ^{32}P
   c. Whole abdomen radiation therapy

4. Advanced disease may be managed with

   a. Systemic chemotherapy
      i. Cisplatin (Platinol)
      ii. Cyclophosphamide (Cytoxan)
   b. Intraperitoneal chemotherapy
   c. Biologic response modifiers
   d. Autologous bone marrow transplantation
   e. Hormonal therapy

5. Palliative therapies include

   a. Surgery to debulk the tumor
   b. Radiation
   c. Drainage of ascites or plerual effusion

6. Follow-up usually involves:

   a. Serial CA125 levels to assess disease process
   b. May include follow-up laparotomy to assess for residual disease

VI. PROSTATE CANCER[8, 12, 19, 20]

A. General comments/Predisposing factors

1. Most common nonskin malignancy
2. Second most common cause of cancer mortality in men
3. Increased incidence in

   a. Men over the age of 50
   b. African American descent

    c. Those with a family history of
      i. Prostate cancer
      ii. Breast cancer
      iii. Endometrial cancer
      iv. Colon cancer
    d. Men with a personal history of
      i. Colon cancer
      ii. High-fat diet consumption
      iii. Occupational exposure to cadmium or rubber

4. Green tea, selenium, and vitamin A, B_6, C, and E may decrease prostate cancer risk.
5. Prostate-specific antigen (PSA) screening should be offered annually to men age 50 or older.
6. Awareness of the patient's consumption of the following medication(s)/herbs is important because they can lower PSA levels and produce a normal level PSA in some cases of early prostate cancer. They include:

    a. Finasteride (Proscar or Propecia)
    b. Androgen-receptor blockers
    c. Saw palmetto
    d. PC-SPES

B. Subjective findings

1. Initially, usually asymptomatic
2. Local symptoms: Rapid onset usually due to urinary tract obstruction and include

    a. Nocturia
    b. Urgency
    c. Frequency
    d. Hesitancy

3. Regional symptoms

    a. Lower extremity edema
    b. Hematuria

4. Systemic symptoms

    a. Low back pain due to lumbar sacral spinal metastasis
    b. Weakness
    c. Weight loss

C. Physical examination findings

1. Digital rectal examination (DRE) findings

    a. Prostatic nodule
    b. Induration
    c. Enlargement
    d. Asymmetry

2. DRE can be normal.
3. The patient may present with

   a. Hydronephrosis
   b. Adenopathy
   c. Back pain due to metastasis
   d. Biopsy revealing "adenocarcinoma of unknown primary"

D. Laboratory/Diagnostic findings

1. PSA > 4 ng/mL = abnormal
2. Age-specific normal reference ranges for PSA for men are based on having had a previous PSA of < 4 ng/mL and are as follows:

   a. Age 40–49, < 2.5 ng/mL
   b. Age 50–59, < 3.5 ng/mL
   c. Age 60–69, < 4.5 ng/mL
   d. Age 70–79, < 6.5 ng/mL

3. Normal PSAs are present in approximately 40% of cases of prostate cancer.
4. Prostatic acid phosphatase (PAP) may be used to evaluate for nonlocalized disease.
5. Bone scans generally are not indicated with PSA < 10 ng/mL and no bone pain.
6. Transrectal ultrasonography (TRUS) is used to evaluate the prostate for biopsy.
7. Transrectal biopsy or aspiration with biopsy is required for diagnosis.
8. Lymph node biopsy may be obtained.

   a. Incisional biopsy or
   b. Fine-needle aspiration

9. A present-free PSA may be ordered for borderline range PSA values. A low percent free-PSA suggests the presence of cancer and suggests the need for biopsy.
10. The following may be ordered for cancer staging:

    a. CT
    b. MRI
    c. Radionuclide bone scan

11. The most common prostate cancer grading system is the Gleason system, ranging from 1 to 5.

    a. The primary and secondary grades are summed to yield 2–10.
    b. The higher the score, the poorer the prognosis.

E. Major treatments

1. Localized prostate cancer

  a. "Watchful waiting"
     i. Palliative therapy for symptomatic/metastatic progression
  b. Radical prostatectomy is reserved for patients with >10-year life expectancy.
     i. Radical retropubic approach
     ii. Perineal approach
  c. Radiation therapy is reserved for high-grade malignancy and poor surgical candidates.
     i. External beam radiation
     ii. Brachytherapy (internal radiation)
  d. Cryotherapy (new therapy)

2. Regional or metastatic prostate cancer

  a. Palliative therapy includes
     i. Transurethral resection/incision of the prostate (TURP/TUIP)
     ii. Stents
     iii. Hormonal therapy
     iv. Bilateral orchiectomy
     v. Medical orchiectomy
     vi. Radiation therapy
     vii. Chemotherapy

3. Follow-up: 3–6 month intervals with DRE and PSA
4. For clinical guidelines for specific therapies related to stages of prostate cancer, see the American Cancer Society web site at www.cancer.org, or the National Comprehensive Cancer Network web site at www.nccn.org.

VII. BLADDER CANCER[2, 12, 19]

A. General comments/Incidence/Predisposing factors

1. The fourth most common cancer in males in the U.S. and eighth among women
2. Mean age at diagnosis is 65
3. Reduced levels of serum carotene and serum retinol are seen in patients with bladder cancer.
4. Increased incidence associated with

  a. Cigarette smoking
  b. Exposure to industrial dyes or solvents
  c. High dietary fat

5. Reduced incidence associated with

  a. Soy protein and garlic
  b. Vitamin A, B_6, C, E, and selenium administration

6. Nonsteroidal anti-inflammatory drugs may inhibit the development of bladder cancer.

B. Subjective findings

1. May be asymptomatic in early disease
2. Hematuria

   a. Gross or microscopic
   b. Chronic
   c. Intermittent

3. Irritative voiding symptoms such as urinary frequency and urgency

C. Physical examination findings

1. Masses detected on bimanual examination
2. Hepatomegaly or supraclavicular lymphadenopathy may be present in metastatic disease.
3. Lymphedema of lower extremities may be present owing to metastases to pelvic lymph nodes.
4. Pyuria, occasionally

D. Laboratory/Diagnostic findings

1. Urinalysis may show hematuria in the majority of cases.
2. Azotemia associated with ureteral obstruction
3. Anemia may be present owing to blood loss.
4. Urine tests to detect recurrent bladder cancer after treatment

   a. Urine cytology—Very effective in detecting high-grade bladder cancers, but will miss many papillary urothelial neoplasms of low malignancy.
   b. BTA (a new tumor marker)—Looks for specific proteins in the urine indicative of recurrent bladder cancer cells.
   c. NMP22 (a new tumor marker)—Also looks for protein specific to recurrent bladder cancer cells.
   d. BTA and NMP22 are more sensitive than urine cytology in detecting low-grade cancers such as papillary urothelial neoplasms.
   e. Other new markers under testing include HA-HAase, CYFRA21-1, and an antibody to whole cells called Immunocyt.

5. Exfoliated cells from normal and abnormal urothelium are seen in voided urine specimens.

   a. Cytology is sensitive to detection of exfoliated cells but may be enhanced by flow cytometry.

6. Filling defects may be detected by

   a. Intravenous urography
   b. Ultrasound

   c. CT
   d. MRI

7. Diagnosis and staging of cancer confirmed by

   a. Cystoscopy
   b. Biopsy
   c. Transurethral resection

8. Grading based on

   a. Size
   b. Pleomorphism
   c. Mitotic rate
   d. Hyperchromatism

9. Staging based on

   a. Extent of regional metastases
   b. Distant metastases

E. Major treatments

1. Surgical treatment

   a. Transurethral resection (TUR)
     i. Initial form of treatment
     ii. Muscle-infiltrating cancers require more aggressive therapy.
   b. Partial cystectomy
     i. Solitary lesions
     ii. Bladder diverticulum
   c. Radical cystectomy removes
     i. In men
       (1) Bladder
       (2) Prostate
       (3) Seminal vesicles
       (4) Surrounding fat
       (5) Peritoneal attachments
     ii. In women
       (1) Uterus
       (2) Cervix
       (3) Urethra
       (4) Anterior vaginal vault
       (5) Ovaries
       (6) Bladder
     iii. Bilateral pelvic lymph node dissection may be accomplished at the same time in both men and women.
     iv. Urinary diversion may also be performed.

2. Intravesical immunotherapy—agents delivered directly into the bladder by a urethral catheter.

3. Intravesical chemotherapy
4. Chemotherapy

   a. A cisplatin-based combination chemotherapy is commonly used.
   b. Chemotherapy may be used prior to surgery or postoperatively in an attempt to preserve the bladder.

5. Radiotherapy

   a. External beam radiotherapy is generally well tolerated.
   b. Ten to fifteen percent of patients develop bladder, bowel, or rectal complications.

6. Decision algorithms for bladder cancer are anticipated to be available in 2001 on the American Cancer Society web site, www.cancer.org, and at the National Comprehensive Cancer Network web site, www.nccn.org.

VIII. ENDOMETRIAL CANCER[10, 14, 15]

A. General comments/Predisposing factors

1. Cancer of the endometrium is the most common cancer of the female reproductive organs.
2. Increased incidence with

   a. Women 50–70 years old
   b. Menopause (75%)
   c. Obesity, especially upper body fat
   d. Unopposed exogenous estrogen
   e. History of infertility or nulliparity
   f. Diabetes
   g. Polycystic ovaries with prolonged anovulation
   h. Extended use of tamoxifen for the treatmnet of breast cancer
   i. Personal or family history of ovarian or breast cancer
   j. Higher socioeconomic status
   k. Prior pelvic radiation therapy

3. Whites are 70% more likely to develop endometrial cancer than are African Americans.

4. The 5-year survival rate is 84% for all types of endometrial cancer, collectively.

B. Subjective findings

1. Postmenopausal bleeding should be treated as endometrial cancer until proven otherwise.
2. Abnormal bleeding is the presenting sign in 80% of cases.
3. Lower abdominal pain or pressure
4. Back pain (rare)

5. Lower extremity edema may manifest secondary to metastasis.
6. Weight loss

C. Physical examination findings

1. Usually findings are normal on examination of

   a. Vagina
   b. Uterus
   c. Cervix

2. Enlarged uterus or pelvic mass may be present with advanced disease.
3. Cervical stenosis
4. Pyometra
5. Mucosanguinous vaginal discharge may be present in cervical and vaginal metastases.
6. Bladder or rectal mass may be a presentation of regional metastasis.

D. Laboratory/Diagnostic findings

1. Endometrial biopsy (EMB) is a first-line procedure in the office and may consist of

   a. Endocervical sampling
   b. Endometrial sampling

2. EMB provides an adequate sample in 90–95% of cases.
3. Dilatation and curettage (D&C) has a higher sensitivity especially when combined with EMB; the detection rate approaches 100%.
4. Transvaginal uterine ultrasonography (TRUS) determines the thickness of the endometrium.
5. Hysteroscopy with directed biopsy may be required for staging of occult cancer.
6. Routine Pap smear

   a. May detect cancer as "endometrial cells"
   b. Insensitive diagnostic tool

7. Serial serum CA125 may be used to determine cancer recurrence.

E. Major treatments

1. Extrafascial total abdominal hysterectomy with wide vaginal cuff

   a. Salpingo-oophorectomy
   b. Retroperitoneal lymph node sampling

2. Radical hysterecotomy
   a. Salpingo-oophorectomy
   b. Retroperitoneal lymph node dissection when there is cervical involvement
3. Radiation may be used in the uterine cavity or externally before surgery in grade 3 or greater lesions
4. Radiation also is used for recurrences
5. In advanced or recurrent disease:
   a. Continuous nonestrogenic progesterone derivatives are used and evaluated every 3 months.
   b. Hydroxyprogesterone, 1g, 1–7 times per week IM, may also be used.
6. Common follow-up schedules include
   a. Every 2 months for the first year
   b. Every 3 months for the second year
   c. Every 4 months for the third year
   d. Every 4 months for the fourth year
   e. Every 6 months for the fifth year
   f. Then, annually
   g. Breast examination every 6 months
   h. Mammogram annually
   i. Cytologic smears from the vaginal apex
      i. Every 6 months for 5 years
      ii. Then, annually
      iii. May require vaginal lubrication and plastic vaginal dilator, particularly if radiation has been used.
7. Decision algorithms for endometrial cancer are anticipated to be available in 2001 on the American Cancer Society web site, www.cancer.org, and at the National Comprehensive Cancer Network web site, www.nccn.org.

References

1. Baldini, E.H., & Strauss, G.M. (1997). Women and lung cancer. Waiting to exhale. *Chest, 112,* 229S–234S.
2. [Bladder Cancer—American Cancer Society] http://www3.cancer.org/cancerinfo/load_cont.asp?st=tr&ct=44&language=english.
3. [Breast Cancer—American Cancer Society, Version 1 March 2000] http://www.cancer.org.
4. Burke, W., Daly, M., Garber, J., Botkin, J., Kahn, M.J.E., Lynch, P., McTiernan, A., Offit, K., Perlman, J., Petersen, G., Thomason, E., & Varricchio, C. (1997). Recommendations for follow-up care of individuals with an inherited predisposition to cancer: II. BRCA1 and BRCA2. *Journal of the American Medical Association, 277,* 997–1003.
5. [Cervical Cancer—American Cancer Society] http:www3.cancer.org/cancerinfo/load_cont.asp?st=tr&ct=8&language=english.
6. [Colon and rectal cancer treatment guidelines for patients, Version 1, March 2000] http://www.cancer.org.

7. Chestnutt, M.S. (2000). Lung. In L.M. Tierney, Jr., S.J. McPhee, & M.A. Papadakis (Eds.). *Current medical diagnosis & treatment* (39th ed.) (pp. 264–350). Stamford, CT: Appleton & Lange.

8. Davis, D.L. (1998). Prostate cancer treatment with radioactive seed implantation. *AORN Journal, 68,* 15–48.

9. Dewar, M.A. (1996). Breast cancer. In R.E. Rakel (Ed). *Saunders manual of medical practice* (pp. 408–410). Philadelphia: W.B. Saunders.

10. [Endometrial Cancer—American Cancer Society] http//www3.cancer .org/cancerinfo/main_cont.asp?st=pr&ct=11

11. Giuliano, A.I. (2000). Breast. In L.M. Tierney, Jr., S.J. McPhee, & M.A. Papadakis (Eds.). *Current medical diagnosis & treatment* (39th ed.) (pp. 678–702). Stamford, CT: Appleton & Lange.

12. Kamat, A.M., & Lamm, D.L. (1999). Chemoprevention of urological cancer. *Journal of Urology, 161,* 1748–1760.

13. [Lung Cancer—American Cancer Society] http://www3.cancer.org/ cancerinfo/load—cont.asp?st=tr&cr=26&language=english.

14. MacKay, H.T. (2000). Gynecology. In L.M., Tierney, Jr., S.J. McPhee, & M.A. Papadakis (Eds.). *Current medical diagnosis & treatment* (39th ed.) (pp. 723–757). Stamford, CT: Appleton & Lange.

15. Mayeaux, E.J., Jr. (1996). Endometrial Cancer. In R.E. Rakel (Ed). *Saunders manual of medical practice.* (pp. 408–410). Philadelphia: W.B. Saunders.

16. McQuaid, K.R. (2000). Alimentary tract. In L.M. Tierney, Jr., S.J. McPhee, & M.A. Papadakis (Eds.). *Current medical diagnosis & treatment* (39th ed.) (pp. 553–655). Stamford, CT: Appleton & Lange.

17. Nuovo, J. (1996). Cervical cancer. In R.E. Rakel (Ed). *Saunders manual of medical practice* (pp. 408–410). Philadelphia: W.B. Saunders.

18. [Ovary Cancer—American Cancer Society] http://www3.cancer.org/ cancerinfo/load—cont.asp?st=tr&ct=8&language=english.

19. Presti, J.C., Jr., Stoller, M.L., & Carroll, P.R. (2000). Urology. In L.M. Tierney, Jr., S.J. McPhee, & M.A. Papadakis (Eds.). *Current medical diagnosis & treatment* (39th ed.) (pp. 917–958). Stamford, CT: Appleton & Lange.

20. [Prostage cancer—American Cancer Society guidelines for patients, Version 1, June 1999] http://www.cancer.org.

Management of Patients with Immunologic Disorders

HIV/AIDS AND OPPORTUNISTIC INFECTIONS

David A. Miller, MD, FCCP

Current therapy for HIV infection and its major complicating secondary illnesses (opportunistic diseases), as well as for prevention of these secondary illnesses, undergoes frequent changes in current standards of care. The provider of care to these patients is cautioned to check the most current standards. The Centers for Disease Control and Prevention issues updates to guidelines for care on a regular basis; these are available in printed media and on the Internet (see the references at the end of this chapter).

I. HIV INFECTION[1, 7]

A. Etiology/Incidence

1. HIV infection and AIDS are common; approximately 30–40 million individuals, including men, women, and children, are infected worldwide.
2. The incidence among groups of HIV infection varies.

   a. Heterosexually acquired HIV infection is high in Africa and Asia, although the incidence of heterosexually acquired HIV infection is rising rapidly in Western societies as well.
   b. In Western nations, men who have sex with men, injecting drug abuse, and congenital spread have been responsible for most HIV infections to date.

B. Course of infection and important pathophysiologic markers

1. Retroviral infection by one of the strains of the human immunodeficiency virus
2. HIV infects cells that express the CD4 receptor, including

   a. Macrophages
   b. CD4+ T lymphocytes
   c. Langerhans cells of the skin
   d. Macrophages in the central nervous system
   e. Others

3. HIV infection is chronic and progressive.

   a. Initially, there is a rapid increase in the number of viral particles in the blood.
   b. During a period of clinical latency, which can be pro-

longed, the number of viral particles in each mL of blood (the viral load) is low.

c. During the development of symptomatic HIV disease and AIDS, the viral load increases and the number of CD4+ lymphocytes measurable in the blood decreases.

4. Therapy against HIV infection may alter the rate of progression to advanced immunodeficiency.

a. Recent data suggest that persons with HIV disease and AIDS live longer than in the past and that medications and appropriate management have reduced the mortality from HIV disease and AIDS.[1]

II. DOCUMENTING HIV DISEASE[7]

A. The medical history

1. Significant risk factor review[10]

a. Documented risk factors for viral transmission
   i. Males who have sex with males
   ii. Sexual partners of HIV-infected individuals. Note that sexual transmission through rectal, vaginal, and oral sex has been documented.
   iii. Persons who share injecting drug use equipment
   iv. Receipt of a blood transfusion in the early or mid 1980s, prior to screening of the blood supply
   v. Placental transmission from an infected mother to her unborn child
   vi. Transmission at the time of delivery
   vii. Transmission during breast-feeding, both to the infant from an infected mother and to the mother from an infected baby
   viii. Transmission via blood in health care settings, including
      (1) Accidental needle stick
      (2) Splashing of blood onto wounds
      (3) During dental procedures

b. No other evidence of transmission has occurred during the pandemic.

2. Current symptoms[1, 7]

a. The acute retroviral syndrome
   i. Flu-like illness
      (1) Fever
      (2) Chills
      (3) Fatigue
      (4) Diffuse erythematous rash

    ii. Serologic tests for HIV may be indeterminate, negative, or positive, depending on the length of time after the infection.

    iii. HIV viral load measures are clearly elevated, and the CD4+ T lymphocyte count is within normal limits or slightly reduced.

    iv. Often missed clinically because of rapid resolution without the need for acute medical care

    v. When documented, clearly dates the onset of infection

b. Latent HIV infection

    i. Few or no symptoms or signs referable to HIV-related illness; the patient may have persistent generalized lymphadenopathy.

    ii. Positive ELISA and Western blot for HIV infection

    iii. Variable HIV viral load and CD4+ T lymphocyte count

c. Symptomatic HIV disease (formerly AIDS-related complex)

    i. Fever, chills, diarrhea, weight loss (unintended)

    ii. Appearance of non-AIDS–defining infections that are normally kept quiescent by an intact immune system, including

        (1) Shingles (herpes zoster)

        (2) Thrush (candidiasis)

            (a) Oral

            (b) Mucocutaneous

            (c) Vaginal

        (3) Frequent bacterial infections

    iii. Laboratory evidence of declining CD4+ T lymphocyte count and/or increasing HIV viral load

d. AIDS

    i. Measurable immunodeficiency, with the appearance of one of many AIDS indicator illnesses, or opportunistic infections (see Section VI. Prophylaxis Against Opportunistic Infections)

    ii. The CD4+ T lymphocyte count is typically below 500/mL.

    iii. AIDS is diagnosed in the absence of opportunistic disease if the CD4+ T lymphocyte count is below 200/mL.

e. Advanced HIV infection[7]

    i. A category of HIV disease in which the CD4+ T lymphocyte count is below 50/mL

    ii. Symptoms include

        (1) Wasting

        (2) Periodic fevers

        (3) Fatigue

    iii. Single or multiple opportunistic infections may occur.

    iv. If this phase is documented during therapy for HIV infection, the prognosis is poor.

III. CLINICAL EVALUATION OF THE PATIENT AT RISK FOR HIV INFECTION

A. Serologic testing[1]

1. Screening tests

   a. The enzyme-linked immunosorbent assay (ELISA) for HIV

     i. A prepackaged test that looks for at least one of the known antibodies against HIV

     ii. On repeat testing, the test should be repeatedly reactive.

   b. Rapid screening tests, with results known in less than 30 min, have been used in other countries, and recently have been released for use in the United States.

     i. In general, these tests are not as reliable as the standard ELISA owing to a higher rate of false-positive results.

     ii. However, they are most useful in urgent care situations.

       (1) Hospital emergency rooms

       (2) After HIV exposure in health care settings

       (3) When the patient is not likely to return for screening results

     iii. These tests include

       (1) A saliva test (Orasure)

       (2) A urine test (Calypte HIV Urine EIA)

       (3) Both are available only to health professionals.

     iv. These tests have not replaced the ELISA in the screening for HIV infection, although all are reasonably sensitive and specific.

   c. One kit is available for patients to use at home.

     i. Home Access Express Test

     ii. Counseling is given by telephone to those with positive results.

2. Confirmatory tests for HIV infection[1, 7]

   a. Western blot test for the presence of antibodies against HIV

     i. Relies on the detection of several different antibodies, and to be interpreted as positive should include at least one from each of the following groups:

     ii. Antibodies against envelope proteins of the HIV. To be considered indicative ("positive") for HIV infection, at least two of the following should be present:

       (1) gp160/120

       (2) gp41

       (3) p24

    iii. "Indeterminate" tests, in which only one antibody is measurable, may be re-evaluated in 4–6 weeks.

  b. Or, they may be rechecked by determination using the HIV DNA by polymerase chain reaction (PCR) or HIV RNA by PCR (quantitative). These tests require more time (days) and are more costly.

B. Current and past health history, along with

1. Complete physical examination
2. Prior medication intolerance and allergies

C. Initial laboratory evaluation of the HIV-infected patient[7]

1. Complete blood cell count
2. CD4+ cell count (the CD4+ T lymphocyte is a target cell for HIV infection) and CD8+ T lymphocyte count (often termed "AIDS lymphocyte subsets")
3. HIV RNA level, quantitative ("viral load")

  a. Inflammatory processes, including other infections, may increase the viral load.

  b. Interpretation of the viral load must always take that fact into consideration, *including* during repeat viral load testing *after* therapy has begun.

4. Syphilis testing (VDRL or rapid plasma reagin [RPR])
5. Hepatitis screening (A, B, and C)
6. Serum chemistry evaluation, including lipid profile and liver profile
7. Tuberculosis skin test (results are positive if ≥5 mm induration)
8. Pap smear/gynecologic evaluation
9. Chest x-ray
10. Other testing[7]

  a. Toxoplasmosis serology (to assist in the differential diagnosis of central nervous system lesions)

  b. Cytomegalovirus (CMV) serology, especially for those at apparent low risk for CMV infection (CMV is a blood-borne pathogen)

  c. Glucose-6-phosphate dehydrogenase levels (especially in men of Mediterranean background and possibly in men of African background as well) prior to dapsone, primaquine, and sulfonamide therapy, which is associated with severe hemolysis in G6PD-deficient individuals)

  d. Varicella antibody testing to determine prior infection (in patients unable to recall prior disease) with chicken pox or shingles in the event that a significant exposure occurs in the future

IV. INITIATION OF HIGHLY ACTIVE ANTIRETROVIRAL THERAPY (HAART)[1, 2, 5–9, 11]

A. Asymptomatic patients

1. HIV RNA >20,000 mL by polymerase chain reaction (PCR) or >10,000 mL by branched-chain DNA (bDNA) assay, *or* CD4+ cell count <500/mL

   a. Offer treatment and initiate if patient accepts and is likely to adhere.
   b. Individuals with ongoing drug abuse behavior should receive rehabilitation prior to initiation of therapy, if possible.

2. HIV RNA <20,000 mL by PCR or < 10,000 mL by bDNA, and CD4+ count over 500/mL: Treatment may be offered.

B. Symptomatic patient (with or without AIDS defining illness; acute retroviral syndrome)

1. Treat regardless of CD4+ cell count or viral load measurement

V. ANTIRETROVIRAL THERAPY (HIGHLY ACTIVE ANTIRETROVIRAL THERAPY [HAART])

A. Initial regimens
Initial regimens involve one choice from column A and one from column B in Table 66–1. These recommendations are evolving, and caregivers should check current recommendations.

1. Alternatively, some experts suggest that, if the patient is unlikely to adhere to a multiple-pill-per-day regimen, that three nucleoside analogs (e.g., zidovudine [Retrovir], lamivudine [Epivir], and didanosine [Videx], or zidovudine, lamivudine, and abacavir sulfate [Ziagen]) could be administered without risk of immunologic deterioration.

   a. Individualization is needed in any treatment regimen.
   b. Consultation with an experienced HIV clinician may be needed.

2. Similarly, a regimen containing two nucleoside analogs with a non-nucleoside reverse transcriptase inhibitor, thus again sparing the protease inhibitor class for later therapy, may be beneficial and effective (Table 66–2).

   a. Long-term data on these combinations is lacking (see Table 67–2 for doses and common side effects).
   b. This regimen may require the patient to use only five pills per day (e.g., Combivir [lamivudine, 150 mg, and zidovudine, 300 mg], 1 pill b.i.d., and Sustiva [efavirenz], 3 pills, 200 mg/pill, or 600 mg, at bedtime).

TABLE 66-1. ANTIRETROVIRAL THERAPY: INITIAL REGIMENS

COLUMN A: PROTEASE INHIBITORS, WITH DOSES AND COMMON SIDE EFFECTS	COLUMN B: NUCLEOSIDE ANALOG REVERSE TRANSCRIPTASE INHIBITORS, WITH DOSES AND COMMON SIDE EFFECTS
Crixivan (indinavir) 400 mg p.o. q8h (on an empty stomach or with a snack containing <2 g fat) Kidney stones, from precipitation of the drug in the urine, are a relative contraindication. Adequate hydration is mandatory.	**Retrovir (AZT; zidovudine) + Videx (ddI; didanosine)** 300 p.o. b.i.d. + 200 mg b.i.d. AZT: Nausea, headache at initiation of therapy; anemia and myopathy are possible. ddI: Peripheral neuropathy and pancreatitis; antacid content may interfere with absorption of other medications.
Viracept (nelfinavir) 750 mg p.o. t.i.d. (taken with food). Diarrhea is frequent and may be treated with calcium supplements.	**Zerit (stavudine, d4T) + Hivid (zalcitabine, ddC)** 20–40 mg b.i.d. + 200 mg b.i.d. d4T; Peripheral neuropathy not uncommon. ddC: peripheral neuropathy common; oral ulcers are less frequent.
Norvir (ritonavir) 600 mg p.o. q12h Nausea and diarrhea are common.	**Retrovir + Hivid (zalcilabine, ddC)** 300 mg p.o. b.i.d. + 0.375–0.75 mg b.i.d.
Fortovase (saquinavir, soft gel cap) 1200 mg p.o. t.i.d. (with a fatty meal) Well tolerated.	**Retrovir + Epivir (lamivudine) as Combivir** 1 pill p.o. b.i.d.
Agenerase (amprenavir) 1200 mg p.o. b.i.d. Nausea, diarrhea, and rash are the more commonly encountered side effects.	**Zerit + Epivir (lamivudine)** Lamivudine: 40 mg b.i.d. + 150 mg b.i.d. Well tolerated.
	Ziagen (abacavir) + Retrovir/ Epivir (Combivir) 300 mg b.i.d. (Ziagen); 1 pill p.o. b.i.d. Combivir: Hypersensitivity reaction, while uncommon, can be severe, with fever and a rash. Discontinue drug if occurs and do not rechallenge patient with the drug.

TABLE 66–2. NON-NUCLEOSIDE REVERSE TRANSCRIPTASE INHIBITORS WITH DOSES AND COMMON SIDE EFFECTS

Sustiva (efavirenz)	600 mg p.o. at bedtime; dizziness and transient rash
Viramune (nevirapine)	200 mg p.o. once daily for 2 weeks, then 200 mg b.i.d. or 400 mg q.d.; transient rash and drug-induced hepatitis
Rescriptor (delavirdine)	400 mg p.o. t.i.d.; transient rash

B. Contraindicated combinations of antiretroviral agents[9]

1. Antagonistic combinations

   a. The two thymidine-containing nucleoside analogs, zidovudine (formerly azidothymidine, AZT) and stavudine (d4T), are antagonistic.
   b. Indinavir and saquinavir are antagonistic in laboratory settings, and their concomitant use is not advisable.

2. Risk of neuropathy

   a. Concomitant use of didanosine (dideoxyinosine, ddI) and zalcitabine (dideoxycytidine, ddC) increases the risk of peripheral neuropathy.
   b. Stavudine similarly but less frequently can cause neuropathy.

3. Combinations of non-nucleoside reverse transcriptase inhibitors are not recommended at present owing to insufficient data.

C. Follow-up of initial HAART

1. CD4+ cell count and HIV viral load determination one month after initiation and every 3–6 months. A half log rise in the viral load or a significant drop in the CD4+ cell count warrants consideration for revision of the HAART.
2. Patient counseling about the need to faithfully adhere to the prescribed medication regimen and to scheduled follow-up visits is mandatory.

   a. The need for adherence and follow-up visits should be reiterated at each visit.
   b. Prophylaxis against opportunistic infections (OIs) should be continued once started.
   c. Current recommendations may alter prophylaxis recommendations if the patient has significant immunologic stability and/or improvement in immunodeficiency (see Section VI. Prophylaxis Against Opportunistic Infections).

D. Treatment for patients deteriorating during HAART therapy

Deterioration is measured by deteriorating CD4+ cell count, a verified half log rise in the viral load, or the appearance of an OI during HAART therapy.

1. Drug resistance testing may be used to determine if a patient's dominant HIV strain is still sensitive to current antiretroviral therapy.

   a. Genotypic testing looks for known patterns of mutations in the reverse transcriptase and/or the viral protease genes.[9]
   b. This testing may therefore guide changes in antiretroviral therapy if needed.
   c. The test is currently expensive and requires several weeks to complete.
   d. However, improved drug selection in "rescue" regimens results from this testing.[1, 2]

2. Two new nucleoside analogs and a new protease inhibitor (consider amprenavir [Agenerase], 1200 mg p.o. q12h)
3. Two new nucleoside analogs and a non-nucleoside reverse transcriptase inhibitor (Note: All three non-nucleoside reverse transcriptase inhibitors exhibit drug cross resistance)

E. All patients changing HAART medication regimens in general should have two new drugs added at the time the change is made, along with follow-up CD4+ cell count and viral load testing approximately 4 weeks after beginning the new regimen.

VI. PROPHYLAXIS AGAINST OPPORTUNISTIC INFECTIONS (OIs)

A. Strongly recommended

1. Tuberculosis, based on a positive purified protein derivative test (≥ 5 mm), on recent exposure to a person infected with active TB, or on previously inadequately treated TB: Isoniazid, 300 mg p.o., with pyridoxine, 50 mg p.o., q.d. for 9 months
2. *Pneumocystis carinii*, based on a rapidly declining CD4+ cell count or an absolute CD4+ cell count of <200/mL:

   a. Trimethoprim-sulfamethoxazole (TMP/SMX) DS, 1 p.o. daily, or dapsone, 100 mg daily, if allergic to sulfa (assessing for G6PD deficiency first)
   b. Patients whose CD4+ T lymphocyte counts rise above 200/mL for 6 months may stop primary prophylaxis (i.e., no prior *P. carinii* pneumonia [PCP]).
   c. Secondary prophylaxis (i.e., patients with a prior history of PCP) should continue prophylaxis.

3. Toxoplasmosis, based on CD4+ count < 100/mL *and* positive IgG serology

   a. TMP/SMX as above for PCP; dapsone, 50 mg q.d., plus pyrimethamine, 50 mg every week, with leucovorin, 25 mg every week

   b. Patients whose CD4+ T lymphocyte counts rise above 100/mL for 6 months may stop primary prophylaxis against toxoplasmosis.

   c. Secondary prophylaxis should continue indefinitely.

4. *Mycobacterium avium*, based on CD4+ cell count <50/mL

   a. Azithromycin (Zithromax), 1200 mg once per week, *or* clarithromycin (Biaxin), 500 mg b.i.d.

   b. Patients whose CD4+ T lymphocyte count is over 100/mL for 6 months may stop primary prophylaxis against *M. avium*.

   c. Patients who have had active *M. avium* infection, especially bacteremia, should complete the therapy of their primary infection and then receive secondary prophylaxis, as listed in 4b. While some clinicians would stop this secondary prophylaxis as in 4b, others would treat indefinitely. Until further studies are done, no firm recommendation beyond the use of secondary prophylaxis for 6 months can be made at this time.

B. Vaccinations recommended

1. Hepatitis B, based upon finding anti-hepatitis B core antigen negative

   a. Recombivax HB, 10 μg IM, *or* Engerix-B, 20 μg IM, on three separate occasions, at 3, 6, and 12 months

   b. Assess antibody response, especially if CD4+ counts rise above 200/mL.

2. Influenza vaccine (all patients): 0.5 mL IM annually in October or November

   a. Note: This may cause the viral load to increase temporarily.

   b. Viral load determinations should be done prior to administering the vaccine or after waiting several weeks after the vaccine.

3. Hepatitis A vaccination, for all patients with chronic hepatitis C infection[1]

   a. Havrix, 0.5 mL IM on two occasions 6 months apart

   b. The CDC has recommended Havrix for all men who have sex with men who are seronegative for hepatitis A.[4]

4. Pneumococcal vaccine (for all patients), 0.5 mL IM once

   a. Revaccination can be recommended for those patients whose initial CD4+ T lymphocyte count was <200/mL and rises above that level.
   b. Revaccination should be considered 5 years after the initial vaccination.

VII. AIDS INDICATOR CONDITIONS[3]

An HIV serology screening should be done in all patients presenting with the conditions listed in this section. *Note:* Major symptoms and signs are given only for more commonly encountered OIs; see text references at the end of the chapter for others.

A. Candidiasis of the esophagus, trachea, bronchi, or lungs

1. Symptoms are referable to the region of the body affected.
2. Severe disease may require IV therapy: Amphotericin B, 0.5–1 mg/kg/day; fluconazole (Diflucan), 200–400 mg/day.
3. Milder disease may respond to fluconazole, 200 mg/day po.

B. Cervical cancer, invasive
C. Coccidioidomycosis, extrapulmonary
D. Cryptococcosis, extrapulmonary

1. Meningitis

   a. Manifestations may include fever, headache, and altered level of consciousness.
   b. Treatment: Amphotericin B, 1 mg/kg/day IV, followed by fluconazole, 400 mg/day p.o. for 10 weeks, followed by secondary prophylaxis at 200–400 mg/day

2. Pulmonary/disseminated disease

   a. Fluconazole, 200–400 mg/day, followed by secondary prophylaxis at 200 mg/day

E. Cryptosporidiosis, with diarrhea for over 1 month
F. Cytomegalovirus of any organ, excluding liver, spleen, and lymph nodes
G. Herpes simplex mucocutaneous outbreak lasting over 1 month, or of the bronchi, lungs, or esophagus

1. Treatment of severe disease: Acyclovir (Zovirax), 15–30 mg/kg IV daily for 7–10 days; 800 mg, five times daily p.o. for 7 days
2. Secondary prophylaxis should be offered to those patients with recurrences of herpes outbreaks: Acyclovir, 400 mg b.i.d., unless concomitantly receiving ganciclovir (Cytovene) or foscarnet (Foscavir) for active CMV infection

H. Histoplasmosis, extrapulmonary
I. HIV-associated dementia
J. HIV-associated wasting
K. Isosporosis, with diarrhea for over 1 month
L. Kaposi's sarcoma in a patient <60 years old
M. Lymphoma, brain, in a patient <60 years old
N. Lymphoma, non-Hodgkins, of B-cell origin, or immunoblastic lymphoma
O. *Mycobacterium avium* or *M. kansasii* infection with dissemination
P. *Mycobacterium tuberculosis* infection, disseminated
Q. *Mycobacterium tuberculosis* infection, pulmonary

1. For symptoms, findings, diagnosis, and treatment, see Chapter 25.

R. Nocardiosis
S. *Pneumocystis carinii* pneumonia

1. Moderately high (e.g., 103°F) fever, nonproductive cough, and dyspnea, often out of proportion to radiographic findings; may progress to respiratory failure with acute respiratory distress syndrome
2. Diagnosis, definitive: Silver stains of bronchial washings or biopsies. Some clinicians elect to treat empirically.
3. Treatment

   a. Trimethoprim, 15 mg/kg/day, with sulfamethoxazole, 75 mg/kg/day IV, in four divided doses, changing to oral TMP/SMX (two double-strength tablets t.i.d.) for a total of 21 days of therapy.
   b. Corticosteroids (prednisone, 40 mg b.i.d., or Solu-Medrol, 40 mg IV q12h) are indicated for moderately severe or severe disease (PaO$_2$ <70 on room air), tapering the dose as the disease responds to antimicrobial therapy.

T. Pneumonia, recurrent bacterial
U. Progressive multifocal leukoencephalopathy
V. *Salmonella* septicemia, recurrent (non-typhoid)
W. Strongyloidosis, outside the gut
X. Toxoplasmosis, internal organ
Y. CD4+ cell count <200/mL

References

1. Bartlett, J.G., & Gallant, JE. (2000). *2000–2001 Medical management of HIV infection.* Baltimore: Port City Press, 2000. [Updates on care of HIV infected individuals are at the Johns Hopkins AIDS Service web site: http://www.hopkins-aids.edu.]
2. Carpenter, C., Cooper, D.A., Fischl, M.A., Gatell, J.M., Gazzard, B.G., Hammer, S.M., Hirsch, M.S., Jacobsen, D.M., Katzenstein, D.A., Montaner, J.S., Richman, D.D., Saag, M.S., Schechter, M., Schooley, R.T.,

Thompson, M.A., Vella, S., Yeni, P.G., & Volberding, P.A. (2000). Antiretroviral therapy in adults: Updated recommendations of the International AIDS Society–USA panel. *Journal of the American Medical Association, 283,* 381–390.

3. Centers for Disease Control and Prevention (1992). 1993 Revised classification system for HIV infection and expanded surveillance case definition for AIDS among adolescents and adults. *MMWR. Morbidity and Mortality Weekly Report, 40,* 1–94.

4. Centers for Disease Control and Prevention (1999). Prevention of hepatitis A through active or passive immunization: Recommendations of the Advisory Committee on Immunization Practices (ACIP). *MMWR. Morbidity and Mortality Weekly Report, 48,* 27.

5. Centers for Disease Control and Prevention. The most current updates to guidelines on HIV treatment and management of OIs are found at http://www.hivatis.org.

6. Cohen, O.J. (2000). Antiretroviral therapy: Time to think strategically (editorial). *Annals of Internal Medicine, 132,* 320–322.

7. Dolin, R., Masur, H., & Saag, M. (Eds.) (1999). *AIDS therapy.* New York: Churchill Livingstone.

8. Henry, K. (2000). The case for more cautious, patient-focused antiretroviral therapy. *Annals of Internal Medicine, 132,* 306–311.

9. Schutz, M., & Wendrow, A. (2000). Quick reference guide to antiretrovirals. January 1, 2000. www.medscape.com, http://hiv.medscape.com/updates/quickguide.

10. Staprans, S.I., & Feinberg, M.B. (1997). Natural history and immunopathogenesis of HIV-1 disease. In M.A. Sande & P.A. Volberding (Eds.), *The medical management of AIDS* (pp. 29–55). Philadelphia: W.B. Saunders.

11. Ungvarski, P.J. (1999). Adolescents and adults: HIV disease care management. In P.J. Ungvarski & J.H. Flaskerud (Eds.), *HIV/AIDS: A guide to primary care management* (4th ed.) (pp. 131–193). Philadelphia: W.B. Saunders.

AUTOIMMUNE DISEASES

67

Sally K. Miller, MS, RN, CS, ACNP, ANP, GNP, CCRN

I. GIANT CELL ARTERITIS

A. Definition

1. Systemic, panarteritis of the medium and large arteries, usually the temporal artery and/or aorta
2. Believed to represent the extreme spectrum of polymyalgia rheumatica

   a. A clinical diagnosis based on pain and stiffness of the shoulders and pelvis
   b. Associated with weight loss, fever, and malaise

3. Considered a medical emergency

   a. Untreated temporal arteritis may result in irreversible blindness.
   b. Untreated aortic arteritis may result in the serious or life-threatening sequela of aortic occlusion.

B. Etiology/Incidence/Predisposing factors[1]

1. Vascular endothelial cells become "activated" and

   a. Act as antigen-presenting cells and sources of cytokine production
   b. Interact with immune-competent cells
   c. Express adhesion molecules, promoting leukocyte binding and aggregation

2. Occurs most commonly in adults over age 50
3. Slightly more common in women than in men
4. Approximately 50% of patients with giant cell arteritis also have polymyalgia rheumatica.

C. Subjective findings[2, 4, 5]

1. Persistent headache
2. Localized scalp tenderness on palpation
3. Jaw claudication
4. Visual impairment
5. Tongue claudication
6. Anorexia
7. Weight loss
8. Malaise

9. Symptoms consistent with vertebrobasilar transient ischemic attack

   a. Vertigo
   b. Deafness
   c. Tinnitus
   d. Ataxia

D. Physical examination findings[2, 5]

1. Difficulty talking
2. Fever
3. Temporal artery may be large, nodular, or pulseless.
4. Blindness

E. Laboratory/Diagnostic findings[2, 4]

1. Normal white blood cell count between 6000–10,000/mL
2. Elevated erythrocyte sedimentation rate (ESR) greater than 100 mm/h
3. Biopsy of the affected artery is the gold standard.

   a. Positive biopsy result confirms the diagnosis.
   b. False-negative biopsy result can occur; if clinical suspicion is strong, the patient should be treated regardless of the negative result.

4. Aortogram as indicated by clinical presentation of arotic aneurysm or occlusion

F. Management[2, 4]

1. Should begin immediately upon clinical diagnosis

   a. Do not wait for biopsy.
   b. Biopsies obtained 1–2 weeks after initiation of prednisone are reliable.

2. Prednisone, 1–2 mg/kg/day (typically 60 mg), for 6 weeks to 2 months
3. Prednisone may be tapered after 6 weeks to 2 months if symptoms have subsided.
4. Falling ESR may be used as a guide to begin tapering, but tapering should not begin less than 6 weeks after initiation of therapy regardless of ESR.
5. Educate patient regarding signs and symptoms of recurrence; patients are at greater risk for recurrence.

II. SYSTEMIC LUPUS ERYTHEMATOSUS (SLE)

A. Definition[2]

1. A chronic, inflammatory, autoimmune disorder that may affect multiple body systems

2. Clinical signs and symptoms are caused by trapping of antigen-antibody complexes in capillaries or visceral structures and/or autoantibody-mediated destruction of host cells.
3. Clinical course is manifested by exacerbations and remissions; the disease may be mild or rapidly fatal.

B. Etiology/Incidence/Predisposing factors[2, 3]

1. A variety of stimuli are thought to trigger aberrant function of T- and B-cells in a genetically predisposed host.
   a. Sex hormones
   b. Ultraviolet radiation
   c. Infection
   d. Stress
   e. A variety of drugs and chemicals, including
      i. Hydralazine
      ii. Procainamide
      iii. Isoniazid
      iv. Methyldopa
      v. Chlorpromazine
2. Autoantibody and immunoglobulin production is increased.
3. Eighty-five percent of patients with SLE are women.
4. SLE occurs more often in African American women.
5. There is an increased familial risk.

C. Subjective findings[2, 3]

1. Fatigue
2. Myalgias, arthralgias
3. Pleuritic chest discomfort
4. Pericarditis
5. Dyspnea
6. Hemoptysis
7. Headaches
8. Neuropathies
9. Photophobia
10. Transient blindness
11. Raynaud's phenomenon—Present in only 20% of patients, but when it occurs, it is one of the earliest manifestations.
12. Abdominal pain

D. Physical examination findings[2-4]

1. Malar or butterfly rash of cheeks, forehead, chin, bridge of nose
2. Pericardial friction rub
3. Adenopathy
4. Edema
5. Periungual erythema
6. Splinter hemorrhages

7. Cardiac dysrhythmias
8. Arterial and/or venous thrombosis
9. A variety of neurologic findings

   a. Deficits consistent with cerebrovascular infarction
   b. Seizures
   c. Cognitive deficits
   d. Psychosis

E. Laboratory/Diagnostic findings[2–4]

1. Serum antinuclear antibody (ANA) is present in virtually all patients and is sensitive but not specific; titers $< 1:160$ are usually false-positives.
2. A variety of other laboratory tests may demonstrate abnormalities, but not with 100% frequency.

   a. Anemia (hemoglobin $< 12g/dL$)
   b. Leukopenia (white blood cell count $< 5000/mL$)
   c. Positive anticardiolipin antibody test
   d. Positive direct Coombs' test
   e. Proteinuria
   f. Hematuria
   g. Presence of antinative DNA

3. No specific test is diagnostic; a collection of subjective and objective findings and laboratory tests are the basis of diagnosis.

F. Management

1. Treatment is supportive; no curative management strategies are currently available.
2. Sunscreen for photosensitivity
3. Topical corticosteroid creams or lotions for rashes
4. Nonsteroidal anti-inflammatory drugs (NSAIDs) for minor joint symptoms.
5. Hydroxychloroquine, 400 mg/day, for joint symptoms not responsive to NSAIDs
6. Prednisone, 40–60 mg/day, for serious manifestations—taper to low doses during disease inactivity
7. Pulse therapy for life-threatening exacerbations

   a. Methylprednisolone, 500–1000 mg daily for 3–6 days, followed by 60 mg oral prednisone daily
   b. Requires consultation with a specialist

8. Calcium supplementation, 1000 mg/day, along with multivitamin containing vitamin D for patients on long-term systemic corticosteroid therapy.
9. Warfarin (Coumadin) to an INR of 3.0 for patients with anticardiolipin antibodies
10. Cytotoxic drugs for serious/life-threatening manifestations; requires specialty consultation

11. Patient education
    a. Rest/activity balance
    b. Sun avoidance or appropriate protection
    c. Smoking cessation

References

1. Calabrese, L.H., & Duna, G.F. (1998). Vasculitis syndromes. In J.H. Stein (Ed.), *Internal Medicine* (5th ed.) (pp. 1218–1226). St. Louis: Mosby.
2. Hellmann, D.B., & Stone, J.H. (2000). Arthritis and musculoskeletal disorders. In L.M. Tierney, Jr., S.J. McPhee, & M.A. Papadakis (Eds.), *Current medical diagnosis and treatment* (39th ed.) (pp. 807–859). Stamford, CT: Appleton & Lange.
3. Kahl, L.E. (1996). Systemic lupus erythematosus. In J. Noble (Ed.), *Textbook of primary care medicine* (2nd ed.) (pp. 1130–1139). St. Louis: Mosby.
4. Lefkowith, J.B., & Kahl, L.E. (1998). Arthritis and rheumatologic diseases. In C.F. Carey, H.H. Lee, & K.F. Woeltje (Eds.), *The Washington manual of medical therapeutics* (29th ed.) (pp. 456–474). Philadelphia: Lippincott-Raven.
5. Skarf, B. (1996). Neuro-ophthalmology. In J. Noble (Ed.), *Textbook of primary care medicine* (2nd ed.) (pp. 1502–1516). St. Louis: Mosby.

Management of Patients with Miscellaneous Health Problems

INTEGUMENTARY DISORDERS

68

Sylvia R. Love, MED, MSN, RN, CS, ACNP, ANP

I. GENERAL

A. History[6, 7, 9, 12]

1. Presenting complaint

   a. Presenting lesion
   b. Onset and progression

2. Past and present systemic disorders
3. Family history

   a. Blood relatives (genetic or infectious diseases)
   b. Are household contacts affected similarly—include information regarding pets in the home environment

4. Drug history (Table 68–1)

   a. Question carefully about medications that have been taken within the last month, as well as commonplace routine medications taken on a regular basis that otherwise may be forgotten.
   b. Question which treatments have already been tried, including over-the-counter remedies, and how successful they were.

5. Occupation and leisure activities, in particular any activities that have been adopted recently or near time of onset of symptoms
6. Travel—within or out of the country

B. Morphology[6, 9]

1. Skin lesions are categorized according to the configuration of the lesions or identifying characteristics (Fig. 68–1).
2. Various terms are applied to skin changes (Table 68–2).
3. Skin eruptions or exanthems are divided into three groups

   a. Macular and maculopapular lesions
   b. Vesicular or bullous lesions
   c. Pustular, petechial, or purpuric lesions
   d. Figure 68–2 describes various types and shapes of skin lesions.

C. Physical examination[6, 9]

1. It is necessary to examine *entire* skin including nails, scalp, palms, soles, and mucous membranes. The patient is examined undressed in an area with good lighting.

TABLE 68–1. ASSOCIATION BETWEEN SOME CUTANEOUS DISORDERS AND DRUGS

DISORDER	DRUGS
Urticaria	Aspirin, penicillin, serum, toxoid, vaccines, imipramine
Systemic lupus erythematosus	Hydralazine, isoniazid, penicillamine, procainamide
Purpura	Quinine, quinidine, meprobamate, cytotoxic drugs
Photosensitivity	Tetracycline, sulfonamides, nalidixic acid, amiodarone
Eczematous dermatitis	Sulfonamides, phenylbutazone, methyldopa, antibiotics
Exfoliative dermatitis	Gold, phenylbutazone, indomethacin, allopurinol
Pigmentation	Heavy metals, chloroquine, mepacrine
Acne	Corticosteroids, isoniazid
Bullous lesions	Barbiturate overdose, sulfonamides, penicillamine
Erythema multiforme	Salicylates, sulfonamides, penicillin, hydantoins, sulfonylureas, barbiturates
Lichenoid eruption	Mepacrine, chloroquine, quinine, thiazides, quinidine, chlorpropamide
Psoriasiform rash	Methyldopa, gold
Erythema nodosum	Sulfonamides, contraceptives

(From Mir, M.A. [1997]. *Atlas of clinical skills* [p. 208]. Philadelphia: W.B. Saunders, with permission.)

2. Most important part of the assessment in relation to skin cancer or moles.
3. Identify morphology, configuration, and distribution of any lesions.
4. Use a magnifying glass to view the surface of lesions.
5. Examine for secondary changes of skin lesions (Table 68–3).

II. DERMATITIS MEDICAMENTOSA (DRUG ERUPTION)

A. Definition[2, 5, 12]

1. Also referred to as adverse cutaneous drug reaction

   a. Drug eruptions are caused by immunologic or nonimmunologic mechanisms.
   b. Eruptions are provoked by systemic or topical administration of a drug.

2. True allergic drug reactions involve prior exposure to the offensive drug and require minimal doses to elicit a reaction.
3. Most allergic reactions have skin manifestations.

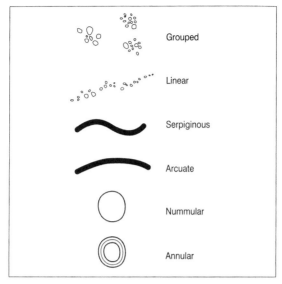

Figure 68–1. Various configuration of skin lesions. (From Mir, M.A. [1997]. *Atlas of clinical skills* [p. 214]. Philadelphia: W.B. Saunders, with permission.)

B. Incidence/Predisposing factors[2, 5, 9, 12]

1. See Table 68–1 for reactions associated with particular drug classes.
2. Classification of adverse cutaneous drug reactions

   a. Type I—Immediate-type immunologic reaction: IgE-mediated; manifested by urticaria and angioedema of skin or mucosa and edema of other organs and fall in blood pressure (anaphylactic shock).
   b. Type II—Cytotoxic reaction: Drug or causative agent causes lysis of cells such as platelets or leukocytes or may, by combination with another drug, cause antibodies (immune complexes) that cause lysis or phagocytosis.
   c. Type III—Serum sickness, drug-induced vasculitis: IgG or, less commonly, IgM antibodies are formed against a drug; manifested by vasculitis, urticaria-like lesion, arthritis, nephritis, alveolitis, hemolytic anemia, thrombocytopenia, and agranulocytosis.
   d. Type IV—Morbilliform (exanthematous) reaction: Cell-mediated immune reaction; sensitized lymphocytes react with the drug, releasing cytokines that bring on a cutaneous inflammatory response.

TABLE 68–2. USUAL TERMS APPLIED TO SKIN CHANGES

Macule	A flat, circumscribed area of skin discoloration
Patch	A large macule, more than 2 cm in diameter
Papule	A circumscribed, palpable elevation of the skin, less than 1 cm in diameter
Nodule	A circumscribed, palpable area of the skin which is more than 0.5 cm in diameter, and is either in part or wholly in the dermis
Plaque	A circumscribed, disk-shaped elevated area of the skin, more than 1 cm in diameter
Vesicle	A visible accumulation of fluid beneath the epidermis (less than 0.5 cm in diameter)
Bulla	A large vesicle, more than 0.5 cm in diameter
Pustule	A visible collection of pus
Ulcer	A loss of epidermis and part or whole of the dermis
Weal	A circumscribed, elevated area of cutaneous edema
Purpura	Extravasation of blood in the skin causing macules and papules (about 2 mm in diameter); larger spots are called ecchymoses
Stria	A streak-like, linear, atrophic, pink, purple, or white lesion caused by stretching of the skin
Telangiectasia	A visible dilatation of a small cutaneous blood vessel

(From Mir, M.A. [1997]. *Atlas of clinical skills* [p. 209]. Philadelphia: W.B. Saunders, with permission.)

3. Beta-lactams cause the most frequently encountered allergic skin reactions.
4. Cephalosporins are associated with reactions in 5–15% of penicillin-sensitive patients. Third-generation cephalosporins may be less likely to react than first-generation cephalosporins.
5. "Red man" syndrome associated with vancomycin often responds to slowing of infusion rate.
6. Angiotensin-converting enzyme (ACE) inhibitors are associated with chronic cough and angioedema.
7. Beta-blockers can precipitate asthma and should not be given to patients at risk for anaphylaxis, because beta blockers may block the action of epinephrine.
8. Anticonvulsants are a frequent cause of maculopapular rashes.
9. Radiocontrast media and opioids may simulate mast cell histamine release by a non–IgE-mediated mechanism. Only 20–30% have repeat reactions.

C. Subjective findings[2, 5, 12]

1. Abrupt onset
2. Usually with bright confluent erythema
3. May have facial edema or central facial involvement

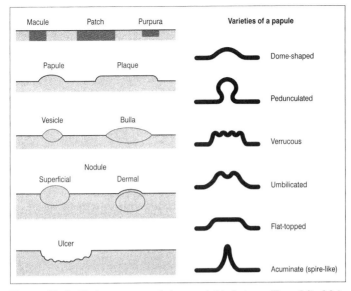

Figure 68–2. Various types and shapes of skin lesions. (From Mir, M.A. [1997]. *Atlas of clinical skills* [p. 209]. Philadelphia: W.B. Saunders, with permission.)

TABLE 68–3. SECONDARY CHANGES ASSOCIATED WITH SKIN LESIONS

Crust	Accumulated dried exudate
Excoriation	A superficial (epidermal) abrasion caused by scratching
Lichenification	An area of increased epidermal thickening with exaggerated skin markings, caused by constant rubbing (e.g., atopic eczema)
Scar	An area of fibrous tissue replacing the lost epidermis
Scales	Visible and often palpable, whitish flakes due to aggregation of dried/diseased shed epidermal cells
Comedone	A plug of keratin and sebum wedged in a dilated pilosebaceous orifice

(From Mir, M.A. [1997]. *Atlas of clinical skills* [p. 213]. Philadelphia: W.B. Saunders, with permission.)

4. May have swelling of the tongue
5. Often with itching
6. Fever may be present
7. Skin reaction usually symmetrical in distribution
8. May have arthralgias or arthritis symptoms
9. May have accompanying shortness of breath, wheezing, hypotension
10. False history of drug reaction may be due to patient misunderstanding, such as

   a. Specific drug reactions are not inherited.
   b. Undetermined reactions of childhood may not be reproducible in adult life.
   c. Common side effects such as nausea or weight gain may be mistaken for allergy.
   d. When a true allergic reaction has not actually occurred, the patient's records should be corrected.

11. A detailed, accurate account of a drug reaction should be documented.

D. Physical findings[2, 5, 12]

1. Bright confluent erythema is the common presentation.
2. Urticaria and angioedema imply mast cell degranulation. If an IgE-mediated mechanism was the cause, a repeat reaction is likely.
3. May have morbilliform (exanthematous) eruptions—the most common type of cutaneous drug reaction. May develop exfoliative dermatitis, especially if drug is not discontinued
4. May have eczematoid rash
5. May have photodermatitis
6. Reactions involving other systems that may occur include

   a. Hemolytic anemia
   b. Liver or kidney dysfunction
   c. Serum sickness (rash, fever, malaise)

E. Laboratory/Diagnostic findings[2, 5, 12]

1. Diagnosis is usually made on clinical findings alone.
2. Routinely ordered blood work is usually of no value in diagnosis.
3. Eosinophil count $>1000/\mu L$: lymphocytosis with atypical lymphocytes
4. Consider ordering:

   a. Liver function tests (not usually done)
   b. Skin biopsies (may be of value in making diagnosis)
   c. Allergy skin testing (should not be done while skin is flared—may give false positive results)

   d. Patch and photo testing (may reveal contact or photodermatitis—not commonly done)

   e. Challenge dosing, preferable orally, of the drug, if an anaphylactic reaction seems unlikely

   f. Serum level and hepatic/renal monitoring when indicated

F. Management[2, 5, 12]

1. Withdrawal of the drug may be the only treatment necessary.
2. Treatment is aimed at symptoms.
3. Epinephrine 1:1000, 0.3 to 0.5 mL subcutaneously, may give
rapid temporary relief from urticaria and angioedema. Dosage may be repeated in 20 minutes.
4. Give oral or intravenous (IV) antihistamine. Diphenhydramine (Benadryl), 25–50 mg, may follow epinephrine.
5. Corticosteroids are generally not indicated if the offending
agent is discontinued. When indicated, prednisone, 70 mg,
tapering by 10 mg or 5 mg daily over 1–2 weeks.
6. Wheezing may be treated by use of inhaled bronchodilators.
7. Treatment of the dermatitis present varies according to stage
of presentation, ranging from topical application comfort
measures to hospitalization for extensive blistering eruptions, such as toxic epidermal necrolysis resulting in erosions and superficial ulcerations requiring hospitalization
care as for burns.
8. For more serious anaphylactoid reactions, see Chapter 75,
Management of the Patient in Shock.
9. Morbilliform rashes and serum sickness may require 1–2
weeks of treatment with antihistamines and/or systemic corticosteroids.
10. Corticosteroid use in Stevens-Johnson syndrome is controversial.
11. Prevention of drug reactions

   a. Use alternative drug in a different class.

   b. Premedication does not prevent true IgE-mediated reactions but may be successful for non–IgE-mediated reactions, for example:

     i. Prednisone, 50 mg at 13 h, 7 h, and 1 h prior to radio-
contrast media

     ii. Diphenhydramine, 1 mg/kg 1 h prior to drug

     iii. Some sources indicate cimetidine, 4 mg/kg and/or
ephedrine, 25 mg 1 h prior

   c. Desensitization may be successful but may be temporary.

12. Follow-up

   a. Patient education: A written list of drugs most likely to
cause problems should be given to the patient.

b. Avoid unnecessary medications.
c. Medical warning bracelet should be worn by the patient who has a history of life-threatening reactions, and he or she should have an epinephrine injection kit.

III. CELLULITIS

A. Definition[1, 4]

1. An acute infection of the skin and subcutaneous tissues
2. An infection of the deeper layers of the skin

B. General comments/Incidence/Predisposing factors[1, 4]

1. A break in the integrity of the skin almost always precedes this infection.
2. The cellulitis may be in proximal tissue adjacent to a necrotic area such as an abscess.
3. The following predispose to cellulitis:

    a. Prior trauma
    b. An underlying skin lesion
    c. Diabetes
    d. Pedal edema
    e. Venous and lymphatic compromise

4. Cellulitis has a predilection for the lower extremities.
5. Cellulitis predisposes to recurrent infection.
6. Cellulitis of the lower extremities of the elderly is often complicated by deep vein thrombosis.
7. Group A beta-hemolytic streptococci are responsible for most lower extremity cellulitis; occasionally *Staphylococcus aureus* is responsible, though gram-negative rods such as *Escherichia coli* may also be responsible.
8. Gram-negative bacilli, such as *Serratia, Proteus, Enterobacter*, and fungi (*Cryptococcus neoformans*), often cause cellulitis in neutropenic and immunosuppressed patients.
9. *Haemophilus influenzae* is usually responsible for facial or upper extremity cellulitis, especially in children.
10. Streptococci and staphylococci are predominant agents in patients with diabetes mellitus, but if associated with an infected ulceration of the skin, probably will also have anaerobic bacteria and gram-negative rods.
11. Occupational exposure to cellulitis of the hands occurs in fish and meat handlers.

    a. *Erysipelothrix rhusiopathiae* for fish, meat, or poultry handlers
    b. *Aeromonas*—A gram-negative bacillus; freshwater exposure
    c. *Vibrio*—saltwater exposure

C. Subjective findings[1, 4]

1. The trauma site within several days exhibits

    a. Tenderness
    b. Pain
    c. Swelling
    d. Erythema
    e. Warmth

2. Symptoms intensify rapidly and spread.
3. Fever, chills, and malaise may be present.

D. Physical findings[1, 4]

1. Erythema with indistinct margins; warmth and tenderness of the skin
2. Enlargement and tenderness of regional lymph nodes are common.
3. Linear streaks of erythema and tenderness indicate lymphatic spread.
4. Patches of erythema and tenderness may occur a few centimeters proximal to the edge of infection.
5. Lymph node enlargement and lymphatic streaking confirm the diagnosis of cellulitis.

E. Laboratory/Diagnostic findings[1, 4, 5]

1. Identification of the infecting organisim is usually not obtained and may not be necessary.
2. Blood and clysis culture of the leading edge of infection rarely yield the pathogen.
3. Blood cultures and skin site cultures may be taken when patients

    a. Fail to respond to standard therapy
    b. Have serious other medical problems
    c. Have ulcers or abscesses

F. Management[1, 4, 5]

1. Antibiotic coverages of both streptococci and staphylococci are generally appropriate choices. For the outpatient without concomitant serious illness or comorbid conditions, the following may be given:

    a. A penicillinase-resistant oral penicillin, such as dicloxacillin (Dynapen), 500 mg to 1 g q.i.d., *or*
    b. A first-generation cephalosporin, such as cephalexin (Keflex), 500 mg q.i.d.
    c. An alternative antibiotic for penicillin-allergic patients is erythromycin, 500 mg q.i.d.
    d. Ceftriaxone (Rocephin), 1g IM daily for the first few days may be given for sicker patients.
    e. Therapy should be given for 10–14 days.

2. Patients who appear toxic or who have underlying diseases causing impaired immune response should be hospitalized. Inpatient therapy, when intravenous (IV) antibiotics are used, may include such antibiotic choices as:

    a. Nafcillin (Nafcil, Unipen), 1 to 2 g IV q4h

    b. Cefazolin (Ancef), 2 g IV q6h

    c. For immunocompromised patients

       i. Ticarcillin/clavulante (Timentin), 3.1 g q6h

      ii. Cefoxitin (Mefoxin), 1 g q6h

3. When specific causative agents are suspected, therapy may include

    a. *Erysipelothrix:* Penicillin

    b. *Vibrio* species: Aminoglycosides and tetracyclines

    c. *Aeromonas hydrophila:* Aminoglycosides and chloramphenicol

4. Immobilization and elevation of the affected limb may be helpful initially.

5. Moist heat may help localize the infection.

6. Follow-up is necessary to ensure eradication of infection.

7. When an accompanying tinea skin infection is present, topical antifungal creams such as miconazole, terbinafine hydrochloride, and ketoconazole should be used.

8. Long-term, low-dose antibiotic therapy may be indicated in select patients who have recurrences of cellulitis: for example, penicillin G, 250–500 mg orally b.i.d.

IV. HERPES ZOSTER (SHINGLES)

A. Definition[5, 7, 10, 11]

1. The reactivation of latent varicella-zoster virus (VZV), usually of the sensory neurons

2. Characterized by unilateral pain and a vesicular or bullous eruption limited to a single dermatome or may involve two or three dermatomes

B. Incidence/Predisposing factors[5, 7, 10, 11]

1. Patient is usually >50 years of age.

2. Impaired immune system, therapeutic radiation, local trauma, surgery stress, spinal cord tumors, lymphoma, fatigue, and age are predisposing factors.

3. Postherpetic neuralgia (PHN) increases with age; severe prodromal pain or severe pain on the first day of rash is predictive of severe PHN.

C. Subjective findings[5, 7, 10, 11]

1. Prodromal symptoms of pain ("stabbing," pricking, sharp, boring, penetrating, lancinating, shooting), burning, itching,

or a dull ache in the affected dermatome precede eruptions by 3–5 days (range 1–14 days).
2. Malaise, fever, and headache are present in about 5% of patients.
3. The patient may experience allodynia, a heightened sensitivity to mild stimuli.
4. The patient may be afebrile or have low-grade fever.

D. Physical examination findings[5, 7, 10, 11]

1. Lymphadenopathy may occur 1–2 days before development of vesicles.
2. Grouped vesicles appear on an erythematous, tender base usually along a sensory nerve group unilaterally. Two or more contiguous dermatomes may be involved. Noncontiguous dermatomal zoster is rare.
3. Occasionally, one to three vesicles may cross the midline or appear in other areas.
4. Papules appear in 24 h and progress to vesicles and bullae by 48 h, then to pustules in 96 h. Crusts form in 7–10 days.
5. New lesions continue to appear for up to 1 week.

E. Laboratory/Diagnostic findings[5, 7, 10, 11]

1. ECG is ordered during prodromal phase to rule out ischemic heart disease.
2. Additionally, imaging studies are ordered in prodromal phase to rule out organic, pleural, pulmonary, or abdominal disease.
3. VZV antigen detection: Clinical findings are confirmed by direct fluorescent antibody obtained from vesicle base or fluid.
4. Tzanck's test is positive in 75% of cases.
5. Viral culture may require up to 2 weeks and is positive in 44% of cases.
6. Polymerase chain reaction technique, when clinically available, can be final in 24h; collected on unstained slide made for Tzanck's smear.
7. Antibody testing takes too long for clinical usefulness; does establish cause.

F. Management[5, 7, 10, 11]

1. Ophthalmic zoster is heralded by vesicles on the side and tip of the nose.

   • When ophthalmic zoster is encountered, an *ophthalmologist should always be consulted* owing to potential complications.

2. High-risk groups with need for physician referral include patients with Hodgkin's disease or AIDS.

3. Acyclovir (Zovirax) 800 mg p.o. q.i.d. for 7–10 days, can accelerate healing of skin lesions and decrease the duration of acute pain, particularly if given within 48 h of the onset of the rash.

4. Severely immunocompromised patients should receive IV acyclovir, 10 mg/kg q8h for 7–10 days, ideally started within 48 h of onset.

5. Alternative drugs include

   a. Famciclovir (Famvir), 500 mg p.o. three times a day for 7 days

   b. Foscarnet (Foscavir) for immunocompromised patients who do not respond to acyclovir

   c. Vidarabine (Vira-A) is occasionally used at 15 mg/kg/day over 12 h IV for 7 days.

   d. Leukocyte interferon used to reduce severity and duration of new lesions; can cause reduced granulocyte counts, fever, and neurasthenia

   e. Varicella vaccine recommendations are pending.

6. Minimizing pain with narcotic analgesics is indicated.

   a. Intractable pain may warrant suicidal precautions.

   b. Non-narcotic analgesics such as acetaminophen may reduce the pain of zoster.

7. Application of moist dressing (water, saline, Burow's solution) 15 min q.i.d. or soothing baths with baking soda added to the water aids in alleviating pain.

8. Oral corticosteroids, such as prednisone, early in the course may elicit benefits.

9. Hydroxyzine (Atarax), 25–50 mg p.o. t.i.d. may be used for relief of pruritus.

10. Postherpetic neuralgia pain management includes

    a. Tricyclic antidepressants such as doxepin, 10–100 mg p.o. at bedtime or amitriptyline, 10–25 mg daily, may reduce postzoster discomfort

    b. Capsaicin cream q4h

    c. Topical anesthetic such as EMLA cream or lidocaine gel

    d. Patch or nerve block for allodynia

    e. Analgesics

11. Health care workers with no immunity or pregnant women should avoid exposure to active cases. Contagion rate is low, but can elicit chicken pox in contacts who have never been exposed.

12. Follow patients until pain is resolved—usually by 1 year.

V. SKIN CANCER

A. Definition[2, 3, 5, 6, 13]

1. Basal cell carcinoma (BCC) is locally invasive, slowly evolving, and destructive, but has a limited capacity to metastasize.
2. Squamous cell carcinoma (SCC) is a malignant tumor of epithelial keratinocytes (skin and mucous membrane) with the capacity to metastasize. SCC is usually the result of exogenous carcinogens.

B. Etiology/Incidence/Predisposing factors[2, 3, 5, 6, 13]

1. BCC is the most common form of cancer.

    a. Sun exposure before age 14 predisposes to development of BCC.
    b. Arsenic exposure increases risk for superficial multicentric BCC 30–40 years later.
    c. BCC is rare in brown- and black-skinned persons.
    d. Usually develops in sun-exposed areas, especially face and neck.

2. Squamous cell carcinoma (SCC) is the second most common skin cancer in whites and the most common skin cancer in African Americans.

    a. Male to female ratio 2 : 1
    b. Smokers have an increased risk for lip involvement
    c. Occurs more frequently on the legs of females
    d. Slow-evolving cancer
    e. Penile SCC is more common (20%) in developing countries, with only 1% in the United States
    f. Human papillomavirus is associated with increased incidence of SCC.

3. Commonalities of BCC and SCC include

    a. Occur most frequently on skin with highest degree of sun exposure
    b. White-skinned persons with poor tanning capacity are at highest risk for development of these cancers, but BCC and SCC can appear in other skin types.

C. Subjective findings[2, 3, 5, 6, 13]

1. BCC may manifest as bumps, patches, or scabbed lesions.
2. BCC when on the back, frequently appears as erythematous, somewhat shiny, scaly plaques.
3. SCC should be suspected in any lesion that is scaly, red, or crusty, or does not heal.
4. SCC is usually asymptomatic.

D. Physical examination findings[2, 3, 5, 6, 13]

1. BCC can present in several forms.

   a. Nodule-ulcerative tumor
      i. Small, pearly or translucent, waxy papule that enlarges peripherally and develops a central depression that may be ulcerated or scaly.
      ii. Borders are translucent, elevated, and shiny with fine telangiectasias.
   b. Superficial BCC: Erythematous scaly macule or patch with an elevated thread-like border

2. SCC tumors

   a. Appear as firm, skin-colored to reddish-brown nodules on damaged skin
   b. May arise out of actinic keratoses
   c. Central ulceration may be present.
   d. Scaling and crusting may be present.
   e. Seventy percent are on the head and neck.
   f. Lesions on the lower lip appear as firm, whitish macules (leukoplakia) with possible central ulceration.
   g. Lip, oral cavity, tongue, and genital SCC have greater rates of metastasis, and require special management.

E. Laboratory/Diagnostic findings[2, 3, 5, 6, 13]

1. Suspected BCC or SCC lesions should be biopsied, shaved, or punch biopsied.
2. Confirmation of the diagnosis is made histologically.

F. Management[2, 3, 5, 6, 13]

1. Curettage and electrodesiccation for BCC lesions <1 cm in diameter and in nonfacial area

   a. The technique of three cycles of curettage and electrodesiccation is the gold standard.
   b. This is not indicated for head and neck lesions.
   c. Appropriateness for use with SCC varies in the literature.

2. Cryosurgery: For superficial BCC lesions except around nose, ears, eyelids, forehead, and temples. It is not appropriate for SCC.
3. Tissue must be microscopically evaluated to ensure clear borders and is appropriate for both BCC and SCC when removed by excision.
4. Radiotherapy infrequently used in BCC. Usually reserved for very large lesions. Recurrent lesions after radiation are generally more aggressive and difficult to treat.
5. *Referral for fresh tissue microscopically controlled excision (Mohs') surgery is indicated* for head/neck or cosmetically prominent

location or area difficult to treat such as eyelids, inner canthus, nose, or ears. Indicated for both SCC and BCC.

6. Systemic agents are not indicated for treatment of uncomplicated BCC or SCC.

7. Prophylaxis therapy for BCC includes

   a. 5-Fluorouracil, topically to affected area b.i.d. daily for 2–4 weeks; may be repeated twice yearly. Avoid sun exposure; or,
   b. Low-dose isotretinoin, 10 mg/day.
      i. Caution with pre-existing renal or hepatic disease.
      ii. Contraindicated in pregnancy

8. Follow up BCC patients to detect new or recurrent lesions for 5 years.

9. Topical application of sunscreen is recommended for prevention.

VI. MELANOMA

A. Definition[2, 5, 8]

1. A tumor characterized by dark pigmentation
2. Malignant melanomas develop from benign melanocytic cells.

B. Etiology/Incidence/Predisposing factors[2, 5, 8]

1. Malignant melanoma is the leading cause of death from skin disease.
2. Prevention is the key to cure—avoidance of blistering solar radiation and the use of sunscreen especially during adolescent years.
3. The worldwide incidence of melanoma increases with proximity to the equator.
4. Highest incidence is between ages 30 and 50. Median age at diagnosis is 45.
5. Family history of melanoma in parents, children, or siblings increases risk.
6. Increased risk if a person has fair skin, freckling, blue eyes and blond hair.
7. Twice the risk if sunburned at young age.
8. Those with increased number of nevi are at greatest risk.
9. The most common sites in males are head, neck, and trunk; lower extremities the most common site in females.

C. Subjective findings[2, 5, 8]

1. May manifest with any change in pigmented lesion including

   a. Bleeding
   b. Scaling

    c. Texture change
    d. Size change
    e. Development of inflammation
    f. Ulceration
    g. Color change
    h. Itching

D. Physical examination findings[2, 5, 8]

1. Six signs of malignant melanoma (ABCDE changes):

    a. *A*symmetrical shape
    b. *B*order irregularity
    c. *C*olor variegation
    d. *D*iameter is usually large (>6 mm)
    e. *E*levation is almost always present
    f. *E*nlargement or increase in the size of the lesion is probably the most important sign.

2. Primary malignant melanomas may be classified into the following types:

    a. Superficial spreading malignant melanoma
        i. The most common type
        ii. Primarily a disease of whites
    b. Lentigo maligna melanoma (on sun-exposed skin, older individuals)
    c. Nodular malignant melanoma
    d. Acral-lentiginous melanoma
        i. On the palms, soles, and nail beds
        ii. More common on darkly pigmented people
    e. Malignant melanoma on mucous membranes
    f. Miscellaneous forms
        i. Amelanotic (nonpigmented) melanoma
        ii. Melanomas arising from blue nevi (rare)
        iii. Congenital and giant nevocytic nevi

E. Laboratory/Diagnostic findings[2, 5, 8]

1. Surgical biopsy is the only form of appropriate diagnostic procedure.

    a. A full-thickness total excisional biopsy must be sent for pathologic specimen.
    b. The melanoma should never be curetted, electrodesiccated, or shaved.

2. Lesions are staged by the pathologist (Clark's staging):

    a. Level 1—confined to epidermis (in situ)
    b. Level 2—invasion of papillary dermis
    c. Level 3—invasion of interface of papillary and reticular dermis

d. Level 4—invasion of reticular dermis
e. Level 5—invasion of subcutaneous fat

3. Lesion may also be staged by the pathologist using Breslow staging;

   a. Thin: <0.75 mm depth of invasion
   b. Intermediate: 0.76–3.99 mm depth of invasion
   c. Thick: >4 mm depth of invasion

4. Elective lymph node dissection in the absence of clinical involvement is controversial.
5. Sentinel node biopsy is used for staging melanoma patients.

E. Management[2, 5, 8]

1. Suspicion of malignant melanoma should *always be referred to a dermatologist* owing to the potential for metastasis and resultant death.
2. Follow up every 3–6 months with skin examinations.
3. Patient should be instructed to self-examine skin weekly.
4. Treatment of melanoma is based on stage.

   a. Melanoma <1.0 mm thick: Wide excision with a 1.0-cm margin. Routine elective lymph node dissection is not usually recommended for this group.
   b. Melanoma measuring 1.0–4.0 mm in thickness and/or Clark's Level IV lesions of thickness: Recommended to have wide excision with 2.0 cm margins. Nodal biopsy is usually recommended.
   c. Melanoma measuring >4.0 mm in thickness: Recommended to have at least 2.0 cm margins.

5. Adjuvant therapy (chemotherapy, radiotherapy, immunotherapy, and isolated limb perfusion)
6. Alpha-interferon and vaccine therapy may be indicated for high-risk melanomas.
7. Strong recommendation for referral of intermediate-risk and high-risk patients to centers with expertise.

References

1. Andreoli, T.E., Bennett, J.C., Carpenter, C.C.J., & Plum, F. (1997). *Cecil essentials of medicine* (4th ed.) (pp. 663–676, 715–719). Philadelphia: W.B. Saunders.
2. Berger, T.G. (1999). Skin and appendages. In L.M. Tierney, Jr., S.J. McPhee, & M.A. Papadakis (Eds.), *Current medical diagnosis and treatment* (38th ed.) (pp. 116–180). Stamford, CT: Appleton & Lange.
3. DuPree, M. (1996). Basal and squamous cell carcinoma. In R.E. Rakel (Ed.), *Saunders manual of medical practice* (pp. 936–938). Philadelphia: W.B. Saunders.
4. Ellis, C.L. (1996). Cellulitis. In R.E. Rakel (Ed.), *Saunders manual of medical practice* (pp. 862–863). Philadelphia: W.B. Saunders.

5. Fitzpatrick, T.B., Johnson, R.A., Wolff, K., Polano, M.K., & Suurmond, D. (1997). *Color atlas and synopsis of clinical dermatology* (3rd ed) (pp 208–214). New York: McGraw-Hill.

6. Goldsmith, L.A., Lazarus, G.S., & Tharp, M.D. (1997). *Adult and pediatric dermatology: A color guide to diagnosis and treatment.* Philadelphia: F.A. Davis.

7. Hooper, B.J., & Goldman, M.P. (1999). *Primary dermatologic care.* St. Louis: Mosby.

8. Jakob, H.A. (1996). Melanoma. In R.E. Rakel (Ed.), *Saunders manual of medical practice* (pp. 942–943). Philadelphia: W.B. Saunders.

9. Mir, M.A. (1997). *The skin: Atlas of clinical skills* (pp. 203–217). Philadelphia: W.B. Saunders.

10. Robertson, V.E. (1996). Varicella infections. In R.E. Rakel (Ed.), *Saunders manual of medical practice* (pp. 864–867). Philadelphia: W.B. Saunders.

11. Slaughter, A.R. (1996). Herpes zoster infection. In R.E. Rakel (Ed.), *Saunders manual of medical practice* (pp. 956–957). Philadelphia: W.B. Saunders.

12. Smith, D.L. (1996). Drug allergy. In R.E. Rakel (Ed.), *Saunders manual of medical practice* (pp. 727–728). Philadelphia: W.B. Saunders.

13. Woolliscroft, J.O. (1998). *Handbook of current diagnosis and treatment: A quick reference for the general practitioner* (2nd ed.). Philadelphia: C.V. Mosby.

ECTOPIC PREGNANCY AND SEXUALLY TRANSMITTED DISEASES

JoAnn Broadus, MSN, RN, CS, FNP

I. ECTOPIC PREGNANCY

A. Definition

1. Implantation of the fertilized ovum in tissue other than the endometrium.
2. The most common implantation site is the fallopian tube.[1, 10]

B. Etiology/Incidence/Predisposing factors[1, 2, 17, 18]

1. Any condition that prevents or retards the passage of the fertilized ovum into the uterus, such as

   a. Pelvic inflammatory disease, sexually transmitted diseases (STDs), especially *Neisseria gonorrhoeae* and *Chlamydia trachomatis* salpingitis
   b. History of endometriosis
   c. Prior tubal or uterine surgery related to adhesions
   d. Use of a contraceptive intrauterine device (IUD)
   e. Congenital anomalies associated with diethylstibestrol (DES)
   f. Tubal tumors
   g. Infertile women treated with ovulation-inducing drugs, such as clomiphene citrate (Clomid)
   h. Postabortal and puerperal infections
   i. Prior tubal pregnancy
   j. Previous tubal sterilization
   k. Cigarette smoking

2. Most common cause of maternal mortality in the first trimester
3. Second leading cause of maternal mortality in the United States. Two of every 100 women who were known to conceive had an ectopic pregnancy.

C. Subjective findings[1]

1. Early

   a. Missed or delayed menses, followed by continuous intermittent vaginal spotting, generally dark in color
   b. The nature, duration, and intensity of pain vary considerably
   c. Sudden, sharp, and stabbing abdominal pain, diffuse pelvic pain, referred neck and/or shoulder pain

651

2. Late
    a. Fainting, vertigo, dizziness
    b. Nausea, vomiting, diarrhea

D. Physical examination findings with rupture and intra-abdominal hemorrhage[1]

1. Palpation of adnexal mass
2. Uterine size is generally normal; uterus is sometimes displaced to the side.
3. Signs of hypovolemic shock, that is, hypotension, skin pallor, tachycardia
4. Pelvic examination is very painful with movement of uterus and cervix
5. Temperature may or may not be changed.
6. Ecchymotic blueness around umbilicus (Cullen's sign)
7. Marked abdominal tenderness with rebound

E. Laboratory findings/Diagnostic findings[1]

1. Decreased hemoglobin and hematocrit with mild leukocytosis
2. Transvaginal ultrasound: The absence of an intrauterine gestational sac is suggestive of ectopic pregnancy.
3. Positive human chorionic gonadotropin (beta-hCG) test
4. Culdocentesis (aspiration of the cul-de-sac) when ultrasound is not available. Aspiration of nonclotting blood is considered positive.
5. Pregnancy test: Beta-hCG radioimmunoassay is usually decreased in ectopic pregnancies.

F. Management[7, 10]

1. Thinking "ectopic" in any woman of childbearing age with an acute abdomen should be a major priority concern for the acute care nurse practitioner.
2. Salpingectomy: Per outpatient laparoscopy
3. Linear salpingostomy: Unruptured tube >2.0 cm
4. Outpatient nonsurgical treatment using methotrexate (amethopterin) therapy. Methotrexate is a folic acid antagonist.
    a. Criteria
        i. <6 weeks pregnant
        ii. Unruptured tubal mass <3.5 cm
        iii. No embryonic cardiac motion
        iv. No active renal or hepatic disease
        v. No evidence of thrombocytopenia or leukopenia
        vi. Hemodynamic stability
    b. Pretreatment medical workup should consist of baseline laboratory values for
        i. Transvaginal ultrasound to determine the presence or absence of extrauterine gestational sac

      ii. Quantitative: Beta-hCG level

      iii. Liver function (SGOT)

      iv. Renal function (BUN) creatinine

      v. Blood type Rh factor and presence of antibodies

      vi. Complete blood count (CBC)

      vii. Bone marrow function tests

  c. Contraindications

      i. Unstable or noncompliant patient

      ii. History of renal disease

      iii. History of hepatic disease

      iv. Current thrombocytopenia

      v. Hemodynamically unstable

  d. Dosage of methotrexate: 50 mg/m^2 IM single dose, follow up on day 4 and 7, then weekly

  e. Additional management

      i. Central venous line if unstable hemodynamically for Ringer's lactate or normal saline and run at rate appropriate for patient's hemodynamic condition

      ii. Blood transfusions, packed red blood cells (RBCs) as indicated for low hemoglobin/hematocrit

      iii. Maintain urinary output at 30 mL/h.

      iv. Iron dextran (InFeD) IV 2mL (100 mg) test dose. Use cautiously in patients with a history of allergies or asthma. Give 0.5 ml (25 mg) epinephrine at bedside for anaphylaxis.

      v. Cefoxitin (Mefoxin) 2 g IV single dose

      vi. Oxycodone/acetaminophen (Percocet) q4–6h p.r.n. for pain. Give morphine, 15 mg, with a hospitalized patient high-dose patient-controlled analgesia (PCA) pump

      vii. NPO

      viii. Rh$_0$(D)-negative unsensitized patient to receive IM injection of Rh$_0$(D) immune globulin (RhIG), 300 μg

      ix. Biweekly hCG is required (with a drop in hCG after 7 days); a 1500 mIU/mL beta-hCG is considered normal.

      x. Stop ingestion of vitamins with folic acid with methotrexate therapy.

II. PELVIC INFLAMMATORY DISEASE (PID SALPINGITIS)

A. Definition

Acute or chronic bacterial inflammation of the upper female genital tract[2–6, 11, 16, 18]

B. Etiology/Incidence/Predisposing factors

1. 2.5 million cases of PID reported in United States annually
2. Polymicrobial causation

3. Most common causative organisms are *N. gonorrhoeae* and *C. trachomatis* (exogenous)
4. Other etiologic agents[4]

   a. Normal vaginal flora
      i. Anaerobes
      ii. *Gardnerella vaginalis*
      iii. Streptococci
      iv. Enteric gram-negative rods
      v. *Mycoplasma hominis*
   b. Trauma
   c. Surgery

5. Predisposing risk/factors

   a. Sexually active women with multiple partners
   b. Age <25 years
   c. Sexual exposure to a partner with urethritis
   d. Use of contraceptive intrauterine device (e.g., IUD)
   e. Douching
   f. Menses: Incidence increases with onset or cessation of menses
   g. Smoking: Alters the protective nature of cervical mucus
   h. Substance abuse
   i. Pelvic surgery
   j. Prior history of PID or cervicitis

6. Complications: Infertility, tubal pregnancy, chronic pelvic pain due to adhesions, recurrent PID, tubo-ovarian abscess, and pelvic abscess and rupture
7. Infectious perihepatitis (Fitz-Hugh–Curtis syndrome)

C. Subjective findings[4, 10–13]

1. Early (up to 1 week)

   a. Clinical presentation varies widely; many women have atypical or no symptoms.
   b. Lower abdominal pain
   c. Menstrual cramping
   d. Low-grade fever
   e. Malaise

2. Late symptoms

   a. Sever lower abdominal pain
   b. Temperature greater than 101.4°F (38.6°C)
   c. Increased foul, purulent vaginal discharge
   d. Dyspareunia and painful defecation

D. Physical examination findings[3, 4, 6, 12]

1. Mucopurulent cervical or vaginal discharge

2. Friable cervix (bleeding)
3. Uterine and cervical motion tenderness (Chandelier's sign: Marked tenderness of the cervix, uterus, and adnexa)
4. Abdominal rebound tenderness and/or guarding
5. Infectious perihepatitis, Fitz-Hugh–Curtis syndrome (i.e., right upper quadrant abdominal pain)

E. Laboratory findings/Diagnostic findings

1. Assessment of last normal menstrual period (LNMP), STD history, contraceptive use, sexual history
2. Centers for Disease Control (CDC) Diagnostic Criteria for PID (1998)[4]

   a. Minimum criteria for diagnosing PID (CDC 1998)
      i. Direct (abdominal) tenderness
      ii. Adnexal tenderness
      iii. Cervical motion tenderness
   b. Additional criteria
      i. Oral temperature >101°F (>38.3°C)
      ii. Elevated erythrocyte sedimentation rate (ESR)
      iii. Elevated C-reactive protein
      iv. Laboratory evidence of gonococcal or chlamydial infection
      v. Leukocytosis (white blood cell count [WBC] >10,000/mm^3)
   c. Definitive criteria for diagnosing PID (CDC 1998)
      i. Histopathologic evidence on endometrial biopsy
      ii. Tubo-ovarian abscess on transvaginal sonography
      iii. Laparoscopic abnormalities consistent with PID (diagnosis confirmed in 60% of cases)

F. Management[4, 6, 11, 14]

1. Early detection and aggressive treatment of STDs and lower genital tract infections essential in prevention of PID
2. CDC Treatment Guidelines for treatment of acute PID

   a. Parenteral inpatient treatment
      i. Regimen A
         (1) Cefoxitin sodium (Mefoxin), 2 g IV q6h or cefotetan disodium (Cefotan), 2 g IV q12h *plus*
         (2) Doxycycline (tetracycline), 100 mg IV or orally q12h for 10–14 days
      ii. Regimen B
         (1) Clindamycin hydrochloride (Cleocin), 900 mg IV q8h *plus*
         (2) Gentamicin sulfate (Garamycin) loading dose IV or IM (2 mg/kg body weight) followed by a maintenance dose (1.5 mg/kg q8h until discharge)

iii. The regimens are continued until at least 48 hours after significant clinical improvement. Then follow-up with doxycycline (tetracycline), 100 mg p.o. q12h for 10–14 days or clindamycin, 450 mg p.o. q.i.d. for 10–14 days

b. 1998 CDC recommended regimens for outpatient treatment of PID

i. Regimen A

(1) Ofloxacin (Floxin), 400 mg p.o. b.i.d. for 14 days *plus*

(2) Metronidazole (Flagyl), 500 mg p.o. b.i.d. for 14 days

ii. Regimen B

(1) Cefoxitin sodium (Mefoxin), 2 g IM plus probenecid (Benemid), 1 g p.o. in a single dose concurrently; or ceftriaxone sodium (Rocephin), 250 mg IM or other parenteral third-generation cephalosporin (e.g., ceftizoxime sodium [Cefizox] or cefotaxime sodium [Claforan]) *plus*

(2) Doxycycline (tetracycline), 100 mg p.o. b.i.d. for 14 days (include this regimen with one of the above regimens)

3. CDC 1998 recommendations for hospitalization[4]

a. Surgical emergencies; rule out ectopic pregnancy or appendicitis

b. Coexisting pregnancy; HIV infected with low CD4 counts; adolescent; immunosuppressed; nausea, vomiting, fever; dehydration; pelvic and tubo-ovarian abscess suspected

c. Unable to tolerate or follow an outpatient regimen

d. Failed to respond clinically to oral antimicrobial therapy within 72 h

4. Additional considerations

a. Notification and prompt treatment of sexual partners

b. Counseling on safer sex practices and high-risk behaviors

c. Screen for other STDs

d. Testing for cure within 7 days of completing therapy

e. Rescreening in 4–6 weeks for *C. Trachomatis* and *N. gonorrhoeae*

f. Removal of IUD

g. Testing for HIV

5. Other treatments

a. Warm sitz baths 10–15 min as needed for pain

b. Use sanitary napkins

c. Avoid sexual intercourse

d. Promote bed rest in a semi-Fowler's position

e. Over-the-counter pain medications, such as acetaminophen (Tylenol)
f. Adequate hydration (6–8 glasses of water per day)

III. *CHLAMYDIA TRACHOMATIS* INFECTION

A. Definition

Chlamydia is a parasitic sexually transmitted infection that
produces serious reproductive tract complications in either
sex.[3, 8, 11, 14, 16]

B. Etiology/Incidence/Complications[8–10, 13, 14]

1. Etiology

   a. Causative organism, *Chlamydia trachomatis*, is an obligate,
   intracellular parasite. This bacteria can only live inside of
   cells; therefore, a transfer of body fluids is necessary for
   transmission.
   b. Poorly defined incubation period

2. Incidence

   a. Over three million new cases occur annually
   b. Age: Commonly <25 among either sex in the general population
   c. Age: Commonly 15–19 among women
   d. Annual screening recommended for the following women:
       i. Sexually active adolescents
       ii. Nonusers of contraceptive devices
       iii. Those who have had one or more sexual partners
       within the last 3 months
       iv. Pregnant
       v. Those who are undergoing abortion

3. Complications

   a. Women
       i. Pelvic inflammatory disease (PID)
           (1) Pelvic abscess (ovarian)
           (2) Involuntary infertility
           (3) Ectopic pregnancy
       ii. Abnormal Pap smear with mucopurulent cervicitis
       iii. Late-onset postpartum endometritis
   b. Men
       i. Epididymitis
       ii. Reiter's syndrome (primarily young men). Includes ure-
       thritis, conjunctivitis, arthritis, and skin lesions
   c. Newborn
       i. Conjunctivitis
       ii. Pneumonia

C. Subjective findings[3, 8, 10, 13, 14]

1. Female

   a. Often asymptomatic (70–80%)
   b. Intramenstrual spotting
   c. Postcoital bleeding
   d. Lower abdominal pain
   e. Painful urination (dysuria)
   f. Painful intercourse (dyspareunia)
   g. Mucopurulent endocervical discharge

2. Male

   a. Often asymptomatic (25–50%)
   b. Painful urination (dysuria)
   c. Thick, cloudy penile discharge
   d. Unilateral testicular pain and swelling

D. Physical examination findings[14, 15]

1. Vital signs: Temperature >100°F (37.7°C) when infection has progressed to PID

   a. Abdominal assessment
      i. Guarded referred pain
      ii. Rebound tenderness
   b. External genitalia inspection
      i. Edema
      ii. Ulcerations
      iii. Lesions
      iv. Excoriations
      v. Erythema
   c. Speculum examination
      i. Vaginal walls reddened
      ii. Cervical erythema and friability
      iii. Mucopurulent cervical discharge may or may not be present.
      iv. Cervical erosion (cervical lips inflamed and eroded)
   d. Bimanual examination
      i. Cervical motion, tenderness (i.e., Chandelier's sign)
      ii. Adnexal tenderness and fullness
      iii. Uterine tenderness
   e. Male inspection
      i. Scanty mucoid discharge
      ii. Meatus edge red, everted, and edematous
      iii. Unilateral testicular pain

E. Laboratory/Diagnostic findings[3, 8, 10, 14]

1. McCoy cell culture gold standard for diagnosis

   a. Advantages

      i. Most specific (100%) with acceptable sensitivity (70–80%)
     ii. Detects infection with small numbers of organisms present
    iii. Findings positive if mature inclusion bodies found in cells on microscopic examination

  b. Disadvantages
      i. Method technically difficult
     ii. Specific transport and storage requirements for test
    iii. Takes 2–6 days to obtain results

2. Nonculture tests

  a. Advantages
      i. Sensitivity of test is 70–90%.
     ii. Results available sooner than culture test
    iii. Less influenced by storage and transport

  b. Disadvantages
      i. Most are <99% specific
     ii. False positives in low-risk populations

  c. Types available
      i. Direct immunofluorescent monoclonal antibody stain
     ii. Enzyme-linked immunosorbent assay (ELISA)
    iii. Nucleic acid hybridization test (DNA probe). Sensitivities and specificities vary.
    iv. Rapid enzyme immunoassay (EIA) (e.g., Chlamydiazyme).

  d. Other relevant laboratory tests
      i. Wet mount: Polymorphonuclear (PMN) cells present
     ii. If history indicates, testing for syphilis and gonorrhea (coinfection high)
    iii. HIV testing
    iv. Hepatitis B testing

F. Management[4, 14, 15]

1. 1998 CDC Recommended Regimens for Adolescents and Adults

  a. Azithromycin (Zithromax), 1 g single-dose p.o. Safety for persons <15 years of age and in pregnancy not established
  b. Doxycycline (tetracycline), 100 mg p.o. b.i.d. for 7 days

2. Alternative regimens

  a. Erythromycin base (E-Mycin), 500 mg p.o. q.i.d. for 7 days
  b. Erythromycin ethylsuccinate (EES), 800 mg p.o. q.i.d. for 7 days
  c. Ofloxacin (Floxin), 300 mg p.o. b.i.d. for 7 days. Not active against *Treponema*

3. 1998 CDC Recommended Regimens for Pregnancy

    a. Erythromycin base (E-Mycin), 500 mg p.o. q.i.d. for 7 days

    b. Amoxicillin (Amoxil), 500 mg p.o. t.i.d. for 7 days

4. Alternative regimens for pregnancy

    a. Erythromycin Base (E-Mycin), 250 mg p.o. q.i.d. for 14 days

    b. Erythromycin ethylsuccinate (EES), 400 mg p.o. q.i.d. for 14 days

    c. Azithromycin (Zithromax), 1 g p.o. in a single dose. Will probably become treatment of choice in pregnancy

5. 1998 CDC Follow-up Guidelines

    a. If symptoms persist or reinfection is suspected. Advise sexual partners of need for treatment.

    b. Test of cure not routinely required per CDC guidelines, but if done should be 3 weeks after treatment

    c. Consider retesting 3 weeks after completion of treatment with erythromycin

    d. Avoid sexual activity until cured.

    e. Use condoms containing Nonoxynol-9.

6. Report positive tests according to state regulations.

IV. HERPES

A. Definition[4, 9, 13, 15, 16]

1. Recurrent, incurable, viral infection of the genital or orofacial skin or epithelia characterized by vesicular eruptions on a lightly raised erythematous base.

2. There are two strains of the herpes simplex virus (HSV), HSV-1 and HSV-2. The strains are quite different (50% difference in genome). Differences include

    a. Sensitivity to viral drugs, and

    b. Ability to cause specific disease in other organs.

B. Etiology/Incidence/Predisposing factors[9]

1. Etiology: Organism is a double-stranded DNA virus. Both HSV-1 and HSV-2 may be excreted by asymptomatic persons. Can cause oral or genital lesions.

    a. HSV Type 1: Commonly causes herpes labialis (cold sores) and herpes keratitis

        i. Acute gingivostomatitis: Occurs in both children and adults.

        ii. Causes 25% of primary genital infections (oral sex, kissing)

        iii. Incubation period ranges from 2–10 days; lesion heals within 3 weeks

    iv. Milder recurrences that diminish in frequency

    v. HSV-1 is more common; tends to occur earlier in life.

  b. HSV Type 2[1]:

    i. Cause of 90% of genital herpes infections

    ii. Tends to cause more severe and recurrent episodes and occurs later in life

    iii. Incubation period is from 4–7 days; lesion heals in 2–3 weeks

    iv. Recurrent episodes vary greatly from person to person.

    v. Symptoms vary from person to person

    vi. Most recurrent infections are milder, and lesions heal faster

2. Incidence

  a. Use of HSV-2 specific antibody test shows that one third of sexually active adults have serologic evidence of HSV-2.

  b. Less than 5% have past history of HSV.

  c. Up to one million new HSV-2 infections may be transmitted each year in the United States.

  d. Approximately 45 million individuals are infected with HSV-2.

3. Predisposing factors/Causes

  a. Caused by close physical contact, usually sexual (vaginal, anal, and/or oral) with infected individual

  b. Multiple sexual partners

  c. Use of alcohol or drugs prior to and during sexual activity

  d. Improper use of condoms

C. Subjective findings: Genital herpes (primary infection)

1. Fever, fatigue, headache, pharyngitis, myalgias, backache (flu-like symptoms)

2. Itching, pain, urinary retention, constipation, lower extremity weakness

3. Dysuria

4. Hyperesthesia (unusual sensitivity to sensory stimuli)

D. Physical examination findings

1. Genital herpes (primary infection):

  a. Small, painful vesicles or pustules distributed over external genitalia

  b. More common in genital area are painful ulcerating papules; white-gray area of necrosis on cervix. *All* lesions are contagious

  c. Inguinal lymphadenopathy

  d. Vaginal discharge

  e. Extragenital cutaneous lesions on hips and buttocks

2. Recurrent genital herpes

    a. Precipitated by trauma, menses, stress, illness, fever, over-exposure to sun
    b. Prodrome of local burning, itching, or tingling
    c. Recurrent disease symptoms generally milder
    d. Eruption of lesions over course of 3 days and resolve in 7–10 days
    e. Viral shedding occurs around days 4–7
    f. Recurrences are due to reactivation of virus already present in the nerve endings

E. Laboratory/Diagnostic findings[13, 15]

1. Tzanck smear

    a. Immediate diagnosis: 85–95% sensitivity and 95% specificity
    b. Collecting specimen
        i. Unroof vesicular lesion and scrape
        ii. Transfer specimen to glass slide; fix immediately
        iii. Positive smear shows giant cells with eosinophilic inclusion bodies

2. HSV culture (confirmatory test of choice)

    a. Results available in 3–7 days
    b. Expensive and time-consuming

3. ELISA and Western blot are highly accurate
4. Differentiate HSI-1 from HSV-2 antibiodies

F. Management: Recommendations of the CDC: Palliative management options[4]

1. No cure for disease; duration of symptoms and infectivity are reduced by drug therapy.
2. First primary episode

    a. Acyclovir (Zovirax), 400 mg p.o. t.i.d. for 7–10 days or until healing is complete. Contraindicated in patients with acute or chronic renal involvement
    b. Extensive counseling regarding
        i. The natural history of genital herpes, sexual transmission
        ii. Methods to reduce sexual transmission, i.e., use of condoms to prevent transmission of virus even in the absence of lesions because of viral shedding
        iii. Potential recurrent episodes
        iv. Asymptomatic viral shedding: Extremely infectious
    c. Acyclovir (Zovirax), 400 mg p.o. 5 times a day for 10 days for first episode of herpes proctitis and oral infection

including stomatitis or pharyngitis, or until healing is complete

3. Recurrent infections

   a. Acyclovir is *not* routinely indicated in immunocompromised patients.
   b. If used, institute during prodrome or within 2 days of onset of lesions
   c. Recommended regimens for episodic recurrent infection:
      i. Acyclovir (Zovirax), 400 mg p.o. t.i.d. for 5 days, *or*
      ii. Acyclovir (Zovirax), 200 mg p.o. 5 times a day for 5 days, *or*
      iii. Acyclovir (Zovirax), 800 mg p.o. b.i.d. for 5 days, *or*
      iv. Valacyclovir (Valtrex), 500 mg p.o. b.i.d. for 5 days, *or*
      v. Famciclovir (Famvir), 125 mg p.o. b.i.d. for 5 days
   d. Suppressive treatment is often offered to clients with >6 episodes per year of herpes infection
   e. Suppressive therapy with acyclovir (Zovirax), 400 mg b.i.d. daily for up to 12 months
      i. Laboratory evaluation of liver function and blood urea nitrogen (BUN). Should be done at end of 1 year of suppressive therapy
      ii. Provision for effective contraception should be made.

4. Complications

   a. Secondary infections
   b. Keratitis (keep fingers away from eyes)
   c. Meningitis
   d. Encephalitis
   e. Pneumonitis
   f. Hepatitis

5. Follow-up: As needed
6. Education: Always use acyclovir (Zovirax) in full doses to avoid resistance

V. SYPHILIS[4, 9, 16]

A. Definition

A systemic STD that progresses through distinct stages: Primary, secondary, latent, and tertiary.

B. Etiology/Incidence/Predisposing factors

1. Causative organism is the bacterium *Treponema pallidum*, a strict anaerobic spirochete
2. Incubation period varies, generally 10–90 days, average 21 days
3. Case rate of 3 per 100,000 people in the United States

4. Incidence: 200,000 new cases reported annually; rates have increased
5. This type of bacterium is capable of infecting any organ or tissue in the unborn and is transported to various sites via the bloodstream.
6. Infection occurs at the site of inoculation: A small abrasion or sore results.

C. Subjective findings

1. Primary syphilis

   a. Chancre: The classic finding is a painless and indurated ulcer, "sore" or lesion; usually appears about 3–4 weeks postexposure; heals spontaneously from 1–5 weeks
   b. Regional lymphadenopathy

2. Secondary syphilis (stage of dissemination)

   a. Flu-like symptoms (low-grade fever, headache, sore throat, malaise); generalized arthralgia
   b. Maculopapular rash on palms and soles of feet 2–6 weeks after infection, which heals spontaneously in 4–10 weeks
   c. Patchy alopecia
   d. Condyloma lata (wart-like lesions) occur in mouth, throat, and cervix
   e. Genital lesions are highly infectious and transmitted by direct contact.
   f. Untreated lesions resolve in 3–12 weeks.

3. Latent syphilis: Often asymptomatic and lasts 5–20 years

   a. Early latency: Infection of <1 year may be infectious
   b. Late latency: Infection of >1 year that is noninfectious
   c. Blood test remains positive for antibodies to *T. pallidum*

4. Tertiary (late) syphilis may take the form of gummatous syphilis (soft granulomatous tumor of the tissues), cardiovascular syphilis (rare), or neurosyphilis.

D. Physical examination findings

1. Primary: A classic chancre—rounded painless indurated ulcer with serous exudate; may be genital or extragenital; regional lymphadenopathy
2. Secondary: Maculopapular rash covering entire body; condyloma lata
3. Latent: Asymptomatic
4. Tertiary: Symptoms depend on which organ system is affected

E. Laboratory/Diagnostic findings

1. Positive darkfield microscopic examination and direct fluorescent antibody test of lesion exudate are definitive tests for diagnosing early syphilis.

2. Nontreponemal serologic test (VDRL-RPR) can be negative in up to 30% of patients at an initial visit for primary syphilis.

   a. Venereal Disease Research Laboratory (VDRL) and rapid plasma reagin (RPR) become positive 1–2 weeks after chancre formation.

   b. Treponemal specific test: Treponemal antibody absorption test (FTA-ABS) or microhemagglutination assay for antibodies to *T. pallidum* (MHA-TP) are positive. False-positive test occurs in Lyme disease.

   c. Most commonly used test; patient remains positive indefinitely after treatment. All reactive serologic tests require confirmation with a treponemal test. Both nontreponemal and treponemal test become reactive within 3 weeks after chancre has occurred.

3. Secondary: All serologic tests are positive.
4. Latent: serologic tests are positive.
5. Treponemal tests remain positive for life.

F. Management: Treatment is stage-specific

1. Early primary, secondary, and early latent: Benzathine penicillin G (Bicillin), 2.4 million units IM, single dose
2. Late latent syphilis or syphilis of unknown duration: Benzathine Penicillin G (Bicillin), 7.2 million units IM given as 2.4 million units per week for 3 weeks
3. Tertiary disease, excluding neurosyphilis: As for latent disease
4. Neurosyphilis: Penicillin G sodium (sterile), 12–24 million units/day IV (2–4 million units q4h) for 10–14 days, procaine penicillin G (Bicillin), 2.4 million units per day IM plus probenecid, 500 mg p.o. q.i.d. for 10–14 days
5. Exposure (sexual contact with persons with infectious syphilis): As for early disease
6. If penicillin allergy exists, desensitize, then treat with penicillin (see 1998 CDC guidelines[4])
7. Follow-up

   a. Clinical and serologic follow-up at 3 and 6 months after treatment

   b. If symptoms persist or recur with a sustained fourfold increase in the nontreponemal test titer compared with baseline or previous titer, suspect either failed treatment or reinfection: retreat after HIV testing.

   c. Some experts recommend cerebrospinal fluid (CSF) examination

   d. Recommended retreatment regimen: Procaine penicillin G (Bicillin), 2.4 million units IM given 1 week apart for 3 consecutive weeks unless CSF examination indicates neurosyphilis is present

8. Management of sex partners: Treat presumptively.
9. Report positive test according to state regulations.

VI. GONORRHEA[4, 9, 11, 16]

A. Definition

A classic bacterial STD that prefers columnar and pseudostratified epithelium and can be symptomatic or asymptomatic in men and women

B. Etiology/Incidence/Predisposing factors

1. Causative organism is *N. gonorrhoeae*, a gram-negative, intracellular, nonmotile, diplococcal bacterium cultured from the genitourinary tract, oropharynx, and/or anorectum of men and women.
2. The Centers for Disease Control reports that in the United States an estimated 650,000 new infections with *N. gonorrhoeae* occur each year.
3. Incidence in the population is about 1–2% (1.3 million per year).
4. Incubation period averages 3–5 days with a range of 1–14 days.
5. Male to female transmission is 80–90% after exposure; female to male transmission is as low as 20% after exposure.
6. Possible serious complications include pelvic inflammatory disease, ectopic pregnancy, involuntary infertility, perihepatitis (Fitz-Hugh–Curtis syndrome), disseminated gonococcal infection, and epididymitis.

C. Subjective findings

1. Females: 80% asymptomatic

   a. Early symptoms: Dysuria and frequency; malodorous and mucopurulent vaginal or urethral discharge; labial pain and swelling; lower abdominal discomfort; and pharyngitis
   b. Later symptoms: Fever, abnormal menstrual periods, increased dysmenorrhea, nausea and vomiting, joint pain and swelling

2. Males: Usually symptomatic

   a. Early symptoms: Dysuria with frequency, whitish urethral discharge, and pharyngitis
   b. Later symptoms: Yellow-greenish, profuse, purulent urethral discharge with meatal edema and erythema; epididymitis; and lower abdominal pain (proctitis)

D. Physical examination findings

1. Fever often present

2. Abdominal examination: Guarding, referred pain, rebound pain, and hyperperistalsis
3. Pelvic examination (women)

   a. Inspect Bartholin's and Skene's glands for tenderness, enlargement, or discharge
   b. Urethral discharge
   c. Vaginal wall discharge or redness
   d. Cervix: Mucopurulent discharge and friability; most frequent site of infection in women
   e. Adnexal tenderness and masses, uterine tenderness, and cervical motion and tenderness per bimanual examination

4. Throat and endocervical culture, if oral and vaginal sex practiced
5. Men

   a. Inspect for erythema and edema in the penile shaft
   b. Purulent urethral discharge
   c. If anal sex is practiced, perform rectal examination for tenderness and discharge

E. Laboratory/Diagnostic findings

1. Endocervical and throat culture for *N. gonorrhoeae* using modified Thayer-Martin media is cornerstone of diagnosis
2. Cervical culture or antigen detection of *C. trachomatis*
3. Test all patients for syphilis
4. Offer HIV testing
5. Differential diagnoses: Chlamydia, appendicitis, ectopic pregnancy, pelvic inflammatory disease
6. Elevated WBC
7. Elevated ESR
8. Examine male patient at least 1 hour after voiding

F. Management

1. CDC 1998 recommendations for treatment of adults with uncomplicated gonococcal infections of cervix, urethra, throat, and rectum

   a. Ceftriaxone (Rocephin), 125–250 mg single dose IM, *or*
   b. Cefixime (Suprax), 400 mg p.o. single dose, *or*
   c. Ciprofloxacin (Cipro), 500 mg p.o. single dose

2. Treatment for coexisting *C. trachomatitis:* Doxycyline (tetracycline), 100 mg p.o. b.i.d. for 7 days.
3. Patients should be instructed to refer sex partners for evaluation and treatment.
4. All sex partners of patients whose last sexual contact with the patient was within 60 days before onset of symptoms or diagnosis of infection should be evaluated and treated for *N. gonorrhoeae* and *C. trachomatis* infections.

5. Patients should be instructed to avoid sexual intercourse until cure is established.
6. Follow-up

   a. Test for cure *not* is recommended by CDC unless symptoms recur, exacerbate, or do not resolve.
   b. Any gonococci isolated should be tested for antimicrobial susceptibility.
   c. Report positive tests according to state regulations.

7. Persons with disseminated gonococcal infection should be hospitalized for initial therapy.

   a. Ceftriaxone (Rocephin), 1 g IM or IV q24h for 2 days or until improvement begins, at which time therapy may be switched to a regimen to complete a full week of therapy: Cefixime (Suprax), 400 mg p.o. b.i.d. for 7 days, or ciprofloxacin (Cipro), 500 mg p.o. b.i.d. for 7 days.

References

1. Seoggin, J., & Morgan, G. (1997). *Practice guidelines for obstetrics and gynecology.* Philadelphia: J.B. Lippincott.
2. Larson, E.B., & Ramsey, P.G. (1998). *Medical therapeutics* (3rd ed.). Philadelphia: W.B. Saunders.
3. Johnson, C.A., Johnson, B.E., Murry, J.L., & Apgar, B.S. (1996). *Women's health care handbook.* Philadelphia: Hanley and Belfus, Inc.
4. Centers for Disease Control and Prevention. (1998). *1998 Guidelines for treatment of sexually transmitted diseases. Morbidity and Mortality Weekly Report*, J47:RRI (No. RR = 1). Available online at http://www.cdc.gov/
5. Star, W.L., Lommel, L.L., & Shannon, M.T. (1995). *Women's primary health care protocols for practice.* Washington, DC: American Nurses Pub.
6. Mott, A.M. (1998). Preventions and management of pelvic inflammatory disease by primary care providers. *American Journal for Nurse Practitioners, 2,* 7–15.
7. Maiolatesi, C.R., Peddicord, K. (1996). Methotrexate for nonsurgical treatment of eetopic pregnancy: Nursing implications. *Journal of Obstetric, Gynecologic, and Neonatal Nursing, 25,* 205–208.
8. Alexander, L.L., Freiman, K., & Clarke, P. (1996). National survey of nurse practitioner chlamydia knowledge and treatment practices of female patients. *The Nurse Practitioner: The American Journal of Primary Health Care, 2,* 48–54.
9. Sharts, N.C. (1997). STD's in women: What you need to know. *American Journal of Nursing, 97,* 46–53.
10. Lowdermilk, D.L., Perry, S.E., & Bobak, L.M. (1997). *Maternity and Women's Health Care* (6th ed.). St. Louis: CV Mosby.
11. Miller, H.S., McEvers, J., & Griffith, J.A. (1997). *Instructions for Obstetric and Gynecologic Patients* (2nd ed.). Philadelphia: W.B. Saunders.
12. Allen, K.M., & Phillips, J.M. (1997). *Women's health across the lifespan: A comprehensive perspective.* Philadelphia: J.B. Lippincott.
13. U.S. Preventive Services Task Force. (1996). *Guide to clinical preventive services: Report of the U.S. Preventive Services Task Force* (2nd ed.). Baltimore: Williams & Wilkins.

14. Terreira, N. (1996). Sexually transmitted *Chlamydia trachomatis. Nurse Practitioner Forum, Current Topics and Communications, 7,* 40–46.

15. Hawkins, J.W., Roberto-Nichols, D.M., & Stanley-Haney, J.L. (1997). *Protocols for nurse practitioners in gynecologic settings* (6th ed.). New York: The Tiresras Press.

16. Youngkin, E.Q., Sawin, K.J., Kissinger, J.F., & Israel, D.S. (1999). *Pharmacotherapeutics: A primary care clinical guide.* Stamford, CT: Appleton & Lange.

17. Flemming, M.E., Quilan, G.M., Johnson, R.E., Nahmias, A.J., Aral, S.O., Lee, F.K., & St. Louis, M.E. (1997). Herpes simplex virus type 2 in the United States, 1976–1994. *New England Journal of Medicine;* 337: 1105–1111.

18. Cunningham, F.G., MacDonald, P.C., Gant, N.F., Leveno, K.J., Gilstrap, L.G., Hankins, G.D.V., & Clark, S.L. (1997). *Williams' obstetrics* (20th ed.) (pp. 607–633). Stamford, CT: Appleton & Lange.

EYE, EAR, NOSE, AND THROAT DISORDERS

Carolyn G. White, MSN, RN, CS, FNP, PNP, CCRN, and Diantha D. Miller, MSN, RN, CS, ACNP, ANP, CEN

I. CONJUNCTIVITIS

A. Definition[1, 2, 9, 10]

1. Common, generally acute, painful inflammation of the conjunctiva (palpebral and/or bulbar), but not involving the cornea or deeper structures of the eye
2. Can be chronic, but most cases are acute, and many are infectious

B. Etiology/Predisposing factors[2, 3, 10–12, 15, 16]

1. Spread by direct inoculation via fingers or droplets
2. Bacteria

   a. *Staphylococcus aureus*
   b. *Diplococcus*
   c. *Haemophilus influenzae*
   d. *Streptococcus pneumoniae*
   e. *Pseudomonas* (most common)

3. Viruses

   a. Commonly adenovirus
   b. Herpesvirus (may be vision-threatening)

4. Allergens/hypersensitivity to

   a. Pollen
   b. Dust
   c. Contact lenses
   d. Dyes
   e. Ophthalmic drops

5. Trauma (chemical and ultraviolet flash burns)
6. Parasitic infestation (pediculosis pubis)
7. Systemic infections

   a. Reiter's syndrome
   b. Behçet's syndrome
   c. Temporal arteritis

8. May accompany other eye disorders

   a. Keratitis
   b. Uveitis
   c. Acute angle-closure glaucoma

C. Subjective findings[3, 5, 6, 9]

1. Redness and/or excessive tearing (sense of a foreign body in eye)
2. Swelling and/or itching
3. History of allergenic/infectious/traumatic exposure
4. Discharge

D. Physical examination findings[4, 6, 9, 10, 13]

1. Visual acuity (See Laboratory/Diagnostic findings)
2. Edema of external eye and lid
3. Extraocular movement (EOM), visual fields, pupillary response, cornea, and anterior chamber are usually normal.

   • The presence of photophobia rules out conjunctivitis.

4. Conjunctival injection/swelling/foreign body

   a. Wearing gloves, evert the upper lid by rolling it externally along the cotton end of a swab.
   b. Examine for obvious foreign body.

5. Drainage may be purulent or serous.

   • If intent is to culture, specimen should be taken before the instillation of drops or irrigation.

E. Laboratory/Diagnostic findings[6, 7, 9, 10]

1. Decreased visual acuity may indicate a more serious condition.
2. Consider culture of secretions: Giemsa's stain for possible infection with *Chlamydia* and/or gonorrhea

F. Management[4, 5, 9, 13]

1. To rule out corneal abrasion or foreign body

   a. Instill topical anesthetic (two drops tetracaine [Pontocaine], 0.5%, or proparacaine, 0.5%).
   b. Stain the eye with fluorescein using drops or paper.

2. Bacteria

   a. Topical antibiotic ophthalmic solutions or ointments
      i. Gentamicin, 3 mg/mL solution or 3 mg/g ointment, 1–2 drops q4h while awake for 5 days, or if severe may be increased to 2 drops every 1–2 hours
      ii. Neomycin (Neosporin), polymixin, or sulfacetamide sodium (Sodium Sulamyd), 10% solution, 1–2 drops into affected eye every 2–3 h while awake for 5–7 days
      iii. Ocuflox 0.3% solution: 1–2 drops into affected eye for 2 days then q.i.d. for up to 5 days more (total 7 days)
   b. Note: A 15% potential for adverse reaction to neomycin-containing products (Neosporin) has been reported.

3. In the presence of other systemic disease, treat the underlying condition accordingly (e.g., otitis media: amoxicillin, 500 mg p.o. t.i.d. for 10 days).
4. *Chlamydia*/gonorrhea: Erythromycin ointment q.i.d. for 7 days
5. Allergy

    a. Over-the-counter naphazoline, 0.05%, or antazoline 0.5% (Albalon-A, Vasocon-A), 2 drops q2–4h and as needed.
    b. Oral prescription antihistamine (loratidine [Claritin], 10 mg q.d.) or over-the-counter diphenhydramine (Benadryl), 25–50 mg p.o. q6–8h.

II. CORNEAL ABRASION

A. Definition[2, 6, 12, 13]

Disruption of the epithelium of the cornea (the clear, anterior covering of the eye)

B. Etiology/Incidence/Predisposing factors[5, 9, 10]

1. Usually associated with chemical, burn, or mechanical trauma (including foreign body)
2. Very common
3. Result of outdoor activity, occupational hazards (e.g., welding, painting, construction)

C. Subjective findings[5, 6, 9, 13]

1. Intense pain secondary to the vast sensory nerve supply of the eye
2. A sense of foreign body in the eye
3. Report of redness and/or discharge of the conjunctiva
4. History of decreased visual acuity
5. Complaint of tearing

D. Physical examination findings[3, 9, 10, 13, 15]

1. Decrease in visual acuity

    a. Except in trauma involving emergency need for irrigation of the eye, the visual acuity should be the initial measure of vision.
    b. When a Snellen chart is unavailable, gross evaluation such as a finger count can be used.
    c. Instill a topical anesthetic such as tetracaine (Pontocaine) ophthalmic drops (1–2 drops).
    d. Avoid repeated use of eye anesthetic, which may result in further injury and delayed healing.

2. Inspect for other signs of trauma (foreign body) by everting the lid.

    a. Note positive findings with location.

b. See preceding, Conjunctivitis, D, 4, for lid eversion procedure.

3. Fluorescein staining of the cornea

a. May reveal disruptions in the corneal epithelium
b. Appears as increased uptake (pooling) of dye when illuminated by a Wood's lamp or blue light.

E. Management[2, 5, 13, 17, 18]

1. Apply antibiotic ointment (preferred by many clinicians) or solution such as

a. Gentamycin ophthalmic, 3 mg/g ointment, b.i.d. or t.i.d., or solution, 3 mg/mL drops, 1–2 drops into affected eye q2–3h while awake, or
b. Sulfacetamide sodium, 10% ointment, apply a small amount to affected eye q3–4h and at bedtime for 5–7 days, or solution, 1–2 drops q2–3h, for 1–3 days

2. Apply a soft eye patch.
3. Update tetanus immunization if indicated.
4. Re-evaluate in 24 h, at which time healing should be complete.
5. Refer to ophthalmologist for removal of foreign bodies or failed initial management.

III. DIABETIC RETINOPATHY

A. Definition[2, 17]

Ocular disease of the retina resulting from systemic diabetes

B. Etiology/Incidence/Predisposing factors[2, 3, 17, 18]

1. Most common cause of blindness in the United States
2. Inhibition of aldose reductase pathways results in increased blood flow and pressure, diminishing the integrity of the blood/retina barrier.

a. Entry of large cells into the extracellular space of the retina causes macular edema.
b. Microaneurysms, intraretinal microvascular leaking, and hemorrhage may result.

C. Subjective findings[2, 13, 16]

1. Symptoms that may be present

a. Flashing lights in peripheral visual fields
b. Blurred vision
c. "Cobwebs"
d. Black spots
e. Sudden loss of vision

D. Physical examination findings[17]

1. Funduscopic examination may reveal exudates (hard or soft) and microaneurysms seen as dot and flame hemorrhagic markings.
2. Hard, bright yellow markings may be noted arising from lipid transudation via leaky capillaries.
3. Soft exudates produced by infarcted nerve tissue appearing as pale yellow, irregular, cotton-wool spots may be present.

E. Laboratory/Diagnostic findings[17]

1. Retinopathy is associated with poor glycemic control.
2. Sustained glucose levels over 130 mg/dL have been associated with an increase in microvascular complications.

F. Management[2, 17]

1. Refer to ophthalmologist.

   a. Macular edema can only be ascertained via a stereoscopic examination or by fluorescein angiography.
   b. Visual acuity is not a sufficient indicator of retinopathy.

2. Laser photocoagulation for focal macular edema
3. Vitrectomy and laser therapy as indicated
4. Control of blood glucose is paramount.

IV. RETINAL DETACHMENT

A. Definition[2]

Separation of the neural retina from the choroid following trauma, hemorrhage, increased intraocular pressure, or transudation of fluid

B. Etiology/Incidence/Predisposing factors[2, 3]

1. Trauma
2. Intraocular/intracerebral mass
3. Uveitis (inflammation of the iris)
4. Annually 10 per 100,000 persons suffer a retinal detachment without rhegmatogenous tear.
5. One to three percent of patients undergoing cataract surgery suffer a retinal detachment.
6. Associated with chronic disease

   a. Diabetes mellitus
   b. Sickle cell anemia

C. Subjective findings[1, 2, 12, 13]

1. Painless visual changes, floaters, blurred vision, light flashes
2. As detachment becomes pervasive, a "curtain" may obscure part or all of the field of vision.

3. Large detachments may produce a Marcus Gunn pupil (afferent pupil that reacts more consensually than directly).

D. Physical examination findings[3]

1. Elevations of the retina related to tears
2. Exudative, bullous elevation without tears

E. Management[2, 3, 13, 17]

1. Immediate referral to ophthalmologist for possible treatments

   a. Diathermy
   b. Cryotherapy
   c. Scleral buckling
   d. Photocoagulation

2. If the detachment is a result of traumatic insult, patch the eye with a metal shield (e.g., Fox's eye shield).

V. CENTRAL RETINAL ARTERY OBSTRUCTION

A. Definition

1. An abrupt blockage of the central retinal artery causing sudden visual loss or loss of visual fields
2. Permanent partial or complete visual loss may ensue without immediate intervention.

B. Etiology/Predisposing factors

1. Causes

   a. Thrombosis
   b. Embolism
   c. Arteritis of the central retinal artery

2. Associated with

   a. Migraine
   b. Advancing age
   c. Use of oral contraceptives
   d. History of vasculitis

C. Subjective findings[2, 3, 13, 17]

1. Sudden, painless, visual loss
2. Visual loss may be central (if fovea is affected) or peripheral.

D. Physical examination findings[2, 3, 13, 17]

1. Partial dilation of pupil, which is sluggishly reactive to direct light, but may have a normal consensual response
2. Funduscopic exam

   a. May reveal a pale, opaque fundus and characteristic "cherry-red spot" at the fovea
   b. Arterial vessels may appear pale and bloodless.

E. Laboratory/Diagnostic findings[17]

1. Elevated erythrocyte sedimentation rate associated with giant cell arteritis
2. Hyperlipidemia is associated with venous occlusions.
3. Presence of antiphospholipid antibodies

F. Management[2, 13, 14, 17]

1. Immediate consultation with an ophthalmologist
2. Intermittent digital massage of the anterior chamber by gentle pressure over the eyelid may be sight-saving.

   • If an embolus can be dislodged, retinal ischemia can be relieved.

3. Consider rebreathing CO_2 per airtight mask or bag to decrease alkalosis.
4. Consider IV anticoagulant (e.g., heparin, 10,000 units)

VI. GLAUCOMA

A. Definition[1, 2, 13, 17, 18]

1. A disorder of progressive visual loss
2. Often caused by increased intraocular pressure leading to partial or complete blindness

B. Etiology/Incidence/Predisposing factors[2, 9, 13, 17, 18]

1. Primarily of two types

   a. Chronic open-angle (wide) (most common) or
   b. Acute or chronic closed-angle (narrow)

2. Primary open-angle glaucoma accounts for nearly two-thirds of all cases.
3. Two other types exist

   a. Congenital glaucoma (primary)
   b. Secondary or induced glaucoma, resulting from
      i. Prolonged steroid use
      ii. Uveitis
      iii. Cataracts
      iv. Tumor

4. Obstruction of the outflow of aqueous humor from the ciliary body through the trabecula and canal of Schlemm produces increased intraocular pressure, which leads to atrophy of the optic nerve head.
5. Affects approximately 2% of the population
6. Risk factors

   a. Advancing age
   b. Heredity

    c. Myopia
    d. African American ethnicity

C. Subjective findings[1-3, 9, 13, 16-18]

1. In open-angle glaucoma, visual changes occur slowly, with decreasing peripheral vision noted over time.
2. Photophobia and visual blurring may occur.
3. Headache and halos around lights are atypical, although a unilateral headache in conjunction with visual changes on the same side as the headache may occur.
4. In secondary glaucoma, such as with ophthalmic corticosteroid use, elevated intraocular pressure may be produced in just 2 weeks.
5. In acute closed-angle glaucoma, symptoms develop rapidly.

    a. The patient complains of intense eye pain and visual disturbances (halos around lights), with nausea and vomiting.
    b. Note: While pain is common with closed-angle glaucoma, there are painless variants distinguished only by a fixed pupil.

D. Physical examination findings[1-3, 9, 13, 15, 17, 18]

1. Inspect for external signs such as redness, tearing, lid deformities, proptosis, or ptosis, and for corneal clouding.
2. A ''hard eye'' may be palpated in acute glaucoma.
3. Observe changes in pupillary response, reactivity, symmetry, and accommodation.
4. Visual acuity may remain normal.
5. Examine for increased intraocular pressure (IOP) by measuring IOP with Schiøtz's tonometer or Goldmann's applanation tonometer.

    a. Never apply the tonometer to an infected or possibly infected eye.
    b. Increased IOP is defined as >23 mmHg.[8]
    c. In acute angle-closure glaucoma, IOP may be in the 40–80 mmHg range.

6. Observe for decreased peripheral vision with confrontation test.
7. Funduscopy

    a. Optic disk may appear irregular with notching of the physiologic cup or ''cupping.''
    b. Observe for increased cup-to-disk ratio.

E. Management[5, 12, 13, 15, 17, 18]

1. Immediate referral to an ophthalmologist

2. Open-angle glaucoma may respond well to laser surgery or to medical treatment.

    a. Timoptic ophthalmic solution, 0.25–0.5%, 1 drop in affected eye(s) b.i.d., or

    b. Pilocarpine (Ocusert), one wafer q 7 days, or solution, 1–2 drops up to 6 times q.d., or

    c. Acetazolamide (Diamox), 250–1000 mg p.o., in divided doses

3. Other treatment options include possible laser surgery and/or trabeculectomy.

4. *Closed-angle glaucoma is an ophthalmologic emergency.*

    a. Immediate pressure-reducing IV antiglaucoma medications can be eye-saving.

       i. Acetazolamide, 500 mg IV, followed by 250 mg p.o. q.i.d.

      ii. Oral glycerol or IV mannitol at 1–2 g/kg can be used if initial diuretic treatment is unsuccessful.

    b. Consult an ophthalmologist as soon as the diagnosis is suspected.

VII. BELL'S PALSY

A. Definition[16]

1. A sudden onset of unilateral facial paralysis
2. Generally self-limiting, with restoration of health in a matter of weeks

B. Etiology/Incidence/Predisposing factors[2, 3, 14, 16–18]

1. Idiopathic
2. Probably involves inflammation of cranial nerve VII near the stylomastoid foramen
3. Affects individuals across the life span without gender preference
4. Affects 25 in 100,000 persons in the U.S. annually
5. Clinical appearance often correlates with periods of stress, viral infection, or fatigue.
6. Familial tendency
7. Increased incidence in

    a. Late pregnancy
    b. Hypertension
    c. Diabetes
    d. Ramsay Hunt syndrome
    e. Herpes zoster
    f. Demyelinating disease
    g. Sarcoidosis
    h. Lyme disease

8. May be related to cold exposure

C. Subjective findings[3, 17, 18]

1. Unilateral paralysis of the face

   a. Affects the eyebrow, eyelid, and/or mouth
   b. Although the paralysis may mimic symptoms of cerebro-vascular accident, only facial muscle involvement is seen.

2. Taste impairment
3. Ipsilateral pain of ear, cheek, and face

D. Physical examination findings[3, 14, 17]

1. Weakness of upper and lower face
2. Inability to close the eyelids
3. May be drooling secondary to mouth paralysis
4. Abnormal corneal reflex on the affected side
5. Hyperacusis (increased hearing sensitivity)
6. Normal facial sensation
7. Taste disturbance

E. Laboratory/Diagnostic findings[2, 3, 11, 17, 18]

1. Diagnostic testing is nonspecific; diagnosis is one of exclusion.
2. A lumbar puncture is not typically needed, but may reveal elevated levels of cerebrospinal fluid protein and cells.
3. Consider tests to confirm other diagnoses such as

   a. CT, MRI (tumor)
   b. Lyme titer (if history of tick exposure)
   c. Audiogram to rule out cranial nerve VIII involvement (not associated with Bell's palsy)

4. The corneal reflex (blink test) is abnormal in 100% of cases.

F. Management[3, 8, 14, 17, 18]

1. Eye care, including moisturizers such as Artificial Tears or Tears Naturale, as needed
2. Eyelids may require taping closed to prevent external trauma.
3. Consider referral to a physical therapist for evaluation, exercise, and stimulation.
4. The use of steroids is indicated to decrease inflammation around cranial nerve VII.

   a. In the early stages of illness (prior to day 10 of onset)
   b. Typically, methylprednisolone (Medrol Dosepak), 21 4.0-mg tablets
     i. Day 1: 2 tablets p.o. t.i.d.
     ii. Day 2: 2 tablets p.o. AM and PM, and 1 tablet at bedtime

   iii. Day 3: 2 tablets p.o. b.i.d.
   iv. Day 4: 2 tablets p.o. AM and 1 tablet p.o. PM
   v. Day 5: 1 tablet p.o. b.i.d.
   vi. Day 6: Last tablet p.o. in AM

5. Explain to the patient that the disorder is usually self-limiting, with most cases resolving in 4–6 weeks.

VIII. OTITIS EXTERNA

A. Definition[2, 4, 16]

1. Painful inflammation of the external auditory canal and auricle.
2. Commonly known as swimmer's ear

B. Etiology/Incidence/Predisposing factors[2, 7]

1. Five times more common in swimmers
2. More common in humid, warm environments
3. Bacteria

   a. *Pseudomonas aeruginosa*
   b. *Staphylococcus aureus*
   c. *Proteus vulgaris*
   d. *Streptococci*

4. Fungi
5. Trauma: Scratching of the external canal with bobby pins, ear plugs, or other foreign objects

C. Subjective findings[2, 4, 12, 17]

1. Pain: Severity increases with manipulation of the tragus or the pinna.
2. Decreased hearing
3. Fever
4. Lymphadenitis (generally pre-/postauricular and anterior cervical triangle)
5. Tympanic membrane is normal.

D. Physical examination findings[2, 4, 12, 17]

1. Canal edema
2. Otorrhea, which may be

   a. Purulent
   b. Bloody
   c. Serous
   d. Yellow/orange

E. Management[9, 10, 15, 17, 18]

1. Gentle suction and removal of debris from the external canal
2. Once the ear canal is free of debris, administer appropriate drops.

a. Combined antibiotic and steroid solution such as Cortisporin Otic, 4 drops in affected ear t.i.d. to q.i.d. or Cipro HC otic, 3 drops b.i.d. for 7 days

b. Antifungal and antibacterial solution such as TobraDex, 2 drops b.i.d. for 7 days

c. Zoto-HC drops 3 drops b.i.d. for 7 days

3. A cotton gauze wick may be inserted into the canal if severe edema is present (remove within 2–3 days of insertion).

4. Oral antibiotic

a. Amoxicillin–clavulanate (Augmentin), 500 mg b.i.d., or

b. Loracarbef (Lorabid), 200–400 mg p.o. b.i.d. for 7–10 days

5. Warm compresses to outer ear

6. A 50/50 combination of rubbing alcohol and white vinegar may be applied to the affected ear following swimming or bathing.

7. Consider corticosteroids (Medrol Dosepak), 5 day tapering dose, to reduce edema and pain.

8. Oral analgesics, such as acetaminophen (Tylenol #3) q4–6h as needed, may be given for pain.

IX. OTITIS MEDIA

A. Definition[2, 4, 16]

1. Infectious or inflammatory process within the middle ear

2. May be acute, suppurative, or serous in nature

B. Etiology/Incidence/Predisposing factors[3, 4, 10]

1. Eustachian tube dysfunction or congestion that prevents effective drainage of the middle ear

2. Infectious causative agents typically are bacteria

a. *Streptococcus pneumoniae*

b. *Haemophilus influenzae*

c. *Moraxella catarrhalis*

3. Common in children under 2 years of age, but may be seen in adults

4. Individuals with cleft palate, Down syndrome, or allergic rhinitis may be at high risk.

5. A neoplasm may occlude the eustachian tube, causing a build-up of serous fluid.

C. Subjective findings[2, 4, 12, 17]

1. Throbbing pain

2. Hearing loss (conductive)

3. Vertigo and nausea

4. Severe ear pain with sudden relief usually indicates tympanic membrane rupture with immediate release of fluid in the middle ear cavity.

5. Otorrhea may be pulsatile

D. Physical examination findings[2, 4, 12, 17]

1. Red, dull, bulging tympanic membrane (serous fluid may be amber in color)
2. A fine, black line (fluid meniscus) indicates a partially filled cavity.
3. Air bubbles may be visible beyond the tympanic membrane.
4. Bony landmarks are obscured.
5. Hole in tympanic membrane in severe cases

E. Management[4, 9, 10, 15, 17, 18]

1. Antibiotics (oral course for 10 days).

   a. Amoxicillin (Amoxil), 250–500 mg p.o. t.i.d.
   b. If allergic to penicillin, trimethoprim–sulfamethoxazole (Bactrim), 80/400 mg ii tablets p.o. b.i.d. for 10 days, or Azithromycin (Zithromax) 500 mg p.o. on 1st day followed by 250 mgm p.o. days 2–5

2. If perforation exists, Cortisporin Otic, 4 drops topically, t.i.d. for 7 days
3. Analgesics as needed for pain
4. For serous otitis media, decongestants and/or antihistamines may be given as well as corticosteroids to decrease inflammation of the eustachian tube (Claritin-D, one p.o. q24h).

X. VERTIGO

A. Definition[2, 4, 16]

1. A false sensation of movement usually associated with disequilibrium
2. Disequilibrium is a sense of light-headedness or of being off-balance without movement.

B. Etiology/Incidence/Predisposing factors[3, 4, 10]

1. Viral syndromes (e.g., vestibular neuronitis)
2. Labyrinthitis
3. Labyrinthine hydrops (Ménière's disease)
4. Vascular disease/spasm—May occur from thrombosis or disruption in an artery or vein
5. Damage to cranial nerve VIII

   a. Meningitis
   b. Trauma
   c. Tumors

6. Damage to brain stem nuclei

   a. Encephalitis
   b. Brain abscess

    c. Hemorrhage
    d. Multiple sclerosis

7. Metabolic conditions

    a. Syphilis
    b. Intoxication
       i. Drugs
      ii. Alcohol
    c. Hypoglycemia
    d. Thyroid disorders
    e. Anemia
    f. Diabetes mellitus

8. Cerebellar (vertebrobasilar)

    a. Transient ischemic attack
    b. Cerebrovascular accident

C. Subjective findings[4, 6, 11, 12]

1. Sensation of movement/rotation
2. Light-headedness/"faint feeling"
3. Sense of floating, swimming
4. Tinnitus
5. Hearing impairment
6. Nausea, vomiting
7. "Full" sensation in ear

D. Physical examination findings[4, 9, 11, 12]

1. Nystagmus
2. Carotid bruits
3. Positional hypotension
4. Conductive hearing loss
5. Positive Romberg's sign
6. Note: There may be no objective findings.

E. Laboratory/Diagnostic findings[9, 10, 12, 17, 18]

1. Thyroid stimulating hormone (TSH) to rule out hypothy-roidism
2. Hematocrit to rule out anemia
3. Fasting blood sugar (FBS)
4. Electrolytes and therapeutic drug levels
5. Consider alcohol level, drug screen.
6. Venereal disease research laboratory (VDRL) or rapid plasma reagin (RPR)
7. Audiogram/tympanogram evaluation
8. Refer to specialist for possible inner ear testing.
9. Consider CT or MRI of the brain, carotid Doppler studies, Holter monitor.

F. Management[5, 7, 9, 10, 17, 18]

1. Treat symptomatically.
2. Bed rest during acute attacks
3. Vestibular exercises to facilitate central nervous system compensation
4. Vestibular suppressants

    a. Meclizine (Antivert), 12.5–25 mg p.o. t.i.d., for daytime
    b. Diazepam (Valium), 2.5–5 mg p.o., at bedtime
    c. Scopolamine (Transderm Scope patch), apply one patch every 3 days

5. Low salt diet in combination with diuretics if Ménière's disease is suspected
6. Antiemetics—Promethazine (Phenergan), 12.5–25 mg q4h as needed, for nausea and vomiting p.o. (tablet) or per rectum (suppository).

XI. ALLERGIC RHINITIS

A. Definition[2, 4, 16]

1. An IgE-mediated reaction to an antigen (allergen) that develops after previous exposure to the same substance
2. May be seasonal or perennial

B. Etiology/Incidence/Predisposing factors[3, 4, 10]

1. Seasonal

    a. Occurs at the same time every year
    b. Varying pollens depending on geographic region
    c. Common offenders
       i. Trees
      ii. Grasses
     iii. Ragweed

2. Perennial

    a. Occurs year-round
    b. Associated with indoor inhalants
    c. Common offenders
       i. Dust mites
      ii. Mold spores
     iii. Animal dander

3. Other aggravating factors

    a. Cigarette smoke
    b. Temperature changes
    c. Chemical irritants
       i. Perfume

    ii. Candles
    iii. Industrial chemicals
  d. Air pollutants
  e. Foods

C. Subjective findings[4, 6, 10, 12]

1. Clear nasal drainage
2. Nasal congestion/pressure
3. Sneezing
4. Excessive postnasal drainage causing sore throat and cough
5. Facial swelling
6. Itching of nose and eyes
7. Headache
8. Decreased smell and taste

D. Physical examination findings[4, 5, 11, 12]

1. Clear rhinorrhea
2. Pale, edematous mucous membranes
3. Enlarged, blue-boggy turbinates
4. Mouth breathing
5. "Allergic shiners"—Dark circles under the eyes
6. "Allergic salute"—Rubbing of the nose upward, causing a horizontal crease
7. Allergic conjunctivitis

E. Laboratory/Diagnostic findings

Consider referring to an allergist for antigen testing.

F. Management[5, 6, 9, 17, 18]

1. Avoidance of allergens
2. Antihistamines (all as needed or for exacerbations)

  a. Cetirizine (Zyrtec), 10 mg, one p.o. q.d.
  b. Loratidine (Claritin), 10 mg, one p.o. q.d.
  c. Fexofenadine (Allegra), 60 mg, one p.o. b.i.d., or 180 mg, one p.o. q.d.

3. Topical corticosteroid sprays

  a. Fluticasone (Flonase), 2 sprays q.d. for exacerbations
  b. Beclomethasone (Vancenase, Beconase), 1 spray b.i.d.

4. Consider ipratropium (Atrovent) 2 sprays in each nostril up to t.i.d. for immediate relief.
5. Avoid oxymetazoline (Afrin)

  a. When used for more than 3 days, can cause adverse rebound nasal congestion
  b. Addictive

6. May use a corticosteroid (dexamethasone [Decadron]), LA long-acting 8 mg IM, or Medrol Dosepak for acute episodes

7. Oral decongestants may be used in conjunction with antihistamines.
8. Provide environmental counseling.

XII. EPISTAXIS

A. Definition[1, 3, 12]

1. Spontaneous bleeding from the nose
2. May be minor or an indication of a serious disease process
3. Commonly seen from Kiesselbach's plexus in the anteroinferior septum

B. Etiology/Incidence/Predisposing factors[3, 4, 10]

1. Ninety percent of cases occur at Kiesselbach's plexus.
2. Occurs more frequently in winter months
3. Forceful expiration

   a. Sneezing
   b. Coughing

4. Trauma

   a. Blow to the nose
   b. Fractures
   c. Picking the nose
   d. Foreign bodies

5. Drying or thinning secondary to oxygen use, nasal sprays
6. Infectious/allergic sinusitis, rhinitis, systemic infection
7. Nasopharyngeal fibroma, angioma, malignant tumors
8. Hypertension
9. Coagulopathies
10. Change in atmospheric pressure.

C. Subjective findings[4, 6, 10, 11]

1. History of bleeding from the nose
2. May be none

D. Physical examination findings[4, 6, 10, 11, 17]

1. Acute bleeding from nasal fossa and/or posterior nasopharynx
2. Site of bleeding

   a. Anterior bleed—Kiesselbach's plexus
   b. Posterior bleed—Inspect for active bleeding from the posterior oropharynx.
   c. There may be multiple oozing points.

3. Ulcerations or erosions of tissue
4. Blood pressure may be normal or elevated.

E. Laboratory/Diagnostic findings[9, 11, 12, 17, 18]

1. Sinus series to rule out sinusitis, tumor, angiofibroma
2. May consider complete blood count, prothrombin time/partial thromboplastin time, or bleeding time studies to rule out coagulopathy
3. Other laboratory studies as indicated for suspected underlying diseases

F. Management[5, 6, 9–11, 17, 18]

1. Position the patient with head erect and elevated.
2. Provide reassurance.
3. Clear blood from nostrils.

   a. Remove clots with suctioning.
   b. Observe closely for foreign object.

4. Saturate a cotton ball with oxymetazoline (Afrin) and gently insert it into the site of the bleeding.
5. Apply gentle pressure by compressing the nasal alae together.
6. Examine nostril for bleeding site.
7. Apply topical Xylocaine anesthetic, then touch the site with a silver nitrate stick until the vessel ends are completely cauterized.
8. If unable to cauterize, insert nasal packing.
9. If the bleeding is uncontrollable or from a posterior site, consult an ear, nose, and throat specialist.

   • Posterior bleeding can be difficult to control and may require surgical intervention.

XIII. SINUSITIS

A. Definition[2, 4, 16]

1. Infection/inflammation of the paranasal sinus mucous membrane
2. May be acute or chronic (occurring three or more times a year)

B. Etiology/Incidence/Predisposing factors[3, 4, 10]

1. Viruses cause one fifth of cases.
2. One to three percent of upper respiratory infections involve sinusitis.
3. Common organisms

   a. *Haemophilus influenzae*
   b. *Streptococcus pneumoniae*
   c. Various anaerobes

4. Recurrent disease may be due to irritants, allergens, or fungi.

5. Anatomic blockage of sinus openings
6. Nasal polyps, masses, or neoplasms
7. Prolonged nasal intubation and/or prolonged use of nasogastric tubes

C. Subjective findings[4, 6, 10, 12]

1. Pain/pressure over face, nose, cheeks, teeth (molars)
2. Often confused with toothache
3. Purulent/blood-tinged nasal drainage
4. Headache, increased pain in supine or bending positions, sense of "fullness" in the head
5. Nasal congestion
6. Generalized malaise

D. Physical examination findings[4, 6, 10, 12]

1. Fever
2. Localized tenderness over the sinuses
3. Facial edema
4. Swollen, reddened turbinates
5. May be nasal septal deviation
6. Foul smelling nasal or postnasal drainage

E. Laboratory/Diagnostic findings[9, 10, 12, 17, 18]

1. Sinus series reveals clouding or thickening of sinus cavity; may see air-fluid levels.
2. For chronic sinusitis and/or for hospitalized patients, a CT of sinuses is indicated.
3. In chronic manifestation, culture the drainage to determine the causative organism.

F. Management[8, 9, 17, 18]

1. Antibiotics

   a. Amoxicillin, clavulanate (Augmentin), 500 mg p.o. t.i.d. for 10–14 days
   b. Clarithromycin (Biaxin), 500 mg p.o. b.i.d. for 10–14 days
   c. Cefaclor (Ceclor), 250–500 mg p.o. t.i.d. for 10–14 days

2. Oral decongestants/antihistamines—Loratidine/pseudo-ephedrine (Claritin-D), one tablet p.o. q12–24h
3. Analgesics

   a. Acetaminophen (Tylenol), 650 mg p.o. q4h
   b. Propoxyphene/acetaminophen (Darvocet-N 100), one or two tablets p.o. q4–6h

XIV. PHARYNGITIS

A. Definition[2, 4, 16]

1. Inflammation of the pharynx

2. Usually associated with tonsillitis
3. Can be acute or chronic

B. Etiology/Incidence/Predisposing factors[3, 4, 10]

1. Viral

   a. Influenza A and B
   b. Adenovirus
   c. Epstein-Barr virus
   d. Enterovirus

2. Bacterial

   a. Group A beta-hemolytic streptococcus
   b. *Haemophilus influenzae*
   c. *Neisseria gonorrhoeae*
   d. *Chlamydia trachomatis*
   e. *Mycoplasma*

3. Fungal: *Candida albicans* is commonly seen in immunosuppressed patients.
4. Pharyngitis may be associated with

   a. Esophageal reflux
   b. Allergic rhinitis
   c. Sinusitis
   d. Thyroiditis
   e. Carcinoma

C. Subjective findings[2, 4, 12]

1. Sore or painful throat
2. Dysphagia
3. Fever/chills
4. Malaise/myalgia

D. Physical examination findings[4, 6, 10, 12]

1. Viral

   a. Edema of lymphoid tissue in the posterior oropharyngeal wall—Elevated oval islands
   b. Pale, boggy mucosae of the posterior pharynx
   c. Painful ulcers/blistering in oral cavity/pharynx

2. Streptococcal

   a. Bright red, edematous pharyngeal mucosa
   b. White or yellow exudate

3. Candidal

   a. Shiny, white, raised patches located on the
      i. Posterior pharynx

    ii. Tongue

    iii. Buccal mucosa

  b. Patches may have erythematous rims.

4. Lymphadenopathy may be present with all types.

E. Laboratory/Diagnostic findings[9, 10, 12, 17, 18]

1. Throat culture to identify the offending pathogen
2. White blood cell and cell differential counts
3. Monospot test to rule out infectious mononucleosis

F. Treatment[5, 6, 9, 14, 17, 18]

1. Benzathine penicillin (Bicillin L-A), 1.2 million units IM single dose, *or* penicillin V (Pen-Vee K), 250 mg p.o. t.i.d for 7–10 days.
2. Erythromycin (ERYC, E-Mycin) may be given to patients with penicillin sensitivity.
3. Doxycycline (Vibramycin), 100 mg p.o. b.i.d. for 7 days
4. Consider corticosteroids such as dexamethasone (Decadron LA), 8 mg IM, or Medrol Dosepak tapering dose.
5. Consider antiulcers for gastric reflux.

  a. Ranitidine (Zantac), 150 mg p.o. b.i.d.

  b. Lansoprazole (Prevacid) 30 mg p.o. q.d.

6. Analgesics as needed, such as acetaminophen (Tylenol), 650 mg p.o. q4h
7. For *Candida*

  a. Nystatin (Mycostatin), swish and swallow q.i.d., or

  b. Fluconazole (Diflucan), 200 mg p.o. initially, then 100 mg daily for at least 2 weeks

XV. EPIGLOTTITIS

A. Definition[2, 4, 6, 16]

1. Inflammation of the mucous membrane of the epiglottis
2. A life-threatening condition
3. Swelling of the laryngeal entrance obstructs the air flow to and from the lungs.

B. Etiology/Incidence/Predisposing factors[3, 4, 6, 10]

1. Commonly caused by *Haemophilus influenzae* infection
2. Seen more often in males
3. Recent upper airway infection

C. Subjective findings[4, 6, 10, 12, 17, 18]

1. Change in voice
2. Dysphagia
3. Dyspnea

D. Physical examination findings[4, 6, 10, 12]

1. Anxious—The patient may appear exhausted or lethargic.
2. High fever—Greater than 101.3°F
3. Stridor
4. ''Tripod'' position preferred—Mouth held slightly open with neck slightly extended
5. Drooling
6. Do *not* examine the pharynx until

   a. Lateral soft tissue x-rays have been obtained and
   b. Emergency airway equipment is available (to prevent or treat laryngospasm).

7. Substernal retractions

E. Laboratory/Diagnostic findings[7, 10, 12, 17, 18]

1. Lateral soft-tissue neck x-ray (taken with caution) reveals a swollen epiglottis that is posteriorly displaced.
2. CT scan of the neck may be needed.
3. Arterial blood gas analysis
4. Chest x-ray
5. Complete blood cell count
6. Direct laryngoscopy by a specialist

F. Treatment[6, 10, 12, 17, 18]

1. *Consult an otolaryngologist and an anesthesiologist immediately.*
2. Protect the airway.

   • Airway access may be best obtained in the operating room with administration of anesthesia.

3. Prepare for possible surgical opening of the airway.
4. Agents active against *H. influenzae*

   a. Ampicillin (Omnipen-N), 1–2g IV q4–6h
   b. Ceftriaxone (Rocephin), 1–2g IV q12–24h
   c. Cefotaxime (Claforan), 1–2g IV q4–6h, *or*
   d. Cefuroxime (Zinacef), 0.75–1.5 g IV q8h

XVI. TEMPOROMANDIBULAR JOINT DISORDER

A. Definition[16]

A group of symptoms involving pain of the temporomandibular joint (TMJ), decreased range of motion, and jaw clicking, especially with chewing

B. Etiology/Incidence/Predisposing factors[2, 3, 14]

1. Rheumatoid arthritis
2. TMJ synovitis
3. Trauma

4. Ill-fitting dentures
5. Intra-articular disk disease
6. Approximately half of the population is affected although most are untreated.
7. Oromandibular dysfunction

C. Subjective findings[2, 3, 17]

1. TMJ pain
2. TMJ clicking or popping with movement
3. Headache
4. Jaw locking/spasm of masseter muscles
5. Earache

D. Physical examination findings[3, 17]

1. TMJ tenderness
2. TMJ click with range of motion
3. Cervical or cranial tenderness
4. Dental malocclusion
5. Dental erosion from bruxism (teeth grinding)

E. Laboratory/Diagnostic findings[3, 14]

1. In advanced cases, consider x-rays of the TMJ, which may demonstrate bone abnormalities.
2. CT, MRI, and arthrography all may demonstrate soft tissue and bony changes at an earlier stage than x-rays.
3. A positive test for rheumatoid arthritis factor (RAF) may rule out a diagnosis of TMJ disorder.

F. Management[3, 5, 14]

1. NSAIDs

   a. Ibuprofen, 200–600 mg q.i.d. for 5 days
   b. Naproxen, 500 mg p.o. initially, followed by 250 mg p.o. t.i.d.–q.i.d.
   c. Oxaprozin, 600–1200 mg p.o. q.d.

2. Local heat as needed
3. Soft diet
4. Consider referral for surgery in severe conditions.
5. Consider referral for trigger point anesthesia and/or arthroscopy.

XVII. TRIGEMINAL NEURALGIA (Tic Douloureux)

A. Definition[2, 3]

1. Neuralgia (pain, pressure) along the fifth cranial nerve
2. The trigeminal nerve arises from the pons and is a mixed nerve with many branches.
3. Symptoms depend on the branch affected.

B. Etiology/Incidence/Predisposing factors[2, 3, 16]

1. Idiopathic
2. Surgery and autopsy suggest a compressive etiology.
3. Affects 16 out of 100,000 persons annually.
4. Both genders are affected, but most sources note a female preference.
5. Increased incidence after age 50
6. Pain occurs in paroxysms and may last for hours.
7. The right side is most often affected.
8. May be triggered by ordinary events such as brushing the teeth, chewing, and exposure to wind and/or cold

C. Subjective findings[2, 3, 16, 17]

1. Intense bouts of pain along the affected track
2. Symptoms tend to be unilateral.
3. Intractable lip, cheek, gum or facial pain
4. Pain described as "lightening flashes"
5. Facial flushing
6. Salivation
7. Headache

D. Physical examination findings[2, 3, 13, 17]

1. Usually the neurologic examination is normal.
2. Occasionally, a sensory defect is found in cranial nerve V.

E. Laboratory/Diagnostic findings[3, 13, 17]

1. CT to rule out neoplasm
2. MRI for cranial nerve V abnormalities

F. Management[2, 3, 5, 13, 17]

1. Carbamazepine (Tegretol), 100–1200 mg/day (monitor liver enzymes and serum drug levels)
2. If the patient is unable to tolerate carbamazepine: Phenytoin, 200–400 mg/day.
3. Adjunctive therapy with baclofen, 5–20 mg t.i.d.–q.i.d. (maximum dose: 80 mg/day)
4. Consider surgical consultation for possible exploration in patients who fail to respond to pharmacologic management.
5. Recently, posterior fossa exploration has revealed anomalous vascular structures resulting in nerve compression. Relief of symptoms has occurred with decompression and release.

References

1. Andreoli, T., Bennett, J., Carpenter, C., & Plum, F. (1997). *Cecil Essentials of Medicine* (4th ed.). Philadelphia: W.B. Saunders.
2. Berdow, R., & Beers, M. (1999). *Merck manual* (17th ed.). Rahway, NJ: Merck & Co., Inc.

3. Dambro, M.R. (1997). *Griffith's 5 minute clinical consult.* Media, PA: Williams & Wilkins.

4. DeGowin, R.L. (1994). *Diagnostic examination* (6th ed). New York: McGraw-Hill.

5. DiGregorio, J.G., & Barbieri, E.J. (1999). *Handbook of commonly prescribed drugs* (14th ed.). West Chester, PA: Medical Surveillance Inc.

6. Emergency Nurses Association. *Emergency nursing core curriculum* (4th ed) (1994). Philadelphia: W.B. Saunders.

7. Ferri, F. (1999). *Ferri's clinical advisor* (1st ed.). St. Louis: Mosby.

8. Hektor Dunphy, L. (1999). *Management guidelines for adult nurse practitioners.* Philadelphia: F.A. Davis.

9. Hoole, A.J., Tickard, C.G., Ouimette, R., Lohr, J.A., (1999). *Patient care guidelines for nurse practitioners* (5th ed.). Philadelphia: J.B. Lippincott.

10. Kelley, W.N. (1994). *Essentials of internal medicine.* Philadelphia: J.B. Lippincott.

11. Lanros, N., & Barber, J. (1997). *Emergency Nursing.* Stamford, CT: Appleton & Lange.

12. Millonig, V.L. (1999). *Adult nurse practitioner certification review guide* (3rd ed). Potomac, MD: Health Leadership Associates, Inc.

13. Rakel, R.E. (1995). *Rakel textbook of family practice* (5th ed.). Philadelphia: W.B. Saunders.

14. Rakel, R.E. (1996). *Saunders manual of medical practice.* Philadelphia: W.B. Saunders.

15. Tarascon (1999). *Pocket pharmacopoeia.* Loma Linda, CA: Tarascon Publishing.

16. Thomas, C.L. (1996). *Taber's cyclopedic medical dictionary* (18th ed). Philadelphia: F.A. Davis Co.

17. Tierney, L.M., McPhee, S.J., & Papadakis, M.A. (2000). *Current medical diagnosis & treatment* (39th ed.). Stamford, CT: Appleton & Lange.

18. Uphold, C.R., & Graham, M.V. (1999). *Clinical guidelines in family practice.* Gainesville, FL: Barmarrae Books.

HEADACHE

Sylvia R. Love, MED, MSN, RN, CS, ACNP, ANP

I. HEADACHE

A. Definition[8, 11]

1. The subjective sensation of pain involving the scalp, cranium, or cerebrum, with or without associated symptoms
2. Head pain may be explained as a result of distortion, stretching, inflammation, or destruction of pain-sensitive nerve endings.

B. Etiology/Predisposing factors[1, 8, 11–13]

1. Most common headaches are benign.

   a. Ninety percent may be attributed to vascular, tension, or other causes.
   b. Ten percent are secondary to organic disorders.

2. About one third of patients with brain tumors present with chief complaint of headache.
3. Headache ranks ninth among causes of office visits.
4. Headaches are an almost universal symptom.
5. Headache occurs at any age but primarily during the peak productive years of ages 25–55 for both men and women.
6. Three categories of headaches[12]

   a. Acute new-onset headaches or uniquely severe headaches may be caused by
      i. Acute angle-closure glaucoma
      ii. Infection
      iii. Central nervous system mass lesion
         (1) Hemorrhage
         (2) Abscess
         (3) Tumor
      iv. Metabolic causes
      v. Benign causes, e.g.
         (1) Hangover
         (2) Caffeine withdrawal
         (3) Eyestrain
      vi. Subarachnoid hemorrhage
   b. Intermittent discrete headaches may be caused by
      i. Cervical spondylosis
      ii. Pseudotumor cerebri

iii. Tic douloureux

iv. Central nervous system mass lesions (as in the preceding section)

c. Chronic persistent headaches may result from the same causes as intermittent discrete headaches.

7. Danger signals in headache[12]
For danger signals in headache, see Table 71–1.

8. Critical causes of acute headaches[12]
For critical causes of acute headaches, see Table 71–2.

9. Management of subarachnoid hemorrhage[8]
For management of subarachnoid hemorrhage, see Table 71–3.

10. International Headache Society classification[12]
For the International Headache Society classification of headaches, see Table 71–4.

C. Subjective findings[1, 6, 11, 13]

1. Obtain the individual's headache attack profile.

a. Prodromal symptoms (preceding the headache)
b. Time of peak severity of symptoms
c. Duration of symptoms
d. Precipitating factors
e. Associated symptoms
f. Alleviating symptoms

2. Obtain the history of prior headaches.

a. Variables (as in the headache attack profile)
b. Family history of headaches

TABLE 71–1. DANGER SIGNALS IN HEADACHE

DANGER SIGNALS	POSSIBLE CAUSES
Headache during exertion/straining	Leaking berry aneurysm, increased ICP
Headache with fever	Meningitis, encephalitis
Headache when neck is not perfectly supple	Meningitis, encephalitis
Headache in a drowsy, confused patient	Increased ICP (encephalitis, meningitis, metabolic)
Headache with abnormal examination (pupil size, fundus, EOM reactivity, facial asymmetry, reflexes)	Subdural
Headache in a patient who looks ill	Critical causes

ICP, intracranial pressure; EOM, extraocular movement
(From Reddy, M.J. [1996]. Headache. In R.E. Rakel [Ed.], *Saunders manual of medical practice* [p. 1031]. Philadelphia: W.B. Saunders, with permission.)

TABLE 71-2. CRITICAL CAUSES OF ACUTE HEADACHE

CAUSE	ADVERSE OUTCOMES	SIGNS	DIAGNOSTIC TESTS
Acute angle-closure glaucoma	Blindness	Ocular HTN, dilated pupils, eye pain	Ocular HTN, C/D ratio in fundus
Temporal arteritis	Blindness	Tenderness, temporal area, older patient >50, signs of polymyalgia	Sedimentation rate (>50), temporal arteritis biopsy, at least 5 cm required
Meningitis	Increased morbidity and mortality	Nuchal rigidity, fever, Kernig's, Brudzinsky's signs	LP, rapid antibiotic therapy
CVA	Mortality, neurologic deficits	Neurologic signs	Clinical or radiologic
CNS mass lesion: tumor, abscess	Mortality, neurologic deficits	Papilledema, mental status change	CT scan/MRI
Subarachnoid hemorrhage	Mortality, neurologic deficits	Worst ever	CT scan/LP
Malignant HTN	End-organ damage	Papilledema, elevated blood pressure systolic >210, diastolic >120	Vital signs, funduscopy, UA micro, ECG, cardiologic examination
Pheochromocytoma	End-organ damage	Classic presentation	CT of adrenals, urinary metanephrines
Toxic exposure	—	Confusion, nausea	See env/occ chart
HIV	Increased morbidity	HIV risks, opportunistic infections: cryptosporidiosis, CMV, toxoplasmosis	HIV test, LP, CT/MRI
Acute sinusitis	Intracranial extension	Fever, toxic, sinus tenderness	Sinus radiographs, CT

HTN, hypertension; C/D, cup to disk; LP, lumbar puncture; CVA, cerebrovascular accident; CNS, central nervous system; UA, urinalysis; ECG, electrocardiogram; CMV, cytomegalovirus

(From Reddy, M.J. [1996]. Headache. In R.E. Rakel [Ed.], *Saunders manual of medical practice* [p. 1028]. Philadelphia, W.B. Saunders, with permission.)

TABLE 71–3. SUMMARY OF
SUBARACHNOID HEMORRHAGE

Etiology	Craniocerebral trauma
	Cerebral aneurysm rupture
	Cerebral arteriovenous malformation
	Clotting abnormalities
Signs and Symptoms	"Worst headache of my life" with sudden onset, no precipitating factors, no relief with OTC analgesia
	Altered consciousness
	Mental status changes
	Stiff neck
	Nausea and vomiting
	Photophobia
	Seizures
	Cranial nerve abnormalities
	Motor or sensory deficits
Diagnosis	If you suspect an SAH, the first test to obtain is a CT scan of the brain. If negative, a lumbar puncture must be obtained to look for the presence of blood.
	Routine serum blood work includes CBC, BUN, creatinine, glucose, electrolytes, PT, aPTT.
	Upon diagnosis of SAH and in the absence of cranial trauma, a cerebral angiogram is required to ascertain the source of the bleeding.
Treatment	The goals of treatment are to prevent rebleed and prevent secondary complications (most commonly hydrocephalus and cerebral vasospasm).
	"Triple H therapy" to prevent vasospasm:
	Hypertension to SBP = 150
	Hemodilution to hematocrit 31–33 mL/dL
	Hypervolemia which aids in maintaining blood pressure and hematocrit in desired ranges
	Routine medications include:
	Colace, 100 mg p.o. b.i.d.
	Codeine, 30–60 mg SC q4h as needed
	Nimodipine (Nimotop), 60 mg p.o. q4h for 21 days
	Phenobarbital, 30–60 mg p.o./SC q6h as needed for sedation
	Dilantin, 100 mg p.o. t.i.d. (although the use of anticonvulsants as seizure prophylaxis is controversial)
	SAH precautions include
	Dimly lit, quiet, private room
	No stress, limited visitors
	Complete bed rest
	Avoid Valsalva maneuver—Straining to have bowel movement, coughing

OTC, over-the-counter; SAH, subarachnoid hemorrhage; CT, computed tomography; CBC, complete blood count; BUN, blood urea nitrogen; PT, prothrombin time; aPTT, activated partial thromboplastin time; SBP, systolic blood pressure.

(From Keiser, M.M. [1999]. Neurologic disorders. In A. Gawlinski & D. Hamwi [Eds.], *Acute care nurse practitioner: Clinical curriculum and certification review* [p. 299]. Philadelphia: W.B. Saunders, with permission.)

TABLE 71–4. INTERNATIONAL HEADACHE
SOCIETY CLASSIFICATION

PRIMARY CODE	HEADACHE TYPE
1	Migraine
2	Tension-type headache
3	Cluster headache and chronic paroxysmal hemicrania
4	Miscellaneous headache unassociated with structural lesion
5	Headache associated with head trauma
6	Headache associated with vascular disorders
7	Headache associated with nonvascular intracranial disorder
8	Headache associated with substances or withdrawal
9	Headache associated with noncephalic infection
10	Headache associated with metabolic disorder
11	Headache or facial pain associated with disorder of face/cranium
12	Cranial neuralgias
13	Headache not classifiable

(From Reddy, M.J. [1996]. Headache. In R.E. Rakel [Ed.], *Saunders manual of medical practice* [p. 1029]. Philadelphia, W.B. Saunders, with permission.)

   c. Correlation or relationship of headaches to particular events/activities

D. Physical findings[1-3, 7, 11, 13, 14]

1. No gold standard exists for diagnosis of the more common headache categories; diagnosis is based on clinical assessment.
2. Criteria for diagnosis of migraine without aura

   a. Duration of 4–72 h
   b. Two of the following:
      i. Unilateral location—Can be generalized
      ii. Pulsating quality
      iii. Moderate to severe intensity
      iv. Aggravation by routine physical activity
   c. At least one of the following:
      i. Nausea and/or vomiting
      ii. Photophobia and phonophobia
   d. At least five attacks fulfilling criteria listed in a, b, and c, preceding
   e. No evidence of organic disease

3. Criteria for diagnosis of migraine with aura

   a. Pain is preceded by at least one of the following neurologic symptoms:

i. Visual: Combination of field defects and luminous visual hallucinations
    (1) Scintillating scotoma
    (2) Fortification spectra
    (3) Unformed light flashes—photopsia
ii. Sensory
    (1) Paresthesia
    (2) Numbness
    (3) Clumsiness
    (4) Weakness in a circumscribed area
    (5) Speech disturbance
b. No evidence of organic disease

4. Criteria for diagnosis of tension-type headache

a. At least two of the following:
    i. Pressing/tightening (nonpulsating) quality
    ii. Bilateral
    iii. Not aggravated by routine physical activity
b. Both of the following:
    i. No nausea or vomiting
    ii. Photophobia and phonophobia absent or only one present
c. No evidence of organic disease

5. Criteria for diagnosis of cluster headache

a. Severe unilateral, orbital, supraorbital, and/or temporal pain lasting 15–180 min
b. At least one of the following on the headache side:
    i. Reddened conjunctiva
    ii. Facial sweating
    iii. Lacrimation
    iv. Miosis
    v. Nasal congestion
    vi. Ptosis

E. Management of common headaches[8]

For management of common headaches, see Table 71–5.

F. Additional agents[2, 4, 5]

1. Triptans should be used only in patients who are not at risk for coronary disease.

a. Zolmitriptan (Zomig): For acute migraines with or without aura
    i. Initially give 2.5 mg or lower p.o.; increase to 5 mg per dose as needed.
    ii. A second dose may be administered 2 h after the initial dose if the headache returns.

TABLE 71-5. MANAGEMENT OF COMMON HEADACHE SYNDROMES*

HEADACHE SYNDROME	PHARMACOLOGIC MANAGEMENT	NONPHARMACOLOGIC MANAGEMENT
Tension	Acetaminophen Aspirin NSAIDs	Supportive care to monitor stress levels and coping mechanisms. Lifestyle modification (e.g., weight loss, cessation of substance abuse, nutritional diet) has shown to decrease episodes in frequent headache sufferers. Follow-up in 2 weeks to monitor progress. Consultation with a physician if conservative treatment fails or clinical depression is suspected.
Migraine	*Acute attack* (must be taken at onset of symptoms or aura to be effective) Sumatriptan (Imitrex), 6 mg SC, may repeat in 1 hour as needed—No more than two doses/day. Cafergot (ergotamine maleate 1 mg + caffeine 100 mg), 1–2 tablets, may repeat 1 tablet q30min up to 6 tablets (if attack includes nausea/vomiting, Cafergot suppositories, ergotamine tartrate inhalers [0.36 mg per puff], and ergotamine SL 2-mg tablets are available) Dihydroergotamine mesylate (DHE 45), 0.5–1 mg IV or 1–2 mg SC/IM, repeat q1h as needed to maximum of 3 mg	Diet counseling—See Table 71-6. Lifestyle modification (i.e., weight loss, smoking cessation, nutritional diet) has shown to decrease episodes in frequent migraine sufferers. During attacks, patient should stay in a dark, quiet environment and rest. Warm baths may help patient to relax. Follow-up at regular intervals to assess effectiveness of treatment (initially every 2 weeks for 2 months, then every month for 6 months, and as needed if treatment successful). Consultation with physician if patient does not respond to traditional management or condition worsens.

Table continued on following page

701

TABLE 71–5. MANAGEMENT OF COMMON HEADACHE SYNDROMES* *Continued*

HEADACHE SYNDROME	PHARMACOLOGIC MANAGEMENT	NONPHARMACOLOGIC MANAGEMENT
	Midrin (a combination drug containing isometheptene mucate 65 mg, dichloralphenazone 100 mg, acetaminophen 325 mg), 2 tablets p.o., may repeat q1h until relief, maximum of 5 tablets/day	
	Prophylaxis (should be considered if patients have attacks more than two or three times per month)	
	Aspirin, 650–1950 mg/day	
	Propranolol (Inderal), 80–240 mg/day	
	Imipramine (Tofranil), 10–150 mg/day	
	Ergonovine maleate, 0.6–2 mg/day	
	Cyproheptadine (Periactin), 12–20 mg/day	
	Clonidine (Catapres), 0.2–0.6 mg/day	
	Methysergide (Sansert), 4–8 mg/day	
	Verapamil (Calan), 80–160 mg/day	
Cluster	*Acute attack*	Lifestyle modification and supportive care are of limited benefit for these patients, as there are few known precipitating factors for a bout of attacks.
	Sumatriptan (Imitrex), 6 mg SC (see above)	
	Dihydroergotamine mesylate (DHE 45), 1–2 mg SC/IM (see above)	

Ergotamine tartrate aerosol (0.36 mg/puff)—up to 6 puffs/attack

100% oxygen inhalation (7 L/min for 15 min)

Butorphanol tartrate nasal spray (Stadol NS), 10 mg/mL—one spray in one nostril, repeat q3–4h

Prophylaxis

Ergotamine tartrate
   Suppository 0.5–1 mg at bedtime or b.i.d.
   Orally 2 mg/day
   Subcutaneous 0.25 mg t.i.d. 5 days a week
Propranolol (Inderal), 80–240 mg/day
Amitriptyline (Elavil), 10–150 mg/day
Cyproheptadine (Periactin), 12–20 mg/day
Methysergide (Sansert), 4–6 mg/day
Verapamil (Calan), 240–480 mg/day
Lithium carbonate (Eskalith), 150–600 mg/day
Prednisone, 20–40 mg q.d.–q.o.d. for 2 weeks followed by gradual withdrawal

During a bout, some patients report that alcohol, stress, glare, or ingestion of certain foods will precipitate an attack, but this is highly individual—patients are certainly advised to avoid anything that they feel worsens their condition.

Follow-up at regular intervals during treatment; spacing of visits will vary depending on the patient's pattern of remissions and bouts.

---

* In the management of all headaches, narcotic or addictive medications should be avoided, as these patients have a tendency to overmedicate due to the duration of symptoms.

NSAIDs, nonsteroidal anti-inflammatory drugs.

(From Keiser, M.M. [1999]. Neurologic disorders. In A. Gawlinski & D. Hamwi [Eds.], *Acute care nurse practitioner: Clinical curriculum and certification review* [pp. 300–301]. Philadelphia: W.B. Saunders, with permission.)

      iii. Maximum dose: 10 mg/24 h

      iv. Highly effective in menstrual migraine

  b. Rizatriptan (Maxalt, Maxalt-MLT): For acute migraines with or without aura

      i. Available in regular tablet or rapidly dissolving form

      ii. In acute migraine, give 5–10 mg p.o.

      iii. May repeat in 2 h if necessary.

      iv. Maximum dose: 30 mg/24 h

      v. Patients also on propranolol (Inderal) should use 5 mg, with maximum 15 mg/24 h.

  c. Naratriptan (Amerge): For acute migraines with or without aura

      i. Lasts longer; good for prolonged attacks

      ii. In acute migraine, give 1–2.5 mg p.o.; may repeat in 4 h if necessary.

      iii. Maximum dose: 5 mg/24 h

      iv. Patients with mild or moderate renal or hepatic impairment should not exceed 2.5 mg/24 h.

  d. The various triptans are similarly effective. If one does not work, another may.

2. A stratified approach for pharmacologic management is recommended.

  a. Start low and build up slowly with a course or full trial lasting 1–2 months.

  b. Such an approach allows the patient to choose among several treatment options, depending on the severity of the attack.

TABLE 71–6. FOOD/FOOD ADDITIVE PRECIPITANTS OF MIGRAINE

SUBSTANCE	MAJOR FOOD SOURCE
Nitrates/nitrites	Reddened (colored with additives) meats (e.g., hot dogs)
Phenylethylamines (e.g., tyramine)	Aged cheeses, red and blush wines, champagne, chocolates, certain nuts
Monosodium glutamate (MSG)	Many prepared foods, Oriental foods
Caffeine (by withdrawal)	Coffee, tea, sodas, and cola beverages
Other	Fruits, dairy products, shellfish

(From Stevens, M.B. [1996]. Migraine headache. In R.E. Rakel [Ed.], *Saunders manual of medical practice* [pp. 1032–1033]. Philadelphia: W.B. Saunders, with permission.)

3. Consider[9]

   a. Administering tricyclic antidepressants if depression is associated with headaches
      i. The patient may see improvement without evidence of depression.
      ii. Use standard dosing.
   b. Avoid calcium channel blockers in patients of childbearing age (these drugs may induce infertility).

G. Food/food additive precipitants of migraine[13]

For foods and food additives that may preciptate migraine, see Table 71–6.

References

1. Aminoff, M.J. (1997). Nervous system. In L.M. Tierney, Jr., S.J. McPhee, & M.A. Papadakis (Eds.), *Current medical diagnosis & treatment* (36th ed.) (pp. 892–948). Stamford, CT: Appleton & Lange.
2. Bartleson, J.D. (1999). Treatment of migraine headaches: Concise review for clinicians. *Mayo Clinic Proceedings, 74*, 702–708.
3. Bruehl, S., Lofland, K.R., Semenchuk, E.M., Rokicki, L.A., & Penzien, D.B. (1999). Use of cluster analysis to validate IHS diagnostic criteria for migraine and tension-type headache. *Headache, 39*, 181–189.
4. Ferrari, M.D. (1999). Rizatriptan: A new milestone in migraine treatment. *Headache, 39* (Suppl 1), 1.
5. Goadsby, P.J. (1999). Understanding migraine pathophysiology through studying the mechanism of action of rizatriptan. *Headache, 39* (Suppl 2), 2–8.
6. Graham, J. R. (1996). Headaches. In J. Noble (Ed.), *Textbook of primary care medicine* (2nd ed.) (pp. 1283–1319). St. Louis: Mosby.
7. Green, M.W. (1999, June). Migraine: Effective management in the female patient. In American Academy of Nurse Practitioners 1999 National Conference, Atlanta, GA.
8. Keiser, M.M. (1999). Neurologic disorders. In A. Gawlinski & D. Hamwi (Eds.), *Acute care nurse practitioner: Clinical curriculum and certification review* (pp. 295–304). Philadelphia: W.B. Saunders.
9. Landy, S., McGinnis, J., Curlin, D., & Laizure, S.C. (1999). Selective serotonin reuptake inhibitors for migraine prophylaxis. *Headache, 39*, 28–32.
10. Plum, F., & Posner, J.B. (1997). Disorders of sensory function. In T.E. Andreoli, J.C. Bennett, C.J. Carpenter, & F. Plum (Eds.). *Cecil essentials of medicine* (4th ed.) (pp. 818–824). Philadelphia: W.B. Saunders.
11. Posner, J.B. (1996). Disorders of sensation. In J.C. Bennett & F. Plum (Eds.). *Cecil textbook of medicine* (20th ed.) (pp. 2030–2036). Philadelphia: W.B. Saunders.
12. Reddy, M.J. (1996). Headache. In R.E. Rakel (Ed.). *Saunders manual of medical practice*. (pp. 1028–1031). Philadelphia: W.B. Saunders.
13. Stevens, M.B. (1996). Migraine headache. In R.E. Rakel (Ed.). *Saunders manual of medical practice*. (pp. 1032–1033). Philadelphia: W.B. Saunders.
14. Torelli, P., Cologno, D., & Manzoni, G.C. (1999). Weekend headache: A retrospective study in migraine without aura and episodic tension-type headache. *Headache, 39*, 11–20.

Common Problems in Acute Care

FEVER

Amy E. Sayler, MSN, RN, CS, ACNP

I. FEVER

A. Definition[2, 4]

1. An increase in body temperature above normal limits (normal body temperature: 36–37.8°C or 98.6°F), which is induced by the regulatory processes of the nervous system
2. The elevated body temperature is attributed to an increase in internal heat production as well as to a decrease in the loss of heat.
3. The monitoring of body temperature is routinely used to determine the presence or absence of infection.

B. Cause[4]

1. Endogenous and exogenous pyrogens stimulate the release of prostaglandins, which then act on the hypothalamus to increase body temperature.
2. The primary source of pyrogenic cytokines is phagocytic monocytes or macrophages.

   a. Disease processes such as infections, tumors, and immunologic reactions cause the secretion of pyrogenic cytokines from macrophages.
   b. It is important to note that many different diseases follow the same final pathway to the diagnosis of fever.
   c. This fact is important when considering fever of unknown origin as the diagnosis.

C. Other causes for increased body temperature[1, 4]

1. Exercise
2. Heat stroke
3. Malignant hyperthermia: A rare hereditary disease that occurs in association with general anesthesia
4. Neuroleptic malignant syndrome: A syndrome associated with antipsychotic drugs such as haloperidol (Haldol)

II. FEVER OF UNKNOWN ORIGIN (FUO)

A. Definition[4]

1. Fever of at least 3 weeks' duration, which makes the presence of a self-limiting disease unlikely
2. The patient must have been carefully examined and have had laboratory work and a chest x-ray to rule out other causes.

3. Fever should be significant on several occasions (above 101°F).

B. Causes[4]

1. Factitious fever

    a. Occurs in patients who are about to undergo extensive or invasive procedures

    b. Most common among young people in the health professions

    c. Consider the presence of psychiatric problems.

2. Infections

    a. Bacterial diseases

        i. Abscesses

           (1) Most commonly located intra-abdominally

           (2) Must be considered in patients with FUO

        ii. Tuberculosis: Infections that tend to manifest as FUO occur in

           (1) Kidneys

           (2) Female genitalia

           (3) Mesenteric lymph nodes

        iii. Hepatobiliary infections

           (1) Causes of FUO include

               (a) Acute cholecystitis

               (b) Bacterial hepatitis

           (2) Alkaline phosphatase levels are high in these patients.

        iv. Urinary tract infection (UTI): Rarely causes FUO

        v. Endocarditis

           (1) Rarely causes FUO

           (2) Failure to diagnose may be owing to

               (a) Lack of heart murmur

               (b) Negative blood cultures

        vi. Osteomyelitis

        vii. Other bacterial diseases

           (1) Brucellosis is the most important bacterial cause.

           (2) Common cause of FUO in Latin America and the Mediterranean region

    b. Viral diseases

        i. Herpesvirus

           (1) Cytomegalovirus and Epstein-Barr virus can cause prolonged febrile illnesses.

           (2) Lymph node enlargement may be minimal and missed on examination.

        ii. HIV

           (1) Prolonged fever may be caused by

               (a) Opportunistic infections

          (b) Lymphomas
          (c) HIV itself
      (2) Imaging studies are needed.
  c. Other infectious causes
      i. Fungi: Antibiotics, immunosuppression, and intravascular devices expose patients to opportunistic fungi such as *Candida*.
      ii. Parasites
          (1) Toxoplasmosis should be considered.
          (2) It may be difficult to diagnose because of the slight lymph node enlargement.
          (3) Rising IgM levels confirm the diagnosis.
      iii. *Chlamydia: Chlamydia psittaci* infection should be considered in patients who have a history of contact with birds.
      iv. Rickettsia

3. Neoplastic diseases

  a. Lymphomas
      i. Both Hodgkin's and non-Hodgkin's lymphomas cause
          (1) Fever
          (2) Night sweats
          (3) Weight loss
      ii. Diagnosis may be delayed if tumor is difficult to detect.
  b. Malignant histiocytosis: Associated with
      i. High fevers
      ii. Night sweats
      iii. Weight loss
  c. Leukemias
      i. Bone marrow aspirate alone may not reveal the proper diagnosis.
      ii. Bone marrow biopsy is necessary.
  d. Solid tumors
      i. Hypernephroma is the most common tumor associated with FUO.
      ii. Myxoma
          (1) Rare tumor of the heart
          (2) Patients have
              (a) High erythrocyte sedimentation rate
              (b) Anemia
      iii. These rare tumors are easily detected by echocardiogram.

4. Collagen, vascular, and autoimmune diseases

  a. Systemic lupus erythematosus
  b. Rheumatoid arthritis
  c. Rheumatic fever

5. Granulomatous diseases

   a. Giant cell arteritis
      i. Occurs in people over age 60
      ii. Signs and symptoms include
         (1) Headache
         (2) Tender temporal arteries
      iii. Patients have
         (1) Anemia
         (2) High erythrocyte sedimentation rate
   b. Regional enteritis: Crohn's disease is the most common gastrointestinal cause of FUO.
   c. Sarcoidosis: Sarcoidosis should be considered in the presence of fever and malaise without lymph node or pulmonary involvement.
   d. Granulomatous hepatitis
      i. In some patients, a specific diagnosis cannot be found.
      ii. Elevated alkaline phosphatase levels are present.
   e. Idiopathic granulomatosis
      i. Etiology is unclear.
      ii. These granulomas involve multiple organs.
      iii. They are associated with fever and other nonspecific signs and symptoms.
      iv. Typical therapy involves treatment with corticosteroids.

6. Miscellaneous causes

   a. Inherited diseases such as
      i. Mediterranean fever
      ii. Hypertriglyceridemia
      iii. Fabry's disease
   b. Drug fevers: Most often caused by drugs such as
      i. Quinidine
      ii. Procainamide
      iii. Methyldopa
      iv. Isoniazid

C. Diagnostic approach to FUO in adults[1, 3, 4]

1. History

   a. Collect information about symptoms involving all major organ systems.
   b. Observe for such general complaints as
      i. Weight loss
      ii. Chills
      iii. Fever
      iv. Night sweats
      v. Arthralgias
      vi. Myalgias

    c. Inquire about any previous surgery, including dental.

    d. Obtain any history of psychiatric disorders.

    e. Evaluate

        i. Family history

        ii. Immunization status

        iii. Recent travel

        iv. Nutrition

        v. Sexual history

        vi. Recreational habits

2. Physical examination

    a. Take the patient's temperature more than once.

    b. Be aware of

        i. Any new rashes

        ii. Abdominal tenderness

        iii. Cardiac murmurs

        iv. Lymph node enlargement

    c. Specific physical signs and symptoms of fever include:

        i. Flushed, warm skin

        ii. Diaphoresis

        iii. Tachypnea

        iv. Tachycardia

        v. Chills

        vi. Altered mental status

3. Basic laboratory tests and procedures

    a. Complete blood count (CBC): May show anemia or leukocytosis with a shift to the left

    b. Urinalysis (UA): To rule out UTI and tumors of the urinary tract

    c. Kidney and liver function studies

    d. Cultures that may be needed to determine source of infection

        i. Blood

        ii. Urine

        iii. Sputum

        iv. Stool

        v. Cerebrospinal fluid

        vi. Peritoneal fluid

        vii. Liver

        viii. Bone marrow

        ix. Lymph nodes

    e. Tuberculosis skin test

    f. Serologic tests

        i. For the most part, serologic tests are of limited diagnostic value.

        ii. They may be used to diagnose causes of FUO such as

            (1) Cytomegalovirus

            (2) Infectious mononucleosis

      (3) HIV

      (4) Chlamydial diseases

  g. An increased procalcitonin level usually follows fever.

      i. Measurement of procalcitonin may help in the early diagnosis of a bacterial infection.

      ii. However, this test has a decreased sensitivity in cases of gram-positive bacteremia.

  h. Imaging

      i. Chest x-ray or abdominal ultrasound

      ii. To look for tumors or abscesses

  i. CT scans

      i. Used if an ultrasound examination does not reveal anything in a patient with signs and symptoms suggestive of an intra-abdominal process

      ii. Intravenous pyelogram may be more sensitive in some instances.

      iii. Since there is no reason to perform both an MRI and a CT scan on these patients, an MRI is not recommended.

  j. Endoscopy

      i. To look for

        (1) Crohn's disease

        (2) Biliary tract diseases

        (3) Gastrointestinal tumors

      ii. A barium enema or upper gastrointestinal series may also be needed.

  k. Radionuclide studies

      i. Ventilation-perfusion scans are needed to diagnose a pulmonary embolus.

      ii. Some cases may require pulmonary angiography.

  l. Echocardiography: Helps to diagnose cardiac tumors or endocarditis

  m. Invasive procedures and biopsy are the final method of diagnosing a fever of unknown origin.

      i. Biopsies may be taken from enlarged, accessible lymph nodes or from the bone marrow.

      ii. An exploratory laparotomy may be indicated when noninvasive testing indicates an intra-abdominal process.

D. Treatment[2, 4, 5]

1. When caring for a critically ill patient who is febrile, the health care provider must determine whether or not to treat the fever.

  a. Fever may prove to be beneficial in some cases by increasing the host defense response.

b. However, studies show that fever is associated with increased cardiovascular demands and an increased metabolic rate.

c. Therefore, patients with congestive heart failure or coronary artery disease may not tolerate these increased demands, and should be treated.

2. If the caregiver determines that the fever should be treated, recommendations for therapy include:

a. Antibiotics rarely produce favorable results and may lead to superinfection or drug toxicity.

   i. However, in patients with persistent fever, amphotericin B, 0.3–1.5 mg/kg/day IV, is administered empirically to treat or prevent any hidden fungal infections.

   ii. Amphotericin B lipid complex, 5 mg/kg/day IV, is preferred over conventional amphotericin B because it is more effective in preventing breakthrough fungal infections and nephrotoxicity.

b. Corticosteroids are used as initial empiric therapy.

c. It is important to avoid continued fever, chills, and sweats.

   i. Cooling blankets are often used to treat fever in the critically ill, although there is little research to support this practice.

   ii. When using these blankets, cooler temperatures may not always be the most effective for promoting heat loss.

   iii. Colder temperatures have a tendency to decrease the blood flow to the skin, thus decreasing heat loss.

   iv. Also, patients are more comfortable when the blankets are set for a higher temperature.

   v. For extreme cases of hyperthermia, patients may be immersed in an ice water bath until their body temperature decreases to the normal range.

3. Antipyretic drug therapy

a. Acetaminophen, 500–1000 mg p.o. q4–6h as needed

   i. Critically ill patients have decreased GI function; consider this, as Acetaminophen is metabolized by the liver.

   ii. In addition, studies show that fever also decreases the function of the gastrointestinal system.

   iii. These two factors may contribute to an alteration in the pharmacokinetics of antipyretics such as acetaminophen.

   iv. Nevertheless, when rectal and gastric absorption were compared in a study, the plasma concentration was higher, and the peak concentration earlier, when

administration of acetaminophen was by nasogastric tube.
  b. NSAIDs (e.g., ibuprofen), 200–400 mg p.o. q4–6h as needed
    i. NSAIDs may be used.
    ii. However, the maximum change in temperature occurred earlier with acetaminophen than with ibuprofen.
  c. Aspirin, 650 mg p.o. q4–6h as needed

References

1. Davis, A.T. & Phair, J.P. (1997). Temperature regulation, the pathogenesis of fever, and the approach to the febrile patient. In S.T. Shulman, J.P. Phair, L.R. Peterson, & J.R. Warren (Eds.), *The biologic and clinical basis of infectious diseases* (5th ed.) (pp. 64–73). Philadelphia: W.B. Saunders.
2. Henker, R. (1999). Evidenced-based practice: Fever-related interventions. *American Journal of Critical Care, 8,* 481–489.
3. Ruokonen, E., Nousiainen, T., Pulkki, K., & Takala, J. (1999). Procalcitonin concentrations in patients with neutropenic fever. *European Journal of Clinical Microbiology Infectious Diseases, 18,* 283–285.
4. Tauber, M.G. (1998). Fever of unknown origin. In J.H. Stein, J.M. Eisenberg, J.J. Hutton, J.H. Klippel, P.O. Kohler, N.F. LaRusso, R.A. O'Rourke, H.Y. Reynolds, M.A. Samuels, M.A. Sande, & N.J. Zvaifler (Eds.), *Internal Medicine* (5th ed.) (pp. 1375–1380). St. Louis: Mosby.
5. Walsh, T.J., Finberg, R.W., Arndt, C., Hiemenz, J., Schwartz, C., Bodensteiner, D., Pappas, P., Seibel, N., Greenberg, R.N., Dummer, S., Schuster, M., & Holcenberg, J.S. (1999). Liposomal amphotericin B for empirical therapy in patients with persistent fever and neutropenia. *New England Journal of Medicine, 340,* 764–771.

PAIN

Alice S. Bohannon, PhD, ARNP,
and Sara C. Majors, PhD, CRNA

I. PAIN

A. Definition[3, 10]

1. Pain is a word used to describe a subjective perception of distress.
2. The physiologic process of pain begins with a series of neurologic steps beginning with stimulation of peripheral nerves and transmission through the spinal cord tracts to the brain where impulses are interpreted and experienced as pain.
3. Because pain historically has been undertreated, many new patient education publications have been developed that include a list of rights for patients with pain.

B. Types of pain[3, 6, 10]

1. Acute pain: Generally caused by tissue damage; duration is usually short (<6 months). This pain normally subsides with appropriate interventions and as healing or resolution of tissue damage occurs.
2. Chronic pain: Generally prolonged duration (>6 months) and may be continual or episodic; usually produces significant negative changes in an individual's life, and treatment aims at improving or stabilizing the patient's status. Frequent re-evaluation is required, and combination therapy is usually used.
3. Cancer pain: Most commonly caused by direct tumor involvement of sensory receptors in cutaneous and deep tissues. Pain decreases if there is a response to chemotherapy or radiation. Combination drug therapy (opioids and nonsteroidal anti-inflammatory drugs [NSAIDs] for bone pain) and surgery are useful for cancer pain. Low doses of tricyclic antidepressants may be helpful for neuropathic pain.

C. Pain location[4, 7, 10]

1. Cutaneous: Localized on skin or body surface
2. Visceral: Poorly localized, originating in internal organs
3. Somatic: Nonlocalized, originating in muscle, bone, nerves, blood vessels, and supporting tissue
4. Neuropathic (may be referred to as somatic): Specifically caused by nerve injury or spinal cord compression, frequently caused by a tumor

D. Subjective findings[3, 6, 11]

1. The most reliable indicator of the existence and intensity of acute pain is the patient's self-report; therefore, pain can be perceived only by the person experiencing it. Pain is what the experiencing person says it is.
2. Many times the experience of pain is expressed on a continuum from using descriptive words to moaning, groaning, facial grimacing, crying, and screaming.
3. Pain can be described in many ways: ranging from sharp knife-like pain to dull, prolonged pain.
4. Intensity can be mild to severe, or it can be constant or intermittent.
5. Psychological and cultural factors influence a person's interpretation and response to pain.

E. Physical examination findings[1, 2, 5]

1. Elevated heart rate, respiratory rate, and blood pressure (in particular systolic); temperature (over time); decreased O_2 saturation; guarding a particular area or tenderness to palpation; acute tissue damage, such as trauma, burns, or surgery

F. Diagnostic tests[7]

1. These tests may include complete blood count, electrolytes, biochemical tests for liver, kidney, and pancreatic function, electrocardiography, x-rays, ultrasound, upper/lower gastrointestinal series, magnetic resonance imaging, computed tomography, and biopsy.

G. Pain assessment[1, 3, 5, 10]

1. Comprehensive approach to pain assessment requires evaluation of the following:

   a. Patient's self-report
   b. Physiologic and behavioral responses

2. Consider asking the patient experiencing pain the following questions:

   a. What is the location of pain, intensity, quality of pain, onset, duration, variations or rhythms, manner of expressing pain?
   b. What relieves the pain and causes the pain?
   c. What effects has the pain had on your life?
   d. What other comments about your pain have not been discussed?

3. Three frequently used self-report pain assessment tools for use with adults and children are

   a. A numerical rating scale (NRS) (Fig. 73–1): Scales from 0–10 with 0 being "no pain" and 10 being "worst pain"

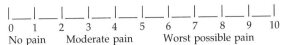

0   1   2   3   4   5   6   7   8   9   10

No pain   Moderate pain   Worst possible pain

Figure 73–1. 0–10 Numeric Pain Intensity Scale

    b. A visual analog scale (VAS) (Fig. 73–2): Pictures that show some visual representation of pain feelings
    c. An adjective rating scale (ARS) (Fig. 73–3): Descriptive words chosen by the patient to indicate type and intensity of pain

4. Pain should be assessed and documented

    a. Routinely and at regular intervals, as determined by the severity of pain
    b. A suitable interval after each analgesic intervention (30 min after parenteral drug therapy, and 1 h after oral analgesics)

H. Pain management[1–3, 5, 6, 8, 9, 11, 12, 14]

1. Each institution should develop the resources necessary to provide the best and most modern pain relief appropriate to its patients and should designate who and/or which departments are responsible for the required activities.
2. Optimal application of pain control methods depends on cooperation among different members of the health care team throughout the patient's course of treatment.
3. To ensure that this process occurs effectively, formal means must be developed and used within each institution to assess pain management practices and to obtain patient feedback to gauge the adequacy of pain control.
4. The institution's quality assurance procedures should be used periodically to assure that the following pain management practices are being carried out.

    a. Nonpharmacologic
       i. Relaxation
      ii. Biofeedback
     iii. Guided imagery
     iv. Music distraction
      v. Deep, slow, rhythmic breathing
     vi. Application of heat or cold
    vii. Massage

No pain   Pain as bad as it could possibly be

Figure 73–2. Visual Analog Scale (VAS)

|_____|_____|_____|_____|_____|
None   Mild   Moderate pain   Severe   Very severe   Worst possible pain

Figure 73–3. Simple Descriptive Pain Intensity Scale

    viii. Exercise
     ix. Immobilization
      x. Transcutaneous electrical nerve stimulation
  b. Pharmacologic (Fig. 73–4): Pain should be treated as type
    and severity of pain indicates, beginning with nonopioid
    analgesics and increasing to opioid analgesics. Adjuvant
    drug therapy may be added at the start of therapy.
     i. WHO analgesic ladder
       (1) Begin with nonopioid analgesics and an adjuvant
         (NSAIDs) (Table 73–1).
       (2) With persisting or increasing pain, add an opioid
         for mild to moderate pain plus adjuvant drugs
         (Table 73–2).

Text continued on page 728

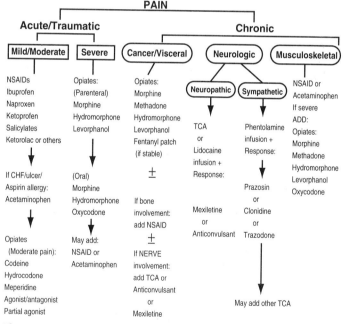

Figure 73–4. Medication section in the treatment of pain. (Redrawn from Reisner-Keller, L.A. [1996]. Pain management. In E.T. Herfindal & D.R. Gourley [Eds.], *Textbook of therapeutics: Drug and disease management* [6th ed.]. Baltimore: Williams & Wilkins, with permission.)

TABLE 73–1. DOSING GUIDELINES FOR ADJUVANT ANALGESICS COMMONLY USED FOR CHRONIC PAIN

DRUGS/ROUTES	USUAL STARTING DOSE (MG/DAY)	USUAL EFFECTIVE DOSE RANGE (MG/DAY)	DOSING SCHEDULE	COMMENTS
Anticonvulsants				
Carbamazepine (Tegretol) PO	200	600–1200	q6–8h	
Clonazepam (Klonopin) PO	0.5	0.5–3	q8h	
Divalproex sodium (Depakote) PO	500	1500–3000	q8h	
Phenytoin (Dilantin) PO	300	300	hs	Loading doses may be used, e.g., 500 mg × 2.
IV	500–1000	?	?	IV dose used for rapidly escalating neuropathic pain.
Valproate sodium (Depacon) IV	max. 20 mg/kg over 5 minutes	?	?	IV dose used for rapidly escalating neuropathic pain; followed by PO doses.
Gabapentin (Neurontin) PO	100–300	300–3600	q8h	May increase dose daily.
Tricyclic antidepressants				
Amitriptyline (Elavil) PO	10–25	50–150	hs	Traditionally amitriptyline was first line. Due to side effects and recent evidence of comparable analgesia, desipramine is preferred for many patients, especially the elderly; less hypotension with nortriptyline. Evaluate and titrate upward q3–5 days.
Clomipramine (Anafranil) PO	10–25	50–150	hs	
Desipramine (Norpramin) PO	10–25	50–150	hs	
Doxepin (Sinequan) PO	10–25	50–150	hs	
Imipramine (Tofranil) PO	10–25	50–150	hs	
Nortriptyline PO (Aventyl, Pamelor)	10–25	50–150	hs	

Table continued on following page

TABLE 73–1. DOSING GUIDELINES FOR ADJUVANT ANALGESICS COMMONLY USED FOR CHRONIC PAIN *Continued*

DRUGS/ROUTES	USUAL STARTING DOSE (MG/DAY)	USUAL EFFECTIVE DOSE RANGE (MG/DAY)	DOSING SCHEDULE	COMMENTS
"Newer" antidepressants				
Fluoxetine (Prozac) PO	10–20	20–40	qd	"Newer" antidepressants have fewer side effects than tricyclics; less evidence of effectiveness
Paroxetine (Paxil) PO	20	20–40	qd	
Sertraline (Zoloft) PO	50	150–200	qd	
Corticosteroids				
Dexamethasone (Decadron) PO	Low-dose regimen: 1–2 mg	same	qd or bid	In advanced medical illness, long-term treatment with low doses is generally well tolerated; used when pain persists after optimal opioid dosing.
	High-dose regimen: 100 mg then 96 mg in 4 divided doses.	same	qid	High doses used for acute episodes of severe pain unresponsive to opioids.

Local Anesthetics

Mexiletine (Mexitil) PO	150	900–1200	q8h	Mexiletine is safer than tocainide. Plasma concentrations should be followed to reduce risk of toxicity.
Lidocaine IV	2–5 mg/kg	—	—	Brief infusion over 20–30 minutes. Analgesia occurs within 15–30 minutes. May be appropriate for rapidly escalating neuropathic pain.
Subcutaneous, IV	2.5 mg/kg/h	same	—	Continuous infusion.

Others

Baclofen (Lioresal) PO	15	30–200	q8h	Indicated for "shooting" neuropathic pain.
Calcitonin subcutaneous, IV	25 IU	100–200 IU	qd	Calcitonin is indicated for various neuropathic pains; bone pain; and possibly osteoarthritis.
Nasal spray (Miacalcin)	200 IU	200–400 IU	qd	
Clonidine transdermal (Catapres)	0.1	?	qd	Clonidine doses may be increased by 0.1 mg/day q3–5 days.
PO	0.1	?	qd	Multipurpose for chronic pain.

? = unknown, unclear; h = hour; hs = bedtime; q = every; qd = every day

Adjuvant analgesics usually tried first for:
  Continuous neuropathic pain: antidepressants, systemic local anesthetics, gabapentin.
  Lancinating and sudden onset neuropathic pain: anticonvulsants, baclofen.

(From Portenoy, R.K., & McCaffery, M. [1999]. Adjuvant analgesics. In M. McCaffrey & C. Pasero [Eds.], *Pain: Clinical Manual* [pp. 342–344]. St. Louis, Mosby, with permission.)

TABLE 73–2. EQUIANALGESIC CHART: APPROXIMATE EQUIVALENT DOSES OF OPIOIDS FOR MODERATE TO SEVERE PAIN

ANALGESIC	PARENTERAL (IM, SC, IV) ROUTE[1, 2] (MG)	PO ROUTE[1] (MG)	COMMENTS
Mu Opioid Agonists			
Morphine	10	30	Standard for comparison. Multiple routes of administration. Available in immediate-release and controlled-release formulations. Active metabolite M6G can accumulate with repeated dosing in renal failure.
Codeine	130	200 NR	IM has unpredictable absorption and high side effect profile; used p.o. for mild to moderate pain; usually compounded with nonopioid (e.g., Tylenol #3).
Fentanyl	100 μg/h parenterally and transdermally $\cong$ 4 mg/h morphine parenterally; 1 μg/h transdermally $\cong$ 2 mg/24h morphine p.o.	—	Short half-life, but at steady state, slow elimination from tissues can lead to a prolonged half-life (up to 12 h). Start opioid-naive patients on no more than 25μg/h transdermally. Transdermal fentanyl NR for acute pain management. Available by oral transmucosal route.
Hydromorphone (Dilaudid)	1.5	7.5	Useful alternative to morphine. No evidence that metabolites are clinically relevant; shorter duration than morphine. Available in high-potency parenteral formulation (10 mg/ml) useful for SC infusion; 3 mg rectal $\cong$ 650 mg aspirin p.o. With repeated dosing (e.g., PCA), it is more likely that 2–3 mg parenteral hydromorphone = 10 mg parenteral morphine.

Drug	Dose	Comments
Levorphanol (Levo-Dromoran)	2	Longer acting than morphine when given repeatedly. Long half-life can lead to accumulation within 2–3 days of repeated dosing.
Meperidine	75	300 NR	No longer preferred as a first-line opioid for the management of acute or chronic pain due to potential toxicity from accumulation of metabolite, normeperidine. Normeperidine has 15–20 h half-life and is not reversed by naloxone. NR in elderly or patients with impaired renal function; NR by continuous IV infusion.
Methadone (Dolophine)	10	20	Longer acting than morphine when given repeatedly. Long half-life can lead to delayed toxicity from accumulation within 3–5 days. Start p.o. dosing on PRN schedule; in opioid-tolerant patients converted to methadone, start with 10–25% of equianalgesic dose.
Oxycodone	—	20	Used for moderate pain when combined with a nonopioid (e.g., Percocet, Tylox). Available as single entity in immediate-release and controlled-release formulations (e.g., OxyContin); can be used like p.o. morphine for severe pain.
Oxymorphone (Numorphan)	1	10 rectal	Used for moderate to severe pain. No p.o. formulation.

Agonist–Antagonist Opioids

Not recommended for severe, escalating pain. If used in combination with mu agonists, may reverse analgesia and precipitate withdrawal in opioid-dependent patients.

Table continued on following page

TABLE 73–2. EQUIANALGESIC CHART: APPROXIMATE EQUIVALENT DOSES OF OPIOIDS FOR MODERATE TO SEVERE PAIN *Continued*

ANALGESIC	PARENTERAL (IM, SC, IV) ROUTE[1, 2] (MG)	PO ROUTE[1] (MG)	COMMENTS
Buprenorphine (Buprenex)	0.4	—	Not readily reversed by naloxone; NR for laboring patients.
Butorphanol (Stadol)	2	—	Available in nasal spray.
Dezocine (Dalgan)	10	—	
Nalbuphine (Nubain)	10	—	
Pentazocine (Talwin)	60	180	

A GUIDE TO USING EQUIANALGESIC CHARTS

Equianalgesic means approximately the same pain relief.

The equianalgesic chart is a guideline. Doses and intervals between doses are titrated according to individual's response.

The equianalgesic chart is helpful when switching from one drug to another, or switching from one route of administration to another.

Dosages in the equianalgesic chart for moderate to severe pain are not necessarily starting doses. The doses suggest a ratio for comparing the analgesia of one drug to another.

For elderly patients, initially reduce the recommended adult opioid dose for moderate to severe pain by 25–50%.

The longer the patient has been receiving opioids, the more conservative the starting doses of a *new* opioid.

EQUIANALGESIC CHART

Approximate equivalent doses of p.o. nonopioids and opioids for mild to moderate pain

Analgesic	p.o. Dosage (mg)
Nonopioids	
Acetaminophen	650
Aspirin (ASA)	650
Opioids[†]	
Codeine	32–60
Hydrocodone[††]	5
Meperidine (Demerol)	50
Oxycodone[††]	3–5
Propoxyphene (Darvon)	65–100

[1] Duration of analgesia is dose dependent; the higher the dose, usually the longer the duration.

[2] IV boluses may be used to produce analgesia that lasts approximately as long as IM or SC doses. However, of all routes of administration, IV produces the highest peak concentration of the drug, and the peak concentration is associated with the highest level of toxicity, e.g., sedation. To decrease the peak effect and lower the level of toxicity, IV boluses may be administered more slowly, e.g., 10 mg of morphine over a 15 min period or smaller doses may be administered more often, e.g., 5 mg of morphine every 1–1.5 h.

FDA = Food and Drug Administration; NR = not recommended; ≅ roughly equal to

[+] Often combined with acetaminophen; avoid exceeding maximum total daily dose of acetaminophen (4000 mg/day).

[++] Combined with acetaminophen, e.g., Vicodin, Lortab.

[+++] Combined with acetaminophen, e.g., Percocet, Tylox. Also available alone as controlled-release OxyContin and immediate-release formulations.

Selected references

American Pain Society (APS). (1992). *Principles of analgesic use in the treatment of acute pain and cancer pain* (3rd ed.). Glenview, IL: APS.

Kaiko, R., Lacouture, P., Hopf, K., et al. (1996). Analgesic efficacy of controlled-release (CR) oxycodone and CR morphine. *Clinical Pharmacology and Therapeutics, 59*, 130.

Lawlor, P., Turner, K., Hanson, J., et al. (1997). Dose ratio between morphine and hydromorphone in patients with cancer pain: A retrospective study. *Pain, 72*, 79–85.

McCaffery, M., & Portenoy, R.K. (1999). Nonopioids: Acetaminophen and nonsteroidal antiinflammatory drugs. In M. McCaffery & C. Pasero (Eds.), *Pain: Clinical manual* (p. 131). St. Louis: Mosby.

Manfredi, P.L., Borsook, D., Chandler, S.W., et al. (1997). Intravenous methadone for cancer pain unrelieved by morphine and hydromorphone: Clinical observations. *Pain, 70*, 99–101.

Pasero, C., Portenoy, R.K., & McCaffery, M. (1999). Opioid analgesics. In M. McCaffery & C. Pasero (Eds.), *Pain: Clinical manual* (pp. 241–243). St. Louis: Mosby.

Portenoy, R.K. (1996). Opioid analgesics. In R.K. Portenoy & R.M. Kanner (Eds.), *Pain management: Theory and practice* (pp. 249–276). Philadelphia: F.A. Davis.

(From McCaffery, M., & Pasero, C. [Eds.] [1999]. *Pain: Clinical manual*. St. Louis: Mosby; with permission.)

    (3) When pain is persistent, or moderate to begin with, use appropriate doses of a strong opioid and add adjuvants as needed.

  ii. Nonopioid analgesics

    (1) Aspirin (ASA), 650–975 mg q4 h

    (2) Acetaminophen (Tylenol): 650–975 mg q4 h

  iii. Nonsteroidal anti-inflammatory drugs (NSAIDs)

    (1) Ibuprofen (Motrin), 400 mg q4–6 h

    (2) Ketorolac (Toredol), 10 mg IM or IV q6 h; progress to p.o. as soon as possible; relatively contraindicated in patients with renal disease and at risk of coagulopathy

    (3) Naproxen (Naprosyn), 500-mg initial dose, then 250 mg q6–8 h

    (4) Diflunisal (Dolobid), 1000-mg initial dose, followed by 500 mg q12 h

    (5) Etodolac (Lodine), 200–400 mg q6–8h

    (6) Diclofenac (Voltaren), 50–100 mg q6–8h

    (7) Celecoxib (Celebrex), 100–200 mgq 8h. Celecoxib is the first in a new class of painkillers called Cox-2 inhibitors with fewer gastrointestinal upsets.

  iv. Opioid analgesics

    (1) Morphine: Standard agent for opioid therapy
      (a) Oral: 30 mg q3–4h
      (b) Parenteral: 2–10 mg q3–4h

    (2) Hydromorphone (Dilaudid)
      (a) Oral: 7.5 mg q3–4h
      (b) Parenteral: 1.5 mg q3–4h

    (3) Meperidine (Demerol)
      (a) Oral: 300 mg q2–3h
      (b) Parenteral: 25–100 mg q3–4h
      (c) Demerol is contraindicated in patients with impaired renal function or those receiving antidepressants that are monoamine oxidase inhibitors.
      (d) Normeperidine is a toxic metabolite of meperidine, and is excreted through the kidney. Normeperidine is a cerebral irritant, and accumulation can cause effects ranging from dysphoria and irritable mood to seizures.

    (4) Fentanyl patch: 25–300 μg/h. To convert from IM or p.o. morphine, the patch dose must be calculated by calculating the previous 24-h analgesic requirement and convert the morphine dose to an equivalent fentanyl dose (charts are available).

  v. Pain-relief devices: Medication administered via continuous epidural, intrathecal, intrapleural, or peripheral nerve catheters; pain relief devices use local anesthetics and/or narcotics and/or steroids.

(1) Drugs of choice may be fentanyl, morphine (Duramorph), steroids, and local anesthetics (primarily bupivacaine [Marcaine]).

(2) Permanent implantable pain devices may be refilled on an outpatient basis.

(3) Management of catheters or devices for analgesia to alleviate acute postsurgical pain, pathologic pain or chronic pain, including reinjection of medication (following establishment of appropriate therapeutic range) or adjustment of drug infusion rate, should be in compliance with the authorized provider's orders or protocols.

References

1. Agency for Health Care Policy and Research, U.S. Department of Health and Human Services. (1993). *Acute pain management in adults: Operative procedures.* (AHCPR No. 92-00109). Rockville, MD.
2. Agency for Health Care Policy and Research, U.S. Department of Health and Human Services. (1992). *Acute pain management: Operative of medical procedures and trauma; Clinical practice guidelines.* (AHCPR No. 92-0032). Rockville, MD.
3. Agency for Health Care Policy and Research, U.S. Department of Health and Human Services. (1994). *Management of cancer pain: Clinical practice guidelines and trauma.* (AHCPR No. 94-0592). Rockville, MD.
4. Beck, S.L. (1999). Health policy, health services, and cancer pain management in the new South Africa. *Journal of Pain and Symptom Control. 17*, 16–26.
5. Bohannon, A.S. (1995). Physiological, self-report, and behavioral ratings of pain in three- to seven-year-old African-American and Anglo-American children. *Dissertation Abstracts International.* (University Microfilms No. 9540967)
6. Eisenhauer, L.A., & Murphy, M.A. (Eds.). (1998). *Pharmocotherapeutics and advanced nursing practice.* New York: McGraw-Hill.
7. Fauci, A.S. Braunwald, E., Isselbacher, K.J., Wilson, J.D., Martin, J.B., Kasper, D.L., Hauser, S.L., & Longo, D.L. (Eds.). (1998). *Harrison's principles of internal medicine* (14th ed.). New York: McGraw-Hill.
8. *Equianalgesic dosing tables.* (1999). Http://www.mosby.com/PAIN.
9. Kastrup, E., & Hebel, S. (1999). *Drug facts and comparisons* (p. 1395). St. Louis: Facts & Comparisons.
10. McCaffery, M., & Pasero, C. (1999). *Pain: Clinical manual* (2nd ed.). St. Louis: CV Mosby.
11. Miaskowski, C., & Dibble, S.L. (1995). The problem of pain in outpatients with breast cancer. *Oncology Nursing Forum, 22,* 791–797.
12. Miller, R. (1999). *Anesthesia* (pp. 2353–2356). Philadelphia: Churchill-Livingstone.
13. Reisner-Keller, L.A. (1996). Pain management. In E.T. Herfindal & D.R. Gourley (Eds.). *Textbook of therapeutics: Drug and disease management* (6th ed.). Baltimore: Williams & Wilkins.
14. World Health Organization, WHO Expert Committee on Cancer Pain Relief and Active Supportive Care. (1996). *Cancer pain relief: With a guide to opioid availability* (2nd ed.). Geneva: WHO Technical Reports.

PSYCHOSOCIAL PROBLEMS IN ACUTE CARE

CHAPTER 74

Jason A. Jones, EdD, RN, CS, ARNP

I. VIOLENCE

A. Definition
Direct verbal or physical assault of another person

B. Etiology/Predisposing factors

1. Psychosis, mood disorders, substance abuse
2. Anger at health care providers/system
3. Domestic problems
4. Undiagnosed medical problem (e.g., seizures, subdural hematoma)
5. Personal problems

C. Subjective findings

1. Abuser

   a. Increased anxiety, confusion, depression, agitation, verbal threats
   b. Guilty feelings and remorse after a violent episode
   c. Controlling behavior with the abused

2. Abused person

   a. Evasion of questions about injuries
   b. Depression, anxiety, refusal to talk about problems, and fear

D. Physical examination findings[9]

1. Abuser

   a. Pacing
   b. Loud voice
   c. Threatening gestures
   d. Clenched fists
   e. Dilated pupils
   f. Alcohol on the breath

2. Abused person—May have

   a. Scars, lacerations, poorly healed old fractures
   b. Bruises on the inner aspects of the arms and legs
   c. Bite marks

E. Laboratory/Diagnostic findings[3, 11]

1. Abuser

   a. Blood/urine drug screen and blood alcohol level (to rule out substance abuse)
   b. Electrolytes (to rule out fluid and electrolyte imbalance)
   c. CT scan of the head (to rule out subdural hematoma in sudden, unprovoked violent episode)
   d. EEG (to rule out seizures in sudden, unprovoked violence)
   e. X-ray of injured bones to detect fractures in abuse victims

2. Abused person

   a. Assess for life-threatening injury.
   b. X-ray injured areas to detect fractures.

F. Management[1, 7, 14, 15, 20]

1. Abuser

   a. Summon police to control a violent person if the abuser is armed with weapons.
   b. Offer food, beverage, and assistance in resolving problems nonviolently.
   c. Avoid direct eye contact, since many people find eye contact threatening.
   d. Encourage violent individuals to sit down to discuss their concerns.
   e. Hospitalize the abuser if a danger to self or others.
   f. Correct underlying medical problems or seek consultation with a specialist.
   g. Physical restraints
      i. Use (if on protocol) only as a last resort and by trained personnel.
      ii. Time of failed attempts to verbally control behavior before restraints are applied must be documented.
   h. Medication (immediately)[6]
      i. Haloperidol (Haldol), 2–5 mg p.o. or IM, and
      ii. Lorazepam (Ativan), 1–2 mg p.o. or IM STAT
   i. A legal duty exists to warn threatened individuals if a person voices harmful intent against another individual's life, or to notify authorities if a child or an elderly person is abused.

2. Abused person

   a. Problem-solve to encourage the person to avoid being harmed.
   b. Discuss all options, including staying with the abuser, as some individuals will not leave the abuser initially.

    c. Assist to identify resources such as friends, family members, and others who may give aid and shelter.

    d. Refer to social services and/or to a battered person's program.

II. DEPRESSION[3, 11, 13–15, 17, 19, 20]

A. Definition

1. A depressed mood, diminished interest in normal activity, fatigue, feelings of worthlessness, and impaired concentration nearly every day

2. The depressed person may or may not be suicidal or homicidal.

B. Etiology/Predisposing factors/Risk factors

1. Depression is the most common psychiatric diagnosis and may be undertreated.

2. May be caused by

    a. Imbalance in levels of neurotransmitters

    b. Negative perception of life events

    c. General medical disorders/medication side effects

3. Significant indicators of depression

    a. Past family or personal history of depression/suicide attempts

    b. Recent bad news

    c. Chronic or medical conditions with poor prognosis

    d. Old age

    e. Loss of significant others

    f. Lack of a support system

4. Suicidal risk must be assessed.

    a. Elderly white males with medical problems who lack social supports are at greatest risk.

    b. Firearms are the most successful means of suicide.

    c. Good and Nelson (1995) developed a useful way to remember assessment of suicide risk by the following mnemonic—SUICIDAL[8]:

        i. S—*S*ex (Males are more successful at suicide. Females make more attempts.)

        ii. U—*U*nsuccessful attempts (past attempt history, reasons for attempts)

        iii. I—*I*dentified family members with a history of successful suicide

        iv. CI—Chronic *I*llness history

        v. D—*D*epression, drug abuse, and drinking

        vi. A—*A*ge of the patient (The elderly are more successful. Teenagers make more attempts.)

vii. L—Lethal method available (Guns are most lethal, followed by hanging and intentional drug overdose.)

C. Subjective findings

1. Feelings of

   a. Hopelessness
   b. Increased/decreased appetite
   c. Decreased libido
   d. Helplessness
   e. Worthlessness
   f. Guilt

2. Lack of energy
3. Sleep disturbances, particularly

   a. Early morning awakening, or
   b. Oversleeping

4. Psychomotor agitation/retardation
5. Thoughts of death or suicide
6. The patient may have auditory hallucinations.

D. Physical findings

1. Poor physical hygiene, unkempt appearance, poor posture, over/underweight
2. Diarrhea or impaction
3. Only complaints may be abdominal or chest pain without physical cause.
4. Physical symptoms may be over- or under-reported.

E. Laboratory/Diagnostic findings

1. Rule out underlying medical problems.
2. Thyroid function studies to rule out hypothyroidism
3. Vitamin B_{12} and folate levels
4. Blood glucose level to rule out diabetes
5. Complete blood count to detect anemia, infection, or other problems
6. The patient must have an ECG prior to starting tricyclic antidepressants (tricyclics may exacerbate existing conduction problems).
7. A 24-h creatinine clearance test is recommended before starting lithium (lithium is excreted through the kidneys and may reach toxic blood levels if renal function is poor).
8. Drug screen (Drug effects may mimic depressive symptoms.)
9. Blood alcohol level, as appropriate
10. Gastric lavage if appropriate for drug-overdose suicide attempts

F. Management

1. If the patient is a danger to self or others, hospitalize and refer to a psychiatrist.
2. Treat any underlying medical problems.
3. If not suicidal/homicidal/hallucinating, the patient may be referred for outpatient psychotherapy by a mental health professional.
4. Counsel the patient that depression is a very treatable condition.
5. Useful mnemonic for counseling mildly depressed patients or other patients with self-limiting emotional conditions— BATHE[8]

   a. B—Background (Allow the patient time to tell about the problem, with healing expression of feelings.)
   b. A—Affect (Elicit affect/feelings; e.g., "How do you feel about that?")
   c. T—Trouble (Find out the most disturbing thing about the problem by asking, "What was most troubling about the situation?")
   d. H—Handling (Assess coping: "How have you been handling the situation?")
   e. E—Empathy (Acknowledge the difficulty of the situation and commend the patient's strength in handling the problem.)

6. Possible pharmacologic treatment[3, 17]

   a. Selective serotonin reuptake inhibitors (SSRIs)[6]
      i. Sertraline (Zoloft), 50–150 mg daily, or
      ii. Fluoxetine (Prozac), 20–40 mg daily,
      iii. Most commonly prescribed treatment owing to
         (1) Low overdose danger
         (2) Fast symptom response (10–21 days)
         (3) Low cardiac conduction problems
   b. Tricyclic antidepressants and monoamine oxidase inhibitors are not used as often as in the past owing to increased side-effect profiles and high overdose potential.
   c. Bipolar disorder
      i. Treated with lithium carbonate, carbamazepine (Tegretol), or valproic acid alone or in combination with antidepressants
      ii. Treatment with these drugs should be implemented by a psychiatrist or a psychiatric nurse practitioner.

III. SUBSTANCE ABUSE[5, 14–17, 20]

A. Definition

1. Prolonged use of alcohol or other mood-altering substance creating an emotional and/or physical reliance on the substance to deal with normal life stress

2. Substance abuse may result in physical and emotional dependence on the drug.

B. Etiology/Incidence/Predisposing factors

1. The cause of substance abuse may be specific alterations in opiate receptors and neurotransmitters, or genetic predisposition.
2. Alcohol is the most frequently encountered drug of abuse owing to its low cost and high availability.
   a. Alcohol and sedative/hypnotic withdrawal both have potentially fatal outcomes if not managed with care.
   b. Both alcohol and sedative/hypnotic withdrawal are treated by a slow taper with benzodiazepines.
3. Frequently substance abusers mix alcohol with other drugs, which can make withdrawal difficult.
4. Alcohol withdrawal is the most problematic to manage of any drug withdrawal owing to progression into potentially fatal delirium tremens (DTs) if treatment for withdrawal is not initiated.
5. There is a 10% mortality rate in DTs with complications from associated
   a. Electrolyte disturbances
   b. Aspiration pneumonia
   c. Hepatic failure
   d. Pancreatitis
   e. Gastrointestinal bleeding
6. Cannabis, central nervous system stimulants, opiates, hallucinogens, inhalants/solvents
   a. Commonly abused drugs that can be stopped abruptly without life-threatening results
   b. Although opiate withdrawal is mildly uncomfortable physically, it is not fatal.

C. Subjective findings

1. Symptoms vary according to the substance abused.
2. Most persons who abuse drugs look for the mood-altering features of the substance or the recreational/euphoric/hallucinogenic effects.

D. Physical examination findings

1. Physical findings vary according to the substance ingested.
2. Withdrawal syndrome from alcohol is common and a serious medical concern.
   a. Early symptoms of alcohol withdrawal
      i. Elevated temperature, blood pressure, and pulse

    ii. Anxiety
    iii. Diaphoresis
  b. If untreated, the patient may progress to DTs, with
    i. Auditory/visual hallucinations
    ii. Seizures
    iii. Death

3. Currently there is no method to predict which patient will go into DTs other than monitoring vital signs during the withdrawal process.

E. Laboratory/Diagnostic findings

1. Blood/urine drug screen to determine the substance(s) abused, which will govern medical management
2. Blood alcohol level to determine approximate blood alcohol content

  • Individuals abusing alcohol over many years may have high blood alcohol levels, yet still go into withdrawal if they experience a sudden drop in their usual alcohol intake/blood alcohol level owing to tolerance of the substance.

3. Liver function studies (to detect elevated liver enzymes, which indicate liver damage)
4. General chemistry for electrolytes to monitor decreased levels of

  a. Potassium (due to diarrhea)
  b. Sodium (due to diaphoresis)
  c. Magnesium
  d. Other electrolytes

5. Serum amylase levels (to detect pancreatitis)
6. Complete blood count to reveal

  a. Infectious processes
  b. Gastrointestinal bleeding
  c. Anemia

7. Addiction Research Foundation Clinical Institute Withdrawal Assessment (CIWA-Ar) (Fig. 74–1).

  a. The CIWA-Ar is an assessment tool developed to measure potential for withdrawal.
  b. A score of less than 10 is considered to be a mild withdrawal that does not require medication.
  c. A score of more than 10 with or without a history of withdrawal indicates a need for medication.
  d. The tool is not copyrighted and may be used freely.

Addiction Research Foundation Clinical Institute Withdrawal Tool

(CIWA-Ar)*

Patient _____ Date ___/_____/_____   Time _____

Pulse or heart rate, taken for one minute: _____ Blood pressure ___/___

Nausea and vomiting: Ask, "Do you feel sick to your stomach? Have you vomited?" Observation	Tactile disturbances: Ask, "Have you any itching, pins and needles sensations, any burning, any numbness, or do you feel bugs crawling on or under your skin?" Observation.
0 No nausea and no vomiting 1 Mild nausea with no vomiting 2 3 4 Intermittent nausea with dry heaves 5 6 7 Constant nausea, frequent dry heaves and vomiting	0 None 1 Mild itching, pins and needles, burning, or numbness 2 Mild itching, pins and needles, burning, or numbness 3 Moderate itching, pins and needles, burning, or numbness 4 Moderately severe hallucinations 5 Severe hallucinations 6 Extremely severe hallucinations 7 Continuous hallucinations
Tremor: Arms extended and fingertips spread apart Observation	Auditory disturbances: Ask, "Are you more aware of sounds around you? Are they harsh? Do they frighten you? Are you hearing things you know are not there?" Observation
0 No sweat visible 1 Barely perceptible sweating, palms moist 2 3 4 Beads of sweat obvious on forehead 5 6 7 Drenching sweats	0 Not present 1 Very mild harshness or ability to frighten 2 Mild harshness or ability to frighten 3 Moderate harshness or ability to frighten 4 Moderately severe hallucinations 5 Severe hallucinations 6 Extremely severe hallucinations 7 Continuous hallucinations

Figure 74–1. CIWA-Ar Withdrawal Assessment Tool

Illustration continued on following page

Paroxysmal sweats:
Observation

0 No sweat visible
1
2
3
4 Beads of sweat obvious on forehead
5
6
7 Drenching sweats

Anxiety: Ask, "Do you feel nervous?"
Observation

0 No anxiety, at ease
1 Mildly anxious
2
3
4 Moderately anxious, or guarded
5
6
7 Equivalent to acute panic states as seen in severe delirium or acute schizophrenic reactions

Agitation: Observation
0 Normal activity
1 Somewhat more than normal activity
2
3
4 Moderately fidgety and restless
5
6
7 Paces back and forth during most of the interview, or constantly thrashes about

Visual disturbances: Ask, "Does the light appear to be too bright? Is its color different? Does it hurt your eyes? Are you seeing any thing that is disturbing to you? Are you seeing things you know are not there?"
Observation
0 Not present
1 Very mild sensitivity
2 Mild sensitivity
3 Moderate sensitivity
4 Moderately severe hallucinations
5 Severe hallucinations
6 Extremely severe hallucinations
7 Continuous hallucinations

Headache, fullness in head: Ask, "Does your head feel different? Does it feel like there is a band around your head?" Do not rate for dizziness or lightheadedness. Otherwise, rate severity.
0 Not present
1 Very mild
2 Mild
3 Moderate
4 Moderately severe
5 Severe
6 Very severe
7 Extremely severe

Orientation and clouding of sensorium: Ask, "What day is this? Where are you? Who am I?"
0 Oriented and can do serial additions
1 Cannot do serial additions or is uncertain about date
2 Disoriented for date by no more than 2 calendar days
3 Disoriented for date by more than 2 calendar days
4 Disoriented for place and/or person
TOTAL CIWA-Ar Score _____
Max score 67

Figure 74–1 *Continued*

F. Management[3, 14, 17]

1. Possible pharmacologic therapy for alcohol withdrawal

   a. Over 125 regimens for the treatment of alcohol withdrawal have been published.
   b. All patients need consideration of their individual medical status and their vital signs monitored prior to and during withdrawal.
   c. The reader's own institution should be consulted to see whether it has an established withdrawal protocol.

2. IV medication used for DTs

   a. Rehydration up to several liters of saline per day as indicated
   b. Correction of electrolyte imbalance if needed
   c. Hypoglycemia prevention
   d. Thiamine, 100 mg IV daily for at least 3 days
   e. Diazepam (Valium), or chlordiazepoxide (Librium), or lorazepam (Ativan) can be used as a slow IV push both to sedate and to prevent withdrawal seizures.
   f. The following regimen of IV medication is given until the patient is calm:[3, 14]
      i. Chlordiazepoxide, 0.5 mg/kg at 12.5 mg/min
      ii. Diazepam. 0.15 mg/kg at 2.5 mg/min
      iii. Lorazepam, 0.1 mg/kg at 2.0 mg/min
   g. After the patient is calm, doses are individualized according to the patient's needs and tolerance to the effects of the medication, being careful not to depress respirations.
   h. High doses of up to 50–100 mg of diazepam (or its equivalent) per day are not usually given to patients who have a high tolerance for alcohol.

3. Oral medication used for mild withdrawal symptoms

   a. Alcohol withdrawal
      i. Diazepam, 10–20 mg initial loading dose, with repeated 10-mg doses q2h until the patient is sedated
      ii. Often this initial, first day of treatment is adequate, since the drug is slowly eliminated by the liver.
   b. In patients with liver impairment[14, 17]
      i. Oxazepam (Serax), 1–4 mg p.o. q2h may be used, since it bypasses hepatic metabolism.
      ii. However, a slow taper over several days must be used with this drug, owing to its more rapid excretion.
   c. Sedative/hypnotic withdrawal can be accomplished using the same withdrawal methods as for mild alcohol withdrawal.

4. Referral to mental health and 12-step recovery groups (i.e., Alcoholics Anonymous, Narcotics Anonymous) is very important.

IV. ANXIETY[11, 12, 14, 20]

A. Definition

A subjective acute or chronic state of emotional discomfort and apprehension that mobilizes physiologic general adaptation to stress

B. Etiology/Incidence/Predisposing factors

1. Anxiety is caused by a learned emotional response to stress.
2. Anxiety is a common response to medical problems and surgery.

C. Subjective findings

1. Commonly reported symptoms

   a. Restlessness
   b. Problems falling asleep
   c. Fear
   d. Depression
   e. Panic
   f. Guilt
   g. Apprehension
   h. Worry

2. Physical complaints

   a. Diarrhea
   b. Constipation
   c. Indigestion
   d. Vomiting
   e. Muscle stiffness
   f. Headache

D. Physical examination findings

1. Acute manifestations

   a. Trembling
   b. Excess hand perspiration
   c. Tachypnea
   d. Tachycardia

2. Chronic problems

   a. Hypertension
   b. Muscular tension

E. Management[11]

1. First rule out physical causes of anxiety or restlessness, e.g.,

    a. Decreased oxygen saturation
    b. Pain that is insufficiently controlled

2. Listening to a patient's concern can relieve mild anxiety.
3. Benzodiazpines such as lorazepam can be used p.o. or IV to relieve anxiety on a short-term basis.

    a. Hospital protocols should be checked prior to IV benzodiazepine administration, and the patient must be carefully monitored.
    b. Benzodiazepines should be used with caution in the elderly because they may cause confusion.
    c. For anxiety in the Intensive Care Unit, the following is suggested[6]:

       • Lorazepam, 0.044 mg/kg (maximum 2 mg) IV, given slowly over 2–5 min at the lowest dose that relieves anxiety

4. Refer the patient to a mental health specialist for chronic anxiety, which can be treated by cognitive therapy or biofeedback.

V. CRISIS INTERVENTION[3]

A. Definition

1. A method of brief counseling to help individuals, families, and/or groups to cope with stressors
2. Crisis can occur when individuals encounter medical problems or life-threatening situations often present in an Intensive Care Unit environment.
3. Patients, family members, and hospital staff can develop an emotional crisis as a result of being faced with overwhelming issues.
4. Individuals in crisis may or may not have pre-existing mental health problems.

B. Etiology/Predisposing factors/Risk factors

1. Common causes of crisis

    a. Sudden illness
    b. Loss of body parts
    c. Loss of ability to carry out normal life roles
    d. Threat of death
    e. Accidents
    f. Financial problems

2. Individuals with a history of poor coping skills or emotional rigidity are particularly vulnerable to stress.

C. Subjective findings

1. Anger
2. Denial of problem
3. Depression
4. Increased anxiety
5. Slowed thought processes
6. Difficulty with problem solving
7. Anger with medical personnel

D. Management

1. Listen to the patient's concerns. The goal is to encourage using past successful coping skills.
2. Ask about thoughts, feelings, and what the patient's perceptions are about what has happened to cause crisis, which helps vent feelings.
3. Focus on the present and elicit social supports available.
4. Have the patient further clarify and focus on solving the current problem.
5. Discuss who or what agency may assist in meeting the patient's needs. Clarify with the patient what must be done to resolve the problem.
6. Help make a realistic plan for problem resolution, and also contingency plans.
7. Refer to social services or other agencies appropriate to the situation.
8. Medication is not used with individuals without emotional problems owing to its hindering effect on problem solving abilities.

VI. GRIEF[3, 14, 15]

A. Definition

1. An emotional state in response to the actual or perceived loss of a significant person, animal, or object in a person's life
2. Acute grief lasts up to several weeks; however, the grieving process can take years to resolve.
3. Dysfunctional grief occurs when the grieving person cannot carry out normal daily living tasks after three months.

B. Etiology/Incidence/Predisposing factors

1. Most people have experienced grief over a loss.
2. Predisposing factors
   a. Emotional closeness
   b. Quality of a relationship
   c. Prior experience with loss
   d. Support of significant others

3. Chronic stress-related medical problems may worsen.

C. Subjective findings

1. Depression
2. Fatigue
3. Relief over the end of suffering
4. Remorse
5. Guilt
6. Emptiness
7. Sleeping problems
8. Anger
9. Feeling abandoned (common)
10. Anxiety (common)
11. Dreaming (common)
12. Suicidal and homicidal thoughts and psychosis are less common.

D. Physical examination findings

1. Disheveled appearance
2. Poor eye contact
3. Depressed affect

E. Management

1. Listening to the grieving person is the best method of early therapy.
2. Referral to local grief support groups can aid recovery.
3. Medication is not recommended in early grief.
4. Dysfunctional grief sometimes results in depression, and the patient may need a psychiatric referral for antidepressant medication and/or psychotherapy if the condition does not resolve in 3 months and the patient is unable to carry out a normal daily routine.

VII. SEXUALITY

A. Definition
The expression of a person's identification and feelings about intimacy, sexual attraction, and identity as a human being

B. Principles[14, 23]

1. Humans have inherent needs for love and closeness.
2. Both heterosexual and homosexual displays of affection can cause negative reactions, depending on the situation and persons involved.
3. Homosexual orientation is viewed as an optional lifestyle rather than as an illness or disorder. Homosexuality is not recognized as a psychiatric diagnosis by the American Psychiatric Association.[14]
4. Patients may express sexual feelings toward health care providers.

5. Patients may have complex relationships with significant others (e.g., adulterous lovers, homosexual affairs) that may cause guilt, embarrassment, depression, or other feelings.
6. It is important for the health care provider to be nonjudgmental about the patient's relationships or focus of affection.

C. Subjective findings/Physical examination findings

1. Sexual assessment

   a. Discuss whether the patient has any concerns about sexual function.
   b. Inquire about significant others who may be involved with the patient.
   c. Explore whether the person is involved with multiple sexual partners, which may predispose to sexually transmitted diseases (STDs).
   d. Discuss safe-sex and/or contraceptive practices and history of STDs.
   e. Assess whether the patient is comfortable with his or her sexual orientation

2. Symptoms of STDs: Observe for discharges, lesions, or other indications.

D. Laboratory/Diagnostic findings

HIV and other STD testing may require patient consent with provision of counseling if test results are positive.

E. Management

1. Empathy, support, and listening to patients helps facilitate expression of sexual concerns, problems with sexual performance, and other sexuality issues.
2. Referral to an HIV support group and counseling improves survival rates.
3. Refer to an internist, urologist, obstetrician-gynecologist, and/or psychiatrist as needed for workup of sexual dysfunction.

VIII. DELIRIUM[1–4, 6, 7, 10, 11, 14, 18, 21, 22]

A. Definition

1. The *acute* onset of confusion, excitement, incoherent speech, and agitation
2. Delirium is sometimes confused with psychosis, mood disorder, and dementia.

B. Etiology/Incidence/Predisposing factors/Risk factors (Table 74–1)

1. Causes of delirium

   a. Central nervous system disease

TABLE 74–1. COMPARISON OF DELIRIUM
WITH DEMENTIA

	DELIRIUM	DEMENTIA
Onset	Sudden; days or weeks. Associated with a physical stressor	Gradual; months or years
Essential Features	Clouded sensorium, irritability. Misperception of sensory stimuli, possible hallucinations, lucid periods alternating with confusion, suspiciousness, agitation	Memory loss, decreased intellectual functioning (confabulation and circumstantially)
Etiology	Toxins, alcohol/drug abuse, central nervous system or cardiac infarction, trauma, impactions in the elderly, poor nutrition, electrolyte imbalance, anesthesia, infections, tumors, endocrine problems, side effects of medications, hypoxia, hypercapnea	Neurotransmitter deficit, cortical atrophy, ventricular dilation, neurofibrillary tangles, senile plaques, loss of brain cells, possible viral causation, Alzheimer's disease, cerebrovascular accident (multi-infarct dementia)
Age	Any age	Usually older than 60 years

    b. Systemic disease
    c. Either interaction effects or withdrawal or intoxication from drugs or toxic agents (such as mercury or other heavy metals)

2. Approximately 30% of intensive care patients develop delirium.
3. Risk factors for development of delirium

    a. Age older than 60 years
    b. Young children
    c. Pre-existing brain damage
    d. History of alcoholism
    e. Diabetes
    f. Malnutrition
    g. Cancer

4. Estimated mortality rate in 3 months is 23–33%.

C. Subjective findings

1. Onset is acute, and symptoms worsen at night (see Table 74–1, Essential Features).
2. Impaired memory, thinking, and judgment
3. Clouding of consciousness, inattention, and disorientation
4. Also usually present

    a. Perception disturbances
    b. Incoherent speech
    c. Disrupted sleep
    d. Poor insight

D. Physical examination findings

1. Assessment may reveal the underlying medical cause.
2. Findings may include some of the following:

    a. Arrhythmia
    b. Cardiomegaly
    c. Bradycardia
    d. Tachycardia
    e. Fever
    f. Hypotension or hypertension
    g. Carotid bruits
    h. Enlarged thyroid
    i. Liver enlargement
    j. Positive Babinski's sign
    k. Pupil dilation
    l. Papilledema
    m. Neck rigidity
    n. Other symptoms of underlying medical conditions

3. In delirium development of cognitive decline is rapid, as opposed to dementia, where the onset of symptoms is often long and gradual, with a history of progressive mental deterioration obtained from family members.

E. Laboratory/Diagnostic findings[14]

1. Complete blood count with differential, thyroid function studies, STD tests, electrolyte and serum amylase levels, hepatic profile
2. Urinalysis
3. Blood and urine drug screens
4. ECG
5. Chest x-ray
6. EEG (Slowed or focal activity usually indicates delirium.)
7. Lumbar puncture for analysis of cerebrospinal fluid to rule out tertiary syphilis
8. CT scan of the brain to rule out subdural hematoma, or infarcts

9. Mini Mental State examination (a verbal and written screening test for memory, ability to abstract, and motor and cognitive functions)

F. Management[2, 3, 6, 7, 14, 18]

1. Treating the underlying medical condition is vital to resolving delirium.
2. Psychosis
   a. Haloperidol (Haldol) can be used to control psychosis found in delirium.
      i. The FDA has not formally approved haloperidol for IV use; however, clinical and research literature supports haloperidol as successful treatment for agitation and psychosis in patients with delirium.
      ii. Check for institutional protocols for IV haloperidol use.
      iii. Flush the IV line with 2 mL of normal saline before administering haloperidol because many lines are heparinized and the drug can be precipitated by heparin (and also phenytoin).
      iv. The initial bolus dose is 0.5–10 mg according to the following:
         (1) 0.5–2 mg for an elderly patient or a patient with mild agitation
         (2) 5 mg for moderate agitation
         (3) 10 mg for severe agitation
   b. Subsequent doses should be given every hour until the patient is calm and resumed if further agitation occurs.
      i. Ideally, half the first day's dose should be used on subsequent days until the patient is lucid.
      ii. Neuroleptic malignant syndrome and hypotensive episodes have been seen with IV haloperidol but are rare and have usually been associated with hypovolemia.
      iii. Monitoring for progressive Q–T interval widening after the administration of haloperidol is important to alert for the rare development of torsades de pointes ventricular tachycardia.
      iv. Akathesia has been seen in some instances.
      v. Development of restlessness may be encountered after IV haloperidol.
   c. If the patient is lucid, oral forms of haloperidol may be given, ranging from 5–50 mg per day. Management with the lowest effective dose is preferred.[14]
   d. Benzodiazepines may worsen delirium, especially in the elderly, although lorazepam, 0.5–4 mg IV bolus, is sometimes used with haloperidol for delirium.
3. Medical, neurologic, and psychiatric consultations

References

1. Bryant, H. (1998, July). Dementia in the primary care setting. *Advance for Nurse Practitioners, 6,* 28–30.
2. Bulow, K. (1999). Management of psychosis and agitation in elderly patients: A primary care perspective. *Journal of Clinical Psychiatry, 60,* 22–25.
3. Cassem, N.H., Stern, T.A., Rosenbaum, J.F., & Jellinek, M.S. (1997). *Massachusetts General Hospital handbook of general hospital psychiatry.* St Louis: Mosby.
4. Chan, D., & Brennan, N.J. (1999). Delirium: Making the diagnosis, improving the prognosis. *Geriatrics, 54,* 28–42.
5. D'Onofrio, G., Rathlev, N.K., Fish, S.S., & Freedland, E.S. (1999). Lorazepam for the prevention of recurrent seizures related to alcohol. *New England Journal of Medicine, 340,* 915–919.
6. Fuller, M., & Sajatovic, M. (1999). *Drug information handbook for psychiatry.* Cleveland: Lexi-Comp.
7. Gawlinski, A., & Hamwi, D. (Eds.) (1999). *Acute care nurse practitioner: Clinical curriculum and certification review.* Philadelphia: W.B. Saunders.
8. Good, W.V., & Nelson, J.E. (1995). *Psychiatry made ridiculously simple.* Miami: MedMaster.
9. Hattendorf, J., & Tollerud, T.R. (1997). Domestic violence: Counseling strategies that minimize the impact of secondary victimization. *Perspectives in Psychiatric Care, 33,* 14–24.
10. Inouye, S.K., Schlesinger, M.J., & Lydon, T.J. (1999). Delirium: A symptom of how hospital care is failing older persons and a window to improve quality of hospital care. *American Journal of Medicine, 106,* 565–573.
11. Jacobson, J.L., & Jacobson, A.M. (1996). *Psychiatric secrets.* St Louis: Mosby.
12. Lieberman, J., & Kaufman, L. (1996). Stress management. In H.L. Greene (Ed.), *Clinical medicine.* (pp. 760–762). St. Louis: Mosby.
13. Lynch, J.S. (1998). Prescribing medications for mood disorders. *Advance for Nurse Practitioners, 6,* 22–31.
14. Kaplan, H.I., & Sadock, B.J. (1998). *Synopsis of psychiatry* (8th ed.). Baltimore: Williams & Wilkins.
15. Knesper, D.J., Riba, M.B., & Schwenk, T.L. (1997). *Primary care psychiatry.* Philadelphia: W.B. Saunders.
16. Kutlenios, R.M. (1998). Genetics and alcoholism: Implications for advanced practice psychiatric/mental health nursing. *Archives of Psychiatric Nursing, 7,* 154–161.
17. Maxen, J.S., & Ward, N.G. (1995). *Psychotropic drugs fast facts.* New York: W.W. Norton & Co.
18. Maixner, S.M., Mellow, A.M., & Tandon, R. (1999). The efficacy, safety, and tolerability of antipsychotics in the elderly. *Journal of Clinical Psychiatry, 60,* 29–41.
19. O'Tocle, S.M., & Johnson, D.A. (1997). Psychobiology and psychopharmacotherapy of unipolar major depression: A review. *Archives of Psychiatric Nursing, 6,* 304–324.
20. Stern, T.A., Herman, J.B., & Slavin, P.L. (1998). *The MGH guide to psychiatry in primary care.* New York: McGraw-Hill.
21. Tappen, R.M., Williams-Burgess, C., Edelstein, J., Touhy, T., & Fishman, S. (1997). Communicating with individuals with Alzheimer's disease:

Examination of recommended strategies. *Archives of Psychiatric Nursing,* *6,* 249–256.

22. Taft, L., Fazio, S., Seman, D., & Stansell, J. (1997). A psychosocial model of dementia care: Theoretical and empirical support. *Archives of Psychiatric Nursing, 6,* 13–20.

23. Weingourt, R. (1998). A comparison of heterosexual and homosexual long-term sexual relationships. *Archives of Psychiatric Nursing, 7,* 114–118.

MANAGEMENT OF THE PATIENT IN SHOCK

Charlene M. Myers, MSN, RN, CS, ACNP, CCRN

I. SHOCK

A. Definition[5, 8, 11, 12]

1. Acute syndrome of organ and system dysfunction precipitated by failure of the circulation to meet the needs of metabolically active tissues.
2. Inadequate or inappropriately distributed tissue perfusion results in generalized cellular hypoxia.
3. Shock can develop within minutes or hours of an initial insult and, if not promptly reversed, can rapidly progress to death.

B. Pathophysiology[5, 11, 12, 16, 17]

1. The primary physiologic disturbance is impaired cellular function due to decreased nutritional blood flow.
2. Reduced oxygen and nutrient supply → anaerobic metabolism → production of acid (lactic and pyruvic) → decreased adenosine triphosphate (ATP), and decreased energy

   a. Acid depresses cellular function further.
   b. As pH decreases, powerful enzymes (proteolytic) released from the cell destroy the cell membrane and digest the cellular contents.
   c. Once integrity of the cell membrane is lost, cellular changes are irreversible.

C. Etiology[4, 5, 8, 11, 12, 16, 17]

1. Hypovolemia
2. Pump failure
3. Obstruction to blood flow
4. Sepsis
5. Disturbance in nervous system causing poor distribution of cardiac output
6. Anaphylaxis

Each will be discussed separately.

D. Stages of shock[5, 11, 12, 17]

1. Initial stage—Stage I

   a. Early changes occurring at cellular level (nonspecific changes)
   b. No real signs or symptoms

2. Compensatory stage—Stage II
   a. Cardiac output falls dependent on cause.
      i. Decreased cardiac contractility (e.g., acute myocardial infarction, cardiomyopathy, congested heart failure)
      ii. Decreased circulating volume (e.g., hypovolemia, hemorrhage)
      iii. Obstruction of central blood flow due to compression of the heart or great vessels (e.g., pericardial tamponade, aortic dissection, positive end-expiratory pressure (PEEP), pulmonary embolus, tension pneumothorax, aortic/mitral stenosis, abdominal distention, prosthetic valve thrombus, atrial myxoma)
      iv. Altered vascular resistance, such as vasodilation and a decrease in peripheral vascular resistance, resulting in venous pooling and inadequate venous return, which leads to relative hypovolemia (e.g., anaphylaxis, sepsis, neurologic disorders)
   b. Three types of compensatory mechanisms are activated:
      i. Nervous compensation: The decrease in cardiac output (CO) and blood pressure (BP) stimulates the pressoreceptors (baroreceptors) to send impulses to the vasomotor center of the medulla. Here the sympathetic nervous system (SNS) is stimulated, and there is a discharge of norepinephrine:
         (1) Increased activity of sweat glands
         (2) Increased respiratory rate (RR) and depth
         (3) Heart:
            (a) Increased heart rate (HR) and increased force of contraction, which in turn increases CO and BP.
            (b) Vasodilation of coronary arteries helps increase oxygenation to the heart muscle.
         (4) Vasodilation of skeletal muscle vasculature
         (5) Dilation of pupils
         (6) Vasoconstriction of vasculature in skin, gastrointestinal (GI) tract, and kidneys, which increases BP and increases venous return, thus increasing CO and BP. This vasoconstriction shunts blood to priority organs.
      ii. Hormonal compensation
         (1) Sympathetic nervous system stimulation activates the anterior pituitary to release adrenocorticotropic hormone (ACTH).
         (2) The adrenal cortex is activated to increase glucocorticoids in the liver, which increases glycogenolysis and in turn, serum glucose.
         (3) The adrenal cortex also increases the release of aldosterone, which increases Na reabsorption and in turn, H_2O reabsorption.

      (4) This results in increased fluid volume, increased CO, and decreased urine output.

  iii. Chemical compensation

      (1) Pulmonary blood flow is reduced due to decreased CO, resulting in ventilation-perfusion abnormalities: Some alveoli contain O_2 (adequate ventilation) but do not have adequate blood flow through the capillary bed (poor perfusion).

      (2) The low oxygen tension stimulates chemoreceptors in the aorta and carotid arteries leading to increased rate and depth of respirations $\rightarrow$ hyperventilation $\rightarrow$ CO_2 blown off $\rightarrow$ respiratory alkalosis $\rightarrow$ vasoconstriction of cerebral vessels along with decreased O_2 tension $\rightarrow$ cerebral hypoxia and ischemia

  c. Clinical manifestations resulting from compensatory stage:

    i. Blood pressure: Normal or adequate to perfuse vital organs. Mean arterial blood pressure (MAP) may drop 10–15 mmHg.

    ii. Increased HR (101–150)

   iii. Skin: Cool, pale, clammy, sweating

   iv. Urine: Decreased urine output; increased antidiuretic hormone (ADH), which increases urine osmolarity; increased aldosterone, which decreases urine Na

    v. Loss of consciousness: Hypoxia, hypocapnia, and sympathetic catecholamines alter sensorium

   vi. Respirations: Rapid and deep, minute volume is 1½ to 2 times normal

  vii. Bowel sounds: decreased

 viii. Dilated pupils

   ix. Laboratory findings: Hyperglycemia, hypernatremia, hypoxemia, hypocapnia, respiratory alkalosis

3. Progressive stage—Stage III: The compensatory mechanisms begin to fail in maintaining adequate CO:

  a. Cellular function: Arteriolar vasoconstriction $\rightarrow$ decreased capillary blood flow $\rightarrow$ decreased O_2 to cells $\rightarrow$ decreased ATP $\rightarrow$ increased anaerobic metabolism $\rightarrow$ local metabolic acidosis

  b. Capillary dynamics

    i. Capillary hydrostatic pressure increases: Precapillary sphincters dilate in response to acidosis, which allows blood to flow freely into the capillary bed, while the postcapillary sphincter remains constricted, which causes accumulation of blood in the capillaries and pushes fluid into tissues

    ii. Protein leaks out, leading to decreased colloid osmotic pressure.

    iii. The result is decreased intravascular volume → interstitial edema → increased viscosity of blood → increased resistance to flow → capillary sludging → further impairment of flow

    iv. Decreased volume and impaired flow → decreased venous return and decreased CO → decreased BP → decreased coronary artery perfusion → ischemia → arrhythmias or infarction

    v. Decreased CO perpetuates SNS response.

c. Systemic circulation

    i. Blood is shunted to priority organs (i.e., heart and brain).

    ii. Weak or absent pulses and cold extremities reflect severe vasoconstriction.

    iii. Decreased peripheral circulation may lead to ischemia of distal parts, which provides new ports of entry for microbes.

d. Specific organ systems

    i. Brain: Decreased cerebral blood flow leads to decreased level of consciousness (LOC).

    ii. Kidneys: A urine output of <30 mL/h is considered a sign of shock. Urine output decreases due to the reduced renal perfusion → ischemia → acute tubular necrosis → acute renal failure

    iii. GI system: Prolonged decreased perfusion may lead to a paralytic ileus and/or ulceration with an increased incidence of hemorrhage and decreased line of defense → translocation of bacteria into the bloodstream. Decreased perfusion to the GI musculature → slowing of intestinal activity → decreased bowel sounds, distention, nausea, constipation, and high residuals of enteral feedings

    iv. Liver

        (1) Kupffer cells cannot perform phagocytosis → decreased line of defense

        (2) Impaired metabolic activities (such as gluconeogenesis, glucolysis, and fat metabolism)

        (3) Buildup of waste products (ammonia, lactic acid)

        (4) Liver cells eventually become ischemic and die, resulting in increased aspartate aminotransferase (AST), alanine aminotransferase (ALT), lactate dehydrogenase (LDH), bilirubin, and jaundice

    v. Pancreas: Cells become ischemic and release myocardial depressant factor (MDF), which directly de-

presses myocardial contractility. Increased amylase and lipase are caused by pancreatic ischemia
  vi. Lungs
      (1) The most significant respiratory complication is acute respiratory distress syndrome (ARDS)
          (a) Reduced pulmonary blood flow and increased pulmonary vascular resistance → increased pulmonary capillary permeability → increased interstitial edema → atelectasis and alveolar edema (noncardiogenic pulmonary edema)
          (b) Decreased surfactant → atelectasis
      (2) Decreased compliance → hypoventilation and hypoxemia that is refractory to oxygen therapy
  e. Clinical signs of Stage III
      i. Decreased pulse pressure: Systolic blood pressure decreases related to decreased stroke volume (SV), and diastolic blood pressure increases related to increased vasoconstriction (narrowed pulse pressure)
      ii. Increased HR (may exceed >150); weak and thready pulse; decreased filling time and decreased coronary artery perfusion may lead to myocardial ischemia and arrhythmias
      iii. Skin pale or cyanotic, cold and clammy; capillary filling time (CFT) >3 s; possible jaundice
      iv. Decreased urine output
      v. Decreased LOC
      vi. Increased RR, shallow (hypoventilation), rales/rhonchi, resonance leading to dullness
      vii. Bowel sounds decreased or absent; possible paralytic ileus. Bowel sounds may increase if bleeding occurs
      viii. Decreased cellular metabolism leads to decrease in temperature and heat production

4. Refractory stage—Stage IV: The final, irreversible stage of shock resulting in several vicious cycles

  a. Cardiac failure
      i. Coronary perfusion decreases due to increased HR, decreased SV, and decreased BP and lack of perfusion pressure
      ii. Contractility is impaired related to decreased O_2 delivery, MDF, and acidotic state
      iii. CO falls further resulting in decreased coronary perfusion
  b. Acidosis is present related to
      i. Poor tissue perfusion, which results in impaired cellular function
      ii. Poor renal perfusion resulting in retention of waste products

iii. Respiratory failure
iv. Acidosis results in
    (1) Decreased contractility and in turn decreased CO
    (2) Loss of vasomotor tone → fluid shift → relative hypovolemia
    (3) Leads to further impairments in tissue perfusion, renal function, and respiratory function

c. Aberrations in blood clotting
    i. Acidosis, decreased intravascular volume, and sluggish capillary flow → further impairment of flow → more clot formation
    ii. May lead to disseminated intravascular coagulation (DIC) (Table 75–1)

d. Inadequate cerebral blood flow
    i. If cerebral perfusion pressure (CPP) falls <40–50 mmHg, severe ischemia occurs → sympathetic discharge → increased deleterious effects. The patient progresses from being drowsy, confused, and lethargic to unresponsive.
    ii. If ischemia continues, function of brain's vital centers is depressed.
    iii. Vasomotor center fails: Loss of sympathetic tone → severe decrease in BP → decreased HR, lethal decrease in tissue perfusion → decreased cerebral flow → increased cerebral ischemia → death

---

TABLE 75–1. SYMPTOMS OF DISSEMINATED INTRAVASCULAR COAGULATION

Oozing or bleeding from venipuncture sites, incisions, wounds
Bleeding around tubes: endotracheal, nasotracheal or nasogastric, urethral catheters
Bleeding from mucosal surfaces/body orifices: Epistaxis, hematemesis, hemoptysis, melena, hematochezia, hematuria; gingival, scleral bleeding
Skin: Ecchymoses, petechiae, pallor, mottling
Neurologic: Headache, altered level of consciousness, vertigo, lethargy, irritability, confusion, restlessness, focal deficits, seizures, coma
Cardiovascular: hypotension, tachycardia, ST–T wave changes
Renal: Oliguria, hematuria
Gastrointestinal: Abdominal pain, distention, hyperactive or absent bowel sounds
Other: Anxiety, dyspnea, muscle weakness, fatigue, acral cyanosis, acidosis, hematomas, signs of thrombophlebitis

---

(From Hartshorn, J.C., Sole, M.L., & Lamborn, M.L. [1997]. *Introduction to critical care nursing* [2nd ed.] [p. 393]. Philadelphia: W.B. Saunders, with permission.)

E. Laboratory findings/Diagnosis

1. Glucose: Increased early in shock due to sympathetic stimulation, and decreased late in shock due to depletion of body glycogen stores and decreased liver function
2. Total protein and albumin: Decreased due to leakage from capillaries and decreased synthesis in liver cells
3. Blood urea nitrogen (BUN) and creatinine (Cr): Increased due to renal ischemia and development of acute tubular necrosis (ATN)
4. Sodium: Increased early due to increased aldosterone causing renal retention of Na; increased or decreased late due to ATN
5. Potassium

   a. Early: Decreased secondary to increased aldosterone causing renal excretion of K^+
   b. Late: Increased due to acidosis, cell necrosis, and decreased renal function

6. Chloride

   a. Early: Decreased due to alkalotic state and HCO_3 excess
   b. Late: Increased due to acidotic state and HCO_3 deficiency

7. HCO_3

   a. Early: Increased due to alkalotic state
   b. Late: Decreased due to severe metabolic and respiratory acidosis

8. Liver enzymes and bilirubin: Increased due to necrosis of cells
9. Creatine phosphokinase (CPK): Increased due to necrosis of muscle and/or heart cells
10. Amylase/lipase: Increased due to necrosis of pancreatic cells
11. Blood cultures: Positive due to a variety of causative microbes
12. Hemoglobin: Decreased if hemorrhage is present
13. Hematocrit

    a. Early: Increased due to fluid leakage from capillaries (hemoconcentration)
    b. Late: Decreased if there is true blood loss, such as GI bleeding, trauma to liver/spleen; usually does not occur until 6 h after blood loss

14. White blood cell (WBC) count: Increased due to the body's response to infection (if present) and stress response
15. Platelet count: Decreased due to platelet aggregation and microemboli
16. Prothrombin time (PT)/partial thromboplastin time (PTT): Prolonged due to hypercoagulable state (if present)

17. Arterial blood gases (ABGs):
    a. Early: Respiratory alkalosis, due to hyperventilation and CO_2 exhalation
    b. Late: Respiratory acidosis, due to hypoventilation and lactic acid production
    c. Po_2: Decreased due to hypoventilation and hypoperfusion

18. Urine measurements
    a. Creatinine clearance: Decreased due to impaired renal excretion secondary to acute tubular necrosis
    b. Osmolality
       i. Early: Increased due to H_2O retention
       ii. Late: Decreased due to inability of the kidney to concentrate urine
    c. Specific gravity
       i. Early: Increased due to H_2O retention
       ii. Late: Decreased
    d. Sodium
       i. Early: Decreased due to Na reabsorption
       ii. Late: Decreased or increased due to abnormal renal function
    e. Potassium
       i. Early: Increased due to K^+ excretion secondary to aldosterone
       ii. Late: Increased or decreased due to abnormal renal function

19. Chest x-ray: The practitioner should assess for pulmonary edema, tension pneumothorax, and cardiac tamponade. The chest x-ray is helpful in recognizing early ARDS.
20. Electrocardiography (ECG): Note for signs of ischemia such as ST depression

F. Management of shock[5, 8, 11, 12, 16, 17]

1. Maintain airway and ventilation. Monitor respiratory status, O_2 saturation (via pulse oximetry) and ABGs closely. Administer supplemental O_2 for treatment or prevention of hypoxemia. Mechanical ventilation may be necessary for the facilitation of gas exchange.
2. Invasive hemodynamic monitoring is a critical tool for assessment of various types of shock (e.g., arterial line, pulmonary artery catheter). Information can be obtained regarding fluid status, contractility of the heart, and effectiveness of vasoactive agents (Table 75–2).
3. Maintain adequate circulation
    a. Maintain a MAP >60 mmHg or systolic blood pressure >80 mmHg. Some evidence suggests that a MAP of 80 mmHg may be more appropriate

TABLE 75–2. HEMODYNAMIC ALTERATIONS IN SHOCK STATES

PARAMETER/NORMAL RANGE	CARDIOGENIC	HYPOVOLEMIC	OBSTRUCTIVE	DISTRIBUTIVE Septic	DISTRIBUTIVE Anaphylactic Neurogenic
Cardiac output, 4–8 L/min	Low	Low	Low	High then low	Low
Cardiac index, 2.8–4.2 L/min/m²	Low	Low	Low	High then low	Low
Right atrial pressure, 0–8 mmHg	High	Low	High	Low then high	Low
Pulmonary artery diastolic pressure, 4–12 mmHg	High	Low	High	Low then high	Low
Pulmonary capillary wedge pressure, 1–10 mmHg	High	Low	High	Low then high	Low
Systemic vascular resistance, 900–1400 dynes/sec/cm⁻⁵	High	High	Low	Low	Low
Mixed venous oxygen saturation, 60–80%	Low	Low	High	High then low	Low

(From Hartshorn, J.C., Sole, M.L., & Lamborn, M.L. [1997]. *Introduction to critical care nursing* [2nd ed.] [p. 216]. Philadelphia: W.B. Saunders, with permission.)

b. Maintain cardiac index (CI) >2.2 L/min/m²

c. Maintain Svo_2 between 60% and 80%

d. Evaluate skin color and temperature (should be pink, warm, and dry without pallor or cyanosis), capillary refill (CFT <2 s)

e. HR <60–100 beats/min (strong and regular)

f. Nondistended, noncollapsed jugular veins

g. Alert and responsive in those without a head injury

h. Urine output 30–60 mL/h

4. Fluid therapy: Fluid replacement for cellular nutrition and restoration of tissue perfusion. Intravenous (IV) fluids help restore intravascular volume, maintain oxygen-carrying capacity, and establish hemodynamic stability, which is required for optimal tissue perfusion.

   a. Type and amount depend on type of shock, the patient's medical problems, and fluid's availability.

   b. Large-bore IVs (14- or 16-gauge): Minimal of two required.

      i. A central venous catheter is helpful for large volume replacement as well as for monitoring central venous pressure (CVP).

      ii. Triple-lumen catheters allow simultaneous administration of fluid, medications, and blood products.

   c. Generally, patients in shock require 2000–3000 cal/day due to stress state, which depletes nutritional stores and results in protein catabolism.

   d. Fluid challenges are often given to determine patient's response.

      i. Typically a rapid infusion of 250–500 mL of normal saline should be ordered.

      ii. Repeat boluses may be required if blood pressure and hemodynamic parameters remain low.

   e. Monitor Goal is 30–60 mL mL/h.

   f. Be very cautious in the use of IV fluids with patients in cardiogenic shock, as large volumes of fluids overwork the heart that is already failing.

5. Correct acid-base imbalance

   a. Metabolic acidosis: In severe cases (pH < 7.10) $NaHCO_3$ may be administered to increase pH to between 7.20 and 7.25, although this treatment remains controversial. Be careful not to overcorrect the acidosis and precipitate alkalosis

   b. Respiratory acidosis: Mechanical ventilation (to assist in blowing off excessive CO_2) and endotracheal tube (ET) suctioning

c. Respiratory alkalosis: Sedation (in attempt to slow respirations and reserve CO_2) and adjustment of ventilator (decrease set rate on ventilator) settings

6. Pharmacologic treatment: Depends on type of shock. The different drugs are addressed under each type of shock (see later in chapter).
7. No intramuscular (IM) injections should be given due to poor perfusion.
8. Nutritional support

   a. "If the gut works, use it." Early enternal feedings (within 8–12 h after surgery/trauma) have proved to be an inhibitor of intestinal atrophy and subsequent bacterial translocation.
   b. Early nutritional support has been found to preserve the normal immune and defense functions of the GI tract and therefore prevents the movement of bacteria and endotoxin across the mucosal barrier and into the systemic circulation.
   c. Assess bowel sounds and note if the patient has a paralytic ileus or gut stasis prior to initiation of feedings. Monitor residuals every 2–3 h to assess if the patient is tolerating the feeding.

II. TYPES OF SHOCK

A. Hypovolemic[4, 5, 8, 11, 12, 16, 17]

1. Amount of blood volume is inadequate to fill the circulatory system. Caused by exogenous or endogenous loss of circulating volume
2. Associated with a blood volume deficit of at least 15–25%.
3. Internal causes

   a. Third spacing: Ascites, peritonitis, edema
   b. Leakage of fluid from intestinal capillaries into walls and lumen of intestines
   c. Long bone fractures, which can result in a large amount of blood loss
   d. Pooling in extravascular compartments (e.g., ruptured liver/spleen, hemorrhagic pancreatitis, lacerations of great vessels)
   e. Impaired venous return due to obstruction of vena cava

4. External causes

   a. Hemorrhage
   b. GI losses: Vomiting, diarrhea, poor oral intake, large nasogastric tube aspirate, fistulas
   c. Renal losses: Excessive diuresis may occur in certain conditions (e.g., diabetes insipidus, syndrome of inappropri-

ate ADH (SIADH), Addison's disease) or during diuretic therapy

   d. Exudative lesions or burns

   e. Excessive diaphoresis

5. Clinical manifestations specific to hypovolemic shock

   a. Increased HR, decreased BP

   b. Decreased CVP, CO, CI, pulmonary artery pressure (PAP), pulmonary capillary wedge pressure (PCWP)

   c. Positive postural changes (decrease of $\geq$20 mmHg and/or increase of $\geq$20 beats/min

   d. Flat neck veins

6. Up to 10% of blood volume lost: May produce no symptoms due to compensatory mechanisms or slight tachycardia

7. <15% blood volume lost: Patient may exhibit

   a. Slight hypotension

   b. Normal heart rate or <100 beats/min

   c. Capillary filling time <3 s

   d. Anxiety or changes in sensorium

   e. Orthostasis

   f. Urine output adequate (>30 mL/h)

8. 15–30% blood volume lost: Patient may exhibit

   a. Systolic blood pressure usually >90 mmHg

   b. Decreased pulse pressure

   c. Tachycardia >100 beats/min

   d. Cool skin with pallor

   e. Poor capillary filling time (>3 s)

   f. Lethargic, weak

   g. Decreased urine output (<25–30 mL/h)

   h. Increased RR

9. Over 40% blood volume lost: Patient may exhibit

   a. Moderate to severe hypotension (MAP <55 mmHg)

   b. Tachycardia (140 beats/min)

   c. Cold, cyanotic skin

   d. LOC severely compromised

   e. Oliguria

10. Therapy specific to hypovolemic shock:

   a. Vasopressors are contraindicated until circulating volume has been restored

   b. Fluid challenges: 250–500 mL bolus of Ringer's lactate or normal saline. Repeat boluses if BP or CVP remain low.

   c. Fluid replacement

      i. Blood/blood products

         (1) These are clearly indicated in hemorrhagic shock and to maintain hematocrit between 30 mL/dL

and 35 mL/dL in the critically ill. One unit of packed red blood cells (PRBC) will increase the hematocrit by approximately 3 mL/dL and the hemoglobin by 1 g/dL.

(2) Fresh frozen plasma (FFP) may be indicated to replace clotting factors with the exception of platelets. FFP should be ordered to restore coagulation factors when massive transfusions are required.

(3) For every 4–5 units of PRBCs infused, 1 unit of FFP should be infused as well.

(4) Platelets may also be necessary to control bleeding that is a result of a low platelet count (<50,0000/mL).

ii. Crystalloids

(1) Crystalloids are cheap, convenient to use, and free of side effects, but they are rapidly distributed across the cell intravascular and interstitial spaces.

(2) The two most common crystalloid solutions are Ringer's lactate and normal saline.

(3) Ringer's lactate contains physiologic concentrations of sodium, chloride, calcium, potassium, and lactate in water and is effective as a volume expander and buffer in the presence of acidosis.

(4) Normal saline (0.9% NaCl in water) increases the plasma volume and is used most frequently when there has been no loss of red blood cells (RBCs). Usually requires volumes two to four times that of colloid to achieve an equivalent hemodynamic response. Be aware that volume expansion is transient and fluid will accumulate in the interstitial spaces, which may result in pulmonary edema.

iii. Colloids (starches, gelatins)

(1) Colloids produce a greater and more sustained increase in plasma volume with associated improvements in cardiovascular function and O_2 transport.

(2) Plasma protein fractions, such as albumin and plasma protein fraction (Plasmanate), are given when the volume lost is caused by plasma rather than blood, such as in burns, third spacing, peritonitis, and bowel obstruction.

(3) Synthetic plasma expanders, such as hetastarch (Hespan) and dextran, are also effective in increasing plasma volume.

(4) Monitor for adverse side effects such as pulmonary edema, coagulopathies, and anaphylactic reactions. No more than 1 L of dextran and Hespan in a 24-h period is recommended.

d. Military antishock trousers (MAST)

   i. MAST is an external counterpressure device that may be applied to assist with major organ perfusion, although its use is controversial.

   ii. MAST is useful in trauma patients to help splint fractures of the pelvis and long bones and tamponade a bleed. The compression redistributes blood flow from the peripheral circulation, which increases venous return and results in vital organ perfusion.

B. Cardiogenic shock[4, 5, 9, 11, 12, 16]

1. Impaired ability of the heart to pump effectively resulting in decreased SV, CO, and inadequate tissue perfusion. Cardiogenic shock is decreased cardiac output and evidence of tissue hypoxia in the presence of adequate intravascular volume.

2. Results from ineffective contractility due to

   a. Acute myocardial infarction (AMI). (Incidence of cardiogenic shock after AMI is 5–10% with a mortality rate of 50–80%).

   b. Dysrhythmias

   c. Congestive heart failure (CHF)

   d. Pulmonary emboli (PE)

   e. Tension pneumothorax

   f. Cardiac tamponade, myocardial contusion

   g. Dissecting aortic aneurysm

   h. Surgical or spontaneous damage to valves, valvular heart disease (e.g., acute mitral regurgitation, rupture of the interventricular septum, rupture of the free wall, and large right ventricular infarctions)

   i. Myocarditis, end-stage cardiomyopathy

   j. Septic shock with severe myocardial depression

   k. Any form of severe myocardial damage

3. Clinical manifestations specific to cardiogenic shock

   a. Increased PAP, PCWP, SVR. CVP may or may not be elevated, depending on whether the right ventricle is involved, or if volume from the left side of the heart has backed up in to the right side

   b. Decreased SV, CO, and CI. A CI of <1.8 L/min/m^2 indicates cardiogenic shock

   c. Left ventricular ejection fraction (EF) is usually <20–30%

    d. Pulmonary congestion: Rales/rhonchi, decreased Pa_{O_2}, decreased Pa_{CO_2} (early), increased Pa_{CO_2} (late), decreased mixed venous O_2 (MV_{O_2})

    e. S_3/S_4 heart sounds, precordial thrill may be palpable, rapid/faint pulse, a systolic murmur of mitral regurgitation or ventricular septal defect may be heard.

    f. Peripheral edema

    g. Distended neck veins

    h. Signs of decreased tissue perfusion: Oliguria, clouded sensorium, and cool/mottled skin

    i. Cardiogenic shock is diagnosed after documentation of myocardial dysfunction and exclusion or correction of such factors as hypovolemia, hypoxia, and acidosis

4. Diagnostic tests

    a. Electrocardiography should be performed immediately; it provides information on overall and regional systolic function and can lead to a rapid diagnosis of mechanical causes of shock.

    b. Other diagnostic tests usually include chest x-ray, ABGs, electrolytes, complete blood count (CBC), and cardiac enzymes.

    c. Invasive hemodynamic monitoring is very useful to exclude volume depletion, right ventricular infarction, and mechanical complications. Monitor CVP, PCWP, CO/CI, and SVR closely.

5. Treatment specific to cardiogenic shock

    a. Goal is improvement of pump performance and CO.

    b. Oxygenation and airway protection are critical; intubation and mechanical ventilation are often required.

    c. Central venous and arterial access, bladder catheterization, and pulse oximetry are routine.

    d. Initial approach should include fluid resuscitation unless pulmonary edema is present.

    e. Electrolyte abnormalities should be corrected. Hypokalemia and hypomagnesemia are predisposing factors to ventricular arrhythmia, and acidosis can decrease contractile function.

    f. Pharmacologic treatment (Table 75–3)

        i. MSO_4: Relieves anxiety, pain, reduces excessive sympathetic activity, and decreases O_2 demand, preload, and afterload

        ii. Dopamine: 2–10 $\mu g/kg/min$ IV drip for inotropic support; increases myocardial contractility

        iii. Dobutamine (Dobutrex): Positive inotropic agent— 2–20 $\mu g/kg/min$ IV drip

TABLE 75-3. DRUGS COMMONLY USED IN SHOCK

DRUG	ACTION	USE	DOSAGE/ROUTE	STANDARD MIX	SIDE EFFECTS	NURSING IMPLICATIONS
Dopamine	Renal vasodilator	Increases renal perfusion	1–2 μg/kg/min IV drip	400 mg/ 250 mL 5%D/W	Increased heart rate, increased dysrhythmias, increased myocardial oxygen consumption, nausea/vomiting	Do not administer with alkaline solutions. Monitor for myocardial ischemia. Monitor BP at least every 15 min. If IV infiltrates, may cause extravasation. Administer via volumetric pump. Should be tapered gradually. Administer via central catheter if possible.
	Positive inotropic	Increases myocardial contractility	2–10 μg/kg/ min IV drip			Low BP associated with hypovolemia should be treated with aggressive fluid resuscitation prior to drug administration.
	Vasopressor	Increases BP when not caused by hypovolemia	10–20 μg/kg/ min IV drip			

Table continued on following page

TABLE 75–3. DRUGS COMMONLY USED IN SHOCK *Continued*

DRUG	ACTION	USE	DOSAGE/ ROUTE	STANDARD MIX	SIDE EFFECTS	NURSING IMPLICATIONS
Dobutamine	Positive inotropic	Increases BP in low cardiac output states	2–20 μg/kg/ min IV drip	500–1000 mg/ 250 mL 5% D/W or NS	Increased heart rate, increased dysrhythmias, increased myocardial oxygen consumption, headache, tremors, nausea	Monitor for myocardial ischemia. Monitor BP at least every 15 min. Administer via volumetric pump. Should be tapered gradually. Administer via central catheter, if possible.
Norepinephrine	Vasopressor, some positive inotropic effects	Increases BP; refractory to other drugs	2–12 μg/min IV drip	4 mg/250– 1000 mL 5% D/W or NS	Increased myocardial oxygen consumption, increased dysrhythmias, severe vasoconstriction	Monitor for myocardial ischemia. Monitor BP at least every 15 min. Administer via volumetric pump. Should be tapered gradually. Administer via central catheter, if possible. If IV infiltrates, may cause extravasation.

| Nitroglycerin | Venodilator | Reduces preload, pump failure | Start at 5 μg/min and titrate to effect; 50–200 μg/min is range for most patients. An IV bolus dose of 12.5–25 μg may be given prior to infusion | 50–100 mg/250 mL 5% D/W | Headache, hypotension, bradycardia | Monitor BP at least every 15 min. Administer via volumetric pump. Should be tapered gradually. Administer via central catheter, if possible. |
| Nitroprusside | Vasodilator | Reduces preload and afterload | 0.5–10 μg/kg/min IV drip | 50 mg/250 mL 5% D/W or NS | Myocardial ischemia, hypotension, nausea | Monitor for myocardial ischemia. May cause thiocyanate intoxication in large dosages or prolonged administration. Monitor BP at least every 15 min. Administer via volumetric pump. Should be tapered gradually. Administer via central catheter, if possible. |

(From Hartshorn, J.C., Sole, M.L., & Lamborn, M.L. [1997]. Introduction to critical care nursing [2nd ed.] [p. 224]. Philadelphia: W.B. Saunders, with permission.)

   iv. Milrinone (Primacor): 50 μg/kg IV bolus, followed by 0.375–0.75 μg/kg/min IV infusion. Positive inotropic agent

   v. Amrinone (Inocor): 0.75 mg/kg IV bolus; may be repeated in 30 min if necessary, then 5–10 μg/kg/min IV drip. Total daily dose should not exceed 10 mg/kg. Positive inotropic agent

   vi. Isoproterenol (Isuprel): 2–20 μg/min IV drip). May be indicated in patients with low heart rates resulting in decreased CO. Isuprel has positive chronotropic effects and should be given as indicated.

   vii. Norepinephrine (Levophed): 2–12 μg/kg/min IV drip. Is a vasopressor and has some positive inotropic effects

   viii. Diuretics (furosemide [Lasix]), nitroprusside (Nipride), 0.5–10 μg/kg/min IV drip; nitrates (nitroglycerin: begin at 5 μg/min and titrate to desired effect); and morphine sulfate: Agents that may be used in cardiogenic shock to reduce preload. Be careful not to cause extreme loss of volume when these agents are administered. Monitor PCWP, BP, CO/CI, and SVR closely.

   ix. Nitroprusside (Nipride): 0.5–10 μg/kg/min IV drip; may be used to decrease a high afterload which can have deleterious effects on an ischemic heart

   x. Lidocaine (1 mg/kg bolus followed by 1–4 mg/min infusion); may be necessary if there are ventricular dysrythmias resulting in decreased CO

   xi. Be aware that medications proven to improve outcome after AMI, such as nitrates, beta blockers, and angiotensin-converting enzyme inhibitors, may exacerbate hypotension in a patient with cardiogenic shock; therefore, therapy with these medications should be discontinued until the patient stabilizes.

g. Counterpulsation (intra-aortic balloon pump)

   i. Increases pump efficiency

   ii. Augments diastolic pressure

   iii. Increases coronary end-organ perfusion

   iv. Reduces afterload

   v. Reduces myocardial demands

h. Pathophysiologic considerations and clinical trials favor aggressive mechanical revascularization for patients with cardiogenic shock caused by AMI. Patients with successful reperfusion with percutaneous transluminal coronary angiography have much better outcomes, as do those patients in cardiogenic shock who have coronary artery bypass surgery. (Left main artery and three-vessel disease are common in cardiogenic shock.)

C. Distributive shock

1. Includes septic, neurogenic, and anaphylactic shock. All of these types of shock have peripheral vasodilation with a disproportion between the usual circulating volume and the vascular bed. The vasodilation and loss of vasomotor tone result in a massive increase in vascular capacity, venous pooling of blood, and decreased venous return to the heart, which leads to a condition of inadequate tissue perfusion.

2. Septic shock[1, 4, 6, 12, 14–16, 18, 19]

   a. Septic shock is a systemic inflammatory response to an infectious process.
      i. Activation of the complement, clotting, and kinin systems occur as well as the release of vasoactive mediators from damaged tissues.
      ii. The initial manifestation of the infection is overwhelming inflammation followed by a period of immunodepression.
      iii. A systemic cascade is activated by the local release of bacteria, toxins, or other inflammatory mediators.

   b. Causative organisms
      i. Viruses
      ii. Fungal infections
      iii. Bacteria—Gram-negative bacilli (endotoxic shock) most common and most serious
         (1) *Escherichia coli*
         (2) *Klebsiella pneumoniae*
         (3) *Enterobacter*
         (4) *Proteus*
         (5) *Pseudomonas*
         (6) *Serratia*
         (7) Meningococci
      iv. Bacteria—Gram-positive organisms: Incidence has increased significantly almost to that of gram-negative infections
         (1) Staphylococci (*Staphylococcus aureus, S. epidermidis, S. saprophyticus*)
         (2) Streptococci (*Streptococcus pyogenes, S. agalactiae, S. anginosus, S. faecalis, S. bovis, S. viridans, S. pneumoniae*)
         (3) Clostridia (*Clostridium perfringens, C. tetani, C. difficile, C. botulinum*)
         (4) *Bacteroides*

   c. Nosocomial infections in the critically ill are a major cause of sepsis.
      i. Predisposing factors include malnutrition, instrumentation or other invasive procedures, trauma, surgical wounds, advanced age, immunosuppressive therapy

(e.g., cytotoxics, corticosteroids), neoplastic diseases, chronic diseases (e.g., diabetes mellitus and/or renal failure), and long hospital stays.
- ii. Sites of infection include genitourinary (GU) tract (most common cause of sepsis in the elderly), respiratory tract, wounds, invasive lines (IV lines, central lines, etc.), meninges, and the GI tract.
- iii. Increased use of more potent and broader spectrum antibiotics has led to resistant strains of bacteria and increased incidence of infection and sepsis.
- d. Clinical manifestations specific for septic shock
  - i. Hyperdynamic (warm) shock
    - (1) Chills (some patients may actually have rigors)
    - (2) Fever (may not occur in the elderly or chronically ill patient; these patients may possibly have a low temperature)
    - (3) Warm, flushed skin
    - (4) Mental confusion (early sign)
    - (5) BP normal or slightly increased
    - (6) Increased HR and RR (early sign)
    - (7) Decreased PaO_2 despite O_2 therapy
    - (8) Increased SvO_2: less O_2 is utilized by the cell. (SvO_2 is the amount of O_2 delivered to the tissue)
    - (9) Hyperventilation (respiratory alkalosis)
    - (10) Decreased PCWP, CVP and systemic vascular resistance (SVR)
    - (11) CO normal or increased
    - (12) Patient may start having increased residuals if receiving enternal feedings
  - ii. Hypodynamic (cold) shock
    - (1) Cold, clammy skin
    - (2) Tachycardia, decreased BP
    - (3) Decreased PCWP, CO, and an increased SVR
    - (4) Respiratory failure (ARDS)
    - (5) Metabolic acidosis due to lactic acidosis
    - (6) Oliguria
    - (7) May have signs and symptoms of DIC
    - (8) Edema
- e. Diagnostic findings specific to septic shock
  - i. Leukocytosis (with a shift to the left) or neutropenia
  - ii. Thrombocytopenia without evidence of DIC (seen in 50% of septic patients)
  - iii. Abnormal PT and PTT
  - iv. Positive blood cultures: Monitor at 24, 48, and 72 h. Obtain from two or three different sites
  - v. Lactate levels increased
  - vi. Liver function abnormalities
  - vii. Hypoglycemia

      viii. Chest x-ray to rule out pneumonia
       ix. Urine culture and sensitivity to rule out urosepsis
        x. Culture and sensitivity of wounds and/or invasive catheters
       xi. Positive CD10 test result: A rapid new diagnostic test that will be of value in diagnosing sepsis. The major potential benefit is early recognition of developing sepsis in the critically ill.

  f. Therapy specific to septic shock
       i. Treatment is time and dose related; early recognition and treatment are keys to successful management. Look for the source carefully: Look at the chest x-ray to rule out pneumonia; obtain a urine culture and sensitivity to rule out urosepsis; obtain cultures of wounds and/or invasive lines.
      ii. Underlying infection must be treated and tissue perfusion restored.
     iii. Ventilation: Intubation and mechanical ventilation is indicated if arterial O_2 tension is <60 mmHg with F_{IO_2} >60% or RR >35 beats/min. Add PEEP/pressure support if necessary. (See Table 75–4: Indications for Mechanical Ventilation.)
     iv. Volume resuscitation is the mainstay of initial hemodynamic management. Hypovolemia is present in almost all of septic patients, and large amounts of fluid (frequently as many as 10 or more liters) is required until the capillary leak seals.

TABLE 75–4. INDICATIONS FOR MECHANICAL VENTILATION

PARAMETER	NORMAL	VENTILATION
ABGs		
P_{aO_2} (mmHg)	>80	<60
P_{aCO_2} (mmHg)	35–45	>50
pH	7.35–7.45	<7.25
P_{aO_2} = P_{aCO_2}		
Other		
Respiratory rate/min	12–16	>35
Tidal volume (mL/kg)	6–8	<3.5
Vital capacity (mL/kg)	50–60	<10–15
NIF cm/H_2O*	>−25	<−20

*Negative inspiratory force (NIF) is the amount of negative pressure that a patient is able to generate to initiate spontaneous respirations. Normally NIF is −25 cm of H_2O or greater: e.g., −30 cm, −40 cm.

ABG = arterial blood gas.

(From Hartshorn, J.C., Sole, M.L., & Lamborn, M.L. [1997]. *Introduction to critical care nursing* [2nd ed.] [p. 151]. Philadelphia: W.B. Saunders.)

(1) Hemodynamic monitoring is essential and attempts should be made to maintain a PCWP between 10 and 20 mmHg. Assess this carefully in each patient, especially the elderly and those with a history of CHF (monitor for pulmonary edema).

(2) Replace preexisting deficits.

(3) Replace third space losses with balanced solution such as Ringer's lactate. Colloids may be associated with a lower incidence of pulmonary edema.

(4) Blood if hemoglobin or hematocrit is decreased.

g. Pharmacologic treatment (see Table 75–3)

  i. Antibiotics

    (1) Empirical treatment is crucial to survival and should be initiated until source has been identified

    (2) Until culture is identified, a combination of

      (a) Aminoglycoside: Amikacin (Amikin), 5 mg/kg q8h plus

      (b) Agents that will cover suspected areas of infection and/or predisposing factors:

      ☐ Cephalosporin: Cefoxitin (Mefoxin), 1–2 g q6–8h, for suspected pulmonary infection

      ☐ Ampicillin (Ampicin), 1–2 g/day in divided doses q4–6h, to cover enterococci in suspected urinary tract infection (UTI)

      ☐ Add cefotetan (Cefotan), 1–6 g/day IV in divided doses q12h; cefoxitin (Mefoxin), 1–2 g IV q6–8h; clindamycin (Cleocin), 600–1200 mg/day IV in 2–4 divided doses; or metronidazole (Flagyl), 7.5 mg/kg IV q6h to cover anaerobic organisms, plus ampicillin (Ampicin) to cover enterococci for suspected intra-abdominal infection

      ☐ Add nafcillin (Nafzil), 500–1500 mg IV q4h or oxacillin (Bactocill), up to 12–20 g/day IV in divided doses q4–6h to cover staphylococci in suspected skin infections

      ☐ A beta-lactam: Ticarcillin (Ticar), 3 g q3–6h IV or mezlocillin, (Mezlin), 3–4 g q4–6h IV, may be necessary in the neutropenic patient for additional coverage against *Pseudomonas*

      ☐ Once the organism has been identified, adjust the antibiotics to the appropriate coverage

  ii. Steroids

    (1) Controversial: Studies indicate there is no benefit in their use

  (2) Effects rest on microcirculation
  (3) Stabilizes lysosomal membrane in order to de-
      crease capillary leak
  (4) Has been beneficial in suspected adrenal insuffi-
      ciency (hydrocortisone, 100 mg IV q4h)
 iii. Vasopressors: May be indicated when previous mea-
      sures have failed to correct hypotension and PCWP
      has been raised to 15–18 mmHg. Titrate agents to
      raise the MAP to at least 60 mmHg
  (1) Fluid volume: Normal saline or Ringer's lactate
      is essential when using vasopressors.
  (2) Beta-receptor stimulants that have a positive
      inotropic effect and dilate the microcirculation
      may be indicated (e.g., dopamine: Begin at
      5–10 μg/kg/min).
  (3) If dopamine is ineffective at doses of
      10–20 μg/kg/min, other agents such as epi-
      nephrine or norepinephrine may be necessary
      (see Table 75–3).
 iv. Antipyrogenics/cooling blanket will help reduce
     body temperature and metabolic demands.
  v. Closed-space infections require surgical drainage
     (e.g., abscess, infected bowel, infected uterus, in-
     flamed gallbladder).
 vi. Metabolic support is needed. Protein and calorie re-
     quirements are high, and underlying malnutrition is
     prevalent in patients with sepsis. If the gut works,
     use it, even if bowel sounds are diminished or some
     abdominal distention is present. The advantages to en-
     teral feedings as compared with parental feeding in-
     clude gastric buffering, avoidance of the use of
     parenteral-nutrition catheters, preservation of the gut
     mucosa, avoidance of the introduction of bacteria and
     toxins for the GI tract into the circulation, a more
     physiologic pattern of enteric hormone secretion, the
     ability to deliver a complete nutritional source as well
     as fiber, and lastly it is less expensive.
vii. Supportive measures
  (1) Prophylaxis against stress ulcers: H_2 blockers,
      proton-pump inhibitors, or sucralfate (Carafate)
      is indicated in high-risk patients who are being
      mechanically ventilated and cannot be fed enter-
      ally. Carafate is preferred because there is an in-
      creased risk for nosocomial pneumonia in pa-
      tients with elevated gastric pH (i.e., those
      receiving H_2 blockers).
  (2) Deep venous thrombosis (DVT) prophylaxis:
      Fixed-dose unfractionated heparin (Heparin,

5000 units sc q12h), low-molecular-weight heparin (enoxaparin [Levonox], 30 mg sc q12h), and elastic stockings and venous-compression devices, unless contraindicated.

viii. If DIC is present with sepsis, studies reveal that plasminogen activator may be beneficial in lysing the microclots of DIC which may block circulation to organs, causing ARDS and multisystem organ failure (MOF). Unless contraindicated, urokinase, 2200 units/kg bolus in 10 min, followed by 2200 units/kg/h infusion for 24 h, has been proven safe and effective.

ix. Investigational studies include
   (1) Endotoxin-directed therapies: Bactericidal permeability-increasing factor, soluble CD14 receptors, reconstituted high-density lipoproteins
   (2) Anti-inflammatory interventions: Modulation of nitric oxide activity, neutrophil adhesion molecules, infusion of antithrombin III, tissue-factor pathway inhibitors, activated protein C, pentoxyfylline
   (3) Granulocyte colony-stimulating factor: Enhances phagocytic cell function
   (4) Adaptation of molecular biologic techniques: Gene therapy, antisense technology

D. Neurogenic shock (distributive shock)[2, 5, 11–13, 17, 20]

1. Caused by a disturbance in the nervous system causing massive Vasodilation leading to increased vascular capacity as a result of an interruption or loss of sympathetic innervation. Spinal shock, which is frequently seen with neurogenic shock, occurs as a sudden neurophysiologic phenomenon resulting from damage (structural or biochemical) to the spinal cord tissue, causing temporary or permanent, complete or near-complete segmental interruption of neurotransmission (loss of control or reflex activity below the level of the lesion). Duration of spinal shock is usually 24 h up to 12 weeks.

2. Pathophysiology
   a. Loss of sympathetic vasoconstrictor tone
   b. Blood volume is normal but maldistributed
   c. Cardiac function is normal

3. Causes
   a. Injury or disease of the spinal cord or brain stem
   b. High levels of spinal anesthesia
   c. Vasomotor center depression
   d. Drugs that block sympathetic activity
   e. Significant pain or emotional stress

4. Clinical manifestations specific to neurogenic shock

   a. Hypotension: Due to the loss or depression of the autonomic reflex arc that is responsible for maintaining the tension of blood vessel walls resulting in significant vasodilation and producing hypotension

   b. Bradycardia: Caused by loss of sympathetic tone on the heart

   c. Hypothermia

   d. Warm, dry skin due to venodilation, resulting in venous pooling, and loss of sweat response below the level of the lesion

   e. Decreased SVR, stroke volume, and venous return (decreased CVP) due to loss of sympathetic vasoconstrictor tone below the level of the lesion in arterioles, precapillaries, and venules

5. Treatment

   a. Refer to Chapter 3 for detailed management of spinal cord injuries.

   b. Treat or remove cause if possible.

   c. Careful fluid administration ensures adequate tissue perfusion (systolic blood pressure <90 mmHg, urine output <30 mL/h, decreased LOC are indicators of poor perfusion).

   d. It is essential to differentiate neurogenic shock from hypovolemic shock. Both conditions result in hypotension, but patients who are in neurogenic shock manifest warm, dry skin and bradycardia, whereas those in hypovolemic shock have cool, moist skin and tachycardia due to compensatory mechanisms.

   e. Give vasopressors if fluids are not successful (e.g., dopamine, 5–10 μg/kg/min)

   f. For symptomatic bradycardia in which LOC, urine output, and BP are decreased, atropine, 0.5–1.0 mg IV push is indicated.

   g. Treat hypothermia.

   h. As with all shock states, prognosis is dependent on underlying process.

E. Anaphylactic shock (distributive shock)[3, 5, 7, 10–12, 17]

1. The result of an immediate hypersensitivity reaction. The severe antibody-antigen response leads to decreased tissue perfusion and initiation of the general shock response. Anaphylaxis involves one or both of two features: respiratory difficulty and hypotension, which can manifest as fainting, collapse, or unconsciousness.

2. Causes

    a. Foods such as nuts, fish, shellfish, dairy products, legumes, eggs, fruits, and berries

    b. Food additives such as dyes and monosodium glutamate

    c. Diagnostic agents such as allergen extracts, vaccines, radiocontrast media

    d. Blood products

    e. Environmental agents such as latex, pollen, mold spores, animal products, and dust

    f. Drugs, for example, antibiotics, acetylsalicylic acid, narcotics, dextran, anesthetic agents, muscle relaxants, and barbiturates

    g. Venom

3. Clinical manifestations

    a. Cardiovascular: Hypotension, tachycardia, arrhythmias

    b. Respiratory: Bronchospasm, laryngeal edema, lump in throat, dysphasia, hoarseness, dyspnea, stridor, wheezing, rales/rhonchi, hypoxia

    c. Cutaneous: Pruritus, erythema, urticaria, angioedema (swelling)

    d. CNS: Restlessness, uneasiness, apprehension, feeling of impending doom, anxiety, decreased LOC

    e. GI: Nausea and vomiting, diarrhea, abdominal cramps, metallic taste

    f. Hemodynamics: Decreased CO, CI, CVP, PCWP, and SVR

4. Treatment

    a. Speed of treatment is essential.

    b. Immediate administration of epinephrine (adrenaline) IM or SQ (preferably IM): 0.5–1.0 mL of 1:1,000 (1 mg/mL). Further doses may be required if improvement is not evident. Epinephrine should be given to all patients with respiratory difficulty or hypotension.

        i. Inhaled epinephrine is effective for mild to moderate laryngeal edema but would not be given if IM epinephrine has already been given as first-line treatment, and is not a substitute for IM epinephrine.

        ii. Give IV epinephrine if circulation is already compromised in 1:10,000 dilution (1 mg) slow IV push.

        iii. Do not wait to establish IV line; may give via endotracheal tube: 2–2.5 times (2.0–2.5 mg) the usual dose of 1:10,000 epinephrine solution. Use oxygen-valve reservoir bag or "manually bag" patient several sufflations after administration.

        iv. Give 0.1–0.5 mg of 1:10,000 epinephrine; repeat in 10-min intervals until the desired effect is achieved or until side effects occur.

c. Maintain airway: Intubate if necessary and administer supplemental O_2. Tracheostomy may be necessary in those with severe obstruction that makes intubation not possible.

d. Deliver antihistamine (diphenhydramine [Benadryl], 10–50 mg IV/IM single dose; may need up to 100 mg, not to exceed 400 mg/day) to block histamine effects.

e. Give aminophylline and/or albuterol for bronchospasm.

f. Expand vascular volume with Ringer's lactate infusion.

g. Add corticosteroids (hydrocortisone [Hydrocortone], 5 mg/kg IM or slow IV) to aid anti-inflammatory reaction.

h. Inotropic agents (e.g., dopamine) and vasoconstrictor agents may be necessary.

i. The key to management is awareness, early recognition (consider in differential diagnosis), and quick treatment. Anaphylaxis is easily treatable, and patients can make a complete recovery.

III. PREVENTION

A. Once clinical signs are apparent, cellular alterations have already begun to occur.

B. Hypovolemic shock: Careful attention to fluid balance

1. Intake and output

2. Monitor for an increase in HR, decrease in BP, CVP, PCWP, and CO/CI, which all are signs of hypovolemia

3. Hematocrit, hemoglobin, and NA^+ may be high due to hemoconcentration. Hct/Hgb will be low in true blood loss

4. Drainage (tubes, drains, wounds)

5. Insensible losses: Average is approximately 500 mL/day. This will be significantly higher in those with fever and those who are intubated and hyperventilating

6. Daily weights essential in determining fluid status

C. Cardiogenic shock

1. Decrease the workload of heart to minimize infarction size in AMI. Treat the cause (antiarrythmics, pericardiocentisis, etc.)

2. Monitor HR and rhythm, BP.

3. Monitor hemodynamic status: Assess for increase in PCWP/CVP, low CO/CI, and SVR.

D. Neurogenic shock

1. Careful immobilization of spinal cord injuries. After administration of spinal anesthesia, prevent spread of anesthetic agent up cord to medulla. Steroid therapy (methylprednisolone [Solu-Medrol]) may be initiated within the first 6–8 h after injury (see Chapter 3).

E. Anaphylactic shock

1. Good history is imperative. Give IV drugs slowly so that reaction can be detected before an overwhelming dosage is administered.

F. Septic shock

1. Monitor for fever, increased WBCs. Treat infections early. Change central lines, urinary catheters, peripheral lines, and other lines, tubes, and drains as needed. Assess wounds and insertion sites daily for signs and symptoms of infection.

References

1. Astiz, M.E., & Rackow, E.C. (1998). Septic shock. *The Lancet, 351*, 1501–1505.
2. Devinsky, O., Feldmann, E., & Weinreb, H.J. (2000). *Neurologic pearls.* Philadelphia: F.A. Davis Company.
3. Ewan, P.W. (1998). ABC of allergies: Anaphylaxis. *British Medical Journal, 316*, 1442–1445.
4. Ferri, F.F. (1998). *Practical guide to the care of the medical patient* (4th ed.). St. Louis: CV Mosby.
5. Gawlinski, A., McCloy, K., Caswell, D., & Quinones-Baldrich, W.J. (1999). Cardiovascular disorders. In A. Gawlinski, & D. Hamwi (Eds.), *Acute care nurse practitioner clinical curriculum and certification review.* Philadelphia: W.B. Saunders.
6. Hardaway, R.M. (1998). Traumatic and septic shock alias post-trauma critical illness. *The British Journal of Surgery, 85*, 1473–1479.
7. Henderson, N. (1998). Anaphylaxis. *Nursing Standard, 12*, 49–55.
8. Hinds, C.J., & Watson, D. (1999). ABC of intensive care: Circulatory support. *British Medical Journal, 318*, 1749–1752.
9. Hollenberg, S.M., Kavinsky, C.J., & Parrillo, J.E. (1999). Cardiogenic shock. *Annals of Internal Medicine, 131*, 47–59.
10. Hughes, G., & Fitzharris, P. (1999). Managing acute anaphylaxis: New guidelines emphasise importance of intramuscular adrenaline. *British Medical Journal, 319*, 1–2.
11. Jones, K.M., & Bucher, L. (1999). *Critical care nursing.* Philadelphia: W.B. Saunders.
12. McKinley, M.G., Robinson, C.F., & Sole, M.L. (1997). Shock. In J.C. Hartshorn, M.L. Sole, & M.L. Lamborn (Eds.), *Introduction to critical care nursing* (2nd ed). Philadelphia: W.B. Saunders.
13. Nacimiento, W., & Noth, J. (1999). What, if anything, is spinal shock? *Archives of Neurology, 56*, 1033–1035.
14. Palombo, J.D., & Bistrian, B.R. (1999). Early diagnosis of septic shock: A simple test for a complex condition? *Critical Care Medicine, 27*, 465–466.
15. Pedoto, A., Tassiopoulos, A.K., Oler, A., McGraw, D.J., Hoffman, S.P., Camporesi, E.M., & Hakim, T.S. (1998). Treatment of septic shock in rats with nitric oxide synthase inhibitors and inhaled nitric acid. *Critical Care Medicine, 26*, 2021–2028.
16. Stein, J.H. (1998). *Internal medicine* (4th ed.). St. Louis: CV Mosby.
17. Thompson, C.J. (1996). Nursing management of the patient in shock. In S.D. Ruppert, J.G. Kernicki, & J.T. Dolan (Eds.), *Dolan's critical care*

nursing: Clinical management through the nursing process (2nd ed). Philadelphia: F.A. Davis.

18. Tribett, D.L., Wilkens, K., Hardesty, M.T., Davies, J.E., Bates-Jensen, B.M., & Rodgers, K.S. (1999). Infections and common problems in acute care. In A. Gawlinski, & D. Hamwi (Eds.), *Acute care nurse practitioner: Clinical curriculum and certification review*. Philadelphia: W.B. Saunders.

19. Wheeler, A.P., & Bernard, G.R. (1999). Current concepts: Treating patients with severe sepsis. *The New England Journal of Medicine, 340*, 207–214.

20. White, R.J., & Likavec, M.J. (1999). Spinal shock—Spinal man. *The Journal of Trauma, 46*, 979–980.

NUTRITIONAL CONSIDERATIONS

Martha N. Surline, MS

I. NUTRITIONAL ASSESSMENT[1, 2, 4, 5, 8]

A. Laboratory measurements

1. Serum albumin: <3.5 g/dL indicates protein malnutrition; expect edema if <2.7 g/dL. Albumin is a principal drug carrier, and dosage may need adjustment. Albumin has a biologic half-life of 20 days. If evaluation of response to protein therapy is urgent, one should order prealbumin or retinol-binding protein tests.
2. Prealbumin, also known as thyroxine-binding prealbumin or transthyretin, has a half-life of 2 days. It is predictive of nitrogen status as well as carbohydrate intake and is responsive to 7 days of nutritional repletion.
3. Retinol-binding protein has a half-life of 12 hours, and is most reponsive to short-term dietary repletion. It is carried by prealbumin and is altered by vitamin A and carbohydrate levels.
4. Hemoglobin: Low levels (<12 g/dL for women and <13.5 g/dL for men) can indicate lack of iron and/or protein. Inadequate oxygen perfusion to cells results in decreased energy production, affecting many tissue functions including healing and growth.
5. Hematocrit is the percentage of erythrocytes in total blood volume. A low hematocrit confirms low hemaglobin levels.
6. Lymphocyte: Depressed level indicates decreased immune function or increased susceptibility to infection. Steroid use can decrease count.

B. Clinical observations: Use to support laboratory data; not diagnostic

1. Skin—Free of color irregularities, smooth
2. Mucous membranes—Smooth, pink, moist
3. Hair—Shiny, not easily plucked
4. Musculature—Toned, some fat present
5. Skeleton—Erect posture
6. Nails—Regularly shaped, free of ridges
7. Rapid cellular turnover is found in the above six areas, and nutritional deficiencies will become obvious earlier.

C. Dietary evaluation: Use to evaluate food intake; supportive of other data

1. Twenty-four-hour recall: All foods and beverages consumed within the last 24 hours

2. Three-day and 5-day food diaries: List of all food and beverages consumed within the specified time period. Encourage the patient to eat as he or she has previously; can also include occurrence of symptoms
3. Food frequency records: How often one eats a particular food or group of foods
4. Client interviews for diet history: Likes and dislikes, intolerance, allergies, eating patterns, and so on

II. IDEAL BODY WEIGHT (IDBW) CALCULATIONS[1, 2]

A. Men

1. 106 lb allowed for first 5 ft of height
2. 6 lb added for each inch over 5 ft
3. Adjust 10% of total for frame (skeleton) size

   a. Add 10% for large frame
   b. Subtract 10% for small frame
   c. No adjustment for medium or average frame

B. Women

1. 100 lb allowed for first 5 ft of height
2. 5 lb added for each inch over 5 ft
3. Adjust for frame size by 10% as for men

C. Individuals <5 ft in height

1. Consult published tables such as the Metropolitan Life Insurance Company.[7]

III. DETERMINING NUTRITIONAL NEEDS[1, 2, 3, 5]

Stressed patients first receive nutritional support in the hypermetabolic or second stage of the stress response. In the first or acute phase, correct only fluid and electrolyte imbalances.

A. Kilocalories per kilogram of body weight: Use actual or desired weight depending on goal of therapy. Consult dietitian for additional information.

1. Average adult requirement is 30 kcal/kg or 13 kcal/lb of body weight/24 h.
2. Usually, stressed individuals require 25–30 kcal/kg.
3. For weight gain, 35 or more kcal/kg is appropriate.
4. For weight loss, 25 kcal/kg is needed. One pound of body weight is equivalent to 3500 kcal; 1 kg is equivalent to 7700 kcal.
5. Elevated body temperature

   a. Seven percent increase in kcal/24 h required for each degree above 98.6°F

   b. Thirteen percent increase in kcal/24 h for each degree above 37°C

6. One may also use the Harris-Benedict equation for estimating basal energy expenditure (BEE).

   a. Women:

$$BEE = 655 + (9.6 \times wt\ in\ kg) + (1.7 \times ht\ in\ cm) - (4.7 \times age\ in\ years)$$

   b. Men:

$$BEE = 66 + (13.7 \times wt\ in\ kg) + (5 \times ht\ in\ cm) - (6.8 \times age\ in\ years)$$

   c. For activity, add to BEE:
      i. 20%—Sedentary
      ii. 35%—Moderately active
      iii. 50%—Active
   d. For stress, add to BEE:
      i. 10–15% for uncomplicated surgery
      ii. 20–40% for complicated surgery or fractures
      iii. 50–100% for extensive burns
   e. For fever, add to BEE:
      i. 13% per degree Celsius over normal (37°C)
   f. To promote weight gain, add to BEE:
      i. 5% for moderate weight loss
      ii. 10% to 15% for severe weight loss

B. Fluid requirements

1. One mL of fluid/kcal/24 h (30–35 mL/kg body weight) is usual. Water, fruit juices, decaffeinated beverages, popsicles, and flavored gelatin are good sources. Milk is 50% water.
2. Needs increase with elevated vital signs, use of drains, vomiting, diarrhea, and the like. Increase 150 mL/24 h for each degree rise in body temperature above normal.

C. Protein requirements

1. Grams of protein required per day vary from average or normal requirement of 0.8 g/kg of body weight to as much as 2.0 g/kg of body weight for those with extensive burns or surgery.
2. The average for stressed patients is 1.5 g or more per kg of body weight.
3. Renal and hepatic diseases usually necessitate lower levels of protein due to the inability to convert ammonia to urea in the liver, or the inability to excrete urea via the kidneys. Protein is the primary source of all nitrogenous waste products.
4. Consult a dietitian for the optimal amount.

D. Carbohydrate requirements

1. Carbohydrates provide the largest proportion of kilocalories in most diets—approximately 50% of daily need.
2. The metabolism of carbohydrates requires more oxygen (and releases more carbon dioxide) than either protein or fat. Patients with compromised respiratory function benefit from less than average carbohydrate intake.

E. Fat or lipid requirements

1. Fat has the lowest respiratory quotient (i.e., it uses the least amount of oxygen) and produces the least amount of carbon dioxide. If appropriate digestion of dietary fat is a problem (symptom: steathorrhea), a parenteral lipid emulsion is an alternative.
2. Substituting fat for carbohydrate can decrease stress on the respiratory system, particularly if the patient has minimal lung capacity.

F. Vitamins and minerals requirements

1. Use the 1989 Recommended Dietary Allowances (RDA), published by the National Academy of Sciences, as a guide. These guidelines are widely available. Consult a dietitian for individual needs.
2. General guidelines for use in stressed individuals follow:

    a. Zinc promotes wound healing.
    b. The B vitamin group is necessary for energy production; therefore, the need increases with hypermetabolism.
    c. Ascorbic acid or vitamin C is essential for collagen formation, as well as possessing excellent antioxidant capacity.
    d. Vitamin E is an excellent antioxidant.

3. Beware of oversupplementation.

    a. The liver and kidneys must "process" and excrete excessive vitamins.
    b. Ten times the RDA is a megadose, and this amount should be regarded as a medication rather than a supplement.

G. Electrolyte requirements

1. Replace deficits.
2. Beware of excessive amounts (exceeding the RDA), especially in renal disease, or in the first stage of the stress response when acute renal failure may be present.

IV. FOOD GUIDE PYRAMID[9]

A. Definition

Pattern for adhering to Dietary Guidelines for Americans

B. Schematic pyramid of six food groups and recommended numbers of daily servings for each group

1. Bread, cereal, rice and pasta: 6–11 servings—source of complex carbohydates for sustained energy release, and provide fiber to help prevent constipation
2. Vegetables: 3–5 servings—provide fiber and antioxidant vitamins important for gastrointestinal (GI) cancer prevention and cardiovascular health
3. Fruit: 2–4 servings—provide additional vitamins and fiber

   a. The three groups listed above should provide approximately 50% of the total kcal/24 h, primarily carbohydrates, with an energy yield of 4 kcal g.

4. Milk, yogurt, and cheese: 2–3 servings—rich in calcium and protein
5. Meat, poultry, fish, dry beans, eggs, and nuts: 2–3 servings

   a. The last two food groups are primarily protein, needed for tissue growth and maintenance.
   b. They should comprise approximately 20% of the daily kilocalories. Protein is worth 4 kcal/g.
   c. Excessive protein intake increases the amount of nitrogenous waste, or urea, that must be excreted through the urine.
   d. Over a prolonged period of time, additional wear to the kidney nephrons results.

6. Fats, oils, and sweets: Eat sparingly, and when the preceding levels of the Food Guide Pyramid have been satisfied. Fats and oils have 9 kcal/g.

C. Kilocalorie levels

1. The minimum number of servings from each food group is approximately 1600 kcal per day.
2. The maximum number of servings from each food group is approximately 2300 kcal per day.

D. The Food Guide Pyramid is the basic pattern for therapeutic diets.

1. By changing the texture, reducing or increasing the amount of a macronutrient (carbohydrate, protein, fat), amount of a micronutrient (electrolytes such as sodium) or the kilocalorie level, a "regular diet," such as that advocated by the pyramid, becomes a therapeutic diet requiring an order in the hospital setting.

E. Comparison of a client's food intake records with the Food Guide Pyramid provides for a quick dietary assessment.

V. NUTRITIONAL SUPPORT[1-3, 6]

A. Initiation of feeding for the acutely ill patient. Consult with a dietitian.

1. Feeding begins in the hypermetabolic phase for stressed patients.
2. Patients admitted with protein and/or kilocalorie deficits need nutritional support within the first 3–5 days.
3. If protein and kilocalorie intake for the previous 5 days was inadequate, evaluation for nutritional support is necessary (see Nutritional Assessment).
4. The decision regarding the type of nutritional support relies on the following guidelines:

   a. The GI tract is nonfunctional: Parenteral (vascular) feeding is appropriate (see Parenteral nutrition support).
   b. The GI tract is functional: If the client is expected to need support for >6 weeks, use an *enterostomal* tube. If support is for <6 weeks, use a *nasointestinal* tube. If the client is at risk for aspiration, use *duodenal* placement for the tube; if there is no aspiration risk, use a nasogastric tube.

B. Enteral nutrition support

1. Definition: Any feeding employing the GI tract. It is the preferred form of feeding for nutritional support. "If the gut works, use it!"
2. Prevention of transmigration of GI bacteria through the intestinal wall to the bloodstream and resulting sepsis is dependent on the presence of food in the GI tract. Consult the dietitian.
3. Oral support: Feeding administered through the mouth

   a. Clear liquids: Liquids, or foods that become liquid in the mouth, when held to the light are clear or one can see through them.
      i. Clear liquids include flavored gelatin, pulp-free juices, ice, popsicles, carbonated beverages, meat broths, sherbet, sorbets, and tea; neither caffeinated or decaffeinated coffee is included because coffee increases gastric acid production.
      ii. Indications for use are after surgery, for nausea and vomiting, or to maintain minimal GI residue, such as prior to GI surgery.
      iii. This type of feeding is incomplete nutritionally, so it should be used for a minimal time as the only means of nutritional support.
   b. Full liquids: All the foods on a clear liquid diet with the addition of milk and dairy products-fluid milk, plain yo-

gurt, ice cream, cream soups, and hot cereals, such as cream of wheat.

   i. Indications for use include anorexia, previous clear liquid diet, and so on.
   ii. They can be nutritionally complete.
c. Soft foods: These foods are soft in texture and easy to digest, for example, lean, tender meat, potatoes, rice, cooked vegetables, and fruits. Mechanical soft diet usually refers to a puréed or blended diet for those who have difficulty chewing.

   i. Indications for a soft food diet include situations in which energy conservation is important, and previous GI upsets have occurred, including nausea, vomiting, flatus, and cramping.
   ii. A soft food diet can be nutritionally complete.
d. Regular (also called house diet): The house diet follows the guidelines of the Food Guide Pyramid.
e. The four preceding diets are often referred to as "progressive diets" or the "progressive regimen." When a client can tolerate clear liquids, he or she is then advanced to full liquids and with GI toleration, progresses to more complex foods.
f. Supplemental formula feedings: These commercially prepared formulas are offered between meals or as a meal substitute to provide additional kilocalories, or additional amounts of a nutrient, such as protein.

   i. Usually better accepted if served cold and with a drinking straw.
   ii. Should be sipped over a period of at least 20 minutes to avoid GI discomfort.
   iii. Examples of commonly used formulas include Ensure (Ross Products) and Isocal (Mead Johnson).

4. Beginning enteral tube feeding and progression

   a. Consult with the dietitian regarding rates of feeding and formula selection.
   b. Begin feeding when gastric residuals are <300–600 mL/24 h.
   c. Confirm tube placement, preferably by radiographic confirmation.
   d. Begin isotonic (300 mOsm/L) feeding at full strength. Every 8 hours, progress 25 mL until the optimal rate is achieved.
   e. Begin with hypertonic formulas (>300 mOsm/L) diluted to isotonic strength. Advance to full strength. Advance to the optimal rate by 25 mL every 8 hours.

5. Rates of formula flow for tube feedings

   a. Bolus: Usually administered with a large syringe. A volume of 250–500 mL is given over 10–20 minutes every 4–6 hours. Least likely to be well tolerated.

b. Intermittent: a volume of 100–400 mL is allowed to flow by gravity for 20–40 minutes every 2–4 hours. Moderate toleration.
c. Continuous-Requires the use of an infusion pump. Administered over a period of 18–24 hours. Best tolerated.
d. Elevate the head of the patient's bed when administering feedings, and for 30–40 minutes after the feeding.
e. Do not administer iron preparations or insulin through a nasointestinal tube. Consult the pharmacist regarding other medications to avoid drug–nutrient interactions. Flush the tubing before and after giving medications.
f. Most commercial tube feeding formulas contain 80% water by volume. Using the "rule of thumb" of 1 mL of water for every kilocalorie, a 2000 mL/24 h volume would contain 1600 mL of water. The remaining 400 mL must be given additionally. Water used to flush the tubing before and after feeding contributes to the day's allowance.

6. Transintestinal tubes (for short-term use—6 weeks or less).

a. Nasogastric tubes
   i. End of tube is located in the stomach. Most similar to route of normal digestion.
   ii. Acid reflux is common.
   iii. Lack of integrity of the gastric mucosa is a contraindication for use.
   iv. Same products as used for supplemental feedings are usually appropriate.
   v. These products have "intact" nutrients, or are not "predigested," thus requiring a fully functional GI tract.
b. Nasoduodenal tubes: End of tube is located in the duodenum.
   i. Acid reflux or aspiration is less common than with gastric tubes.
   ii. May require a hydrolyzed or elemental formula, that is, one that is at least, partially, "pre-digested."
   iii. Examples are Vivonex Plus (Sandoz Nutrition) and Peptamen (Clintec).
c. Nasojejunal tubes: Tube placement is in the jejunum. Formula type depends on the area of the jejunum to be used—intact nutrient formula for the upper portion and hydrolyzed formula for the mid to lower portion.

7. Enterostomies: Surgically created openings from the exterior to the GI tract. They are for long-term use (>6 weeks) or when a transnasal tube is inappropriate.

a. Esophagostomy: Ostomy in esophagus with tube end located in the stomach. Intact or blenderized formulas are appropriate.

   b. Gastrostomy: Opening into the stomach.
      i. Percutaneous endoscopic gastrostomy (PEG) is created with the use of an endoscope; often the procedure occurs at bedside with a local anesthetic.
      ii. Can be used for feeding within 24 hours. Intact formula is appropriate.
   c. Jejunostomy: Percutaneous endoscopic jejunostomy (PEJ) is extension of PEG—See NJ tube above for formula choice.

8. Complications of enteral support

   a. The "dumping syndrome" is often associated with enteral feedings as well as gastric resections.
      i. A hyperosmolar formula or a hyperosmolar load of partially digested material causes fluid from the intestinal capillaries to rapidly enter the jejunum.
      ii. This action results in increased peristalsis as well as lowered blood volume; hence diarrhea and lowered blood pressure occur.
   b. GI complications such as diarrhea, constipation, cramping, and gastric retention are fairly common.
      i. Manipulate the fiber content of the formula for stool consistency.
      ii. Osmolarity of the formula can also be a factor.
      iii. Formula is best tolerated at room temperature. Ensure that hydration is adequate.
   c. Check regularly for metabolic complications such as hyperglycemia and electrolyte imbalances.
   d. Be aware of the side effects of drugs, and their interactions with nutrients.
   e. The refeeding syndrome can occur in malnourished/food-deprived individuals if they are fed relatively large quantities of nutrients enterally as well as parenterally.
      i. Simply put, the body has adjusted to starvation, and overfeeding overwhelms its capability to metabolize nutrients.
      ii. Electrolyte imbalances, cardiac failure, fluid imbalances, and so on can result.
      iii. Gradual introduction of feedings, with close monitoring of electrolytes and blood glucose, can be preventive.
   f. Consult a dietitian and a pharmacist for additional information or problem solving.

C. Parenteral nutrition support

1. Definition: Use of the vascular system to deliver nutrients. It may be used in conjuction with enteral feedings or as sole nu-

tritional support. Consult the pharmacist for content of the solutions.

2. Choose parenteral nutrition support if the GI tract is not functional, or if additional support beyond the capacity of the GI tract is necessary.

   a. If support is expected to be necessary for >2 weeks, use a central vein; if it will be needed for <2 weeks, a peripheral vein is appropriate.

3. Peripheral parenteral nutrition—also called intravenous or IV nutrition—is limited to 10–14 days because of vein infiltration.

4. Central parenteral nutrition (CPN or TPN) usually administered using the right or left subclavian vein to access the superior vena cava and is indicated for support of >10–14 days.

5. Considerations when administering parenteral support:

   a. Concentrations of dextrose >10% require a central line.
   b. Check blood glucose every 6 hours.
   c. Infuse fat emulsions slowly.
   d. Involve the pharmacist, dietitian, and physician in planning parenteral support.

6. Complications of parenteral nutritional support are many and varied. Metabolic complications, such as hyperglycemia and hypercapnia, may result as well as those involving the GI tract and the liver. Always be aware of the possibility of catheter sepsis.

References

1. Cataldo, C.B., Rolfes, S.R., & Whitney, E.N. (1998). *Understanding clinical nutrition* (2nd ed.) Belmont, CA: West/Wadsworth.
2. Dudek, S. (1997). *Nutrition handbook for nursing practice* (3rd ed.). Philadelphia: Lippincott-Raven.
3. Gawlinski, A., & Hamwi, D. (Eds.) (1999). *Acute care nurse practitioner. Clinical curriculum and certification review.* Philadelphia: W.B. Saunders.
4. Grodner, M., Anderson, S.L., & DeYoung, S. (1996). *Foundations and clinical applications of nutrition—a nursing approach.* St. Louis: Mosby–Year Book.
5. Lutz, C.A., & Przytulski, K.R. (1997) *Nutrition and diet therapy* (2nd ed.). Philadelphia: F.A. Davis.
6. Rombeau, J.L., & Rolandelli, R.H. (1997). *Clinical nutrition—Enteral and tube* feeding (3rd ed.). Philadelphia: W.B. Saunders.
7. Society of Actuaries and Association of Life Insurance Medical Directors of America. (1980). *1979 Build Study.*
8. Williams, S.R. (1997). *Nutrition and diet therapy* (8th ed.). St. Louis: Mosby–Year Book.
9. U.S. Dept. of Agriculture (1992). USDA Human Nutrition Information. Pub. No. 249. Washington, DC: U.S. Government Printing Office.

FLUID, ELECTROLYTE, AND ACID-BASE IMBALANCES

R. Michael Culpepper, MD, FACP

I. HYPONATREMIA

A. Definitions[1]

1. Hyponatremia is a decreased serum sodium concentration: $[Na^+]$ <135 mEq/L; the norm is 135–145 mEq/L.
2. Hypotonic hyponatremia (low serum osmolality): State of body water excess diluting all body fluids. Clinical signs arise from the water excess itself.
3. Isotonic hyponatremia (normal serum osmolality): A laboratory artifact occurring with extreme hyperlipidemia or hyperproteinemia. Body water is normal and patients are asymptomatic.
4. Hypertonic hyponatremia (high serum osmolality): State of dilution of sodium-containing extracellular fluids in presence of high concentrations of nonsodium solute (e.g., hyperglycemia, mannitol), which pulls water from inside cells. Clinical signs arise from primary disorder, not water state.

B. Etiology/Incidence/Predisposing factors[1-8]

1. 1–4% prevalence in hospitalized patients
2. Occurs in states of deficient renal water excretion (either concentration of urine by antidiuretic hormone (ADH) or insufficient formation of free water by renal tubules) plus continued water intake
3. Hypervolemic hyponatremia: State of edema (excess total body sodium content) plus or minus circulatory deficiency (stimulus to ADH secretion)

   a. Congestive heart failure
   b. Hepatic cirrhosis
   c. Nephrotic syndrome

4. Hypovolemic hyponatremia: State of total body sodium deficiency; usually with hemodynamic insufficiency (stimulus to ADH secretion)

   a. Blood loss
   b. Gastrointestinal fluid loss: Suction, emesis, diarrhea
   c. Renal fluid loss: Excess diuresis, aldosterone deficiency
   d. Skin fluid loss: Excess sweating, burns

5. Euvolemic hyponatremia: State of normal body sodium content; edema-free and normal hemodynamic state (autonomous ADH secretion or reduced renal water formation)

   a. Syndrome of inappropriate ADH (SIADH)
   b. Diuretics, especially thiazides in elderly females
   c. Renal failure, acute or chronic
   d. Cortisol deficiency
   e. Hypothyroidism
   f. Primary polydipsia ("psychogenic" water ingestion): Capacity for renal water excretion overwhelmed
   g. "Beer potomania": Inadequate solute (salt) intake; kidney cannot make enough solute-free water to excrete large fluid (beer) intake

C. Subjective findings[8, 11, 12]

1. Neurologic; related to brain swelling from water excess; severity roughly parallels fall in serum [Na^+]; more pronounced with acute (hours to 1–2 days) vs. chronic (>2 days to weeks) development of hyponatremia
2. Serum [Na^+]

   a. Serum [Na^+] 120–125 mEq/L: Acute—nausea, malaise; chronic—none
   b. Serum [Na^+] 110–120 mEq/L: Acute—headache, confusion, lethargy, nausea; chronic—none to mild confusion or lethargy
   c. Serum [Na^+] <110 mEq/L: Acute—nausea, seizures, coma; chronic—occasionally none or greater confusion and lethargy

D. Physical examination findings[8, 11, 12]

1. General neurologic depression; rarely focal neurologic findings
2. Major findings may reflect primary condition causing hyponatremia
3. Cardiovascular focus: Determine volume status—edema, ascites, pulmonary rales, cardiac gallop, standing and lying blood pressure (BP) and pulse, jugular venous distention or collapse, etc.

E. Laboratory/Diagnostic findings[1, 3–8, 11, 12]

1. Hypotonic hyponatremia

   a. Serum [Na^+] <135 mEq/L; serum osmolality <270 mOsm/kg (normal: 280–295 mOsm/kg; serum [Osm] $\approx 2 \times$ [Na^+])
   b. Urine osmolality <100 mOsm/L: Primary polydipsia (may be seen if initial disorder causing ADH secretion has been resolved)

   c. Urine osmolality >100 mOsm/L: ADH effect or decreased renal tubule water formation

   d. Urine [Na$^+$] <20 mEq/L: Circulatory deficiency; seen in either the hypervolemic or hypovolemic state

   e. Urine [Na$^+$] >40 mEq/L: SIADH, diuretics, renal failure, hypothyroidism, adrenal insufficiency

2. Isotonic hyponatremia

   a. Serum [Na$^+$] <135 mEq/L; serum osmolality 270–290 mOsm/kg; seen in extreme hyperlipidemia (triglycerides >1000–1500 mg/dL) or hyperproteinemia (protein >12–15 g/dL), as in multiple myeloma

   b. Plasma water [Na$^+$] (obtained after separation of nonsoluble lipid or protein from serum) normal

3. Hypertonic hyponatremia

   a. Serum [Na$^+$] <135 mEq/L; serum osmolality >290 mOsm/kg; extraosmolar substance in serum (high glucose concentrations in diabetes mellitus, mannitol, glycerol)

   b. For each 100 mg/dL increment in serum [glucose] above 100 mg/dL, measured serum [Na$^+$] falls by 1.6 mEq/L; for example, for a serum [glucose] of 900 mg/dL, serum [Na$^+$] falls (8 × 1.6 mEq/L) 13 mEq/L

F. Management[3–5, 8, 11, 12]

1. Only hypotonic hyponatremia requires treatment directed at serum [Na$^+$] itself. Therapy is guided by symptoms, level of serum [Na$^+$], and rapidity of development. Rate of correction of serum [Na$^+$] is critical; overcorrection or very rapid rise in serum [Na$^+$] may inflict further central nervous system (CNS) injury, as in pontine myelinolysis

2. Seizures or coma with serum [Na$^+$] <115 mEq/L, acute or chronic: 3% hypertonic saline at rate to raise serum [Na$^+$] by 1–2 mEq/L/h until serum [Na$^+$] rises by 12–15 mEq/L or to a level of 120 mEq/L

   a. *Example*: [Na$^+$] required = 0.5 × body wt (kg) × (120 − serum [Na$^+$]); for an 80-kg patient with serum [Na$^+$] of 107 mEq/L, [Na$^+$] required = (0.5 × 40) × (120 − 107) = 520 mEq; about 1000 mL of 3% saline ([Na$^+$] = 513 mEq/L) infused over 6–12 h is needed to correct the acute hyponatremia

3. Lesser symptoms or serum [Na$^+$] <110 mEq/L, especially acute onset: 3% saline as above or treat based on volume status (see below)

4. Mild or no symptoms, hypovolemic state: 0.9% saline (NS) at rate to correct volume deficiency

5. Mild or no symptoms, hypervolemic state: Loop diuretic furosemide (Lasix), 40–80 mg IV or p.o.; NS should be used for any intravenous (IV) fluid use
6. All cases: Restrict water or total fluid intake to ≤1000 mL/24 h
7. Associated hypokalemia: Supplement potassium, especially with diuretics
8. Underlying condition: Hypothyroidism—thyroid replacement; adrenal insufficiency—cortisol therapy; SIADH—demeclocycline, 150–300 mg p.o., q6 h, antagonizes ADH effect in chronic, pathologic ADH release
9. Monitor serum $[Na^+]$ q2–4h in all symptomatic patients

II. HYPERNATREMIA

A. Definition

1. An increased serum sodium concentration; serum $[Na^+]$ >150 mEq/L (normal: 135–145 mEq/L)
2. Hypernatremia always indicates hyperosmolality—a deficit of body water
3. Occurs only when free access to water is limited or thirst is impaired

B. Etiology/Incidence/Predisposing factor[2-8]

1. Primary water loss

    a. Central (pituitary) diabetes insipidus
    b. Nephrogenic (renal) diabetes insipidus
    c. Increased insensible loss in febrile states

2. Water in excess of sodium loss

    a. Renal osmotic diuresis: Glucosuria of diabetes mellitus, mannitol therapy, urea excretion in burns, or relief of urinary obstruction
    b. Gastrointestinal fluid loss: Persistent diarrhea or emesis, drainage
    c. Cutaneous fluid loss: Burns, sweating

3. Hypertonic sodium gain

    a. Hypertonic $NaHCO_3$ with cardiopulmonary resuscitation (CPR)
    b. Hypertonic NaCl IV or NaCl tablets p.o.

4. Occurs in 0.3–1% of hospitalized patients
5. Combination of excess water loss plus inability to acquire water; common in debilitated elderly, debility following cerebrovascular accident (CVA), and infants

C. Subjective findings[8, 12]

1. Mostly neurologic: Related to brain shrinkage from water loss; severity is relative to degree and rapidity of development of hypernatremia
2. Serum [Na$^+$] 155–160 mEq/L: Acute—nausea, weakness, lethargy, confusion, or irritability; chronic—none to mild CNS symptoms
3. Serum [Na$^+$] >160 mEq/L: Acute—stupor, coma; chronic—none to more severe CNS symptoms
4. Thirst/polydipsia: Very common in communicative patients
5. Polyuria/nocturia: Clue for renal basis; either diabetes insipidus or osmotic diuresis (glucosuria in hyperglycemia)

D. Physical examination findings[8, 12]

1. CNS depression, rare focal neurologic findings
2. Hypotension, tachycardia, oliguria in volume-depleted states
3. Major findings reflect primary disorder causing hypernatremia

E. Laboratory/Diagnostic findings[3–8, 12]

1. Serum [Na$^+$] >150 mEq/L; serum osmolality >300 mOsm/L
2. Urine osmolality <300 mOsm/L: Central or nephrogenic diabetes insipidus
3. Urine osmolality 300–400 mOsm/L: Suggests osmotic diuresis
4. Urine osmolality >400 mOsm/L: Gastrointestinal, cutaneous, or insensible fluid (water) loss
5. Serum ADH levels, while in hyperosmolar state
6. Water deprivation test: Withhold all fluid intake, monitor BP, serum [Na$^+$], and urine osmolality; when urine osmolality is near constant, inject aqueous vasopressin 5 units SC; measure serum [Na$^+$] and urine osmolality in 1 h
   a. Central diabetes insipidus: >50% increase in urine osmolality
   b. Nephrogenic diabetes insipidus: Little or no increase in urine osmolality

F. Management[3–5, 8, 12]

1. Rapid lowering of the serum [Na$^+$] indicated for acute, symptomatic hypernatremia; chronic hypernatremia must be treated more slowly
2. Estimate water deficit $\approx 0.4 \times$ body wt (kg) $\times$ {(serum [Na$^+$]/140) $- 1$}
3. Replace water at rate calculated to reduce serum [Na$^+$] by ≈ 1 mEq/L/h in acute hypernatremia; to reduce serum [Na$^+$] by $\approx$ one half of excess above 140 mEq/L/24 h for chronic hypernatremia

4. Oral water preferable replacement in conscious patients
5. Mild volume depletion: IV 5% dextrose in water (D_5W); must avoid hyperglycemia/glucosuria to prevent further renal water loss
6. Moderate volume depletion: IV 0.5 NS; saline component restores extracellular fluid (ECF) volume; free water component repletes body water
7. Severe volume depletion: IV NS; follow with 0.5 NS or D_5W when cardiovascular state stabilized
8. Monitor serum [Na^+]: q2–4 h in acute hypernatremia; q4–6h in chronic hypernatremia
9. Treat diabetes insipidus if present (see Chapter 53)

III. HYPOKALEMIA

A. Definition

1. A decreased serum potassium concentration; usually serum [K^+] <3.5 mEq/L
2. Serum levels may fall from body loss or increased cellular uptake of K^+

B. Etiology/Incidence/Predisposing factors[2–8, 13, 14]

1. Renal potassium loss

   a. Diuretics: Acetazolamide, loop diuretics, thiazides, osmotic diuretics (mannitol, glucose in diabetics)
   b. Mineralocorticoid excess
      i. Aldosterone excess in hypovolemic states
      ii. Primary hyperaldosteronism
      iii. Renovascular hypertension
      iv. Renin-secreting tumor
      v. Cushing's syndrome or adrenal hyperplasia
      vi. Exogenous mineralocorticoid effect; high-dose prednisone therapy, fludrocortisone, authentic licorice ingestion
   c. Renal tubular disorders
      i. Renal tubular acidosis (RTA), Types I and II
      ii. Bartter's and Liddle's syndromes
   d. Hypomagnesemia

2. Nonrenal potassium loss

   a. Emesis and nasogastric suction; both gastrointestinal (GI) and renal losses occur
   b. Diarrhea, especially from laxative abuse and secretory diarrheas

3. Potassium uptake into cells

   a. Insulin therapy; common in treatment of diabetic ketoacidosis

    b. Catecholamine excess; epinephrine or intense beta-adrenergic therapy

    c. Metabolic diseases

       i. Familial periodic paralysis

       ii. Thyrotoxic paralysis

4. Inadequate dietary potassium intake; rare
5. Occurs in up to 20% of hospitalized patients and in from 10–40% of outpatients on diuretics (incidence correlates to diuretic dose)

C. Subjective findings[2, 13, 14]

1. Skeletal muscle cramps, tenderness and weakness; leg weakness may ascend with eventual diaphragmatic paralysis in extreme hypokalemia
2. Paralytic ileus; abdominal distention, nausea, emesis
3. Cardiac palpitations; varied cardiac arrhythmias
4. Polyuria and polydipsia; renal concentrating defect in chronic hypokalemia

D. Physical examination findings[8, 13, 14]

1. Muscle tenderness or weakness
2. Cardiac rhythm changes or extrasystoles

E. Laboratory/Diagnostic findings[3–7, 13, 14, 16]

1. Serum $[K^+]$ <3.5 mEq/L
2. Electrocardiogram: T-wave flattening, appearance of U wave
3. Urinary K^+ excretion: >25 mEq/L/24 h—renal potassium wasting; <25 mEq/L/24 h—nonrenal potassium losses
4. Increased serum $[HCO_3]$: Suggests mineralocorticoid excess
5. Serum $[Mg^{2+}]$ (norm: 1.4–2.2 mg/dL); decreased in up to 40% of hypokalemic patients

F. Management[3–5, 10, 13, 14]

1. Deficits are poorly correlated to serum $[K^+]$; estimate 100 mEq K^+ loss for each 0.3 mEq/L decrease in serum $[K^+]$ <4.0 mEq/L
2. Intravenous KCl: Patients with cardiac arrhythmias (especially on digitalis therapy), hepatic encephalopathy, or unable to take oral potassium

    a. Peripheral vein: Maximum solution concentration 40 mEq/L; central vein maximum concentration, 60 mEq/L

    b. Rate: Maximum 10–20 mEq/h; monitor electrocardiogram (ECG) continuously

3. Oral K^+: Cl^- salt most effective, especially in metabolic alkalosis

    a. KCl (K-Lor and others) 10–40 mEq/day in 1 or 2 doses

    b. KCl Extended Release (K-Dur, Micro-K Extencaps), dose as above

4. Potassium-sparing diuretics; usually in combination with other diuretics

   a. Spironolactone (Aldactone), 25–100 mg p.o. q.d.
   b. Amiloride (Midamor), 5 mg p.o. q.d.

5. High potassium diets: Nuts, dried fruits, tomatoes, potatoes, oranges

IV. HYPERKALEMIA

A. Definition

1. Increased serum potassium concentration; usually serum $[K^+]$ >5.5 mEq/L (normal: 3.6–5.2 mEq/L)
2. Serum levels may rise from decreased renal excretion, decreased cellular uptake, or increased cellular release of K^+

B. Etiology/Incidence/Predisposing factors[2-8, 13, 15]

1. Decreased renal excretion

   a. Renal failure; acute or chronic
   b. Decreased aldosterone synthesis
      i. Adrenal insufficiency
      ii. Heparin therapy
   c. Decreased renal aldosterone effect
      i. Potassium-sparing diuretics
      ii. Certain renal diseases (diabetic, obstructive, sickle cell nephropathies)

2. Renin-angiotensin system disruption

   a. Hyporeninemic-hypoaldosteronism; early diabetic nephropathy most common cause
   b. Angiotensin-converting enzyme (ACE) inhibitor therapy
   c. Nonsteroidal anti-inflammatory drug (NSAID) therapy
   d. Cyclosporine therapy

3. Decreased cell uptake/increased cell release

   a. Insulin deficiency; diabetic hyperglycemic states
   b. Cellular disruption
      i. Hemolysis during venipuncture
      ii. Skeletal muscle ischemia or crush injury
      iii. Tumor lysis syndrome after chemotherapy
   c. Pseudohyperkalemia; occurs in venipuncture tube only
      i. Thrombocytosis, platelet count >500,000/mm^3
      ii. Leucocytosis, white cell count (WBC) >100,000/mm^3
   d. Metabolic acidosis
   e. Digitalis poisoning

4. Increased intake

   a. Oral: K^+ supplements or dietary salt substitutes
   b. IV: Overly aggressive replacement, K^+ salts of drugs

C. Subjective findings[8, 13, 15]

1. Muscle weakness to paralysis
2. Symptoms of underlying disorder often dominate

D. Physical examination findings[8, 13, 15]

1. Muscle weakness
2. Signs of underlying disorder

E. Laboratory/Diagnostic findings[3-7, 13, 15, 16]

1. Serum $[K^+] >5.5$ mEq/L
2. ECG: Progression of peaked T waves, widened QRS complex, disappearance of P wave, fusion of QRS and T to sine wave
3. Blood urea nitrogen (BUN) and serum creatinine to identify renal failure
4. Paired serum renin and aldosterone levels to identify primary or secondary hypoaldosteronism
5. Plasma $[K^+]$; measured in heparinized tube; normal in pseudo-hyperkalemia

F. Management[3-5, 9, 10, 13, 15, 16]

1. Urgency and level of intervention based on absence or severity of ECG changes
2. All cases

   a. Repeat serum (or plasma) $[K^+]$
   b. Seek and limit sources of K^+ intake
   c. Discontinue drugs that limit K^+ excretion

3. ECG normal

   a. Furosemide (Lasix), 40–80 mg IV ± $NaHCO_3$ (50–100 mEq IV); increases renal K^+ excretion
   b. Sodium polystyrene resin (Kayexylate), 40–60 g with osmotic cathartic (70% sorbital or lactulose); increases GI K^+ excretion
   c. Hemodialysis or peritoneal dialysis; augments K^+ removal

4. ECG changes present; monitor ECG until normal.

   a. Absent P wave, QRS widening, or sine waves
      i. Calcium gluconate 10%; 10 mL IV infusion over 1–2 min to antagonize hyperkalemic effect; immediate onset; repeat in 3–5 min if needed to normalize ECG
      ii. Regular insulin (10 units), plus glucose (50 g) if euglycemic, IV over 2–5 min to increase cellular K^+ uptake; effect in 15–30 min; insulin drip plus D_5W may follow
      iii. Albuterol (20 mg) via inhalation over 10 min to increase cellular K^+ uptake; effect in 15–30 min
      iv. $NaHCO_3$ (50 mEq) IV over 1–2 min; may help if metabolic acidosis present; onset over 1 h; variable efficacy
      v. Diuretic, resin, dialysis as above to increase removal

b. Peaked T waves alone
   i. Insulin/glucose and/or albuterol as above to increase uptake
   ii. Diuretic, resin, dialysis as above to increase removal

V. HYPOCALCEMIA

A. Definition

1. A decreased ionized fraction of serum calcium concentration, $[Ca^{2+}_i]$, identified by a decreased total serum calcium concentration $[Ca^{2+}]$; typically $[Ca^{2+}] <8.5$ mg/dL and $[Ca^{2+}_i]$ <4.5 mg/dL (normal: $[Ca^{2+}]$ 8.6–10.1 mg/dL; $[Ca^{2+}_i]$ 4.6–5.3 mg/dL).
2. Allow 0.8 mg/dL decrease in serum $[Ca^{2+}]$ per 1.0 g/dL decrease in serum albumin

B. Etiology/Incidence/Predisposing factors[3–9, 18]

1. Hypoparathyroidism; usually surgical after thyroidectomy
2. Hypomagnesemia; especially with serum $[Mg^{2+}] <1.0$ mEq/L
3. Pancreatitis; 40–70% incidence in acute pancreatitis
4. Vitamin D deficiency

   a. Malnutrition; especially infants and elderly
   b. Fat malabsorption: Pancreatic insufficiency, regional enteritis, jejunoileal bypass, hepatobiliary disease
   c. Chronic renal failure

5. Acute pancreatitis
6. Chronic alcoholism
7. Drugs: Phenytoin, cisplatin, estrogen therapy

C. Subjective findings[9, 18]

1. Mental changes: Depression, anxiety, confusion
2. Extrapyramidal changes: Tremors, ataxia, dystonia
3. Tetany
4. Seizures
5. Weakness

D. Physical examination findings[9, 18]

1. Chvostek's sign: Facial twitch on tapping ipsilateral facial nerve
2. Trousseau's sign: Carpal spasm on inflation of BP cuff to occlude brachial artery for 3 min
3. Proximal muscle weakness
4. Integument: Dry skin, brittle hair and nails

E. Laboratory/Diagnostic findings[4–8, 17, 18]

1. Serum $[Ca^{2+}]$; serum $[Ca^{2+}_i]$ if necessary
2. Serum albumin (normal: 3.5–4.6 g/dL) to correct serum $[Ca^{2+}]$ level

3. Serum $[Mg^{2+}]$ (normal: 1.3–2.2 mg/dL) for hypomagnesemia; about 20% of hypocalcemic patients
4. ECG: Prolonged QTc interval, non specific T-wave changes

F. Management[4–6, 9, 18]

1. Symptomatic, acute (tetany or seizures), or if NPO

   a. Calcium chloride, 10 mL 10% solution IV injection over 3–5 min
   b. Calcium gluconate, 20 mL 10% solution IV injection over 3–5 min
   c. Follow with 10 mL of either solution in 500 mL D_5W or NS over 6 h

2. Asymptomatic, chronic

   a. Calcium carbonate or other calcium salt; 2–3 g elemental calcium/day in divided doses; 12–30 tablets depending on preparation
   b. Vitamin D oral preparations: Calciferol (Drisdol), 750–3000 μg/day; calcifediol (Calderol), 50–200 μg/day; calcitriol (Rocaltrol), 0.5–2.0 μg/day
   c. Thiazide diuretic (e.g., hydrochlorothiazide, 25 mg q.d.)

VI. HYPERCALCEMIA

A. Definition

1. An increased ionized fraction of serum calcium concentration, $[Ca^{2+}_i]$, identified by an increased total serum calcium concentration $[Ca^{2+}]$.
2. Typically $[Ca^{2+}] >10.5$ mg/dL and $[Ca^{2+}_i] >5.0$ mg/dL

B. Etiology/Incidence/Predisposing factors[3–9, 19, 20]

1. Hyperparathyroidism: 10–20% of hypercalcemia; most common cause
2. Malignancy: Most common in hospitalized patients, especially lung, renal, or breast cancer patients

   a. Circulating parathyroid hormone–related peptide (PHRP)
   b. Local bone resorption of metastatic disease

3. Vitamin D intoxication
4. Vitamin A intoxication
5. Sarcoidosis: 15–20% of sarcoid patients develop hypercalcemia
6. Hyperthyroidism: 10–20% of hyperthyroid patients develop hypercalcemia
7. Immobilization: Paralysis or body cast, especially in young people
8. Thiazide diuretic therapy

9. Milk-alkali syndrome; calcium antacids plus milk for peptic ulcer disease

C. Subjective findings[9, 19, 20]

1. Neurologic

   a. Lethargy progressing to coma
   b. Depression and/or memory impairment
   c. Personality changes

2. Gastrointestinal

   a. Nausea and vomiting
   b. Constipation

3. Musculoskeletal

   a. Proximal muscle weakness
   b. Bone pain

4. Renal

   a. Polyuria and/or nocturia
   b. Renal colic (complication of renal calculi)

D. Physical examination findings[9, 19]

1. Global CNS dysfunction
2. Depressed deep tendon reflexes
3. Hypertension; usually in moderate, chronic hypercalcemia
4. Hypotension; in severe hypercalcemia with volume depletion

E. Laboratory/Diagnostic findings[4–8, 16, 19, 20]

1. Serum $[Ca^{2+}]$; serum $[Ca^{2+}_i]$ if necessary
2. Parathyroid hormone (PTH) level
3. Thyroid panel: TSH, free T_4 level
4. Vitamin D levels: 25-OH D_3 and 1,25-$(OH)_2D_3$
5. Radiographic bone survey: changes of hyperparathyroidism or metastases
6. PHRP level, if appropriate
7. ECG: Shortened QTc interval

F. Management[4–6, 9, 10, 19, 20]

1. Severe hypercalcemia; typically in malignancy

   a. IV NS to restore volume and induce diuresis >200 mL/h
   b. Calcitonin (Calcimar, Miacalcin), 4 IU/kg body wt q12h SC or IM; may increase to 8 IU/kg body wt *or*
   c. IV bisphosphonates
      i. Pamidronate (Aredia), 90 mg IV infused over 24 h; not to be repeated for 7 days
      ii. Etidronate (Didronel), 7.5 mg/kg body wt in 250 mL NS over 2–3 h for 3 days *or*

    d. Plicamycin (Mithracin), 25 μg/kg body wt in 1 L D_5W or NS over 24 h

    e. Furosemide (Lasix), 40–80 mg q8–12h IV to maintain urine output 150–200 mL/h (with constant NS or 0.5-NS infusion)

    f. Hemodialysis with low-[Ca^{2+}] bath

2. Chronic hypercalcemia

    a. Prednisone, 40–80 mg/day orally; best for hypercalcemia of sarcoidosis, hypervitaminosis D, or lymphoma

    b. Furosemide (Lasix), 40–80 mg p.o. b.i.d. plus 6–8 g sodium diet

    c. Reduced calcium diet, 750–1000 mg/day

VII. HYPOMAGNESEMIA

A. Definition

1. A decreased serum magnesium concentration; usually serum [Mg^{2+}] <1.4 mEq/L (norm: 1.4–2.2 mg/dL)

B. Etiology/Incidence/Predisposing factors[3–5, 8, 21]

1. Renal Mg^{2+} loss

    a. Diuretics: Especially loop diuretics and thiazides; 20–45% incidence of hypomagnesemia

    b. Chronic alcohol use: 30% incidence of hypomagnesemia

    c. Renal drug toxicity: Aminoglycosides, amphotericin B, cisplatin

2. Gastrointestinal Mg^{2+} loss

    a. Persistent diarrhea or laxative abuse

    b. Malabsorption and inflammatory bowel disease

3. Deficient Mg^{2+} intake

    a. Chronic alcohol use

    b. Protein-calorie malnutrition

4. Cellular uptake

    a. Alcohol withdrawal: 80–85% incidence of hypomagnesemia

    b. Acute insulin therapy: as in diabetic ketoacidosis

C. Subjective findings[4, 5, 8]

1. Muscle weakness
2. Tremors
3. Seizures

D. Physical examination findings[4, 5, 10]

1. Trousseau's sign and Chvostek's sign (see Hypocalcemia)
2. Muscle fasciculations or tremors

E. Laboratory/Diagnostic findings[3-5, 8, 17, 21]

1. Serum $[Mg^{2+}]$ <1.4 mEq/L
2. Serum $[Ca^{2+}]$ and serum $[K^+]$: decreased in severe hypomagnesemia
3. Urinary Mg^{2+} excretion: <3 mEq/24 h denotes body deficiency
4. ECG: Prolonged QTc interval, ventricular arrhythmias

F. Management[3-5, 9-11, 21]

1. Parenteral route preferred if patient symptomatic or has hypocalcemia
2. IV: 50% magnesium sulfate ($MgSO_4$) solution

    a. Mild symptoms: 12 mL $MgSO_4$ in 1 L D_5W over 3–6 h, then 6–10 mL in D_5W over next 12–24 h, goal serum $[Mg^{2+}]$ >0.8–1.0 mEq/L
    b. Severe symptoms (seizure, ventricular arrhythmia): 6 mL $MgSO_4$ in 30–50 mL D_5W over 5–10 min then infusions, as above

3. Oral: 30–40 mEq daily; magnesium chloride (Mag-L-100) 2 tablets t.i.d.; magnesium oxide (Mag-Ox 400) 1 or 2 tablets daily; magnesium lactate (Magtab SR) 2 capsules b.i.d.

VIII. HYPERMAGNESEMIA

A. Definition

1. An increased serum magnesium concentration; usually serum $[Mg^{2+}]$ >2.2 mEq/L.
2. Clinical consequences are unusual at serum $[Mg^{2+}]$ <4.0 mEq/L.

B. Etiology/Incidence/Predisposing factors[2, 5, 8]

1. Decreased renal function; almost always in severe hypermagnesemia
2. Ongoing magnesium intake with renal insufficiency: Antacids—magnesium hydroxide (Maalox and others); cathartics—magnesium sulfate (Epsom salt), magnesium hydroxide (milk of magnesia), or magnesium citrate
3. Massive magnesium intake: IV $MgSO_4$ in eclampsia, oral Epsom salt

C. Subjective findings[2, 5, 8]

1. Weakness progressing to paralysis; difficulty swallowing early
2. Lethargy
3. Nausea and emesis

D. Physical examination findings[2, 5, 8]

1. Hypotension
2. Diminished or absent deep tendon reflexes (serum $[Mg^{2+}]$ 4–5 mEq/L)
3. Weakness to flaccid paralysis, including respiratory muscle paralysis (serum $[Mg^{2+}]$ 8–10 mEq/L)

E. Laboratory/Diagnostic findings[2, 5, 8]

1. Serum $[Mg^{2+}]$
2. BUN and serum creatinine to identify renal insufficiency
3. ECG: Lengthening PR interval, widening of QRS, complete heart block

F. Management[2, 8, 9]

1. All cases: Stop magnesium intake
2. ECG changes: IV 10% calcium gluconate 10–20 mL push over 3–5 min
3. IV furosemide (Lasix), 40 mg plus 0.5NS 50–100 mL/h
4. Hemodialysis; ECG changes; consider for any serum $[Mg^{2+}]$ >4 mEq/L

IX. HYPOPHOSPHATEMIA

A. Definition

1. A decreased serum phosphorus concentration; usually serum [Phos] <2.5 mg/dL
2. Severe when serum [Phos] <1.5 mg/dL (normal: 2.5–4.5 mg/dL)

B. Etiology/Incidence/Predisposing factors[2–4, 8]

1. Urinary phosphorus loss

   a. Diuretics
   b. Diabetic ketoacidosis (DKA)
   c. Hyperparathyroidism
   d. Renal tubule defects; Fanconi's syndrome, amphotericin B toxicity

2. Cellular uptake

   a. Increased glucose utilization: Treatment of DKA or alcohol withdrawal, parenteral nutrition (TPN)
   b. Respiratory alkalosis
   c. Burns

3. Deficient gastrointestinal intake or absorption

   a. Chronic alcohol use
   b. Use of oral phosphate binders: Al^{3+} salts (Amphogel) or Ca^{2+} salts (PhosLo, Os-Cal, and others), polymer gels (Renagel)
   c. Malabsorption syndromes

C. Subjective findings[3, 5, 8]

1. Irritability, confusion, paresthesias
2. Weakness

D. Physical examination findings[3, 5, 8]

1. Muscle weakness

E. Laboratory/Diagnostic findings[3, 5, 8]

1. Serum [Phos] <2.5 mg/dL
2. Hemolysis: Complete blood count (CBC), increased serum free hemoglobin, decreased haptoglobin
3. Rhabdomyolysis: Increased creatine kinase (CK) level, positive urinary myoglobin
4. Metabolic acidosis: Decreased serum [HCO_3^-] and arterial pH

F. Management[3-5, 8-10]

1. Oral: Sodium or potassium neutral phosphorus tablets (Neutraphos, K-Phos Neutral), 1–2 g p.o. daily in divided doses
2. IV: Sodium or potassium neutral phosphorus solution, 2 mg phosphorus/kg in 0.5NS infused over 6 h or 5 mg/kg over 12 h

X. HYPERPHOSPHATEMIA

A. Definition

1. An increased serum phosphorus concentration; usually serum [Phos] >5.0 mg/dL in adults; serum [Phos] >6.0 mg/dL in children
2. Normal: Adults—2.5–4.5 mg/dL

B. Etiology/Incidence/Predisposing factors[3, 5, 8, 22]

1. Deficient renal phosphate excretion

   a. Acute or chronic renal failure; usually when glomerular filtration rate to (GFR) < 25 mL/min; most common cause of persistent hyperphosphatemia
   b. Decreased parathyroid hormone effect; primary hypoparathyroidism or pseudohypoparathyroidism

2. Phosphorus redistribution from cell to extracellular fluids

   a. Tumor lysis syndrome; post-chemotherapy of leukemia or lymphoma
   b. Rhabdomyolysis or crush injury
   c. Acute respiratory acidosis

3. Increased intestinal absorption

   a. Use of phosphate-containing salts or cathartics
   b. Vitamin D therapy, especially in renal insufficiency

C. Subjective findings

1. None or related to secondary hypocalcemia (see Hypocalcemia)

D. Physical examination findings[6, 22]

1. Ectopic tissue calcification; occurs at serum [Phos] × serum [Ca^{2+}] >70
2. Sites
   a. Cornea: Acute conjunctivitis
   b. Skin: Grainy feeling of skin, pruritus
   c. Vasculature: Calcified outlines on radiographs
   d. Cardiac tissue: Possible conduction defects on ECG

E. Laboratory/Diagnostic findings[3, 4, 6, 7, 22]

1. Serum [Phos] >5.0 mg/dL in adults; >6.0 mg/dL in children
2. BUN, serum creatinine, or creatinine clearance for renal insufficiency
3. Serum PTH and vitamin D levels
4. Serum [Ca^{2+}] to calculate [Phos] × [Ca^{2+}] product
5. Arterial pH (hyperventilation), WBC (leukemia), serum CK (crush injury)

F. Management[3, 6, 22]

1. Peritoneal or hemodialysis: In acute or chronic renal failure
2. Dietary phosphorus restriction (800–1000 mg/day)
3. Oral phosphate binders: Ca^{2+} salts (Os-Cal, PhosLo, others), polymer gels (Renagel), or Al^{3+} salts (Amphogel); each dosed 2–4 tablets or capsules t.i.d. with meals and at bedtime

XI. ACID-BASE DISORDERS

A. Definition

1. Disturbances in the processes that, collectively, maintain body hydrogen ion concentration ([H^+]) nearly constant
2. Primary disorder: Pathologic change that, unchecked, would displace [H^+] from normal
3. Compensatory process: Reactive change to primary disorder that allows complementary factors to move [H^+] back toward normal; arterial pH points to primary disorder; e.g., acid pH indicates primary acidosis
4. Mixed disorder: More than one primary disorder occurring together; pH points to dominant disorder; e.g., acid pH indicates dominant acidosis

B. Laboratory/Diagnostic findings[4, 6]

1. pH = −log [H^+]; e.g., pH 7 = 10^{-7} Eq/L [H^+] = 10 μEq/L
   Normal pH 7.35–7.45; in acidemia: pH <7.35; in alkalemia: pH >7.45

2. $[H^+] = 24 \times P_{CO_2}/[HCO_3]$; i.e., P_{CO_2} and $[HCO_3]$ determine the pH
3. Serum anion gap (AG) = $[Na^+]_{serum} - [Cl^-]_{serum} + [HCO_3^-]_{serum}$; normal AG: 8–10 mEq/L

XII. METABOLIC ACIDOSIS

A. Definition

1. A process that increases $[H^+]$ ($\downarrow$ pH); identified by a decrease in $[HCO_3^-]$, usually <22 mEq/L; respiratory alkalosis ($\downarrow$ P_{CO_2}) compensating process
2. Normal AG metabolic acidosis: AG <12 mEq/L; indicates primary HCO_3^- loss or H^+ plus Cl^- gain
3. High AG metabolic acidosis: AG >15 mEq/L; indicates addition to serum of non-Cl^- acid anion; e.g., lactate from lactic acid

B. Etiology/Incidence/Predisposing factors[3–8, 23, 25]

1. Normal AG metabolic acidosis

   a. Gastrointestinal HCO_3^- loss: Diarrhea, pancreatic drainage
   b. Insufficient renal acid excretion
      i. Renal tubule acidosis: Types I, II, and IV
      ii. Mild/moderate renal insufficiency: GFR >20–30 mL/min
   c. HCl intake
      i. Acidifying salts: NH_4Cl, Arginine HCl
      ii. HCl infusion

2. High AG metabolic acidosis

   a. Endogenous acids
      i. Lactic acidosis: Hypoxia, sepsis, circulatory shock
      ii. Diabetic ketoacidosis: Lack of insulin
      iii. Alcoholic ketoacidosis: Drinking binge ending in nausea and vomiting with poor nutrition
      iv. Advanced renal insufficiency: GFR <15–20 mL/min
   b. Exogenous acids
      i. Salicylate poisoning: Salicylic acid, aspirin
      ii. Methanol: Formic acid metabolite
      iii. Ethylene glycol: Glycolic and oxalic acid metabolites

C. Subjective findings[3–5, 8]

1. Anorexia and nausea
2. Weakness, lethargy leading to coma
3. Symptoms of underlying disorder

D. Physical examination findings[3–5, 8]

1. Kussmaul breathing: Rapid, regular deep breathing
2. Hypotension

3. Signs of underlying disorder; e.g., sweet breath in ketoacidosis

E. Laboratory/Diagnostic findings[3-8, 23, 25]

1. Arterial blood gases: pH, PCO_2, and calculated $[HCO_3^-]$
2. Serum $[Na^+]$, $[HCO_3^-]$, and $[Cl^-]$; calculate AG
3. BUN and serum creatinine to identify renal failure
4. Urine pH, if >5.5, suspect renal acidifying defect
5. Serum and urine ketones, positive in ketotic states
6. Serum salicylate, methanol, or ethylene glycol levels

F. Management[3-9, 23, 25]

1. $NaHCO_3$ therapy: IV $NaHCO_3$ infusion controversial

   a. Rarely indicated when pH ≥ 7.10
   b. Diabetic ketoacidosis: Not required or recommended
   c. Lactic acidosis: $NaHCO_3$ may actually increase lactate levels
   d. $NaHCO_3$ injection: Very hypertonic; limit to 1–2 ampules
   e. $NaHCO_3$ isotonic infusion
      i. *Example*: HCO_3^- required = $0.5 \times$ body wt (kg) $\times$ (20 − serum $[HCO_3^-]$); add 3 ampules $NaHCO_3$ (150 mEq) to 1 L of D_5W, infuse over 6–12 h
   f. Shohl's solution (BiCitra and others): 1 mL (1mEq)/kg body wt/day

2. Primary disorder treatment

   a. Stop or limit GI HCO_3^- losses
   b. Methanol or ethylene glycol ingestion: Ethanol infusion to maintain 100–150 mg/dL blood level; limits acid metabolites
   c. Salicylate poisoning: Alkalinize urine; isotonic $NaHCO_3$ infusion (see earlier) to maintain urine pH ≥ 8
   d. Diabetic ketoacidosis: IV NS and insulin infusions (see Chapter 47)
   e. Alcoholic ketoacidosis: IV glucose (D_5W or 5% dextrose in NS at 100–150 mL/h) plus thiamine (100 mg)
   f. Lactic acidosis: Maintain tissue perfusion; IV NS more effective than IV $NaHCO_3$

XIII. METABOLIC ALKALOSIS

A. Definition

1. A process that decreases $[H^+]$ ($\uparrow$ pH)
2. Identified by an increase in $[HCO_3^-]$, usually >28 mEq/L
3. Respiratory acidosis ($\uparrow PCO_2$) compensating process

B. Etiology/Incidence/Predisposing factors[3-8, 24]

1. Gastrointestinal hydrogen loss

   a. Vomiting
   b. Nasogastric aspiration

2. Renal hydrogen loss

   a. Secondary hyperaldosteronism from volume contraction
     i. Diuretic therapy
     ii. Vomiting or nasogastric aspiration
     iii. Potassium depletion $\pm$ magnesium deficiency
   b. Hyperaldosteronism with normal or expanded volume
     i. Primary aldosteronism
     ii. Cushing's syndrome
     iii. Renal artery stenosis

3. Bicarbonate gains; more likely in renal insufficiency

   a. $NaHCO_3$ administration
   b. Massive organic anion infusion: Citrate (Blood or fresh frozen plasma transfusion), acetate (TPN, dialysis solutions)

C. Subjective findings[3-5, 8]

1. CNS symptoms: Headache, lethargy ending in coma
2. Tetany or seizure: May be associated with $\downarrow [Ca^{2+}_i]$

D. Physical examination findings[3-5, 8]

1. Postural hypotension and/or tachycardia
2. Respiratory depression
3. Signs of primary disorder

E. Laboratory/Diagnostic findings[3-9, 24]

1. Arterial blood gases: pH, P_{CO_2}, and calculated $[HCO_3^-]$
2. Serum electrolytes, especially decreased $[K^+]$, $[Mg^{2+}]$, and/or $[Ca^{2+}_i]$
3. Urine $[Cl^-]$: Marker of volume status

   a. Urine $[Cl^-]$ <20 mEq/L: Vomiting, low NaCl intake, diuretic use after drug stopped
   b. Urine $[Cl^-]$ >40 mEq/L: Aldosterone excess (1° or 2°), active diuretic use

F. Management[3-9, 24]

1. Volume-depleted states: IV NS at 100–150 mL/h
2. KCl replacement for all potassium-depleted or -losing states (see Hypokalemia)
3. Acetazolamide (Diamox); 250–500 mg IV or p.o. b.i.d; especially useful in volume-expanded states
4. Spironolactone (Aldactone); 25–50 mg p.o. t.i.d–q.i.d; especially useful in aldosterone excess states with hypokalemia
5. HCl infusion: 0.1 M solution (100 mEq/L $[H^+]$); infuse slowly into central vein; total infusion $\approx 0.2 \times$ body wt (kg) $\times$ ($[HCO_3^-]$ − desired $[HCO_3^-]$)

a. *Example*: For 70-kg person to go from serum $[HCO_3^-]$ 38 to 28 mEq/L would require $(0.2 \times 70) \times (38 - 28) = 140$ mEq H^+ or 1.4 L of 0.1 M HCl

XIV. RESPIRATORY ACIDOSIS

A. Definition

1. A process that increases $[H^+]$ ($\downarrow$ pH)
2. Identified by an increase in arterial P_{CO_2}, usually >45 mmHg
3. Metabolic alkalosis ($\uparrow [HCO_3^-]$) compensating process

B. Etiology/Incidence/Predisposing factors[3-8]

1. Acute hypoventilation

   a. CNS depression: Narcotics, sedatives
   b. CNS injury: Brain stem injury, CVA
   c. Neuromuscular disease: Myasthenia gravis, Guillain-Barré syndrome, poliomyelitis
   d. Airway obstruction: Mucus/foreign body, severe broncho-spasm of status asthmaticus, bronchitis, emphysema
   e. Chest disorders: Flail chest, pneumothorax, kyphoscoliosis

2. Chronic hypoventilation

   a. Chronic obstructive pulmonary disease (COPD)
   b. Obesity: Pickwickian syndrome
   c. Diaphragmatic weakness/paralysis

C. Subjective findings[3-6, 8]

1. Acute respiratory acidosis

   a. Decreased level of consciousness: Drowsiness to coma
   b. Mental changes: Headache, anxiety, confusion, hallucina-tions
   c. Dyspnea

2. Chronic respiratory acidosis

   a. CNS symptoms: Sleep disturbances, memory loss
   b. Neuromuscular changes: Impaired coordination, tremor

D. Physical examination findings[3-6, 8]

1. Acute respiratory acidosis

   a. Blood pressure: Usually elevated
   b. CNS signs: Altered level of consciousness, papilledema
   c. Neuromuscular signs: Tremor, abnormal deep tendon re-flexes

2. Chronic respiratory acidosis

   a. CNS signs: No findings to mild tremor

b. Cardiovascular: Signs of cor pulmonale (right ventricular heave, pulmonary diastolic murmur, cyanosis)

c. Pulmonary: Signs of COPD (increased anteroposterior chest diameter, expiratory wheeze, accessory respiratory muscle use)

E. Laboratory/Diagnostic findings[3-9, 23, 24]

1. Arterial blood gases: pH, P_{CO_2}, P_{O_2}, and calculated $[HCO_3^-]$
2. Serum $[HCO_3^-]$
3. Pulmonary function tests: Decreased FEV_1, increased residual volume

F. Management[3-9, 23, 24]

1. Acute respiratory acidosis

   a. Reverse CNS depression

      i. Naloxone (Narcan), 0.4–2.0 mg IV for narcotic suppression

      ii. Flumazenil (Romazicon), 0.2 mg (2 mL) IV over 30 s for benzodiazepine suppression; observe for seizures

   b. Reverse airway obstruction

      i. Bronchodilator therapy for bronchospasm; albuterol (Ventolin, Proventil), 180 μg inhaled aerosol q6 h; itratropium (Atrovent), 36 μg inhaled aerosol q6 h

      ii. Mechanical extraction of secretions, foreign bodies

   c. Assist ventilation

      i. Face mask for continuous positive airway pressure (CPAP)

      ii. Airway intubation with mechanical ventilation

2. Chronic respiratory acidosis

   a. Avoid respiratory depression, e.g., sedatives, O_2 therapy >3 L/min

   b. Nocturnal CPAP

   c. Vigorous treatment of underlying disorder

XV. RESPIRATORY ALKALOSIS

A. Definition

1. A process that decreases $[H^+]$ ($\uparrow$ pH)
2. Identified by a decrease in arterial P_{CO_2}, usually <36 mmHg
3. Metabolic acidosis ($\downarrow [HCO_3^-]$) compensating process

B. Etiology/Incidence/Predisposing factors[3-8]

1. Acute hyperventilation

   a. CNS disorders: Anxiety, pain, fever, head trauma, salicylates

b. Pulmonary diseases: Decreased lung compliance
   i. Pulmonary edema/congestive heart failure
   ii. Pneumonia
   iii. Pulmonary embolism
   iv. Asthma
c. Sepsis
d. Acute salicylate toxicity

2. Chronic hyperventilation

a. Residence at high altitude
b. Pregnancy
c. Chronic hepatic insufficiency/cirrhosis

C. Subjective findings[3-6, 8]

1. Acute respiratory alkalosis

a. CNS symptoms: Lightheadedness, confusion
b. Neurologic symptoms: Paresthesias, especially around mouth
c. Muscular symptoms: Chest tightness, muscle cramps

2. Chronic respiratory alkalosis: Generally none

D. Physical examination findings[3-6, 8]

1. Acute respiratory alkalosis

a. Hyperactive deep tendon reflexes
b. Carpopedal spasm (tetany): Flexed wrist/ankle with hyper-extended digits

2. Chronic respiratory alkalosis: Generally none

E. Laboratory/Diagnostic findings[3, 9, 23, 24]

1. Arterial blood gases: pH, P_{CO_2}, P_{O_2}, and calculated $[HCO_3^-]$
2. ECG—tachyarrhythmias, ischemic-like ST-T wave changes

F. Management[3, 9, 23, 24]

1. Acute respiratory alkalosis

a. Treatment of underlying cause
b. Anxiety/hyperventilation: Assurance, rebreathing into paper bag

2. Chronic respiratory alkalosis: Generally none required

XVI. INTRAVENOUS FLUID MANAGEMENT

A. Principles of body fluid spaces[4, 6, 7]

1. Total body water (TBW)

a. Volume: 50–60% of body weight (kg); lower value in women and obese individuals; higher value in men and lean individuals

b. Composition: Solute composition varies among compartments but total solute concentration (osmolality) is equal (isotonic) among compartments

2. Intracellular fluid (ICF)

a. Volume: ≈60% of total body water
b. Composition: High concentrations of potassium and phosphate ions; low concentrations of sodium and bicarbonate

3. Extracellular fluid (ECF)

a. Volume: ≈40% of total body water
b. Composition: Primarily sodium salts (NaCl, $NaHCO_3$); low concentrations of potassium and phosphate
c. Extravascular (interstitial) compartment of ECF
   i. Volume: ≈80% of extracellular fluid volume
   ii. Composition: Protein-poor electrolyte solution of ECF
d. Intravascular compartment of ECF
   i. Volume: ≈20% of extracellular fluid volume
   ii. Composition: Protein-enriched electrolyte solution of ECF
   iii. Physiology: Compartment whose volume most reflects and most determines cardiovascular function
   iv. Utility: Compartment into which all therapeutic fluids are administered; distribution to all other body fluid spaces is by diffusion or transport into those compartments

B. Purposes of intravenous fluid administration[6, 26, 27]

1. Extracellular fluid volume repletion and maintenance

a. Signs of ECF volume depletion
   i. Physical: Hypotension, tachycardia, postural fall in blood pressure and/or rise in heart rate, decreased internal jugular vein filling
   ii. Invasive: Decreased central venous pressure (CVP), decreased pulmonary capillary wedge pressure (PCWP)
b. Signs of ECF volume excess
   i. Physical: Hypertension, internal jugular vein distention, edema (peripheral, pulmonary, ascites)
   ii. Invasive: Increased CVP and/or PCWP

2. Body water (osmolality) adjustment or maintenance

a. Signs of water deficit: Hypernatremia or serum hyperosmolality
b. Signs of water excess: Hyponatremia associated with serum hypo-osmolality

3. Delivery of therapeutic agents

a. Electrolytes: Specific adjustment of $[K^+]$, $[Mg^{2+}]$, $[Ca^{2+}]$, $[HCO_3^-]$, phosphate, etc.

b. Nutrition: Supply of calories (glucose, lipids) or nitrogen (amino acids), water-soluble vitamins, or trace elements (Zn^{2+}, Mn^{2+}).

c. Drugs: Multiple water-soluble agents

C. Composition of common intravenous fluids[6, 26, 27]

1. Normal saline (NS, 0.9% NaCl): ≈isotonic to plasma

   a. Distribution: Extracellular fluid volume
   b. Usage
      i. ECF volume expansion; ≈1/3 of infused volume remains in vascular space at full distribution
      ii. Drug delivery: For drugs stable only in saline solution

2. 5% Dextrose in water (D_5W): ≈isotonic to plasma

   a. Distribution: All body water spaces
   b. Usage
      i. Repletion or maintenance of body water (osmolality); equivalent to giving pure water once dextrose metabolized
      ii. Drug delivery: For compatible drugs when ECF volume expansion undesirable (<10% remains in vascular space at full distribution)

3. Ringer's lactate solution (NaCl, KCl, $CaCl_2$): ≈isotonic to plasma

   a. Distribution: ECF compartment, similar to NS
   b. Usage: Mostly in surgical patients for replacement or maintenance of ECF volume when physiologic concentration of K^+ and Ca^{2+} desired

4. Lactated Ringer's (LR, Ringer's + Na lactate): ≈isotonic to plasma

   a. Distribution: ECF compartment, similar to NS
   b. Usage: Mostly as repletion or resuscitation fluid in face of actual or ongoing blood loss; lactate ion metabolized in liver to generate HCO_3^-; supplies extracellular buffer not found in other fluids

5. Half-normal saline (0.5 NS, 0.45% NaCl): Hypotonic to plasma

   a. Distribution: One half of volume equivalent to pure water, distributes into total body water; one half of volume equivalent to NS, distributes into ECF compartment; about one sixth of volume remains in vascular space
   b. Usage
      i. Maintenance fluid (most common use); saline component replaces ongoing NaCl losses, maintains ECF vol-

ume; free water component replaces insensible free-water losses, maintains osmolality

 ii. Replacement fluid; saline component restores ECF volume deficit; free-water component restores water deficit in hyperosmolar (hypernatremic) states

6. Dextrose in saline (D_5NS, $D_50.5NS$, $D_50.25NS$)

 a. Equivalent to corresponding saline solution plus supplying 200 kcal energy per liter of solution

7. Colloid solutions: Solutions of large-molecular-weight particles that are substantially retained in the vascular volume and are used for selective vascular volume expansion and hemodynamic support

 a. 25% Human albumin: Expensive; best given in bolus (25 g/100 mL) in hypoalbuminemic patients

 b. 5% Albumin in saline: Expensive; comparable to NS alone

 c. Dextran (Rheomacrodex) and hetastarch (Hespan): Used only in select conditions such as cardiac surgery or trauma resuscitation

 d. Fresh frozen plasma (FFP): Expensive; should not be used in fluid therapy but only when replacing depleted clotting factors

8. Electrolyte solutions: Solutions used for specific replacement therapy

 a. Sodium bicarbonate: 50 mEq HCO_3^- + 50 mEq Na^+/50 mL ampule; very hypertonic (2000 mOsm/L)

  i. Usage

   (1) Urgent treatment of acidemia: May be given as 1–2 ampules IV push if serum $[Na^+]$ <140 mEq/L

   (2) Maintenance treatment of acidemia: 1, 2, or 3 ampules of $NaHCO_3$ mixed in 1 L of D_5W to yield ≈⅓ isotonic, ≈⅔ isotonic, or isotonic solution, respectively

 b. Potassium chloride (KCl): $[K^+]$ 2 mEq/mL

  i. Usage: Added to any of dextrose or saline solutions in final $[K^+]$ concentration of 10–60 mEq/L

References

1. Oster, J.R., & Singer, I. (1999). Hyponatremia, hyposmolality, and hypotonicity. *Archives of Internal Medicine, 159,* 333.
2. Kelley, W.M., DuPont, H.L., Glick J.H. (1997). *Textbook of internal medicine* (3rd ed.). Philadelphia: Lippincott-Raven.
3. Kokko, J.P., & Tannen, R.L. (1996). *Fluids and electrolytes* (3rd ed.). Philadelphia. W.B. Saunders.
4. Arieff, A.I., & DeFronzo, R.A. (1995). *Fluid, electrolyte, and acid-base disorders* (2nd ed.). New York: Churchill Livingstone.

5. Clochesy, J.M., Breu, C., Cardin, S., Whittaker, A.A., & Rudy, E.B. (1996). *Critical care nursing* (2nd ed.). Philadelphia: W.B. Saunders.
6. Rose, B.D. (1994). *Clinical physiology of acid-base and electrolyte disorders* (4th ed.). New York: McGraw-Hill.
7. Schrier, R.W. (1992). *Renal and electrolyte disorders* (4th ed.). Boston: Little, Brown & Co.
8. Smeltzer, S.C., & Bare, B.G. (1996). *Brunner and Suddarth's textbook of medical-surgical nursing* (8th ed.). Philadelphia: Lippincott-Raven.
9. Chernow, B. (1994). *The pharmacologic approach to the critically ill patient* (3rd ed.). Baltimore: Williams & Wilkins.
10. Hardman, J.G., & Limbird, L.E. (1996). *Goodman & Gilman's The pharmacological basis of therapeutics* (9th ed.). New York: McGraw-Hill.
11. Mulloy, A.L., & Caruana, R.J. (1995). Hyponatremic emergencies. *Medical Clinics of North America, 79*, 155.
12. Fried, L.F., & Palevsky, P.M. (1997). Hyponatremia and hypernatremia. *Medical Clinics of North America, 81*, 585.
13. Mandal, A.K. (1997). Hypokalemia and hyperkalemia. *Medical Clinics of North America, 81*, 611.
14. Gennari, F.J. (1998). Hypokalemia. *New England Journal of Medicine, 339*, 451.
15. Greenberg, A. (1998). Hyperkalemia: Treatment options. *Seminars in Nephrology, 18*, 46.
16. Wong, S.L. (1999). Albuterol for the treatment of hyperkalemia. *Annals of Pharmacotherapy, 33*, 103.
17. Chung, E.K. (1996). Electrolyte imbalance. *Internal Medicine, 17*, 92.
18. Reber, P.M., & Heath, H. (1995). Hypocalcemic emergencies. *Medical Clinics of North America, 79*, 93.
19. Potts, J.T. (1996). Hyperparathyroidism and other hypercalcemic disorders. *Advances in Internal Medicine, 41*, 165.
20. Barrett, M.L. (1999). Hypercalcemia. *Seminars in Oncological Nursing, 15*, 190.
21. Agus, Z.S. (1999). Hypomagnesemia. *Journal of the American Society of Nephrology, 10*, 1616.
22. Drueke, T.B. (1999). Medical management of secondary hyperparathyroidism in uremia. *American Journal of Medical Science, 317*, 383.
23. Androgue H.J., & Madias, N.E. (1998). Management of life-threatening acid-base disorders: Part one. *New England Journal of Medicine, 338*, 26.
24. Androgue H.J., & Madias, N.E. (1998). Management of life-threatening acid-base disorders: Part two. *New England Journal of Medicine, 338*, 107.
25. Ishihara, K., & Szerlip, H.M. (1998). Anion gap acidosis. *Seminars in Nephrology, 18*, 83.
26. Edwards, S. (1998). Hypovolemia: Pathophysiology and management options. *Nursing Critical Care, 3*, 73.
27. Yee, J., Parasuraman, R., & Narins, R.G. (1999). Selective review of perioperative renal & electrolyte disturbances in chronic renal failure patients. *Chest, 115* (Suppl 5), 149S.

POISONING AND DRUG TOXICITIES

Elizabeth A. Vande Waa, PhD

I. ACETAMINOPHEN TOXICITY[4, 8, 9]

A. Examples: Tylenol, Panadol, Liquiprin, Anacin-3

B. Subjective findings

1. Usually asymptomatic early
2. Nausea and vomiting at 24–48 h
3. Right upper quadrant pain

C. Physical examination findings

1. Hepatotoxicity including jaundice, prolonged bleeding time, and hepatic encephalopathy (altered mental status, delirium, asterixis, flapping tremor)

D. Laboratory/Diagnostic findings

1. Draw for blood levels at 4 h after ingestion; toxicity seen with doses >7.5 g (adult) or 140 mg/kg (children)
2. Elevated aspartate transaminase, alanine transaminase levels
3. Prolonged prothrombin time (PT)

E. Management

1. Supportive measures and induced emesis or gastric lavage should be first-line management.

   a. To induce emesis, use 30 mL of syrup of ipecac p.o. followed by 500 mL of water.
   b. Gastric lavage should be done with a large-bore orogastric tube (36–40 French).
   c. Lavage the stomach with boluses of 300 mL of body temperature normal saline until the return is clear.

2. Activated charcoal given in a dose of 50–100 g diluted in water.

   a. Repeat doses of superactivated charcoal (*note:* 30 g of superactivated charcoal is equivalent to 90 g of regular charcoal) may be necessary.
   b. Charcoal should be removed by gastric lavage prior to acetylcysteine administration, as it will prevent its absorbance.

3. *N*-Acetylcysteine (Mucomyst), 140 mg/kg loading dose given p.o. within 8–10 h of overdose; maintenance doses of 70 mg/

kg q4h for a total of 17 doses are indicated for as many doses as the acetaminophen stays in the toxic range (above 20 μg/mL). Check blood levels q4h.

II. ALCOHOL (ETHANOL) TOXICITY[1, 3]

A. Subjective findings

1. Emotional lability
2. Impaired coordination
3. Nausea, vomiting, facial flushing

B. Physical examination findings

1. Respiratory depression
2. Stupor

C. Laboratory/Diagnostic findings

1. Blood levels ranging from 50–100% (mild toxicity), 100–300% (moderate toxicity), to >300% (severe toxicity)

D. Management

1. ABCs (airway, breathing, circulation)
2. Emesis with 30 mL of ipecac, gastric lavage with 150–200 mL of warmed saline via 36–40 French tube. Hemodialysis may also be used to reduce ethanol levels in severe toxicity.
3. Intravenous (IV) glucose, 200–500 mg/kg/dose as 25% dextrose; alcoholics will require pretreatment with thiamine (40 mg p.o. or 5–100 mg IM or IV) and fluids.

III. ANTIARRHYTHMIC DRUG OVERDOSE[8, 10]

A. Examples: Lidocaine, quinidine, procainamide, flecainide
B. Subjective/Physical examination findings

1. Nausea, vomiting, diarrhea, dizziness, blurred vision
2. Bradycardia, hypotension, cardiovascular collapse

C. Laboratory/Diagnostic findings

1. Serum levels may confirm overdose and need for monitorings.
2. Bradycardia with atrioventricular (AV) block
3. Prolonged QRS complex, PR interval, and QT interval
4. Hypoglycemia

D. Management

1. Gastric lavage with 0.9% sodium chloride, 150–200 mL/rinse
2. Supportive care including fluids, positional changes, and monitoring

IV. BARBITURATE OVERDOSE[1, 9]

A. Examples: Amobarbital, meprobamate, pentobarbital, phenobarbital, secobarbital

B. Subjective findings

1. Confusion
2. Central nervous system (CNS) depression

C. Physical examination findings

1. CNS depression, drowsiness, confusion, coma, hypothermia
2. Respiratory depression
3. Absent deep tendon, gag, and corneal reflexes
4. Miosis

D. Management

1. Gastric lavage with 0.9% sodium chloride or activated charcoal, 20–50 g p.o. via gastric tube every 2–6 h
2. Hemodynamic support including dopamine or norepinephrine may be necessary to correct hypotension. Maintenance of airway and ventilation is essential.

V. BENZODIAZEPINE OVERDOSE[1, 9]

A. Examples: Diazepam, clonazepam, flurazepam, clorazepate, prazepam

B. Subjective findings

1. Drowsiness, ataxia, confusion
2. Slurred speech
3. Unsteady gait

C. Physical examination findings

1. Respiratory depression
2. Hypoactive reflexes

D. Management

1. Monitor blood pressure and support respiration.
2. Flumazenil (Romazicon), initial dose 0.2 mg IV over 30 sec; then 0.3 mg over 30 sec, then 0.5 mg over 30 s at 1-min intervals for a total of 3 mg
3. Gastric lavage with 0.9% sodium chloride or activated charcoal, 20–50 g p.o. via 36–40 French tube every 2–6 h may also be used.

VI. BETA BLOCKER OVERDOSE[9, 10]

A. Examples: Propranolol, timolol, atenolol, labetalol, metoprolol, nadolol, pindolol

B. Subjective findings

1. Nausea
2. Vomiting
3. Diarrhea

C. Physical examination findings

1. Bradycardia, hypotension
2. CNS depression or seizures depending on agent
3. Bronchospasm

D. Laboratory/Diagnostic findings

1. Blood levels not very helpful or available
2. Hyperkalemia, hypoglycemia
3. AV block, prolonged QRS complex, asystole

E. Management

1. Activated charcoal, 20–50 g p.o. repeated every 2–6 h
2. Glucagon, 3–5 mg IV or in saline
3. Calcium (10% calcium chloride in a dose of 0.2 mL/kg body weight IV over 5 min) to reverse negative inotropic effects
4. Monitor patient for hyperkalemia and seizure activity. Treat these symptoms should they occur.

VII. CALCIUM CHANNEL BLOCKER OVERDOSE[1, 6]

A. Examples: Diltiazem, nicardipine, nifedipine, verapamil
B. Subjective findings

1. Mental status changes (confusion)

C. Physical examination findings

1. Bradycardia
2. Hypotension
3. Cyanosis

D. Laboratory/Diagnostic findings

1. AV block, prolonged QRS complex, asystole
2. Metabolic acidosis, hyperglycemia

E. Management

1. IV calcium chloride or gluconate (10%) at 0.2 mL/kg up to 10 mL over 5 min
2. Atropine, 0.5–1.0 mg IV; repeat as needed q5min

VIII. CARBON MONOXIDE POISONING[1]

A. Subjective findings

1. Shortness of breath, headache, confusion, clumsiness
2. Nausea, vomiting, diarrhea

B. Physical examination findings

1. Dysrhythmias
2. Heart failure
3. Repiratory depression

C. Laboratory/Diagnostic findings

1. Elevated carboxyhemoglobin levels (COHgb 10–50%)
2. Sinus tachycardia, ST depression, premature ventricular contractions
3. Metabolic acidosis

D. Management

1. 100% oxygen by mask
2. Hyperbaric oxygen if COHgb levels are >25%, or if patient is pregnant or has altered mental status

IX. DIGOXIN TOXICITY[1, 8, 9]

A. Subjective findings

1. Nausea, vomiting
2. Blurred vision, green halos

B. Laboratory/Diagnostic findings

1. AV block with supraventricular tachyarrhythmias, bradyarrhythmias
2. Hyperkalemia in acute overdose
3. Digoxin level of >2.4 ng/mL

C. Management

1. Continuous electrocardiographic (ECG) monitoring.

   a. Monitor and correct serum potassium levels; maintain in the high normal range.
   b. Arrhythmias may be managed with lidocaine or phenytoin.

2. Induce emesis or gastric lavage with 0.9% saline; administer activated charcoal, 20–50 g p.o. q2–6h
3. Digoxin immune Fab (Digibind); dose is serum digoxin concentration (SDC) (ng/mL) × body weight (kg) divided by 100 × 38. If SDC is unavailable, administer 760 mg IV.

X. LITHIUM TOXICITY[7]

A. Examples: Eskalith, Lithobid
B. Subjective findings

1. Nausea, vomiting, diarrhea
2. Muscle weakness, tremor

C. Laboratory/Diagnostic findings

1. Lithium levels >1.5 mEq/L
2. Hyperglycemia
3. AV block, prolonged QT interval
4. Nephrogenic diabetes insipidus
5. Leukocytosis

D. Management

1. Gastrointestinal decontamination with 30 mL of ipecac p.o.
2. Supportive care; diuretics for lithium serum levels >2–3 mEq/L
3. Hemodialysis in acute intoxication (serum levels >4 mEq/L)

XI. SALICYLATE TOXICITY[1, 10]

A. Subjective findings

1. Nausea, vomiting
2. Tinnitus, headache, dizziness

B. Physical examination findings

1. Apnea, cyanosis
2. Metabolic acidosis, respiratory alkalosis
3. Dehydration, hyperthermia

C. Management

1. Induce emesis with ipecac; give activated charcoal, 20–50 g p.o. q2–6h.
2. Sodium bicarbonate (1.0–1.5 mEq/kg IV over 10 min) to correct severe acidosis (pH <7.2)

XII. NARCOTIC TOXICITY[1, 7]

A. Examples: Codeine, heroin, methadone, morphine, opium
B. Subjective findings

1. Hypothermia
2. Drowsiness

C. Physical examination findings

1. Shallow respirations, respiratory depression
2. Pinpoint pupils (miosis)
3. Coma

D. Management

1. Do *not* give emetics. Use gastric lavage with 0.9% saline, activated charcoal (20–50 g q2–6h); ensure adequate ventilation and provide respiratory support.
2. Naloxone (Narcan), 5 μg/kg IV; then 2–20 mg of naloxone if patient is unresponsive

XIII. ORGANOPHOSPHATE (INSECTICIDE) POISONING[6]

A. Examples: Malathion, parathion
B. Subjective findings

1. Nausea, vomiting, cramping, diarrhea, excessive salivation
2. Headache, blurred vision (miosis)
3. Mental confusion, slurred speech

C. Physical examination findings

1. Miosis
2. Coma
3. Bradycardia, conduction defects

D. Management

1. Wash skin thoroughly.
2. Activated charcoal if the insecticide was ingested. Give 20–50 g of activated charcoal p.o. q2–6h.
3. Atropine is the drug of choice for organophosphate toxicity.

   a. Administer atropine, 2 mg IV or IM; repeat in 15 min until atropinization occurs (flushing, dry mouth, dilated pupils).
   b. Doses up to 500–1500 mg/24 h may be necessary.

4. Administer pralidoxime, 1–2 g IV, to reverse nicotinic signs such as muscle weakness and respiratory depression.

XIV. ANTIPSYCHOTIC TOXICITY[7, 9]

A. Examples: Haloperidol, thioridazine, clozapine, loxapine, risperidone

B. Subjective findings

1. Lethargy, deep sleep
2. Dystonias

   a. Rigidity
   b. Stiff neck
   c. Hyper-reflexia

3. Neuroleptic malignant syndrome (increased temperature, rigidity)

C. Physical examination/Laboratory findings

1. Hypotension, AV block, atrial and ventricular arrhythmias

D. Management

1. Activated charcoal, 20–50 g p.o. q2–6h
2. Benztropine mesylate (Cogentin), 1–2 mg t.i.d. for extrapyramidal signs
3. Dantrolene sodium (Dantrium), 1–3 mg/kg IV until symptoms subside; supportive care including cooling blankets for neuroleptic malignant syndrome

XV. ANTIDEPRESSANT TOXICITY[1, 5, 7, 9]

A. Examples: Amitriptyline, fluoxetine, imipramine, nortriptyline, buproprion

B. Subjective findings

1. Hallucinations, confusion, blurred vision
2. Urinary retention

C. Physical examination findings

1. Tachycardia, hypotension, arrhythmias
2. Seizures, hypothermia

D. Management

1. Evidence of CNS or cardiac toxicity within 6 h of antidepressant ingestion is an indication for admission to the intensive care unit.
2. Activated charcoal, 20–50 g q2–6h; gastric lavage with 0.9% sodium chloride; avoid emesis if risk of seizures
3. Sodium bicarbonate IV (0.5–2.0 mEq/L) to offset arrhythmias and to maintain pH >7.45
4. Benzodiazepine (e.g., diazepam [Valium], 0.15–5.0 mg/kg as needed up to 20-mg dose) to control seizures
5. Serotonin syndrome is treated with dantrolene sodium (Dantrium), 1 mg/kg IV; clonazepam (Klonopin) is used to treat rigor (0.5 mg t.i.d.); supprotive measures such as cooling blankets to control temperature

XVI. STIMULANT TOXICITY[6, 10]

A. Examples: Cocaine, amphetamine, dextroamphetamine
B. Subjective findings

1. Increased talkativeness, insomnia, irritability
2. Dry mouth, anorexia

C. Physical examination findings

1. Arrhythmias, anginal chest pain, heart block
2. Seizures

D. Management

1. Induce emesis with ipecac; lavage with sodium chloride or activated charcoal may also be used.
2. Reduce external stimuli.
3. Administer chlorpromazine (Thorazine), 0.5–1.0 mg/kg IM or p.o., or diazepam (Valium), IV 5–10 mg, repeat q15min up to a dose of 30 mg to sedate; beta blockers such as propranolol (Inderal) to offset cardiac signs (10–30 mg p.o. t.i.d.; or IV 1–3 mg, may be repeated after 2 min).

XVII. THEOPHYLLINE TOXICITY[8, 10]

A. Subjective/Physical examination findings

1. Vomiting, sometimes hematemesis
2. Restlessness, agitation, irritability
3. Tachycardia, PVCs, atrial arrhythmias
4. Seizures in severe overdose

B. Laboratory/Diagnostic findings

1. Theophylline levels of 20–60 μg/mL in chronic overdose; levels of 60–100 μg/mL in acute overdose are associated with seizures.
2. Hypokalemia, hyperglycemia, metabolic acidosis

C. Management

1. If seizures have not occurred, induce emesis with 30 mL of syrup of ipecac. Multiple doses of activated charcoal (20–50 g p.o.) repeated every 2–6 h may be used to enhance total body clearance of theophylline.
2. Charcoal hemoperfusion is indicated in acute ingestion with levels higher than 100 μg/mL (serum levels >40 μg/mL), or in patients with seizures or serious arrhythmias.
3. Monitor patient for seizures. Phenobarbital may be administered prophylactically to prevent seizures.

XVIII. ANTICOAGULANT OVERDOSE[2]

A. Examples: Heparin, warfarin

B. Subjective/Physical examination findings

1. Severe hemorrhage

C. Laboratory/Diagnostic findings

1. Heparin: Increased activated partial thromboplastin time (APTT) to 1.5–2.5 times control
2. Warfarin: Increased PT to 1.3–2.0 times control; INR >3.0

D. Management

1. Heparin overdose: Give protamine sulfate, IV 1 mg/100 units heparin; use 0.5 mg/100 units heparin if given >30 min after heparin.

   a. Monitor efficacy until APTT is normal.
   b. Must be administered slowly to prevent anaphylaxis and hypotension

2. Warfarin overdose: Give vitamin K (phytonadione IM, p.o. SC, or IV in dose of 2.5–10 mg until PT time is normal (or check INR every 6 h until normal); give fresh-frozen plasma or whole blood if needed.

References

1. Berkow, R., & Fletcher, A.J. (1997). *The Merck manual of diagnosis and therapy* (17th ed). Rahway, NJ: Merck.
2. Dipiro, J.T., Talbert, R.L., Yee, G.C., Matzke, G.R., Wells, B.G., & Posey, L.M. (1997). *Pharmacotherapy: A pathophysiologic approach* (3rd ed). Stamford, CT: Appleton & Lange.
3. Ferri, F.F. (1999). *Ferri's clinical advisor, instant diagnosis and treatment.* St. Louis: Mosby.

4. Jacobs, D.S., DeMott, W.R., Grady, H.J., Horvat, R.T., Huestis, D.W., & Kasten, B.L. (1999). *Laboratory test handbook.* Cleveland: Lexi-comp.
5. LoCurto, M.J. (1997). The serotonin syndrome. *Emergency Medicine Clinics of North America, 15,* 665–675.
6. Page, C.P., Curtis, M.J., Sutter, M.C., Walker, M.J.A., & Hoffman, B.B. (1997). *Integrated pharmacology.* London: Mosby.
7. Preston, J., & Johnson, J. (1997). *Clinical psychopharmacology* (3rd ed). Miami: MedMaster.
8. Sheehy, S.B., & Lenehan, G.P. (1999). *Manual of emergency care* (5th ed). St. Louis: Mosby.
9. Turkoski, B.B., Lance, B.R., & Janosik, J.E. (1999). *Drug information handbook for nursing.* Cleveland: Lexi-comp.
10. Wilson, J.D., Braunwald, E., Isselbacher, K.J., Petersdorf, R.J., Martin, J.B., Fauci, A.S., & Root, R.K. (1995). *Harrison's principles of internal medicine* (12th ed). New York: McGraw-Hill.

WOUND MANAGEMENT

Jean Smith Temple, MSN, BSN, RN

I. TYPES OF WOUNDS—DEFINITIONS

A. Acute[3, 7]

1. Acute surgical: Clean or contaminated after surgery
2. Traumatic wound: Clean or contaminated

B. Chronic ulcers[4, 10]

1. Arterial: Ischemia secondary to various types of arterial occlusive disease
2. Venous: Related to disorders that affect venous blood return to the central circulation
3. Diabetic: Associated with excessive and prolonged elevations of glucose levels and peripheral neuropathies in diabetic patients
4. Pressure: Underlying tissue damage due to prolonged pressure or shearing resulting in decreased blood and oxygen to capillaries of soft tissue beds

II. KEY FACTORS IN DELAYED HEALING[1–10]

A. Excessive tissue load/pressure

B. Decreased tissue perfusion and oxygenation

C. Urinary or bowel incontinence

D. Infection

E. Systemic diseases such as diabetes mellitus

F. Inadequate or poor nutrition

G. Necrotic tissue

H. Immunosuppression

III. SUBJECTIVE FINDINGS[3, 4, 10]

A. Specific to diminished arterial or venous flow or varying combinations depending on areas involved

1. Pain and tenderness

   a. Arterial: Claudication
   b. Venous: Lower legs and feet ''heavy'' and ''sore'' after prolonged standing

2. Neuropathy

    a. Arterial and diabetic ulcers: "Numbness and tingling"

3. Arterial, venous, diabetic ulcers: Patient report of poor wound healing
4. Stated "foot problems" or trauma

B. Applicable pressure ulcer risk assessment tools, such as the Braden or Norton tools (subjective and objective combinations)

IV. GENERAL PHYSICAL EXAMINATION GUIDELINES FOR WOUND ASSESSMENT[2–4, 7, 8]

A. Acute or chronic etiologic factors as underlying cause

B. Specific anatomic location (see Section V. Wound-Specific Physical Examination Findings)

C. Length and width in centimeters

D. Depth of tissue destruction

1. Superficial
2. Partial thickness

    a. Extension through epidermis and partially into dermis

3. Full thickness

    a. Extension through epidermis and dermis, and some subcutaneous layer involvement
    b. Muscle and bone may be involved.

4. Undermining and tunneling

    a. Depth and direction

5. Sinus tracts

E. Color of wound: Red-yellow-black classification system for wound healing by secondary intention

1. Red: Granulation tissue clean and healthy; color is pink to beefy-red
2. Yellow: Exudate present and cleaning needed; color is beige, creamy or whitish yellow, yellow-greenish
3. Black: Eschar present indicating necrotic tissue; cleaning needed
4. Mixed combination of two or more colors

    a. Identify predominant color (treatment geared toward predominant color)

F. Color, amount, and consistency of drainage

G. Presence of foul odor, indicating infection

H. Appearance and temperature of surrounding skin and tissue

1. Presence of erythema, maceration, induration, or edema

I. Calluses (typically on plantar surface of foot)

J. Wound classification system, such as the Wagner Ulcer Grade Classification System of Staging or the National Pressure Ulcer Advisory Panel (see Section V)

K. Presence of pain

V. WOUND-SPECIFIC PHYSICAL EXAMINATION FINDINGS

A. Arterial and diabetic ulcers[4, 10]

1. Typical locations

   a. Toes and below ankles (general arterial disease)
   b. Plantar surface of feet (diabetic ulcers)

2. Pulse volume is diminished or absent.
3. Shiny, cool lower extremities
4. Leg hair is sparse or absent.
5. Foot and lower legs near ankle are cool
6. Ankle-brachial index of <0.5 (arterial); may exceed 1.0 for diabetic patients
7. Toenails are thickened.
8. Deep ulcers with smooth wound margins; small amount of drainage; cellulitis and necrosis

B. Venous ulcers[4-5, 7-8]

1. Typical location

   a. Lower legs, above ankle

2. Varicosity noticeable
3. Edema of lower legs or feet
4. Warm lower extremities and feet
5. Superficial, ruddy, granulating ulcer with irregular margins; moderate to heavy drainage

C. Pressure ulcers[1-4, 6]

1. Typical locations: Bony prominences (sacrum, heels, occiputus)
2. Ulcer description in terms of general assessment of wound (see Section IV) and a wound classification system for pressure ulcers, for example, the classification description by stages according to the National Pressure Ulcer Advisory Panel

   a. Stage 1: Skin intact with nonblanchable erythema; the heralding lesion of skin ulceration

b. Stage 2: Partial-thickness loss
c. Stage 3: Full-thickness loss; clinically appears deep, crater–like, with or without underlying adjacent tissue
d. Stage 4: Full-thickness loss and extensive destruction; tissue necrosis or muscle/bone/supporting structure damage (tendon, joint capsule)

VI. LABORATORY/DIAGNOSTIC FINDINGS[3, 4, 7]

A. Findings conclusive of absent or diminished arterial or venous flow dynamics

1. Doppler pressure studies

   a. Normal: Pressure gradients <30 mmHg between cuffs

2. Digital plethysmography: Measures systolic toe pressure

   a. Normal toe pressure is 80–90% of brachial systolic pressure.

3. Transcutaneous oxygen measurements ($Tcpo_2$): Measures O_2 delivery to skin tissue

   a. $Tcpo_2$ values >30 mmHg indicate a wound area that will heal.
   b. $Tcpo_2$ values <20 mmHg indicate a wound area that will not heal.

4. Venous Doppler ultrasonography

   a. Conclusive findings may indicate clots or incompetent venous valves.

B. Guidelines for referral to vascular specialist (surgeon or vascular laboratory)

1. Urgent vascular appointments

   a. Presence of gangrene
   b. Visible tendon or bone at ulcer base
   c. Cellulitis
   d. Severe infection
   e. Ankle-brachial index <0.5; indicator of perfusion and measures systolic pressure in ankles

2. Semiurgent vascular appointments

   a. $Tcpo_2$ measurement >30 mmHg and ankle-brachial index >1.0
   b. Weak or absent pulses with ankle-brachial index <1.0
   c. Ankle-brachial index between 0.5 and 0.8
   d. Poor wound healing in presence of normal pulses and aggressive wound care protocols

3. Routine/standard vascular appointment

   a. Ankle-brachial index >0.8

C. Complete blood count: Leukocytosis, decreased red cells and/or hemoglobin

D. Abnormal clotting times: Prothrombin time <11 s; activated partial thromboplastin time; <30 s; partial thromboplastin time <60 s

E. Elevated glucose levels (>150 mg/dL).

F. Decreased albumin levels (3.0 g/dL).

G. Quantitative culture and wound culture and sensitivity (specific to organism)

VII. MANAGEMENT[3, 4, 7, 9]

A. Arterial ulcers[3, 4, 7, 9]

1. Wet-to-moist dressings (saline) 3–4 times a day
2. Enzymatic debridement (no surgical debridement)
3. Calcium alginates
4. Nonocclusive/nonadherent dressing (no occlusive dressings)
5. Analgesics as needed

B. Venous ulcers[4, 5, 7, 9]

1. Elevate leg
2. Wet-to-moist dressings (saline) 3–4 times a day
3. Whirlpool therapy
4. Sharp debridement if cellulitis or infection is present.
5. Enzymatic debridement
6. Oral or intravenous antibiotics as appropriate for local or systemic infections

   a. Systemic, e.g., dicloxacillin, 250 mg p.o. q.i.d., or ciprofloxacin, 500 mg p.o. b.i.d.

7. Compression therapy, in presence of normal pulses
8. Analgesics as needed

C. Diabetic ulcers[4, 8, 9]

1. Increase insulin (routine and sliding scale) and/or oral hypoglycemic dosages to control glucose levels.
2. No weight bearing
3. Incision and drainage as indicated
4. Topical antimicrobial
5. Nonocclusive/nonadherent dressings
6. Enzymatic debridement

7. Bactericidal antibiotics specific to microbiologic findings and wound appearances

   a. Aerobic gram-positive cocci coverage for ulcers limited in extent
      i. Clindamycin, 300 mg IV q.i.d. for 14 days
      ii. Cefazolin, 1.0–1.5 g IV q6h
   b. Polymicrobic (aerobes and anaerobes) coverage for recurrent, chronic, limb-threatening lesions
      i. Cefoxitin, 1–2 g IV q8h
   c. Septic and chronic, limb-threatening
      i. Piperacillin, 3.0 g and tazobactam, 0.375 g IV q4–6h

8. Systemic antibiotics if evidence of osteomyelitis, cellulitis, or septicemia
9. Analgesics, as needed
10. Wet-to-moist saline dressings 3–4 times a day
11. Wet gangrene—Do not debride.

D. Pressure ulcers[1–4, 6–8, 10]

1. Positioning: Order q2h turning of patient to relieve pressure on ulcer
2. Support surfaces: Consider ordering air-fluidized beds for wounds.
3. Skin barrier products (Stages I and II ulcers)

   a. Polyurethane, such as Tegaderm or OpSite per manufacturer's instructions
   b. Hydrogel, such as IntraSite or Vigilon per manufacturer's instructions
   c. Hydrocolloids, such as Duoderm or Restore per manufacturer's instructions

4. Debridement
5. Cleansing

   a. Normal saline for most pressure ulcers
   b. Cleanse wound initially and with each dressing change
   c. Avoid cytotoxic skin cleansers and antiseptic agents, such as povidone-iodine, iodophor, sodium hypochlorite solution (Dakin's solution), hydrogen peroxide, and acetic acid
   d. Irrigation
   e. Whirlpool therapy for thick exudate, slough, or necrotic tissue
      i. Discontinue when wound is clean.

6. Dressing

   a. Select to keep ulcer bed continuously moist while maintaining dry surrounding skin and controlling exudate without desiccating ulcer bed

TABLE 79–1. TREATMENT OPTIONS FOR CHRONIC ULCERS

	TYPE OF ULCER			
	Arterial	Venous	Diabetic	Pressure
Cleaning Debridement	Saline preferred Wet-to-moist saline dressing Enzymatic, no surgical debridement Calcium alginates	Saline preferred Sharp—if cellulitis, infection, or necrotic Wet-to-moist, sharp, or whirlpool to remove moderate amount of debris from fibrotic tissue or eschar Enzymatic debridement	Saline preferred Wet-to-moist saline Sharp, aggressive—if nonischemic Enzymatic, whirlpool, nonaggressive sharp, if ischemic Do not debride if wet gangrene	Saline preferred Wet-to-dry saline
Dressing	Nonocclusive, nonadherent Wet-to-moist saline	Wet-to-moist saline	Nonocclusive nonadherent dressing Gauze dressing to plantar area Occlusive dressing to dorsal area	Depending on amount of debris and drainage: collagen, foams, hydrocolloids, hydrogels, moist impregnated packing, wound fillers per manufacturer's guide
Antibiotic	As indicated by culture and sensitivity of wound	As indicated by culture and sensitivity of wound *Topical:* Silver sulfadiazine *Systemic:* Oral, IV	As indicated by culture and sensitivity of wound *Topical:* Ointment, cream, amorphous hydrogels, antimicrobial *Oral:* Use for localized soft tissue *IV:* Use for systemic, localized bone, osteomyelitis	As indicated by culture and sensitivity of wound *Topical:* Use for clean, nonhealing ulcers or exudate after 2–4 week period; effective against gram-negative, gram positive, and anaerobic organisms *Systemic:* Use for bacteremia, cellulitis, osteomyelitis *Table continued on following page*

TABLE 79–1. TREATMENT OPTIONS FOR CHRONIC ULCERS *Continued*

| | TYPE OF ULCER | | |
	Arterial	Venous	Diabetic	Pressure
Compression therapy	None	In presence of normal pulses, no infection, heart failure, or concurrent arterial disease: Elastic bandages, Unna boot, antiembolytic hose, sequential compression device	None	None

IV, intravenous.

7. Topical antibiotics

   a. For clean, nonhealing ulcers or ulcers producing exudate after 2–4-week period
   b. Should be effective against gram-negative, gram-positive, and anaerobic organisms, such as silver sulfadiazine or triple antibiotic with each dressing change

8. Systemic antibiotics as appropriate

   a. For bacteremia, sepsis, advancing cellulitis, or osteomyelitis

9. Nutrition

   a. Increased protein, high caloric diet
   b. Ascorbic acid supplement, 500 mg b.i.d.
   c. Zinc sulfate, 220 mg daily

10. Analgesics, as needed

VIII. SELECTED TREATMENT OPTIONS

See Table 79–1 for selected treatment options for chronic ulcers.

References

1. AHCPR Panel for the Prediction and Prevention of Pressure Ulcers in Adults (1992, May). *Pressure ulcers in adults: Prediction and prevention.* Clinical Practice Guideline, No. 3. AHCPR Publication No. 92-0047. Rockville, MD: Agency for Health Care Policy and Research, Public Health Service, U.S. Department of Health and Human Services.
2. Bergstrom, N., Bennett, M.A., & Carlson, C.E., et al. (1994, December). *Treatment and management of pressure ulcers.* Clinical Practice Guideline, No. 15. AHCPR Publication No. 95-0652. Rockville, MD: Agency for Health Care Policy and Research, Public Health Service, U.S. Department of Health and Human Services.
3. Hess, C.T. (1998). *Nurse's clinical guide: Wound care* (2nd ed.). Springhouse, PA: Springhouse.
4. Krasner, D., & Kane, D. (1997). *Chronic wound care: A clinical source book for healthcare professionals* (2nd ed.). Wayne, PA: Health Management Publications.
5. Margolis, D.J., Berlin, J.A., & Strom, B.L. (1999). Risk factors associated with the failure of a venous leg ulcer to heal. *Archives in Dermatology, 135*, 920–926.
6. The National Pressure Ulcer Advisory Panel (1989). Pressure ulcers: Prevalence, cost and risk assessment. Consensus development conference statement. *Decubitus, 2*, 24–28.
7. Quinn, D. (1999). The Principles of pressure sore prevention. *Nursing Standard, 13*, 46–47.
8. Sussman, C. & Bates-Jensen, B.M. (Eds.). (1998). *Wound care: A collaborative practice manual for physical therapists.* Gaithersburg, MD: Aspen Publishers.

9. Whitney, J., & Heitkemper, M. (1999). Modifying perfusion, nutrition, and stress to promote wound healing in patients with acute wounds. *Heart & Lung, 28,* 123–133.

10. Woolliscroft, J. (1998). *Handbook of current diagnosis and treatment: A quick reference for the general practitioner* (2nd ed.). St. Louis: Mosby.

INFECTIONS

John A. Vande Waa, DO, PhD

I. HOSPITAL-ACQUIRED INFECTIONS

A. Nosocomial urinary tract infection

1. Definition

   a. Infection of the bladder or upper urinary tract

   b. Most nosocomial urinary tract infections are catheter-associated and are the most common hospital-acquired infections.

2. Etiology/Incidence/Predisposing factors[3, 9]

   a. Duration of catheterization is the most important risk factor.

   b. Incidence is 3–10% per catheterization day.

   c. Perineal flora and catheter/drainage bags are the sources of infecting organisms.

   d. Common pathogens include

       i. *Escherichia coli*

       ii. *Klebsiella pneumoniae*

       iii. *Proteus mirabilis*

       iv. *Pseudomonas aeruginosa*

       v. *Enterobacter* spp.

       vi. Enterococci

       vii. Staphylococci

       viii. Yeast

3. Subjective findings[6, 8]

   a. Most cases are asymptomatic and do not usually require treatment.

   b. Fever, abdominal fullness, urinary urgency, and/or urethral irritation may be reported.

4. Physical examination findings[6, 8]

   a. Usually none or nonspecific

   b. Urethral purulence may be present around the catheter at the entry site.

5. Laboratory/Diagnostic findings[6, 8]

   a. Urinalysis usually reveals pyuria, increased leukocyte esterase, and hematuria.

   b. Urine culture shows at least 100,000 colony-forming units per mL of urine.

6. Management[3, 6, 8, 9]

a. Discontinue catheterization if possible.
b. Change to a new catheter.
c. Switch to condom catheters where appropriate.
d. Use intermittent catheterization.
e. Symptomatic bacteriuria: Oral antibiotic therapy is usually sufficient to treat most cases; intravenous therapy is necessary in selected severely ill patients.
   i. Antibiotic choice is dependent upon the organism identified and susceptibilities determined.
   ii. For empiric therapy, knowledge of organisms in the medical unit is imperative; organisms vary from hospital to hospital and are likely to vary from unit to unit.
   iii. Recommended duration of therapy is 3–7 days in uncomplicated cases and 10–14 days in complicated cases.
   iv. For example:
      (1) Oral trimethoprim-sulfamethoxazole, 160/800 mg q12h, or equivalent IV, or
      (2) Ofloxacin, 200–400 mg, q12h, p.o. or IV
      (3) For urosepsis, where empiric coverage for nosocomial pathogens is needed, a combination of a beta-lactam and an aminoglycoside is often prudent (e.g., ceftazidime, 1–2 g IV q8h, or piperacillin, 3–4 g IV q6h, plus gentamicin, 5 mg IV q24h and adjusted for renal function).
f. Symptomatic candiduria: Change the catheter and treat with amphotericin B bladder irrigation, oral fluconazole, or IV amphotericin B, depending on the species of yeast, azole susceptibilities in the medical unit, and the severity of the patient's illness. For example:
      (1) Fluconazole, 100–200 mg p.o. every day, or
      (2) Amphotericin B, 50 mg/L in D_5W, 1 L/day bladder irrigation over 24 h, or
      (3) Amphotericin B, 0.3–0.5 mg/kg/day IV, for 5–7 days

B. Nosocomial pneumonia

1. Definition

a. Most nosocomial infections of the lower respiratory tract are ventilator-associated, defined as onset of pneumonia 48 h after hospitalization.
b. Nosocomial pneumonia is the second most common hospital-acquired infection.

2. Etiology/Incidence/Predisposing factors[3, 4, 9]

a. Highest mortality rate of all the nosocomial infections
b. Incidence ranges from 7–20%, depending on the ICU setting.

c. Colonization of the upper respiratory tract and endotracheal tubing by bacterial pathogens precedes infection.

d. Organisms usually reach the lower respiratory tract by aspiration into the distal airways.

e. Risk factors
    i. Intubation
    ii. ICU setting
    iii. Antibiotics
    iv. Prolonged surgery
    v. Chronic lung disease
    vi. Advanced age
    vii. Immunosuppression

f. Common pathogens are predominantly the gram-negative bacilli, including
    i. *P. aeruginosa*
    ii. *Enterobacter* spp.
    iii. *Klebsiella* spp.
    iv. *E. coli*
    v. *Haemophilus influenzae*
    vi. *Serratia marcescens*

    • *Staphylococcus aureus* is the most common gram-positive pathogen.

3. Subjective findings[6, 7]

a. Fever

b. Cough (usually productive)

c. Shortness of breath

4. Physical examination findings[6, 7]

a. Rales or dullness to percussion on chest examination

b. New onset or change in character of sputum

c. Tachypnea

5. Laboratory/Diagnostic findings[6, 7]

a. Purulent sputum

b. Isolation of a pathogen from
    i. Sputum
    ii. Transbronchial aspirate
    iii. Bronchial brush
    iv. Bronchoalveolar lavage
    v. Biopsy specimen

c. Organism isolated from blood culture

d. Deterioration in oxygenation or ventilation

e. Chest x-ray shows new or progressing
    i. Infiltrate
    ii. Consolidation
    iii. Cavitation
    iv. Pleural effusion

f. Leukocytosis, often with a left shift

6. Management[3, 4, 6, 7, 9]

a. Hand-washing by health care workers (prevention)
b. Elevate the head of the patient's bed 30–45 degrees (prevention).
c. Discontinue nasogastric tubes when possible (prevention).
d. Give sucralfate for stress ulcer prophylaxis (frequently recommended but remains controversial)
e. Increase sputum clearance with incentive spirometry, chest physical therapy, and frequent suctioning.
f. Empiric antibiotics
   i. It is very important to know the susceptibilities of the nosocomial pathogens in the medical unit.
   ii. Typically, antibiotic coverage is targeted broadly to include resistant gram-negative pathogens (e.g., *P. aeruginosa*) at the onset.
   iii. Once the organism(s) are identified by diagnostic means, usually a narrower-spectrum antibiotic therapy can be utilized. For combination antipseudomonal coverage:
       (1) Antipseudomonal beta-lactam
           (a) Piperacillin, 3–4 g IV q4–6h, or
           (b) Ceftazidime, 1–2 g IV q8–12h, or
           (c) Cefepime, 1–2 g IV q12h, plus
       (2) Aminoglycoside
           (a) Gentamicin or tobramycin, 1.7–2.0 mg/kg IV q8h, or 5 mg/kg IV q24h or
       (3) Quinolone
           (a) Ciprofloxacin, 400 mg IV q12h, or
           (b) Ofloxacin, 200–400 mg IV q12h
   iv. For patients with suspected aspiration pneumonia, anaerobic coverage should be considered.
       (1) By the addition to the preceding regimen of clindamycin, 300–900 mg IV q6–8h, or
       (2) Using a beta-lactam/beta-lactamase inhibitor such as piperacillin/tazobactam, 3.375 g IV q6h
   v. Duration of therapy for nosocomial pneumonia is 14–21 days.

C. Nosocomial bacteremia

1. Definition

a. Laboratory-confirmed bloodstream infection with a recognized pathogen from blood culture or a skin colonizer isolated from multiple blood cultures on separate occasions

2. Etiology/Incidence/Predisposing factors[3, 5]

a. The third most common hospital-acquired infection
b. Mortality ranges from 2–60 %.

   c. Most bacteremias are associated with intravascular catheters.
   d. Sources of microbes are skin or intravascular fluids.
   e. Pneumonia, urinary tract infections, and wound infections are usually the other sources of bacteremia.
   f. Risk factors
      i. Bacterial colonization at catheter site
      ii. Longer duration of catheter insertion
      iii. Older age
      iv. Severe underlying illness
      v. Parenteral nutrition
      vi. Loss of skin integrity
      vii. Use of nonpermeable dressings
   g. Common organisms include
      i. Coagulase-negative staphylococci
      ii. *S. aureus* (including methicillin-resistant *S. aureus*)
      iii. Enterococci
      iv. *Enterobacter* spp.,
      v. *P. aeruginosa*
      vi. *Candida* spp.
   h. Complications
      i. Cellulitis or abscess at the site of catheter insertion
      ii. Septic phlebitis
      iii. Endocarditis

3. Subjective findings[5, 6]

   a. The patient may be asymptomatic.
   b. Fever and/or chills
   c. Pain at the catheter insertion site

4. Physical examination findings[5, 6]

   a. Local erythema, edema, tenderness, and warmth at the catheter site
   b. Exit site may be purulent.
   c. Fever, tachycardia, and/or hypotension may be present.
   d. The patient may have a heart murmur and embolic/septic sequelae.

5. Laboratory/Diagnostic findings[5, 6]

   a. A recognized pathogen isolated from a blood culture (and not related to another site), or
   b. A symptomatic patient with a skin colonizer, e.g. a coagulase-negative *Staphylococcus,* in two blood cultures on separate occasions (and not related to another site)

6. Management[5, 6]

   a. It is of paramount importance to determine the source of the bacteremia/candidemia, i.e., rule out pneumonia, urinary tract infection, wound infection, or endocarditis as the source of infection, as opposed to an intravenous catheter/device. Choice and duration of therapy depend entirely upon the diagnosis.

b. Removal of the catheter is nearly always required.

c. Antibiotic therapy

    i. Gram's stain results (gram-positive compared with gram-negative compared with yeast) from the blood culture will be available prior to identification and susceptibilities and can be used as a guide for empiric antibiotic selection in serious infections.

    ii. Once the organism is identified and susceptibilities are determined, a narrower-spectrum antibiotic regimen can usually be utilized.

    iii. Gram-positive cocci

      (1) Nafcillin, 1–2 g IV q4h, or

      (2) Cefazolin, 1–2 g IV q8h, or

      (3) Vancomycin, 1 g IV q12h when methicillin resistance is suspected

    iv. If methicillin-resistant *S. aureus* has been identified, the patient needs to be placed in contact isolation (gloves and gown if soiling is likely).

    v. If vancomycin-resistant *Enterococcus* is isolated, the patient also needs to be placed in contact isolation.

      (1) Optimal therapy for vancomycin-resistant *Enterococcus* has yet to be determined.

      (2) Possibly effective: Ampicillin (*E. faecalis*), quinupristin/dalfopristin (Synercid) (*E. faecium*), 7.5 mg/kg IV q8h, or linezolid (Zyvox), 600 mg IV q12h

      (3) An infectious disease consultation is critical for the management of these infections under most circumstances.

    vi. Vancomycin is not recommended as treatment in response to a single positive blood culture for coagulase-negative staphylococci.[2]

    vii. Gram-negative bacilli

      (1) Antipseudomonal beta-lactam

        (a) Piperacillin, 3–4 g IV q4–6h, or

        (b) Ceftazidime, 2 g IV q8–12h, or

        (c) Cefepime, 2 g IV q12h, plus

      (2) Aminoglycoside

        (a) Gentamicin or tobramycin, 1.7–2.0 mg/kg IV q8h, or 5 mg/kg IV q24h, or

      (3) Quinolone

        (a) Ciprofloxacin, 400 mg IV q12h, or

        (b) Ofloxacin, 200–400 mg IV q12h

      viii. Yeasts

         (1) Amphotericin B, 0.5 mg/kg IV q24h

         (2) If *Candida albicans* is identified, fluconazole, 400–800 mg IV, q24h may be nearly as effective.

    d. Duration of therapy is usually 14 days.

D. Miscellaneous nosocomial infections

1. *Clostridium difficile* colitis (pseudomembranous colitis)[1, 6]

    a. Diagnosis: Fever, abdominal pain, heme-positive stool, and diarrhea in a patient currently or recently receiving antibiotics, and a stool specimen positive for *C. difficile* toxin.

    b. Treatment

      i. Discontinuation of implicated antibiotic when possible

      ii. Patient should be placed in contact isolation.

      iii. Metronidazole, 500 mg p.o. q8h for 10–14 days, or

      iv. Vancomycin, 125 mg p.o. q6h for 10–14 days, if infection is severe

      v. When oral treatment is not possible, metronidazole, 500 mg IV q8h

      vi. For relapses (frequency 5–50%), repeat above treatment.

2. Surgical wound infections[3, 6]

    a. Diagnosis

      i. Purulence within the surgical wound site

      ii. May be associated with fever, leukocytosis, and sepsis (other nosocomial sources ruled out)

    b. Rates of infection are related to the level of contamination, e.g., clean, clean-contaminated, or contaminated wound.

    c. Source of contamination is dependent on multiple factors, including but not limited to skin flora and the surgical procedure or trauma site involved.

    d. Common pathogens in surgical wound infections

      i. *S. aureus*

      ii. *Enterococcus*

      iii. Coagulase-negative *Staphylococcus*

      iv. *E. coli*

      v. *P. aeruginosa*

      vi. *Enterobacter* spp.

      vii. *Klebsiella* spp.

      viii. *Proteus* spp.

      ix. *Streptococcus* spp.

      x. *Bacteroides fragilis*

    e. Treatment

      i. For most clean procedures/wounds, e.g., cholecystectomy, cardiothoracic and vascular surgery, orthopedic

TABLE 80–1. EMPIRIC THERAPY FOR SELECTED COMMUNITY-ACQUIRED INFECTIONS

INFECTION	ORGANISM	RECOMMENDED PHARMACOLOGIC TREATMENT
Pharyngitis	Primarily concerned about group A streptococcus with possible acute rheumatic fever sequelae. Other pathogens include viral, Neisseria, C. diphtheriae, and upper respiratory tract pathogens.	If the streptococcus screen or throat cultures are positive for group A streptococcus, then oral penicillin, cephalosporin, or erythromycin for 10 days. Consider other pathogens if Group A streptococcus is not found.
Sinusitis	S. pneumoniae and H. influenzae are most common, but viral, Staphylococcus aureus, Moraxella catarrhalis, gram-negatives, and anaerobes also may be responsible	Topical and systemic decongestants plus: Augmentin, 875 mg p.o. b.i.d., or Bactrim DS, p.o. b.i.d. for 10–14 days, are usually recommended empirically. Broader spectrum antibiotics, e.g., cefuroxime, 500 mg p.o. b.i.d., or Levaquin, 500 mg p.o. q day, and sinus x-rays are suggested for refractory cases.
Pneumonia	See Chapter 31.	See Chapter 31.
Meningitis	See Chapter 5.	See Chapter 5.
Urinary tract infection	See Chapter 41.	See Chapter 41.
Skin and soft tissue Cellulitis	Primarily concerned about S. aureus, S. pyogenes, and other gram-positives in immunocompetent hosts, but gram-negatives and anaerobes are occasionally responsible	Cephalexin, 500 mg p.o. q.i.d. or, if serious, cefazolin 1–2 g IV q8h is usually started empirically for most skin and soft-tissue infections. Failure to quickly improve with these agents requires aggressive imaging and tissue and blood cultures to evaluate. Surgical and infectious disease consultation if infection is severe and limb- or life-threatening.

Diabetes or Immunocompromised	Same gram-positive organisms as above, but also gram-negatives, including *Pseudomonas* and anaerobes	Same as above, but add a quinolone or, if infection is limb- or life-threatening, piperacillin/tazobactam, 3.375 g IV q6h
Bite wounds	Staphylococcus, streptococcus, *Eikenella*, *Pasturella*, and anaerobes are usually responsible.	Cleaning and debriding the wound and a tetanus shot are essential. Augmentin, 875 mg p.o. b.i.d., or, if severe, ampicillin/sulbactam, 3 g IV q6h
Surgical wounds	Gram positives > gram negatives or polymicrobial, dependent upon injury	See chapter text.
Gastrointestinal Simple diarrhea	Most cases of diarrhea are self-limiting and do not require antibiotics.	Adequate oral hydration is usually sufficient.
Dysentery	*Shigella*, *Salmonella*, enterotoxigenic *E. coli*, *Campylobacter*, *C. difficile*, and *E. histolytica*. Stool culture, stains, O&P, or toxin for these pathogens are often helpful for identification.	Hydration is critical and may need intravenous therapy. In patients who appear toxic or are immunocompromised, treat with a quinolone such as ciprofloxacin, 500 mg p.o. or IV q12h. If *E. histolytica* or *C. difficile* colitis is suspected, then add metronidazole, 750 mg p.o. or IV q8h and follow up on stool studies to confirm.
Sepsis Source unknown	Gram-positive and gram-negative	Ceftriaxone, 2 g IV q24h, or ampicillin/sulbactam, 3 g IV q6h, or piperacillin/tazobactam, 3.375 g IV q6h, usually with an aminoglycoside (gentamicin or tobramycin, 1 mg/kg IV q8h)
Endocarditis	Gram-positive > gram-negative	Nafcillin, 2 g IV q4h, plus gentamicin, 1 mg/kg IV q8h, and follow-up on blood and tissue cultures Infectious disease consultation is highly recommended.

Table continued on following page

TABLE 80–1. EMPIRIC THERAPY FOR SELECTED COMMUNITY-ACQUIRED INFECTIONS *Continued*

INFECTION	ORGANISM	RECOMMENDED PHARMACOLOGIC TREATMENT
Neutropenia	Gram-positive and gram-negative	Ceftazidime, 2 g IV q8h, or cefepime, 2 g IV q8–12h, plus an aminoglycoside or quinolone (dose as in nosocomial infections in this chapter). Infectious disease consultation is highly recommended.
If vascular device present	Primarily gram-positives, including methicillin-resistant Staphylococcus	Add vancomycin, 1 g IV q12h, and follow-up on blood cultures. Usually requires the removal of a vascular catheter when present (see nosocomial bacteremia)

Notes:

1. Table 80–1 provides a limited selection of common community-acquired infections in adults that practitioners frequently encounter. It is by no means a definitive resource but rather an abbreviated guide for some of the most common organisms and appropriate empiric antibiotic treatment regimens for adults. **Empiric antibiotic therapy is not a substitute for a required diagnostic workup and treatment plan for a patient with a suspected infection.** For all infections, it is imperative to identify in the most prudent way what organism(s) are responsible for the infection and their specific antibiotic susceptibilities. From these results, confirmed effective and usually narrower-spectrum antibiotics should be used.

2. A patient's history and infectious disease risks may dramatically alter the organisms and presentation of infection in an individual and is very important when considering empiric antibiotic regimens beyond the scope of this handbook. Consequently, for any serious or critically ill patient where infection may be present or suspected, these risks need to be considered, and an infectious disease consultation is highly recommended.

3. All antibiotics have the potential for serious allergic reactions and toxicities for a patient, and this potential is critical in choosing an antibiotic regimen. It is essential to know the possible allergic reactions and toxicities of any antibiotic before prescribing them. Please refer to the package inserts of these medications and utilize the pharmacy at your facility or hospital for any additional questions.

4. Note: Vancomycin and aminoglycosides (gentamicin, tobramycin, and amikacin) need serum concentration monitoring (peaks and troughs). Please refer to the package inserts and your pharmacy for the specific recommendations.

surgery, and cesarean section, cefazolin is indicated for prophylaxis and treatment.

  ii. For clean-contaminated procedures/wounds, e.g., colon surgery or penetrating abdominal/pelvic trauma, cefoxitin is indicated for prophylaxis and treatment.

  iii. For postoperative sepsis, broad coverage for nosocomial pathogens is indicated, and it is critical to determine the source.

    (1) Empiric coverage for nosocomial pneumonia or bacteremia as described in the preceding sections is usually appropriate.

    (2) If an abdominal or contaminated wound could be a source of infection, then coverage for gram-negatives and anaerobes is prudent, using piperacillin/tazobactam, 3.375 g IV q6h, plus an aminoglycoside.

II. COMMUNITY-ACQUIRED INFECTIONS (Table 80–1)

See Table 80–1 for various community-acquired infections and their recommended empiric pharmacologic treatments.

References

1. Gerding, D.N., Johnson, S., Peterson, L.R., Mulligan, M.E., Silva, J. (1995). Society for Healthcare Epidemiology of America: Position paper on Clostridium difficile-associated diarrhea and colitis. *Infection Control and Hospital Epidemiology, 16,* 459–477.

2. Hospital Infection Control Practices Advisory Committee (1996). Recommendations for preventing the spread of vancomycin resistance. *Infection Control and Hospital Epidemiology, 16,* 105–113.

3. Hospital Infections Program, CDC (1995). Atlanta, National Nosocomial Infections Surveillance semiannual report. *American Journal of Infection Control, 23,* 377–385.

4. McEachern, R., & Campbell, G.D. (1998). Hospital-acquired pneumonia: Epidemiology, etiology and treatment. *Infectious Disease Clinics of North America, 12,* 761–779.

5. Maki, D.G. (1981). Nosocomial bacteremia: An epidemiological overview. *American Journal of Medicine, 70,* 719–732.

6. Mandell, G.L., Bennett, J.E., & Dolin, R. (1999). *Principles and practice of infectious diseases* (5th ed.). New York: Churchill Livingstone.

7. Mayhall, C.G. (1997). Nosocomial pneumonia. *Infectious Disease Clinics of North America, 11,* 427–457.

8. Warren, J.W. (1997). Catheter-associated urinary tract infections. *Infectious Disease Clinics of North America, 11,* 609–621.

9. Weinstein, R.A. (1991). Epidemiology and control of nosocomial infections in adult intensive care units. *American Journal of Medicine, 91* (suppl. 3B), 179–184.

CHEST, ABDOMINAL, AND EYE TRAUMA

Julie T. Sanford, MSN, RN

I. CHEST TRAUMA

A. Rib fractures[1, 2, 4–7]

1. Definition

   a. Fractures of one or more ribs
   b. Possibly resulting in severe damage to underlying structures
      i. Lungs (e.g., pneumothorax, pulmonary contusion)
      ii. Subclavian artery (SCA)
      iii. Subclavian vein (SCV)

2. Etiology/Incidence

   a. Eighty-five percent of patients with blunt chest trauma experience rib fractures.
   b. Associated with motor vehicle crashes (MVCs), assaults, and falls

3. Subjective/Physical examination findings

   a. Pain, worsening with breathing, coughing, movement, and on palpation
   b. Shallow respirations
   c. Splinting of region
   d. Crepitus
   e. Decreased breath sounds on the affected side

4. Laboratory/Diagnostic findings

   a. Chest x-ray may reveal fractures, atelectasis.
   b. Arterial blood gas analysis (ABGs)
      i. ABGs may reveal respiratory acidosis (increased $Paco_2$ >45 mmHg) if the patient is hypoventilating.
      ii. If the patient is hyperventilating, respiratory alkalosis (decreased $Paco_2$ <35 mmHg) may be seen
      iii. Also, hypoxemia may be observed (Pao_2 <90 mmHg) if severe pulmonary contusion is present.
   c. Complete blood count (CBC) if hemothorax is suspected

5. Management

   a. Rule out underlying structural damage (i.e., lacerated SCA or SCV, pneumothorax, lacerated liver or spleen) by ordering arteriography, x-rays, CT scan.

b. Pain medications
  i. Meperidine (Demerol), 50 mg IM, or 25 mg IV, q 3–4 h
  ii. Morphine sulfate, 4–10 mg IV over 5 min.
  iii. Intercostal nerve blocks (such as lidocaine 1%).
c. Aggressive pulmonary toilet, such as Turn, Cough, Deep Breathe, chest physiotherapy on nonaffected side, incentive spirometry.
d. Consider aerosol therapy with albuterol (Ventolin), 1–2 puffs q4–6h to prevent atelectasis and pneumonia.
e. Monitor oxygen saturation; consider giving O_2 at 2 L per nasal cannula, maintaining $Sao_2 > 92$.

B. Flail chest[2, 4, 6, 7, 9]

1. Definition

   a. Fracture of at least two adjacent ribs at two sites
   b. Results in a "floating" segment

2. Etiology/Incidence

   a. Most serious chest wall injury
   b. High likelihood of underlying structural injury
   c. Caused by blunt force

3. Subjective/Physical examination findings

   a. Pain
   b. Shortness of breath
   c. Paradoxical chest wall movement
   d. Shallow respirations
   e. Tachypnea
   f. Decreased level of consciousness (LOC) secondary to hypoxia
   g. Cyanosis
   h. Tachycardia
   i. Splinting of chest wall
   j. Crepitus
   k. Decreased breath sounds on affected side

4. Laboratory/Diagnostic findings

   a. ABGs: Hypoxia, possible respiratory acidosis
   b. Chest x-ray: Reveals rib fractures

5. Management

   a. Administer O_2, correct possible respiratory acidosis, and consider ventilatory support with positive end-expiratory pressure (PEEP) and pressure support.
   b. Administer crystalloids, such as lactated Ringer's solution.
   c. Consider stabilizing flail segment with sandbags or, if ventilatory restriction is severe, operative stabilization.

d. Pain medications
   i. Meperidine, 25–50 mg IV/IM q3–4h
   ii. Morphine sulfate, 4–10 mg IV over 5 min
e. If lung contusion occurs, the patient may require long-term ventilation.
f. Ventilatory with induced paralysis may also be used.

C. Collapsed lung[2, 4, 5, 7, 8, 10]

1. Pneumothorax

   a. Occurs when air is introduced into the pleural space, causing a complete or partial collapse of the lung
   b. May be caused by blunt trauma, mechanical ventilation, central venous access devices, rib fractures, bleb ruptures

2. Hemothorax

   a. Occurs when blood accumulates in the pleural space; considered massive when drainage exceeds 1.5 L
   b. May be caused by blunt or penetrating trauma, lung cancer, anticoagulant therapy complications

3. Open pneumothorax

   a. Sometimes referred to as "sucking chest wound"
      i. Air flows from atmosphere to pleural space and back again.
      ii. Can lead to tension pneumothorax if covered with an occlusive dressing, or if skin flap does not allow air to escape
   b. May be caused by penetrating trauma, such as gunshot wounds or knife wounds

4. Tension pneumothorax

   a. A collapse of the lung caused by the one-way entrance of air flow into the pleural space
      i. Results in increased pressure on the heart, mediastinal shift to the unaffected side, and eventual circulatory collapse
      ii. Tension preumothorax is a *life-threatening* condition.
   b. May be caused by blunt or chest trauma, open pneumothorax, fractured ribs, mechanical ventilation, clamped chest tube

5. General subjective/Physical examination findings of the collapsed lung

   a. Respiratory distress
   b. Hypoxia
   c. Tachypnea
   d. Decreased LOC

    e. Hypotension
    f. Cyanosis
    g. Tachycardia
    h. Shallow respirations
    i. Chest pain
    j. Decreased or absent breath sounds on affected side
    k. Deviation of the trachea to the nonaffected side
    l. Tension pneumothorax may cause severe respiratory distress, leading to circulatory collapse (i.e., decreased cardiac output, decreased blood pressure).
    m. Open pneumothorax: Sucking sound may be heard on inspiration.

6. Laboratory/Diagnostic findings

    a. ABGs may reveal respiratory acidosis.
    b. Chest x-ray reveals collapsed lung and possible mediastinal shift.
    c. ECG may show heart strain.

7. Management[2, 5, 6]

    a. If tension pneumothorax, rapid insertion of large-bore (14–16-gauge) needle into the 2nd intercostal space, midclavicular line of the affected side
    b. Chest tube insertion of low wall suction (−20 cm)
    c. Consider mechanical ventilation with PEEP.
    d. Open pneumothorax: Apply a dressing leaving one side untaped to allow air to escape.
    e. Massive hemothorax: Fluid resuscitation with lactated Ringer's solution should be considered prior to thoracostomy owing to loss of tamponade effect.

D. Cardiac tamponade: Refer to Chapter 11, Angina/Myocardial Infarction.
E. Aortic rupture[1, 3, 7]

1. Definition

An interruption of the wall of the aorta caused by blunt traumatic deceleration injuries

2. Etiology

    a. MVC—most often without use of seatbelt
    b. Falls
    c. Pedestrian struck by automobile
    d. High mortality rate; most die before reaching the hospital.

3. Subjective/Physical examination findings

    a. Shortness of breath
    b. Weakness

c. Blood pressure and pulse amplitude are greater in upper extremities.
d. Chest or back pain
e. Circulatory collapse

4. Laboratory/Diagnostic findings

   a. Chest x-ray may reveal a widened mediastinum.
   b. Aortogram may reveal a widened mediastinum.

5. Management

   a. Thoracotomy to repair the rupture, with cardiopulmonary bypass
   b. Consider nitroprusside (Nipride), 0.5–8 μg/kg/min, to maintain systolic blood pressuse <140 mmHg until patient can be taken to surgery.
   c. Mechanical ventilation
   d. Fluid resuscitation with lactated Ringer's solution and packed red blood cells

II. ABDOMINAL TRAUMA

A. Lacerated liver[2–4, 7, 8]

1. Definition

   a. A laceration or tear of the liver caused by blunt or penetrating injury that typically rsults in profuse bleeding
   b. Classified according to disruption of the organ, Grades 1–6, with Grade 6 incompatible with survival
      i. Grade 1: Capsular tear <1 cm
      ii. Grade 2: 1–3 cm parenchymal depth, <10 cm in length
      iii. Grade 3: >3 cm parenchymal depth
      iv. Grade 4: Parenchymal disruption of 25–75%
      v. Grade 5: Parenchymal disruption >75%
      vi. Grade 6: Hepatic avulsion

2. Etiology

   a. Blunt trauma: MVC, falls, assaults
   b. Penetrating injury: Stab wounds, gunshot wounds
   c. Mortality is usually due to hemorrhage.

3. Subjective/Physical examination findings

   a. Right upper quadrant pain
   b. Guarding
   c. Signs and symptoms of hypovolemic shock
      i. Decreased blood pressure
      ii. Increased heart rate
      iii. Decreased LOC
      iv. Decreased urinary output
   d. Possible hypoactive or absent bowel sounds

4. Laboratory/Diagnostic findings

    a. Positive peritoneal lavage
    b. Decreased hematocrit
        i. Male: 42–52 mL/dL
        ii. Female: 37–47 mL/dL
    c. Decreased hemoglobin
        i. Male: 14–18 g/dL
        ii. Female: 12–16 g/dL
    d. Elevated liver enzymes
        i. Alanine transaminase: 8–48 IU/L
        ii. Aspartate transaminase: 8–38 IU/L
        iii. Alkaline phosphatase: 30–120 IU/L
    e. Positive abdominal CT scan
    f. Increased prothrombin time (11.0–12.5 s)

5. Management

    a. Stabilize impaled objects and wrap.
    b. Fluid resuscitation—See Chapter 75, Management of the Patient in Shock.
    c. Insert nasogastric tube.
    d. Insert Foley catheter.
    e. Peritoneal lavage
    f. Surgery to ligate tears in hepatic artery or perform resection
    g. Hemodynamic monitoring
    h. Antibiotic administration
        i. Gentamicin (Garamycin), 3 mg/kg in individual doses IV q8h for gram-negative organisms. ALSO
        ii. Cefoxitin (Mefoxin), 1–2 g q6–8h IV for gram-positive organisms

B. Ruptured spleen[2, 6, 8]

1. Definition

    a. A tear to the spleen caused by blunt or penetrating injury
    b. Classified according to disruption of the organ
        i. Grade 1: Capsular tear <1 cm
        ii. Grade 2: 1–3 cm parenchymal depth
        iii. Grade 3: >3 cm parenchymal depth
        iv. Grade 4: >25% of spleen
        v. Grade 5: Completely shattered spleen

2. Etiology

    a. Most often caused by MVCs, gunshot wounds, or stab wounds
    b. May be due to rib fractures

3. Subjective/Physical examination findings

   a. Pain
   b. Kehr's sign—Pain at left scapula caused by palpation of left upper quadrant
   c. Hypovolemic shock (increased heart rate, decreased blood pressure)
   d. Guarding

4. Laboratory/Diagnostic findings

   a. Positive peritoneal lavage
   b. Decreased hematocrit
      i. Male: 42–52 mL/dL
      ii. Female: 37–47 mL/dL
   c. Decreased hemoglobin
      i. Male: 14–18 g/dL
      ii. Female: 12–16 g/dL
   d. Increased WBC count ($>10,000/mm^3$)
   e. Positive CAT scan

5. Management

   a. Stabilize impaled objects and wrap sterile dressing around site.

      • *Do not remove foreign object*—Tamponade effect may be lost.

   b. Fluid resuscitation (with lactated Ringer's solution) for prevention of hypovolemic shock
   c. Insert nasogastric tube.
   d. Insert Foley catheter.
   e. Peritoneal lavage
   f. Laparotomy
   g. Hemodynamic monitoring

C. Renal injuries[4-6]

1. Definition

   a. Injuries to the kidneys resulting in fragmentation, caused by blunt or penetrating injuries.
   b. May also be caused by rib fractures

2. Subjective/Physical examination findings

   a. Pain—Abdominal or flank
   b. Flank bruising (Grey Turner's sign)
   c. Hematuria
   d. Palpable mass in flank region
   e. Possible hemodynamic instability

3. Laboratory/Diagnostic findings
   a. Intravenous pyelogram
   b. CT scan
   c. Kidneys, ureters, bladder
   d. Urinalysis may reveal hematuria.

4. Management
   a. Maintain hemodynamic stability.
   b. Possible nephrectomy (ensure functioning of the remaining kidney)
   c. Insert nasogastric tube.
   d. Insert Foley catheter.
   e. Monitor for renal failure.

III. PENETRATING EYE TRAUMA

A. Definition[2]

Impalement of objects into the globe of the eye

B. Etiology

1. Industrial accidents, failure to use protective eyewear
2. Gunshot wounds, stab wounds

C. Subjective/Physical examination findings[4]

1. Decreased visual acuity or complete vision loss
2. Pain
3. The patient may visualize foreign object.
4. If retinal detachment occurs, the patient may experience light flashes, blurred vision.
5. Small, shrunken eyeball

D. Diagnostic/Laboratory findings[4]

Decrease in intraocular pressure (normal: 8–21 mmHg)

E. Management[4]

1. Ophthalmology consultation
2. Immobilize the impaled object.
3. To decrease intraocular pressure (if >21 mmHg), raise the head of the bed.
4. Patch or bandage both eyes.
5. Use no medications in the affected eye because of possible perforation of the eye.
6. Surgery

References

1. Ahrens, T., & Prentice, D. (1998). *Critical care certification: Preparation, review, & practice exams.* (4th ed.). Stamford, CT: Appleton & Lange.
2. Bayley, E., & Turcke, S. (1992). *A Comprehensive curriculum for trauma nursing.* Boston: Jones and Bartlett Publishers.

3. Carrillo, E., Spain, D., Wohltmann, C., Schmieg, R., Boaz, P., Miller, F., & Richardson, J.D. (1999). Interventional techniques are useful adjuncts in nonoperative management of hepatic injuries. *Journal of Trauma, 46*, 619–624.
4. Emergency Nurses Association. (1991). *Trauma nursing core course* (3rd ed.). Chicago: Award Printing.
5. Laskowski-Jones, L. (1995). Meeting the challenge of chest trauma. *American Journal of Nursing, 95*, 23–29.
6. Lewis, S., Collier, I., & Heitkemper, M. (1996). *Medical-surgical nursing: Assessment and management of clinical problems*. St. Louis: Mosby.
7. Maull, K., Rodriguez, A., & Wiles, C. (1996). *Complications in trauma and critical care*. Philadelphia: W.B. Saunders.
8. Moore, E., Cogbill, T., Jurkovich, G., Shackford, S., Malangoni, M., & Champion, H. (1995). Organ injury scaling: Spleen and liver. *Journal of Trauma, 38*, 323–324.
9. Stamatos, C., Sorensen, P., & Tefler, K. (1996). Meeting the challenge of the older trauma patient. *American Journal of Nursing, 96*, 40–48.
10. Sommers, M. (1998). Missed injuries. *RN, 61*, 28–31.

MANAGING THE SURGICAL PATIENT

Sally K. Miller, MS, RN, CS, ACNP, ANP, GNP, CCRN

I. PREOPERATIVE ASSESSMENT

A. History and physical examination—Special emphasis on identification of undiagnosed cardiopulmonary disease[1-4]

1. Past medical history
2. Past surgical history
3. Family history
4. Psychosocial history
5. Allergies
6. Review of systems
7. Current medications
8. Head-to-toe physical examination

B. Laboratory and diagnostic screening[5, 6]

1. Urinalysis
2. Complete blood count
3. Posteroanterior and lateral chest radiographs
4. Patients >40 years of age

   a. Electrocardiogram
   b. Stool for occult blood
   c. Blood chemistry screening battery

5. Pulmonary function testing[7]

   a. Not routinely obtained
   b. Should be ordered for
      i. Patients having lung surgery
      ii. Patients with a history of smoking >10 pack-years who are having coronary artery bypass grafting (CABG), or upper or lower abdominal surgery

6. Appropriate specific laboratory/diagnostic evaluation of complaints or abnormal physical findings identified during the history and physical examination

C. Assessment of surgical risk[1, 2, 3, 5]

1. Nutritional status

   a. Dietary history
   b. Serum albumin <3 g/dL correlates with prolonged recovery and increased mortality.
   c. Serum transferrin <150 mg/dL correlates with prolonged recovery and increased mortality.

    d. Weight loss >20% caused by illness correlates with pro-
       longed recovery and increased mortality.

2. Immune competence

    a. Total lymphocyte count
    b. Cell-mediated immunity measured by serology
    c. Known immunodeficiency, such as human immunodefi-
      ciency virus (HIV)
    d. Others factors that increase risk of infection
       i. Corticosteroid use
       ii. Immunosuppressive agents
       iii. Cytotoxic drugs
       iv. Prolonged antibiotic therapy
       v. Renal failure
       vi. Irradiation

3. Bleeding risk factors

    a. Patient history
       i. Prolonged bleeding after procedure or injury
       ii. Bleeding 1 day after tooth extraction
       iii. Spontaneous bruising
       iv. Liver or kidney disease
       v. Recent thromobolytics, anticoagulants, nonsteroidal
         anti-inflammatory drugs (NSAIDs), or other drugs that
         prolong bleeding
       vi. Personal (moral, ethical, religious) contraindication to
         transfusion
    b. Physical examination—Consider presence of
       i. Hepatosplenomegaly
       ii. Petechiae
       iii. Ecchymoses
       iv. Findings consistent with anemia
    c. Diagnostic findings
       i. Anemia
       ii. Prolonged prothrombin time or partial thromboplastin
         time (PT/PTT)
       iii. Thrombocytopenia
       iv. Elevated liver function tests (LFT)
       v. Bleeding time

4. Thromboembolic risk increases with

    a. Cancer
    b. Obesity
    c. Age >45 years
    d. Myocardial dysfunction
    e. History of thrombosis
    f. Use of oral contraceptives

5. Patients with coronary artery disease[5]

  a. Reduce systolic BP to <180 mmHg and diastolic BP to <110 mmHg
  b. In low-risk patients
    i. Exercise tolerance test should be conducted when history is unreliable.
    ii. Dipyridamole thallium scintigraphy, stress echocardiography, or ambulatory ischemia monitoring should be performed in patients unable to exercise.
  c. High-risk patients: Postpone surgery unless emergency
  d. Patient should be at least 3 months, and preferably 6 months, post myocardial infarction.

6. Patients with congestive heart failure (CHF)

  a. Should receive medications up to and including day of surgery
  b. Document objective assessment of left ventricular (LV) function (echocardiography).

7. Assessment of pulmonary risk[5]

  a. Chronic lung disease (obstructive and/or restrictive)
  b. Morbid obesity
  c. Tobacco use

D. Control of chronic illness

1. Diabetes mellitus (DM)[8]

  a. Patients who require insulin
    i. Type 1 DM
    ii. Type 2 DM managed with insulin
    iii. Type 2 DM managed with oral agents who are having major procedures
    iv. Methods of insulin administration
      (1) One-half to two-thirds usual dose subcutaneously
      (2) 5–15 units regular insulin in 5–10% glucose at the rate of 100 mL/h (maintain serum glucose <250 mg/dL)
      (3) Infuse insulin via IV drip at 0.5–1.5 units/h; infuse glucose separately to maintain serum glucose <250 mg/dL
      (4) Monitor serum glucose q2–4 h
  b. Patients not requiring insulin
    i. Diet-controlled diabetics
      (1) Avoid glucose solutions the day of surgery.
      (2) Monitor serum glucose q4–6 h during surgery.
    ii. Type 2 DM controlled with oral agents
      (1) Discontinue oral agents the day before surgery.
      (2) Infuse 5% glucose at 100 mL/h.

(3) Monitor glucose q4–6h.

(4) Maintain glucose <250 mg/dL with q6h subcutaneous insulin injection.

(5) Return to oral treatment when baseline diet is resumed.

2. Cardiovascular conditions[1, 8]

a. Coronary artery disease

i. Continue aspirin unless concerns about hemostasis are overriding.

ii. Beta adrenergic blockers, calcium channel blockers, and nitrates should be continued throughout the perioperative period.

3. Anemia[5]

a. Hemoglobin <8 mg/dL is associated with increased perioperative complications.

b. Transfuse preoperatively as indicated by low hemoglobin, presence of cardiopulmonary disease, type of surgery, and anticipated blood loss.

4. Renal disease[1–3, 8]

a. Patients with chronic failure not requiring maintenance: Glomerular filtration rate >15 mg/min; serum creatinine <6 mg/dL

i. Ensure adequate preoperative hydration: Preoperative blood urea nitrogen (BUN) and creatinine should be at patient's baseline.

ii. Transfuse to hematocrit >32 mL/dL.

b. Patients maintained on dialysis

i. Transfuse to hematocrit >32 mL/dL.

ii. Dialyze morning of surgery.

c. Increased risk of bleeding as platelets are inactive in uremic plasma

5. Pulmonary disease[1–3, 7]

a. Cessation of smoking

b. Administer antibiotics for purulent sputum

c. Administration of bronchodilators if patient has a history of pulmonary disease (e.g., albuterol metered-dose inhaler, 2 puffs prior to anesthesia); in severe disease, may be administered IV intraoperatively

E. Physical readiness[1–3, 5, 9]

1. Nutritional status

a. Preoperative supplementation if indicated by physical examination and/or diagnostic evaluation

    b. Preoperative supplementation if prolonged NPO status postoperatively is anticipated

2. Fluid and electrolyte status

    a. Fluid supplementation/diuresis preoperatively as indicated by physical examination/diagnostic studies

    b. Correction of Na^+, K^+, Ca^{2+}, Mg^{2+}, and phosphorus to as normal limits as possible

3. Acid-base balance

    a. Correction of acid-base imbalance as indicated by preoperative condition

    b. Correction of abnormal anion gap to <20

$$Na^+ - (Cl^- + HCO_3^-)$$

4. Anxiety

    a. Accelerates physiologic stress response

    b. Keep patient well-informed—Answer questions.

    c. Nonpharmacologic and pharmacologic anxiety reduction measures as indicated

       i. Guided imagery

       ii. Relaxation exercises

       iii. Medium-length–acting benzodiazepine, such as oxazepam (Serax) to promote sleeping the night prior to surgery

F. Morning of surgery[1-3]

1. Answer patient/family questions and ensure informed consent is signed.

2. Ensure patient has remained NPO since at least 10:00 PM the preceding evening.

3. Ensure preoperative medications are administered.

    a. Antibiotics

    b. Analgesics, sedatives, and other medications ordered by anesthesia provider

    c. Other medications, fluids, and blood products as indicated by preoperative assessment

4. Prepare patient for postoperative period.

    a. Anticipation of

       i. Ventilator support

       ii. Pulmonary artery monitoring

       iii. Nasogastric tube

       iv. Chest tube and/or drains

       v. Foley catheter

       vi. Other drains/monitoring equipment

       vii. Pain

    b. Answer questions and reinforce teaching.

II. POSTOPERATIVE CARE

A. Fluid and electrolytes[1-5]

1. Postoperative fluid replacement—D_5NS solution or lactated Ringer's solution

   a. Maintenance requirements: 1500–2500 mL per 24-h period
   b. Increased needs due to hypercatabolism
   c. Consider losses from drains.
   d. Consider third space losses.
   e. Estimate replacement needs: 30 mL x weight in kg per 24-h period, e.g., a 70-kg patient would need 2100 mL of fluid per 24-h period ($30 \times 70 = 2100$).

2. Electrolyte replacement

   a. Electrolyte measurements are indicated for complicated cases.
   b. K^+ should not be added to IV fluids for the first 24 h after surgery, as there is an intracellular shift during surgery; postoperatively, K^+ will return to the extracellular space, and serum measurements will rise without supplementation.
      i. Exception is replacement fluids lost via nasogastric or gastric drainage.
      ii. Replace 20 mEq for every liter of fluid lost.
   c. Other electrolytes are replaced as assessed on an individual case basis.

B. Pulmonary care[1-3, 5]

1. Encourage deep breathing q1h.
2. Incentive spirometry q2h
3. Mobilization out of bed to chair by postoperative day 1; walking on postoperative day 1 or as soon as tolerated by patient
4. Adequate pain control
5. Instruction regarding splinting with pillows for decreased pain and increased lung expansion

C. Wound care/assessment[1-3, 9]

1. Removal of dressing/handling of wound should be aseptic for first 24 h.
2. Dressings may be removed from dry wounds.
3. Any drainage should be cultured.
4. Skin staples and sutures may be removed on postoperative day 5 or 6; leave in for 2 weeks over creased areas or those closed under tension.
5. Assess for signs of infection.

   a. Erythema
   b. Edema

    c. Heat
    d. Increased pain
    e. Drainage

D. Management of drains[1-3]

1. External portion should be handled with aseptic technique.
2. Attach bag if >50 mL drainage anticipated in an 8-h period.
3. Do not leave Penrose drain in >2 weeks; if continued drainage, replace with rubber catheter such as a Foley catheter.

E. Deep vein thrombosis (DVT) prophylaxis[1-3, 9]

1. Early ambulation
2. Anticoagulation as indicated by procedure
3. Thromboembolic stockings until patient is ambulating or lower extremity edema is no longer present
4. Sequential boots until patient is ambulating

F. Fever[1-3, 5, 9, 10]

1. Most postoperative fever is noninfectious.

    a. Increase lung inflation via turning, coughing, deep breathing, and q2h incentive spirometry, as decreased lung expansion is a major cause of fever in the postoperative course.
    b. Ensure adequate hydration using assessment of vital signs, urine output, BUN/creatinine, and physical examination as indicators.
    c. Rule out reaction to drugs.
    d. Rule out DVT via physical examination.

2. Suspect infectious fever if

    a. Patient feels subjectively unwell.
    b. Pain is worsening.

3. Rule out infection if indicated.

    a. Complete blood count with differential to evaluate leukocytosis/neutrophilia
    b. Culture any purulent drainage.
        i. Incision
        ii. Intravenous lines
        iii. Foley catheter
        iv. Drains
        v. Chest/mediastinal tube drainage
        vi. Sputum
        vii. Stool
    c. Obtain blood cultures.
    d. Begin empirical antibiotic therapy.

G. Bleeding[1–3, 5, 9, 10]

1. Assess for signs of internal bleeding:

    a. Change in vital signs: Tachycardia, hypotension
    b. Localized pain (e.g., abdomen)
    c. Hematoma
    d. Change in mental status
    e. Low or dropping hemoglobin/hematocrit level
    f. Elevated reticuloctye count

2. Management of bleeding

    a. External bleeding usually responds to pressure; may need to apply firm pressure for 20 min
    b. Internal bleeding
        i. Drain hematoma.
        ii. Transfuse as indicated.
        iii. Consider reoperation.

H. Infection (see Section F.3.)

I. Pain[1–3, 5, 9, 11]

1. Must be managed aggressively
2. Limitation of movement secondary to pain can increase risk for

    a. Venous stasis
    b. Thrombosis
    c. Atelectasis

3. Release of stress hormones can promote

    a. Vasospasm
    b. Hypertension

4. Pharmacologic management

    a. Patient-controlled analgesia using a variety of medications, e.g., morphine sulfate, delivering appropriate basal rate and patient-controlled boluses to total an hourly dose appropriate for weight and tolerance
    b. Intramuscular opioids
        i. Peak 1–2 h after injection
        ii. Dose and intervals must be adequate to achieve pain relief
        iii. Observe for signs of respiratory depression
    c. Other agents
        i. Hydroxyzine (Vistaril) potentiates opioids in addition to acting as an antiemetic and an anxiolytic agent.
        ii. Parenteral ketorolac tromethamine (Toradol) has analgesic efficacy equivalent to morphine sulfate.

J. Psychosocial

1. Advise patient of surgical outcomes; answer questions regarding condition.
2. Communicate with family/significant other.

References

1. Way, L.W. (Ed.). (1994). *Current surgical diagnosis and treatment* (10th ed.). Stamford, CT: Appleton & Lange.
2. Sabiston, D.C., Jr., & Lyerly, H.K. (Eds.). (1994). *Essentials of surgery* (2nd ed.). Philadelphia: W.B. Saunders.
3. Schwartz, S.I., Shires, G.T., Spencer, F.C., & Hussler, W.C. (Eds.). (1999). *Principles of surgery* (7th ed.). New York: McGraw-Hill.
4. Schwartz, M.H. (1994). *Textbook of physical diagnosis* (2nd ed.). Philadelpha: W.B. Saunders.
5. Preoperative Assessment and Premedication. (1999). http://www.bconnex.net/~jascah/preop.html
6. Chernecky, C.C., Krech, R.L., & Berger, B.J. (1993). *Laboratory tests and diagnostic procedures*. Philadelphia: W.B. Saunders.
7. Ruppel, G.E. (1997). *Manual of pulmonary function testing* (7th ed.). St. Louis: Mosby.
8. Tierney, L.M., Jr., McPhee, S.J., & Papadakis, M.A. (Eds.). (1999). *Current medical diagnosis and treatment* (38th ed.). Stamford, CT: Appleton & Lange.
9. Carey, C.F., Lee, H.H., & Woeltje, K.F. (Eds.). (1998). *The Washington manual of medical therapeutics* (29th ed.). Philadelphia: Lippincott-Raven.
10. Gomella, L.G. (1993). *Clinican's pocket reference*. Stamford, CT: Appleton & Lange.
11. Eisenhauer, L.A., & Murphy, M.A. (Eds.). (1998). *Pharmacotherapeutics and advanced nursing practice*. New York: McGraw-Hill.

UNIT XIII

Health Promotion

GUIDELINES FOR HEALTH PROMOTION AND SCREENING

Carolyn G. White, MSN, RN, CS, FNP, PNP, CCRN

I. VISIONARY PLAN FOR HEALTH[1-6]

A. Healthy People 2000

1. National health promotion and disease prevention objectives include 376 specific items in addition to sub-objectives for high risk groups.
2. This report, first issued in 1979, outlines three general goals that have been adopted by the World Health Organization for all people.
3. The goals are

   a. To increase lifespan
   b. To reduce health disparities among certain groups
   c. To achieve access to preventive services for all people

4. Healthy People 2000 serves as a dynamic framework for health that has utility for both the provider and the patient.

B. Healthy People 2010

1. In accordance with evolving policy and practice guidelines, the Healthy People 2010 leading health care indicators were released in January 2000 as foundation elements for the understanding and improving of health.
2. Leading health indicators include

   a. Physical activity
   b. Obesity
   c. Tobacco use
   d. Controlled substance use
   e. Sexual practices
   f. Mental health
   g. Accidental and violent injuries
   h. Environmental quality
   i. Immunization
   j. Access to health care

3. These indicators provide the cornerstone for targeted health promotion and preventive practices and should be incorporated into care at all levels from primary prevention to tertiary intervention.

C. Prevention is essential to health maintenance and health promotion at all ages.

Research continues to support the purpose and significance of prevention in primary care as well as in other settings.

D. The role of the advanced practice nurse

1. Advanced practice nurses can play an integral role in achieving wellness, health promotion, and disease prevention via

   a. Holistic assessment of the individual
   b. Appropriate screening for disease
   c. Mutually planned and implemented intervention
   d. Continued monitoring

2. The role of the clinician in prevention and health promotion is defined in the U.S. Preventive Services Task Force report as

   a. Intervention in lifestyle behaviors that place individuals at risk and can be modified
   b. Mutuality in the establishment of individualized plans of care in prevention and health promotion
   c. Judicious use of preventive health care services and screening tests
   d. Shared impetus in the delivery of preventive care to patients.
   e. Selective use of community intervention.

II. PREVENTION AND HEALTH PROMOTION IN CLINICAL PRACTICE[1-5, 7, 8, 11, 12, 14-16]

A. Components

1. Primary prevention

   a. Health promotion that precedes disease or onset of symptoms
   b. Methods of primary prevention may include general health promotion and specific protection from disease such as
      i. Immunizations
      ii. Health education
      iii. Blood pressure measurements
      iv. Genetic screening for sex-linked disorders
      v. Use of seat belts
      vi. Avoidance of second-hand smoke and other environmental pollutants

2. Secondary prevention

   a. Identification and diagnosis, early intervention, and limitation of disability in disease and injury encompass the secondary response to illness.

b. The goal is to shorten or halt the disease process, arresting or preventing complications. Example interventions:

   i. Case finding

   ii. Screening for specific disease (e.g., Pap smear, cholesterol and blood pressure management to prevent cardiovascular disease)

   iii. Isolation to prevent the transmission of communicable diseases

c. Age- and risk-specific cancer screening continue to be effective means for reducing morbidity and mortality.

   i. According to the National Cancer Institute, screening for breast and cervical cancers alone may reduce total cancer deaths by 3% annually.

   ii. While an evidence-based approach to screening should be taken by the practitioner, general guidelines for cancer screening are:

     (1) Breast: Mammography annually after age 50 (baseline at age 40 with frequency of examination during the fifth decade of life determined by risk factors)

     (2) Cervical: Annual Pap smears once sexually active or by age 20

     (3) Colorectal

       (a) Digital rectal examination annually after age 40, with guaiac-based fecal occult blood testing annually

       (b) Flexible sigmoidoscopy every 3–5 years after the age of 50 (consider history of polyps and heritable risk factors)

     (4) Prostate: Although data are inconclusive, a digital rectal examination and/or prostate-specific antigen (PSA) test annually after age 50, and thereafter as findings and risk factors dictate.

     (5) Other: Screening for oral, lung, liver, ovarian, gastric, endometrial, and testicular cancers should be guided by a detailed patient history of heredity, use of tobacco, exposure to infectious disease, and other pertinent factors.

3. Tertiary prevention

   a. The hallmark of tertiary care is the provision of services aimed at restoring and/or arresting disability.

   b. The objective is to return the patient to optimal health within the constraints of the impairment.

c. Utilization of specialized health care teams (e.g., occupational therapy, speech, rehabilitative services) and appropriate referrals for injuries or illnesses such as head and neck injuries and cerebrovascular accidents are examples of tertiary prevention.

B. Periodic Health History and Examination

1. The recommended interval of assessment varies from source to source and should be judiciously individualized to the patient's age, risk, and state of health or illness.

   a. Advanced practice nurses should remain cognizant of the overall health of population aggregates and individuals and know that socioeconomic and educational status are directly linked with the health of populations and of individuals, for virtually all indicators (http://www.cdc.gov).
   b. Although specific guidelines for frequency remain controversial, the periodic health examination is commonly administered to asymptomatic patients in three age groups (Table 83–1).
      i. 11–24 years
      ii. 25–64 years
      iii. 65 and older

2. Additional preventive services

   a. Select screening tests (see Table 83–1)
   b. Immunizations (see Table 83–1). Note that immunization status should be ascertained at every patient encounter and updated.
   c. Chemoprophylaxis, the use of medications or biologicals for the preservation of health or prevention of disease (e.g., vitamin therapy, folic acid supplements for female reproductive health).
   d. Counseling regarding specific health risks or problems
      i. Controlled substance avoidance
      ii. Stress management
      iii. Crisis intervention
      iv. Safety issues

3. Regular surveillance of health risks

   a. General
      i. Lack of physical activity
      ii. Poor nutrition
      iii. Tobacco use
      iv. Premalignant and malignant skin lesions
      v. Domestic violence

  vi. Alcohol and other substance abuse
  vii. Dental disease
  viii. Obesity
  ix. Underuse of known prevention strategies (i.e. breast, cervical, and colorectal cancer screening)
 b. Specific—Age and/or gender related:
  i. Adolescents
   (1) STDs
   (2) Unwanted pregnancy
   (3) Substance abuse
   (4) Depression and/or suicide
   (5) Scoliosis
   (6) Family- or school-related violence
  ii. Elderly
   (1) Peripheral vascular disease
   (2) Thyroid disease
   (3) Inability to perform activities of daily living
   (4) Safety risks (e.g., falling)
  iii. Women who are pregnant or considering pregnancy
   (1) Thyroid disorders
   (2) Blood pressure
   (3) Anemia
   (4) STDs, including HIV
   (5) Rubella
   (6) Hepatitis B
   (7) Urinary tract infections
   (8) Rh typing
   (9) Daily folic acid
   (10) Alcohol, tobacco and other substance use
 c. The CDC's Behavioral Risk Factor Surveillance System is a standardized tracking mechanism that allows health care providers and patients access to current morbidity and risk factor data (http://www.cdc.gov/nccdphp/brfss).
 d. Healthy People 2000 and 2010 offer regular status reports regarding progress on meeting specific goals of health (http://www.health.gov/healthypeople/).
  i. While improvements in insurance coverage for clinical preventive services such as Pap smears, mammograms, and immunizations have occurred, many Americans remain uninsured and thus unaffected by these changes.
  ii. Continued research concerning preventive care and implementation of methods to improve access, reduce barriers, and increase the appropriate use of clinical preventive health services remains the impetus for advanced nursing practitioners in the provision of screening and preventive health care.

TABLE 83–1. AGE-SPECIFIC INFORMATION FOR SCREENING, TESTS, EXAMINATIONS, AND COUNSELING

11–24 YEARS

Immunization/Preventive Care

1. HBV if not done
2. TD once by age 18 and every 10 years thereafter
3. MMR once if not given during preschool period
4. Treat diseases such as diabetes, hypertension, and scoliosis prior to complications. For example, for the early treatment of hyperlipidemia there are three indications for pharmacologic intervention:
   a. LDL over 160 and less than 2 CHD factors.
   b. LDL over 130 and 2 or more factors.
   c. Diagnosed CHD and LDL over 100 mg/dL.

Screening/Tests

1. Height and weight
2. Blood pressure
3. Anemia (CBC)
4. Urinalysis
5. TB
6. Hearing and vision
7. Dental
8. Cancer (breast, testicular, other)
9. Random total HDL and CHD risk factors after age 20 (TCL below 200 mg/dL are considered desirable, 200–239 is moderate, over 239 high). HDL less than 35 is considered an independent coronary risk factor. If patient's levels are high, obtain a fasting TCL and triglycerides (if over 400, measure LDL). LDL, a target measurement, and other risk factors determine treatment course.

Developmental/Age-Related Counseling

1. Injuries
2. STDs including HIV
3. Substance abuse
4. School-, gang-, or domestic-related violence
5. Physical activity
6. Smoking
7. Family planning
8. Oral/dental health
9. Sun exposure
10. Nutrition/obesity
11. Suicide inventory (The HEADS [home, education, activities, drugs, sex and suicide] survey instrument is a commonly used lifestyle questionnaire to identify high-risk teens)
12. Pregnancy prevention; contraception or abstinence
13. Career guidance support

Other

1. Family history and other specific health related risk factors
2. Occupational/environmental/travel outside U.S.

25–64 YEARS

Immunization/Preventive Care

1. TD every 10 years
2. MMR HBV, OPV if needed
3. Pneumovax if needed
4. Multivitamin with folic acid for women of child-bearing age
5. Treatment of hypertension, hyperlipidemia, anemia, depression as indicated.
6. Hormone prophylaxis (peri- and post-menopausal women)

Screening/Tests

1. Height and weight (annually)
2. Blood pressure (annually)
3. Total serum cholesterol (men: age 35–64, women: 45–64)
4. Pap smear annually to every 3 years (women once sexually active or 18 years of age).
5. Mammogram annually after age 50
6. Clinical breast examination annually 18 years and after
7. Fecal guaiac for occult blood annually
8. Sigmoidoscopy annually after age 50 if at increased risk, or every 3–5 years.

Counseling

1. Injury identification (occupational, environmental, domestic violence)
2. Injury prevention: Lap/shoulder belts, helmet use (bicycles, skateboarding, in-line skating, motorcycle and ATV use), water sports safety, smoke and CO detectors, storage and use of firearms
3. Screening sexual history for high risk behaviors, STDs, and unplanned pregnancy
4. Other high risk areas (exposure to TB, chemical exposures, genetic and/or familial risk for health conditions).

Table continued on following page

TABLE 83–1. AGE-SPECIFIC INFORMATION FOR SCREENING, TESTS, EXAMINATIONS, AND COUNSELING *Continued*

25–64 YEARS

Screening/Tests	Counseling

9. Women only:
  a. Folic acid 4.0 mg daily if considering pregnancy
  b. Rubella titer or immunization if of child-producing age.
10. Alcohol and substance abuse inventory (i.e. CAGE questionnaire)
11. Men only:
  a. Clinical testicular examination annually
  b. Digital prostate examination annually after age 40
  c. PSA at age 40 for African American and high risk, age 50 and annually for others
	5. Tobacco, alcohol, illicit drug, and other abuse of substances (including caffeine)
	6. Diet, stress, and exercise: Healthy nutritional habits, limit fat and processed starches and sugars, maintain ideal BMI, emphasize food pyramid, consider calcium supplementation for women, discuss effective coping mechanisms, encourage regular (daily) aerobic exercise.
	7. Smoking cessation intervention.
	8. Professional intervention for substance dependency or abuse.
	9. STD prevention, use of condoms and/or other forms of contraception. High risk behavior avoidance.
	10. Dental hygiene (effective brushing and flossing, regular examinations, need for immediate follow-up).

65 AND OLDER

Immunization/Preventive Care

1. TD booster (every 10 years)
2. Influenza annually
3. Pneumococcal vaccine
4. Women only:
   a. Hormone replacement
   b. Calcium supplementation
5. Consider ASA, vitamin E, folic acid, multivitamin daily

Screening/Tests	Counseling

1. Blood pressure
2. Height and weight
3. Fecal occult blood test and/or sigmoidoscopy
4. Women only:
   a. Pap smear
   b. Mammogram and clinical breast examination annually
5. Hearing and vision
6. Activities of daily living
7. Risk for falls
8. Mental examination (depression, suicide, alcohol and other substance abuse, polypharmacy, memory changes)
9. Signs of elder abuse
	1. Injury prevention (smoke/CO detector, stairs in home, use of seatbelts, helmets, and other protective sports gear)
	2. Safe storage of firearms
	3. Fall prevention
	4. BCLS education for caregiver or family members
	5. Hot water heater set at 120°
	6. Diet and exercise
	7. STD including HIV prevention
	8. Dental health (regular examinations, fluoride toothpaste, flossing)

HBV, hepatitis B virus; TD, tetanus-diphtheria, MMR, measles-mumps-rubella; CHD, coronary heart disease; CBC, complete blood count; LDL, low-density lipoprotein; TB, tuberculosis; TCL, total cholesterol level; STD, sexually transmitted disease; HIV, human immunodeficiency virus; OPV, oral polio vaccine; CO, carbon monoxide; BMI, body mass index; ASA, aspirin; BCLS, basic cardiac life support

References

1. American Cancer Society (1997). *A cancer source book for nurses* (7th ed.). Sudbury, MA: Jones and Bartlett Publishing.
2. Centers for Disease Control and Prevention (1999). Behavioral risk factor surveillance system. [Report posted on the World Wide Web]. Atlanta, GA. Retrieved May 14, 1999 from the World Wide Web: http://www.cdc.gov/nccdphp/brfss.
3. Buttaro, T.M., Trybulski, J., Bailey, P.P., & Sandberg-Cook, J. (1999). *Primary care: A collaborative practice.* St. Louis: Mosby.
4. American Nurses Association (1994). *Clinician's handbook of preventive services.* Washington, DC: American Nursing Publishing.
5. Edelman, C.L., & Mandle, C.L., (1994). *Health promotion throughout the lifespan.* St. Louis: Mosby.
6. Report of the U.S. Preventive Services Task Force (1999). *Guide to clinical preventive services* (2nd ed.). Baltimore: Williams & Wilkins.
7. Hamric, A.B., Spross, J.A., & Hanson, C.M. (1996). *Advanced nursing practice.* Philadelphia: W.B. Saunders.
8. *Healthy people 2010,* conference edition, 2000. USDHHS, Washington D.C.
9. Kane, R.L., Ouslander, J.G., & Abrass, I.B. (1999). *Essentials of clinical geriatrics* (4th ed.). New York: McGraw-Hill, Inc.
10. Knollmueller, R.N. (Ed.) (1993). *Prevention across the lifespan.* American Nurses Association Council of Community Health. Washington, DC: American Nursing Publishing.
11. *Leading Health Indicators for Healthy People 2010,* Second Interim Report, (1999). Institutes of Medicine, National Academy Press [Report posted on the World Wide Web]. Retrieved September 26, 1999 from the World Wide Web: http://www.health.gov/healthypeople/.
12. National Center for Health Statistics (1997). *Healthy People 2000 Review* (1997). Atlanta, GA: U.S. Department of Health and Human Services, Centers for Disease Control and Prevention.
13. National Cancer Institute (1999). *Screening of cancer* [Report posted on the World Wide Web]. Retrieved September 26, 1999 from the World Wide Web: www.nih.gov/clinpdq/screening.
14. Snyder, M. & Mirr, M.P. (Eds.) (1995). *Advanced practice nursing.* New York: Springer Publishing.
15. Socioeconomic Status and Health Chartbook in Health, United States, (1998). Centers for Disease Control and Prevention. [Report posted on the World Wide Web]. Retrieved May 14, 1999 from the World Wide Web: http://www.cdc.gov/nchswww).
16. Uphold, C.R., & Graham, M.V. (1999). *Clinical guidelines in adult health* (2nd ed.). Gainesville, FL: Barmarrae Books.

MAJOR CAUSES OF MORTALITY IN THE UNITED STATES

Barbara S. Broome, PhD, RN

I. LEADING CAUSES OF DEATH IN THE UNITED STATES[2, 3, 5, 10–12]

A. Male and female, all ages (see Tables 84–1 through 84–4)[2, 5, 10, 11]

1. Diseases of the heart
2. Malignant neoplasms
3. Cerebrovascular diseases
4. Chronic obstructive pulmonary disease (COPD)
5. Accidents
6. Pneumonia and influenza
7. Diabetes mellitus
8. Human immunodeficiency virus (HIV)
9. Suicide
10. Chronic liver disease, cirrhosis

II. RISK ASSESSMENT

A. Cardiopulmonary[6, 9, 10, 12, 15]

1. Obesity (20–40% over ideal weight) is a risk-factor for hypertension, stroke, myocardial infarction, and diabetes.
2. Sedentary lifestyle
3. Lower socioeconomic group; poverty is associated with increased health risks.
4. African American race increases cardiovascular risk
5. Assess risk profile using stratifying risk and quantifying prognosis.
6. Smoking
7. Diabetes
8. Family history of cardiac or respiratory disease

B. Malignant neoplasms[10, 11, 14]

1. Use of tobacco
2. Diet high in fat
3. Infection (especially associated with cervical cancer and human papillomavirus)
4. Family history
5. Exposure to toxins in environment/workplace

C. Accidents[10]

1. Alcoholism
2. Drug use

Text continued on page 884

TABLE 84–1. LEADING CAUSES OF DEATH

RANK	HISPANIC	CAUCASIAN	BLACK
1.	Disease hypertension	Diseases of the heart such as rheumatic fever, hypertension	Diseases of the heart such as rheumatic fever, hypertension
2.	Malignant neoplasms	Malignant neoplasms	Malignant neoplasms
3.	Accidents and adverse events: Vehicle accidents, drowning	Cerebrovascular diseases: Hypertension	Cerebrovascular diseases: Hypertension
4.	Cerebrovascular disease	COPD	HIV
5.	HIV	Pneumonia and influenza	Accidents and adverse events
6.	Diabetes mellitus	Accidents and adverse events	Diabetes mellitus
7.	Homicide	Diabetes mellitus	Homicide
8.	Pneumonia and influenza	Suicide	Pneumonia and influenza
9.	Chronic liver disease: Cirrhosis	Alzheimer's disease	COPD
10.	COPD	Nephritis, nephrotic syndrome, and nephrosis	Conditions originating in the perinatal period: Infection, SIDs

SIDs, Sudden infant deaths.
Source: National Vital Statistics 1998; National Center for Health Statistics, 1998.

TABLE 84–2. LEADING CAUSES OF DEATH, FEMALES

RANK	HISPANIC	CAUCASIAN	BLACK
1.	Diseases of the heart	Diseases of the heart	Diseases of the heart
2.	Malignant neoplasms	Malignant neoplasms	Malignant neoplasms: Lung/breast
3.	Cerebrovascular diseases	Cerebrovascular diseases	Cerebrovascular diseases
4.	Diabetes mellitus	COPD	Diabetes mellitus
5.	Accidents	Pneumonia and influenza	Accidents
6.	Pneumonia and influenza	Accidents and adverse events	Pneumonia and influenza
7.	COPD	Diabetes mellitus	HIV
8.	HIV	Alzheimer's disease	COPD
9.	Chronic liver disease	Nephritis, nephrotic syndrome	Nephritis, nephrotic syndrome
10.	Conditions originating in the perinatal period	Septicemia	Septicemia

Source: National Vital Statistics 1998; National Center for Health Statistics, 1998.

TABLE 84–3. LEADING CAUSES OF DEATH, MALES

RANK	HISPANIC	CAUCASIAN	BLACK
1.	Diseases of the heart	Diseases of the heart	Diseases of the heart
2.	Malignant neoplasms: Leading Ca: prostate cancer	Malignant neoplasms	Malignant neoplasms: Prostate cancer: Leading mortality
3.	Accidents	CVA	HIV
4.	HIV	COPD	Accidents
5.	Homicide	Accidents and adverse events	Homicides
6.	Cerebrovascular disease	Pneumonia and influenza	Cerebrovascular disease
7.	Chronic liver disease	Suicide	Pneumonia and influenza
8.	Diabetes mellitus	Diabetes mellitus	Diabetes mellitus
9.	Suicide	Chronic liver disease and cirrhosis	COPD
10.	Pneumonia and influenza	HIV	Certain conditions originating in the perinatal period

CVA, cerebrovascular accident.
Source: National Vital Statistics 1998; National Center for Health Statistics, 1998.

TABLE 84–4. LEADING CAUSES OF DEATH, ALL RACES

RANK	AGE 15–24	AGE 25–44	AGE 45–64	65 PLUS
1.	Accidents	Accidents	Malignant neoplasms	Diseases of the heart
2.	Homicide	Malignant neoplasms	Diseases of the heart	Malignant neoplasms
3.	Suicide	HIV	Accidents/adverse events	Cerebrovascular diseases
4.	Malignant neoplasms	Diseases of the heart	Cerebrovascular disease	COPD
5.	Diseases of the heart	Suicide	COPD	Pneumonia and influenza
6.	HIV	Homicide	Diabetes mellitus	Diabetes mellitus
7.	Congenital anomalies	Chronic liver disease and cirrhosis	Chronic liver disease and cirrhosis	Accidents
8.	COPD	Cerebrovascular disease	Suicide	Alzheimer's disease
9.	Pneumonia and influenza	Diabetes mellitus	HIV	Nephritis, nephrotic syndrome, and nephrosis
10.	Cerebrovascular disease Diabetes mellitus	Pneumonia and influenza	Pneumonia and influenza	Septicemia

Source: National Vital Statistics 1998; National Center for Health Statistics, 1998.

3. Occupational hazards
4. Environmental hazards

D. Diabetes[1, 6, 10]

1. Obesity (>20% over ideal body weight)
2. Age 45 and older
3. Higher in nonwhite race
4. Low high-density lipoproteins (<35 mg/dL) and/or triglyceride level >250 mg/dL
5. Hypertension
6. Family history
7. History of gestational diabetes or delivery of babies over 9 lb

E. HIV[7, 10]

1. Unprotected sex
2. Intravenous drug use/sharing needles
3. Blood transfusions
4. HIV is the leading killer in minority males and females age 25–44.

F. Suicide[6, 9, 10, 13]

1. Catastrophic life events
2. Previous suicidal attempts
3. White male living alone with previous suicide attempts
4. Previous history of depression, alcoholism, or schizophrenia
5. Unemployed
6. Age 60 and older
7. Poor compliance with treatment
8. Psychotic symptoms
9. Assess for risk using rating scale (e.g., Beck Depression Inventory, Structured Clinical Interview for DSM-IV, Schedule for Affective Disorders and Schizophrenia)

   a. Homicide
      i. Young male, ages 15–24
      ii. Young black male, ages 15–24
      iii. Unemployed, limited education
      iv. History of physical or sexual abuse
      v. Substance abuse
      vi. Membership in a violent peer group (gangs)
      vii. Physical agitation and/or anger
      viii. Access to lethal weapons
      ix. Current alcohol or other drug use

G. Chronic liver disease[8, 10]

1. Alcoholism
2. Hepatitis B, hepatitis C
3. History of intestinal bypass surgery

References

1. American Diabetes Association: Clinical Practice Recommendations 1999. (1999). *Summary of Revisions for the 1999 Clinical Practice Recommendations*. Http://diabetes.org/DiabetesCare/Supplement 199/S2 htm.
2. *Centers for Disease Control and Prevention: Deaths/Mortality* (1998) [Electronic data base]. Atlanta: National Center for Health Statistics [Producer and Distributor].
3. *Centers for Disease Control and Prevention: Vital Statistics Report Shows Significant Gain in Health* (1998) [Electronic data base]. Atlanta: National Center for Health Statistics [Producer and Distributor].
4. *Centers for Disease Control and Prevention: New Study for Patterns of Death in the United States* (1998) [Electronic data base]. Atlanta: National Center for Health Statistics [Producer and Distributor].
5. Centers for Disease Control and Prevention (1998, November 10). Deaths and death rates for the 10 leading causes of death in specified age groups, by sex and Hispanic origin and race for non-Hispanic population: Total of 49 reporting States and the District of Columbia. *National Vital Statistics Report* [On-line serial], 47. Available FTP: http://www.wdc.nchswww/fastats/deaths.html.
6. Chest Medicine On-Line. (1999). *The Causes of COPD.* Http://www.priory.com/cmol/diagnosis.htm
7. Community Outreach Health Information System. (1999). *Aids/HIV: Risk factors and methods of transmission.* Http://www.bu.edu/cohis/aids/risk.htm
8. Healthgate (1999). *Cirrhosis.* Http://www/healthgate.com/hic/cirrhosis-liver/index 1. shtml
9. Medicine, Psychiatry, Dental & Veterinary Journals-Priory Lodge Education. (1999). *The Assessment of Risk.* Http://www.priory.com/psych/risk.htm
10. Stanhope, M., & Lancaster, J. (1996). *Community health nursing: Promoting health of aggregates, families, and individuals* (4th ed.). St. Louis: Mosby-YearBook.
11. U.S. Department of Commerce. (1998). *The National Data Book: Statistical Abstract of the United States 1988.* Washington, D.C.: Government Printing Office.
12. U.S. Department of Health and Human Services. (1990). *Healthy People 2000: National Health Promotion and Disease Prevention Objectives.* Washington, D.C.: Government Printing Office.
13. Warren, B., & Keltner, N. (1999). Mood disorder. *In* N. Keltner, L. Schweke, & C. Bostrom (Eds.), *Psychiatric nursing* (3rd ed.). St. Louis: Mosby.
14. World Health Organization (1999). *WHO Cancer Programme—Strategy.* Http://who-pcc.iarc.fr/Strategy/strategy.htm
15. 1999 World Health Organization, International Society of Hypertension and World Hypertension League. (1999). *1999 Who/ISH Hypertension Practice Guidelines for Primary Care Physicians.* Http://www.who.int/ncd/cvd/HT-Guide.html

IMMUNIZATION RECOMMENDATIONS

Teena M. McGuinness, PhD, RN, CS

I. IMMUNIZATION[1, 2]

A. Definition

1. The process of rendering a subject immune (i.e., highly resistant to disease) because of formation of antibodies or development of immunologically competent cells
2. An antigen is any substance capable of inducing a specific immune response.

   a. Antibodies are molecules synthesized in reaction to the antigen that induces its synthesis.
   b. The antigen-antibody reaction begins when the body interprets substances as foreign invaders gaining entrance into the body.

3. Immunization is also called inoculation and vaccination; the original use of word *vaccination* referred to substances used to immunize against smallpox, the very first immunization (see Table 85–1).
4. Active immunity is conferred by antibody formation stimulated by a specific antigen such as

   a. Typhoid fever immunization (dead bacteria)
   b. Salk poliomyelitis injection (dead virus)
   c. Sabin polio vaccine (oral) (live attenuated [less virulent] virus)
   d. Toxoids (altered forms of toxins produced by bacteria, such as immunization against tetanus and diptheria)

5. Active immunity is not without risks and has become an issue among activist parents whose children have suffered injury, primarily due to immunization against pertussis (whooping cough).
6. Passive immunity (Table 85–2) is conferred by the introduction of antibody proteins, such as

   a. Maternal immunity transferred to the fetus
   b. Gamma globulin injections for immunodeficient patients

B. The most important factor in contraindications for vaccine is the recipient's immunocompetence.

1. Severely immunocompromised patients, including HIV-positive persons, usually should not receive live, attenuated vaccines owing to potential lethal risk. These include

TABLE 85–1. ROUTINE ADULT IMMUNIZATIONS TABLE[1-4, 6]

IMMUNIZATION	INDICATIONS	DOSE	CONTRAINDICATIONS
Influenza	>65 years of age; patients at risk from chronic obstructive pulmonary disease, chronic heart disease, renal failure, sickle cell disease, diabetes, immunosuppression	0.5 mL IM every fall	Anaphylactic hypersensitivity to eggs
Pneumococcus	>65 years of age; patients with conditions at high risk for pneumococcal disease, such as HIV infection, diabetes, asplenia, and chronic lung, liver, heart, or renal disease	0.5 mL IM. If age 65, repeat if 5 or more years have passed since first dose.	
Hepatitis A	Travelers to endemic areas, military personnel, food handlers, homosexual males	0.5 mL IM (repeat in 6–18 months for extended immunity)	
Hepatitis B	Health care workers and high-risk patients	1 mL IM in deltoid muscle at 0, 1, and 6 months	

Measles, mumps, rubella (MMR)	Those entering college, health care personnel, U.S. travelers to other countries. Ensure that two doses of MMR are received by adults born since 1956. Those born in 1956 and earlier may be considered immune.	0.5 mL SC	Pregnancy, hypersensitivity to eggs or to neomycin, immunosuppression
Tetanus/diphtheria booster (adult Td)	Those who have not received initial vaccination series should receive complete series.	0.5 mL IM every 10 years (or a single booster at age 50)	Neurologic or hypersensitivity reaction to previous dose
Polio	Those adults not previously immunized should receive primary series of three doses at week 1, weeks 4–8, and a third dose 6–12 weeks after the second dose. Live oral polio vaccine (OPV) and inactivated polio vaccine (EP-IPV) may be used.	Consult package insert	Immunocompromised persons should not be given OPV or exposed to excreted vaccine virus of OPV recipients.

TABLE 85–2. PASSIVE IMMUNIZATION[2, 3, 5]

IMMUNIZATION	INDICATIONS & DOSAGES
Hepatitis A	Postexposure: Within 14 days of known exposure (via sex partners of infected individual, coworkers of infected food handlers, children and staff at day-care centers, and family members of diapered children at those centers), the dose is Havrix: 2 doses separated by 6–12 months. Adults (19 years of age and older)—Dose: 1.0 mL IM.
Hepatitis B	Consult state or local immunization guidelines for post-exposure prophylaxis. Vaccinated health care workers: Check hepatitis B surface antibody titer. If less than 10 IU/mL, give HBIG, 0.06 mL/kg, as well as booster dose of vaccine. If 10 IU/mL or greater, no therapy is indicated.
Hepatitis C	Immune globulin not effective. Occupational health follow-up for baseline and subsequent testing is imperative.
Diphtheria	20,000–100,000 units of diphtheria antitoxin (DAT-equine source) IM after cultures taken. Immunization given in addition to antibiotics.
Measles	Within 6 days of exposure, nonimmune contacts should be given IG, 0.25 mL/kg. Maximum dose is 15 mL for normal host. For immunocompromised patients, give 0.5 mL/kg (also a maximum of 15 mL).
Tetanus	If history of tetanus immunization is unknown or more than 10 years since last dose, give Td (adult tetanus-diphtheria booster) for clean minor wounds. If last dose of Td was within last 10 years and patient has received three or more tetanus immunizations, do not give Td for clean, minor wounds. For other wounds, give tetanus immune globulin (TIG), 250 units IM, in addition to Td if history of tetanus immunization is unknown (give concurrently with Td at separate site).
Rabies	Rabies vaccine is recommended for pre-exposure or postexposure prophylaxis of rabies. Persons at high risk of exposure, including veterinarians and animal handlers, and those with proximity to animals who are potentially rabid should receive the immunization. Postexposure prophylaxis decisions should include consultation with local and state public health officials.

a. Measles, mumps, rubella
b. Oral poliomyelitis
c. Varicella
d. Yellow fever
e. Bacillus Calmette-Guérin (BCG) vaccine
f. Typhoid Ty21a

2. Although killed vaccines may be given to immunocompromised persons, the immune response may be inadequate, and there is no clear evidence of protective efficacy.

C. **Consult manufacturer's recommendations for specific doses, schedules, routes of administration, and potential side effects.**

D. **Documentation on patients' records should include dose, route of administration, manufacturer, and the lot number of the vaccine. Adverse reactions should be reported using forms and instructions in the *Food and Drug Administration Drug Bulletin.***

E. **International travelers may encounter risks when visiting other countries; specific vaccinations are required by different countries.**

1. Recommendations from the Centers for Disease Control and Prevention's automated hotline are accessible by telephone at (404) 332-4559.
2. The same recommendations (also regularly updated) are available at the following Internet address: http://www.cdc.gov. Each clinician is strongly urged to consult the Centers for Disease Control web site for the most current immunization recommendations.
3. Geographic recommendations and disease outbreaks are included in the information available by telephone or at the Internet address.

References

1. Danila, R.N., Lexau, C., Lynfield, R., Moore, K.A., & Osterholm, M.T. (1999). Addressing emerging infections. The partnership between public health and primary care physicians. *Postgraduate Medicine, 106*, 90–105.
2. Fletcher, S.W. (1998). Periodic health examination. In J. Stein (Ed.), *Internal medicine* (5th ed.). (pp. 2254–2256). St. Louis: Mosby.
3. Hutin, Y.J., Bell, B.P., Marshall, K.L., Schaben, C.P., Dart, M., Quinlisk, M.P., & Shapiro, C.N. (1999). Identifying target groups for a potential vaccination program during a hepatitis A communitywide outbreak. *American Journal of Public Health, 89*, 918–921.
4. Nichol, K.L. (1999). Revaccination of high-risk adults with pneumococcal polysaccharide vaccine. *Journal of the American Medical Association, 281*, 280–281.

5. Paunio, M., Peltola, H., Valle, M., Davidkin, I., Virtanen, M., & Heinonen, O.P. (1999). Twice vaccinated recipients are better protected against epidemic measles than are single dose recipients of measles containing vaccine. *Journal of Epidemiology and Community Health, 53,* 173–178.
6. Prevention and control of influenza: Recommendations of the Advisory Committee on Immunization Practices (ACIP).(1999). *MMWR, Morbidity and Mortality Weekly Report, 48* (RR-4), 1–28.

Note: Page numbers followed by the letter f refer to figures; page numbers followed by the letter t refer to tables.